ADVANCES IN CLIMATIC PHYSIOLOGY

Edited by

SHINJI ITOH, M.D.
Professor, Department of Physiology, Hokkaido University School of Medicine

KOREHIRO OGATA, M.D.
Emeritus Professor, Department of Physiology, Institute of Constitutional Medicine Kumamoto University

HISATO YOSHIMURA, M.D.
Emeritus Professor, Department of Physiology, Kyoto Prefectural University of Medicine

SPRINGER-VERLAG BERLIN HEIDELBERG GMBH

PUBLISHERS

© Springer-Verlag Berlin Heidelberg 1972
Originally published by SPRINGER-VERLAG, Berlin · Heidelberg · New York in 1972
Softcover reprint of the hardcover 1st edition 1972

Library of Congress Catalog Card Number 72–78342

ISBN 978-3-642-93012-6   ISBN 978-3-642-93010-2 (eBook)
DOI 10.1007/978-3-642-93010-2

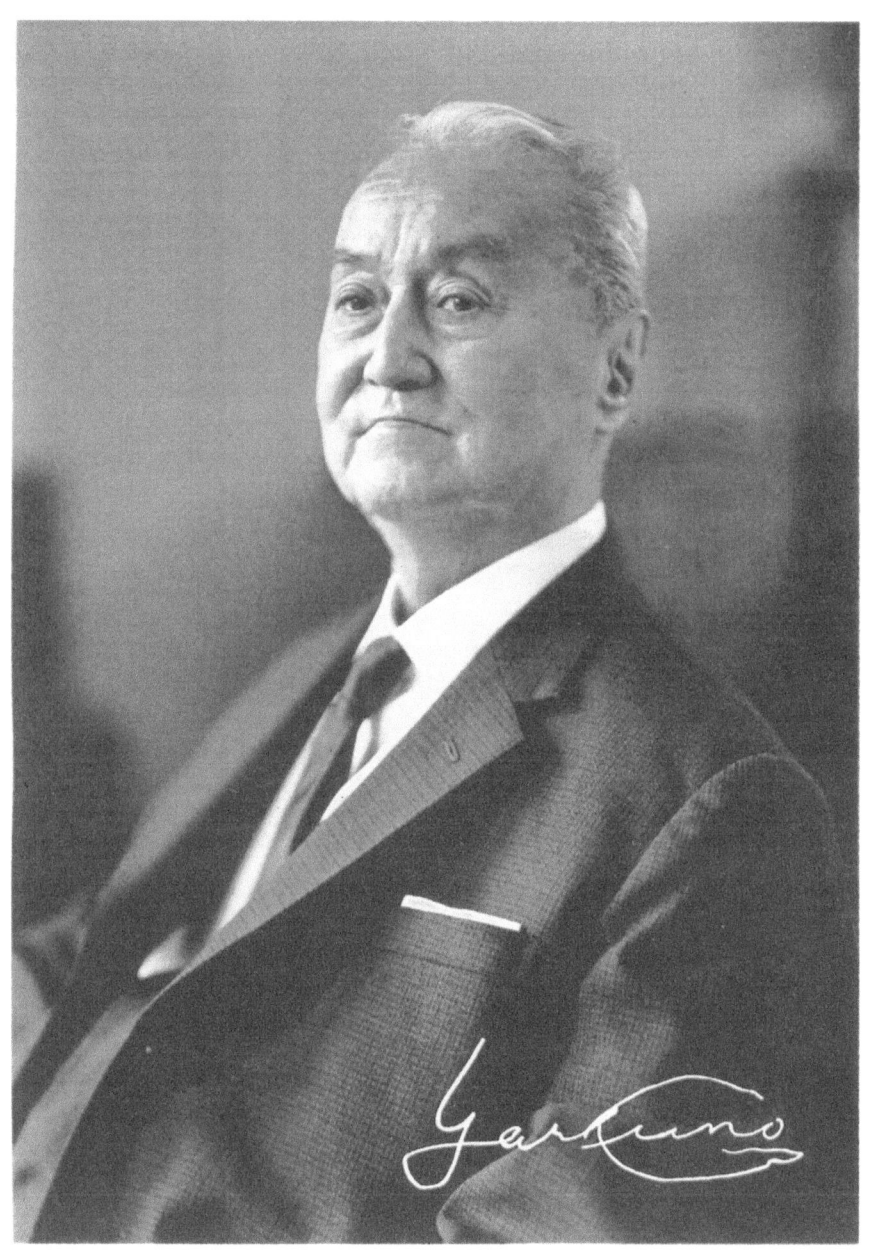

Dr. Yasu KUNO

PREFACE

It is a great pleasure to publish this book in celebration of the 88th birthday on March 3, 1971, of Dr. Yasu Kuno, a member of the Japan Academy and Emeritus Professor of Nagoya University. This celebrated scholar, who is not only respected by those under his direction but who is also a great credit to the medical science of Japan, is a pioneer in the field of physiological research on human perspiration.

The result of his life's work "*The Physiology of Human Perspiration*" (Churchill, London, 1934), to which he devoted all his energies, must be called a monumental work. This book has won worldwide recognition as one of the most authoritative references in this field. Following this work, in 1956, Dr. Kuno published a supplementary volume which contains many of the results of his later research, "*Human Perspiration*" (Charles C Thomas, Springfield, Illinois).

The beginning of his research in perspiration goes back to 1922, when Dr. Kuno was a professor of physiology at Manchuria Medical College. This was also the start in Japan of systematic studies of physiology centering on the study of the regulation of body temperature. Since then, while a professor of physiology at Manchuria Medical College, Kyoto University, Nagoya University and the Mie Prefectural Medical College, and even after cessation of his duties there, Dr. Kuno has not only continued research on his major subject, perspiration, but he has also organized an integrated scientific research group in the Ministry of Education. Its aim is physiological research on climatic variations and reactions to cold. These activities of Dr. Kuno are regarded as the foundation of climatic physiology in Japan. Besides, he plays an important role in the direction of medical research and medical education in Japan.

The brilliant work of Dr. Kuno was recognized by the Japanese government in 1963 when it awarded him its highest decoration in the field of cultural achievements, the Order of Cultural Merits. He also gained honorary membership in the Physiological Society of Great Britain, the American Physiological Society, and the Physiological Society of the Federal Republic of Germany. We Japanese physiologists are proud indeed that his works are held in such high esteem by physiologists throughout the world.

Since olden times, it has been the custom in Japan to honor longevity with celebrations held on certain birthdays. In accordance with this, when Dr. Kuno reached his 77th birthday in 1960, he was honored by those who had once studied under him as well as by fellow Japanese physiologists, with the publication of "*Essential Problems in Climatic Physiology.*" The aim of this publication was additionally to inform physiologists abroad about the state of Climatic Physiology in Japan. We sincerely believe that this aim has been realized.

Now it is our great joy to be able to see Dr. Kuno celebrating his 88th birthday in good health. This birthday is the one traditionally celebrated after the 77th. To mark the occasion, we have planned the publication of "*Advances in Climatic Physiology.*"

It is worthy of note that while the 1960 publication consisted only of articles authored by Japanese physiologists, the present volume includes articles by physiologists throughout the world.

This plan could be realized because of the high international reputation of Dr. Kuno's works, and because of his friendship with scholars abroad. We are indeed grateful that among his numerous friends, twelve physiologists abroad have willingly granted our request to participate in this project. Their contributions will no doubt add important references to the studies of Climatic Physiology, at the same time providing added luster to the birthday celebration of Dr. Kuno.

May we offer this book to Dr. Kuno in honor of his venerable age, while praying for a still longer and happy life.

It is our great pleasure to acknowledge the cordial cooperation of all of the contributors, especially of the foreign prominent scholars for their invariable contributions to this book.

January, 1972   S. ITOH
                                                              K. OGATA
                                                              H. YOSHIMURA

LIST OF CONTRIBUTORS

ADOLPH, E.F.   Department of Physiology, the University of Rochester, Rochester, New York, U.S.A.

ASCHOFF, Jürgen   Max-Planck-Institut für Verhaltensphysiologie, 8131 Erling-Andechs, Germany

DILL, D.B.   Laboratory of Environmental Patho-Physiology, Desert Research Institute, University of Nevada System, Boulder City, Nevada, U.S.A.

EDHOLM, O.G.   Division of Human Physiology, National Institute for Medical Research, London, U.K.

HALBERG, Franz   Chronobiology Laboratories, University of Minneapolis, Minneapolis Minnesota, U.S.A.

HARDY, J.D.   John B. Pierce Foundation Laboratory, and Department of Epidemiology and Public Health, Yale University, New Haven, Conn., U.S.A.

HASEGAWA, Yasuhiro   Department of Physiology, Nagoya City University Medical School, Nagoya, Japan

HEISE, Arend   Max-Planck-Institut für Verhaltensphysiologie, 8131 Erling-Andechs, Germany

HIROSHIGE, Tsutomu   Department of Physiology, Hokkaido University School of Medicine, Sapporo, Japan

HORVATH, Steven M.   Institute of Environmental Stress, University of California, Santa Barbara, California, U.S.A.

IKAI, Kimio   Department of Physiology, Nagoya City University Medical School, Nagoya, Japan

INOUE, Taro   Central Hospital, Aichi Prefectural Colony-Welfare Center for the Mentally and Physically Handicapped, Kasugai, Japan

ITOH, Shinji   Department of Physiology, Hokkaido University School of Medicine, Sapporo, Japan

KAWAKAMI, Masazumi   Second Department of Physiology, Yokohama City University School of Medicine, Yokohama, Japan

KUROSHIMA, Akihiro   Department of Physiology, Hokkaido University School of Medicine, Sapporo, Japan

MOHRI, Motohiko   Second Department of Physiology, Yokohama City University School of Medicine, Yokohama, Japan

MORIMOTO, Taketoshi   Department of Physiology, Kyoto Prefectural University of Medicine, Kyoto, Japan

MURAKAMI, Naotoshi   Department of Physiology, Institute of Constitutional Medicine, Kumamoto University, Kumamoto, Japan

NAKAYAMA, Teruo   Department of Physiology, Nagoya University School of Medicine, Nagoya, Japan

NEGORO, HIDEO   Second Department of Physiology, Yokohama City University School of Medicine, Yokohama, Japan

OCHI, JUNZO   Department of Anatomy, Kyoto Prefectural University of Medicine, Kyoto, Japan

OGATA, KOREHIRO   Department of Physiology, Institute of Constitutional Medicine, Kumamoto University, Kumamoto, Japan

OGAWA, TOKUO   Department of Physiology, Niigata University School of Medicine, Niigata, Japan

OHARA, KŌKICHI   Second Department of Physiology, Nagoya City University Medical School, Nagoya, Japan

SAKAKURA, MUNEKI   Second Department of Medicine, Hokkaido University School of Medicine, Sapporo, Japan

SANO, YUTAKA   Department of Anatomy, Kyoto Prefectural University of Medicine, Kyoto, Japan

SARGENT, FREDERICK, II   Huxley College for Environmental Sciences, Western Washington State College, Bellingham, Washington, U.S.A.

SASAKI, TAKASHI   Department of Physiology, Institute of Constitutional Medicine, Kumamoto University, Kumamoto, Japan

SETO, KATSUO   Second Department of Physiology, Yokohama City University School of Medicine, Yokohama, Japan

SIMON, ECKHART   W.G. Kerckhoff-Institut der Max-Planck-Gesellschaft, Bad Nauheim, Physiologisches Institut der Universitat Gießen, Germany

SMOLENSKY, MICHAEL   School of Public Health, the University of Texas, Houston, Texas, U.S.A.

SUZUKI, MITSUO   Department of Physiology, Institute of Endocrinology, Gunma University, Maebashi, Japan

TAKEBE, KAZUO   Second Department of Medicine, Hokkaido University School of Medicine, Sapporo, Japan

THAUER, RUDOLF   W.G. Kerckhoff-Institut der Max-Planck-Gesellschaft, Bad Nauheim, Physiologisches Institut der Universitat Gießen, Germany

YAMAGUCHI, TADASHI   Second Department of Physiology, Yokohama City University School of Medicine, Yokohama, Japan

YAMAOKA, SADAO   Second Department of Physiology, Yokohama City University School of Medicine, Yokohama, Japan

YOSHIMURA, HISATO   Department of Physiology, Kyoto Prefectural University of Medicine, Kyoto, Japan

YOSHIMURA, KEIICHI   Department of Physiology, Hokkaido University School of Medicine, Sapporo, Japan

YOSHIMURA, MANABU   Department of Physiology, Kyoto Prefectural University of Medicine, Kyoto, Japan

YURUGI, RYOHEI   Airomedical Laboratory, JASDF., Tachikawa, Japan

CONTENTS

Part IV   Seasonal and Circadian Variations of Physiological Activitities

PART I

BODY TEMPERATURE REGULATION

CHAPTER 1

PERIPHERAL INPUTS TO THE CENTRAL REGULATOR FOR BODY TEMPERATURE

J. D. HARDY

John B. Pierce Foundation Laboratory, and Department of Epidemiology and Public Health, Yale University, New Haven, Conn., USA

The early observations of Professor Yasu Kuno [28, 29] and his colleagues [34, 35, 40, 44] on the effects of cutaneous pressure on the pattern of human sweating provided one of the first clear demonstrations of the importance of peripheral nonthermal stimulation in thermoregulation. Although the effects of heat and cold on the skin were recognized as possibly having a stimulatory action through the sensory endings in the skin [2, 31] the role (if any) of these peripheral temperature receptors in the thermoregulatory mechanism has remained debatable [25, 26, 27]. Most of the researches in the past 15 years have been focussed on the problem of the relative roles of the central and peripheral temperature receptors [15, 18] although the characterization of the peripheral receptors by Hensel [26] and the central receptors by Hardy [19] and his colleagues [4, 5, 7, 12, 33] has gone far to clarify much of the physiological data which has been accumulated. The nonthermal stimulation which Professor Kuno discovered to affect sweating has been generally confirmed and accepted although its role in the thermal balance of man is not yet understood.

The dual nature of temperature regulation in the life of the animal has been emphasized in the last decade so that for the unrestrained animal it is supposed that the thermoregulatory response is the result of both behavioral and physiological actions. Thus,

$$R = Be + Ph \tag{1}$$

in which R is the total thermoregulatory response, Be the behavioral component and Ph the physiological action. The total response results in the establishment of thermal balance in such a way as to minimize the total cost to the animal in terms of physiological strains [20]. Thus, if an animal which has been placed in a cold environment is given access to escape routes or sources of heat, it will respond within its capacity in such a way as to minimize shivering. If the behavioral action is made difficult or in some way unacceptable, the animal will use its physiological abilities to establish thermal balance. If the thermal threat cannot be met successfully by the combined behavioral and physiological responses, the animal dies. As Hammel [15] has pointed out in this context, all vertebrates regulate their body temperature to a greater or lesser extent and behavioral regulation is the action that is common to both homoiotherms and poikilotherms. Physiological regulation provides fine control of temperature and is especially well suited to elimination of excess body heat developed during exercise and work.

An idea of man's independence of his thermal environment which is provided by the careful regulation of his body temperature is shown in Fig. 1. To the left in the figure are indicated the Earthly and celestial environments in which man has lived and may explore; to the right are indicated the ranges of environmental temperature for which compensation is possible by physiological and behavioral temperature regulation. A healthy man does not exist with internal body temperature much outside the normal range of 36–38°C although during hard work and in febrile disease he may tolerate for short periods temperatures as high as 40–41°C. Denaturation of vital cellular proteins occurs so rapidly at 44–46°C that pain is evoked and tissue death occurs after a few hours [24]. Man may also tolerate hypothermic states for short times during which his body temperature may be as low as 27–29°C but these temperatures are incompatible with life except under the most careful medical supervision and not even then except for periods of a few days [37]. Man's Earthly environment on the other hand may be at 50°C on a hot day in the desert, 0°C on the high plateau of Australia where the aborigine lives completely unclothed or—60°C on the Antarctic waste lands. By means of protective clothing and heated shelters man can live on the coldest areas of the Earth and in the cold recesses of outer space or a lunar night. Cooling devices permit the exploration of the lunar surface at mid-day and perhaps may allow the penetration of the dense Venusian atmosphere. This great flexibility and freedom in respect to one of the great threats to all life, i.e. environmental temperature, depends primarily upon behavioral control of the body temperatures and is limited only my man's technology.

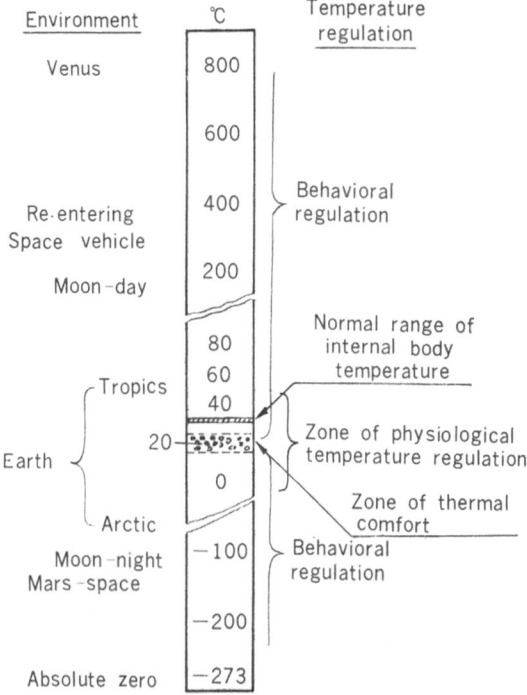

Fig. 1. Thermal environment and human thermoregulation.

Behavioral studies: The interplay between behavioral and physiological temperature regulation has been studied quantitatively by Adair and her associates [1] in the subhuman primate *Saimiri sciureus* (squirrel monkey). These animals were trained to select appropriate amounts of hot (50 °C) and cold (10 °C) air to provide an acceptable ambient temperature, 35 °C. The animals were then implanted with a thermode in the medial preoptic region on one side and with a reentrant tube for thermocouples on the same side. After recovery the animals were again placed in their environmental chamber and allowed to select the environmental temperature. In Fig. 2a

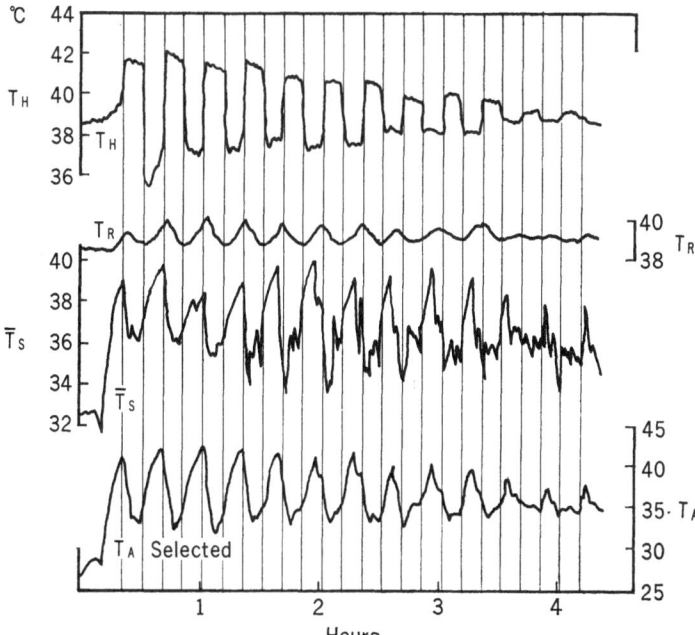

Fig. 2a. Experimental record of changes in rectal temperature (T_R), mean skin temperature (T̄_S) and selected air temperature (T_A) when the temperature of the hypothalamic thermode (T_H) was changed every 10 minutes.

are shown the results of one experiment in which the thermode temperature (T_H) was changed every 10 minutes by decreasing amounts. On being placed in the chamber, the animal began to warm itself by turning on the hot air for a brief period, a behavior generally seen in these animals which are housed in a room at 23 °C. After the initial period, the animal's hypothalamic temperature was raised from 39.5 °C to 41.5 °C and immediately the cold air was turned on. The change in ambient temperature was accompanied by a fall of about 1 °C in rectal temperature. The hypothalamic temperature was then lowered to 35.5 °C and the animal at once switched from cold air to hot; the rectal temperature rose 1.5 °C. The alternate heating and cooling of the preoptic region continued with decreasing temperature displacements for more than four hours at which time the amplitude was ± 0.3 °C from the animal's usual body temperature level. Even these small changes evoked appropriate changes in the monkey's behavior to control its environmental temperature.

In Fig. 2b (top) is another experiment on the same animal and in this case the preoptic temperature was held at 41–42 °C for 90 minutes. During the initial phase of the heating period, the animal cooled its environment thereby causing a drop in its rectal temperature from 39.5 °C to 36.5 °C and its skin temperature from 37.5 °C to 35 °C. At these levels the animal came into a purposeful thermal balance. The clear demonstration that the animal was now "regulating" about a new equilibrium or "set" level is that displacements of the hypothalamic temperature above or below the 41.5 °C level called forth responses from the animal which opposed these changes. For example, when the animal's hypothalamic temperature was *lowered* from 41.5 to 40 °C, the immediate response of the animal was to *heat* itself even though the 40 °C temperature was itself higher than the animal's normal level of 39.5 °C. This be-

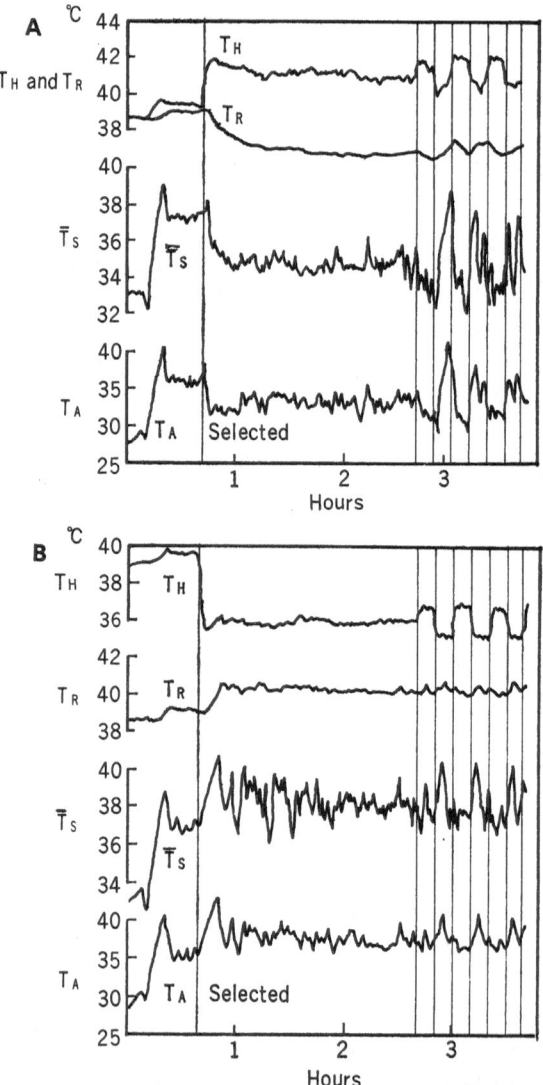

Fig. 2b. Experimental records of thermal clamp experiments at elevated hypothalamic temperature (A) and lowered hypothalamic temperature (B). Note effects of small displacements of T_H about the clamped levels at the end of the experiments. Symbols have same meaning as in Fig. 2a.

havior must indicate that the central regulating system has been "biased," possibly due to the lowering of the peripheral temperatures, a conclusion suggested by Adair et al. [1].

Physiological studies: Data from physiological experiments which indicate that the central regulator is influenced by changes in the temperature of the skin [18] and spinal cord [41] will be discussed elsewhere in this volume and therefore, only one additional physiological experiment will be noted here.

Rawson *et al.* [36] have shown that when electrical heat sources were chronically implanted in the ventral and lateral abdominal cavity of sheep and heated to 43–44°C so as to dissipate 20–22 watts, a rapid increase in respiratory frequency and respiratory water loss was observed as shown in Fig. 3. The delay time was three to five minutes from the beginning of the heating period and the magnitude of the response was approximately a two-fold increase over the control levels. The response was accompanied by a marked fall in the temperature of the hypothalamus of about 0.5°C, a gradual decrease in the vaginal temperature of roughly 0.2°C and an increase of about 1.0°C in the temperature of the skin overlying the heaters. To evaluate the effect of the warm skin, external heat was applied to the same skin areas (EXO in Fig. 3) and the temperature raised 1.5°C. As can be seen from the data there was no effect upon respiration or evaporative water loss from respiration. Rawson and his

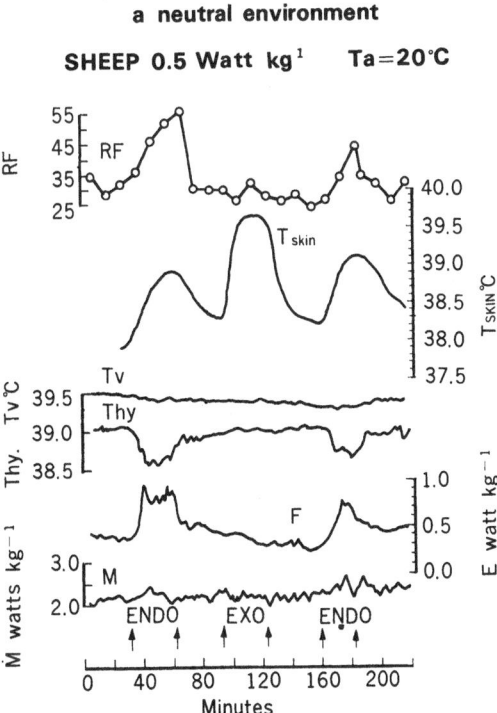

**Response to endogenous heating in
a neutral environment**

SHEEP 0.5 Watt kg^1 Ta=20°C

Fig. 3. Response of 41-Kg sheep to heating of abdominal viscera by electrical heaters implanted along ventral wall of peritoneum (ENDO) and of external heating of overlying skin (EXO). RF, respiratory frequency, in breaths per minute; T_{skin}, skin temperature overlying heaters; T_V, vaginal temperature; T_{HYPO}, hypothalamic temperature; HE, respiratory evaporative heat loss; MR, metabolic rate.

colleagues suggest on the basis of their study that the thermoregulatory effects which they observed may have been due to stimulation by the heating of thermoreceptors in some visceral structures and that these receptors may play a role in the normal regulation of body temperature. Nothing is known at present of the neural connections involved in such a pathway to the central nervous system; however, temperature sensitive neurons have been reported recently by Wood [43]. Recording from single units of the enteric nervous system in Auerbach's plexus of the jejunum of the cat, Wood observed units which discharged in bursts and were spontaneously active at temperatures 32–40 °C. As shown in Fig. 4 (reproduced by permission) both the number of spikes per burst and the frequency of the bursts were increased at high temperature and decreased at low temperatures; the Q_{10} values were given by the author as 3.2 and 15.9 respectively. The data in Figs. 3 and 4 provide evidence for a temperature sensitivity of the viscera which can affect central thermoregulation, although the full importance of this action cannot yet be assessed.

Studies of single units of brain stem: In addition to the physiological and behavioral data which indicate the effects of peripheral stimulation on thermoregulatory centers of the central nervous system there are direct observations of the activity of single

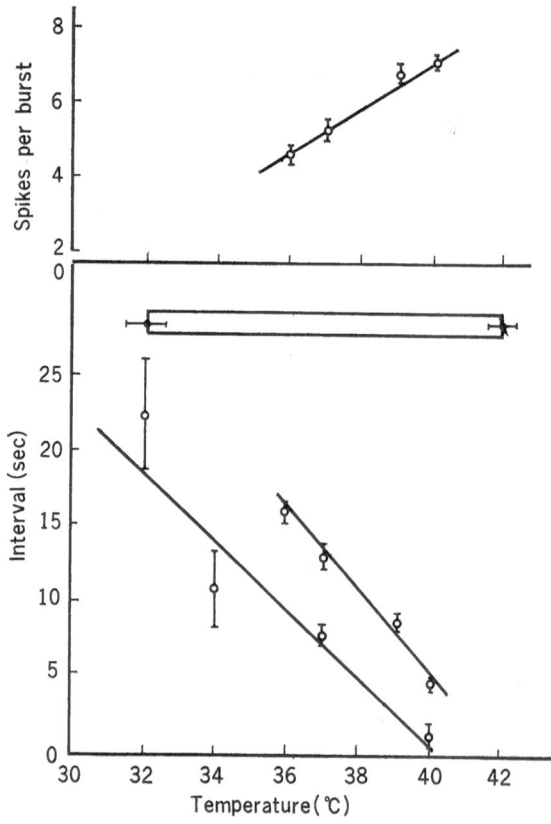

Fig. 4. Temperature sensitivity of single unit in Auerbach's plexus between 32 and 40 °C (Horizontal bar). Lower curve: Interval between bursts of activity as function of temperature of a unit studied between 32 and 40 °C and a second unit 36–40 °C. Upper chart: Temperature effect on spikes per burst of second unit.
(Reproduced by permission of Dr. J. D. Wood).

units of the brain stem which throw light on the interaction of central and peripheral stimuli. These temperature sensitive neurons were first reported by Nakayama *et al.* in 1961 [33] and are discussed in detail elsewhere in this volume. It is the intent here to inquire into the evidence for response of temperature sensitive units of the brain-stem to various peripheral stimuli including temperature change.

Cross and Green [6] in their study of unit activity in the supraoptic nuclei and preoptic region, reported that visual stimulation by flashes of light, auditory clicks and mechanical stimulation of the skin had the effect of altering the discharge rate of neurons in these regions. Also, Stuart *et al.* [39] found that the spontaneous firing rates of cells in the preoptic region were altered during noxious stimulation of the bladder. Murakami *et al.* [32] made a systematic study in the anesthetized and unanesthetized encephale isolé dog of the effects of local peripheral stimulation on the activity of temperature sensitive and insensitive neurons of the preoptic region. Many units were observed to respond to noxious stimuli such as pinching of the skin, touching the skin with a hot object, etc. A total of 259 neurons were studied and in no instance was the activity of any unit altered by the application of moderately warm or cold stimuli to the nose, tongue or shaved areas of the leg or flank. Taken by itself, this observation appears surprising especially when it is a common observation that dogs have marked thermoregulatory responses to environmental thermal stimulation [11, 17]. Indeed, Wit and Wang [42] and Hellon [23] have reported that general heating of the skin of anesthetized cats and unanesthetized rabbits causes alterations in the activity of temperature sensitive neurons of the preoptic region. Also, Nakayama and Hardy [33] have recently shown that marked activity can be evoked in units of the rostral reticular formation by cooling the skin of the anesthetized rabbit. Since units of this region have been shown to affect firing rates of preoptic warm and cold sensitive units, it reasonably can be assumed that cooling as well as heating the skin will affect some preoptic neurons, possibly via the reticular formation. The explantion of Murakami's findings may be that local thermal stimulation of relatively small skin areas did not produce a sufficiently strong effect on the CNS to cause a thermoregulatory action and therefore, could not be observed as an effective stimulus to preoptic neurons. However, since Landgren [30] has shown that even point thermal stimulation of the cat's tongue affects neurons of the thalamus and cortex of the anesthetized animal, it seems that two pathways are available to warm and cold stimuli on the skin and that the one to the preoptic region has a relatively higher requirement for spatial summation. This hypothesis is further strengthened by Murakami's finding that very hot or cold stimuli, at or near noxious levels, had the effect of stimulating and inhibiting spontaneous activity of preoptic units without affecting the thermal sensitivity of the units to local temperature change.

Mechanical stimulation of the skin, such as rubbing the fur affects the activity of temperature sensitive units of both the preoptic region and the midbrain. An example of such a response is shown in Fig. 5 [33], for a cold sensitive neuron located in the rostral reticular formation of the rabbit responding to cooling the midbrain while a constant temperature was maintained in the preoptic region. The unit was silent at brain temperatures above 36 °C but became very active when the midbrain was cooled to 34 °C. The unit was also activated by gentle stroking of the fur of the ipsilateral foreleg but not of the contralateral foreleg. About 45% of the temperature

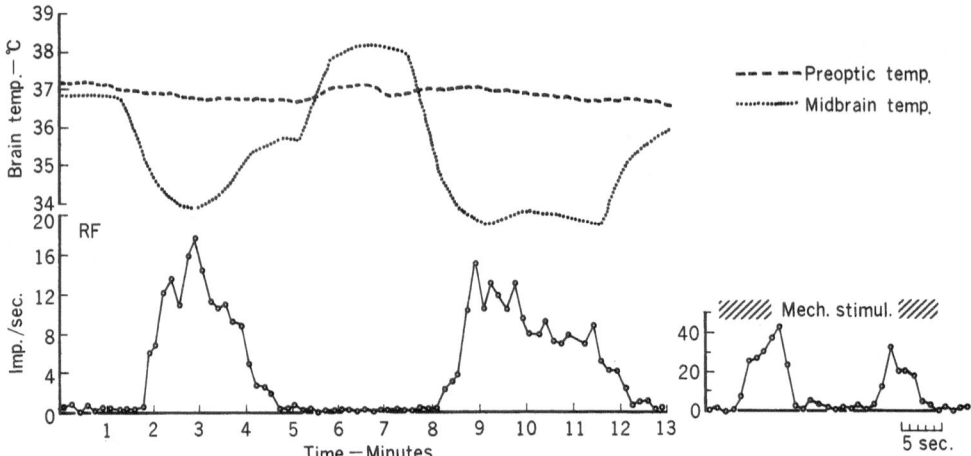

Fig. 5. Neuron in the rostral reticular formation of the urethanized rabbit responding only to local cooling and to rubbing fur of ipsilateral foreleg.

sensitive units reported in the reticular formation responded to peripheral mechanical stimuli and these units generally had nonlinear responses to local temperature change. Many units of the preoptic region which respond nonlinearly to local temperature change are also sensitive to mechanical stimulation of the skin. An example of such a unit is shown in Fig. 6 together with respiratory and vasomotor thermoregulatory responses evoked by temperature changes in the preoptic region and spinal canal [12]. It is seen that the unit responded with increased activity to heating in either of these areas but was unresponsive to cooling and that the unit activity and thermoregulatory responses occurred together. However, the unit was also stimulated by rubbing the animal's foreleg but in this case there was no thermoregulatory response, thus, indicating that this neuron's activity was not essential for thermoregulation. A possible function of the nonthermal stimuli on temperature regulation has been suggested by several authors [14, 33] as providing a background activity for facilitating thermoregulatory responses. Also, it has been suggested that the nonthermal inputs have a role in the thermoregulation during exercise by lowering the "setpoint" so that heat loss mechanisms can be activated without appreciable increase in internal body temperatures [16].

It should be noted that all units with a linear response to local temperature over a wide temperature range (32–42 °C) have been found to be insensitive to mechanical or thermal stimulation of other body regions while highly sensitive to their own temperature. These characteristics have prompted several authors to suggest that these neurons may be the primary temperature "sensors" of the preoptic region. The validity of this assumption seems particularly reasonable in view of the fact that these units are apparently most numerous in the small volume of tissue along the midline which, when heated or cooled, evokes appropriate thermoregulatory responses.

During the past three years our laboratory has focused its attention on the problem of the integration of thermal and other inputs to the temperature sensitive neurons of the preoptic region and the more caudal parts of the brain stem. The general method of experimentation has been to identify units which are sensitive to local temperature change and then while clamping the local temperature at the usual normal level, to observe the change in firing rate when the temperature of other parts of the brain stem,

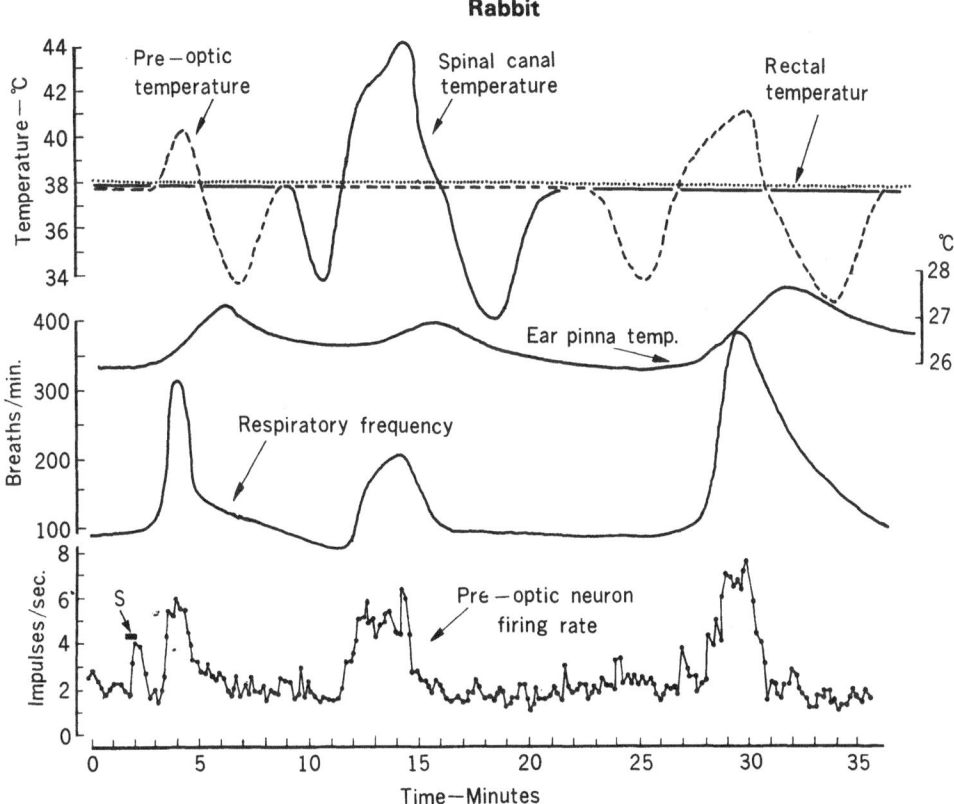

Fig. 6. Response of preoptic neuron to preoptic and spinal cord heating. Unit responded also to rubbing the fur of the ipsilateral foreleg but not to the contralateral leg. Note that heating evokes thermoregulatory response but rubbing leg does not.

spinal cord, viscera, etc. was altered. It immediately became apparent that most of the units had responses which were much more complicated than could be revealed by study of the effects of local temperature alone. A summary of the available data on the preoptic-anterior hypothalamic units is contained in Tables 1 and 2, as reported by Guieu and Hardy [13], who identified at least 22 different types of responses. In the first column is an identifying number for reference to figures and in the next column there is a temperature response diagram which indicates the general type of the reported activity. The species in which the type of unit has been found are listed in the third column and the observers are reported as reference numbers in the last column. The two columns noted as "input" and "output" refer to the effective changes in temperature produced experimentally and the firing rate dependence on temperature respectively. Two examples will serve to illustrate the algebra used to describe the "Estimated Output." Unit #2 responds to temperature changes in hyperthermia only (i.e. $+ \Delta T_{po}$) with a positive temperature coefficient; for temperatures below normal the unit is silent. In order to explain the behavior of this type of interneuron, Murakami *et al.* [32] suggested that the unit was facilitated by the warm sensors and inhibited by some temperature insensitive input firing at a fixed rate, F_o. On this basis the output of unit #2 would be the algebraic sum of the facilitating input from the sensor (i.e.

TABLE 1 Preoptic-anterior hypothalamic units: Positive coefficients for preoptic temperature change

N	Temperature response	Species studied	Effective input temperature	Estimated output (Impulses/sec)	Observer
1	po	Dog, Rabbit Cat, Tiliqua	T_{po}	$+aT_{po}$	4,5,7,8,9,12 22,32,33,42
2	po	Dog, Rabbit Cat, Tiliqua	$(+\Delta T_{po})$	$+aT_{po}-F_o$	4,5,7,8,32
3	po	Cat, Rabbit Dog, Tiliqua	$(+\Delta T_{po})$	$F_o+[a(+\Delta T_{po})]$	4,5,7,8,12,22, 32,33,42
4	po mb	Rabbit	$(+\Delta T_{po}); (+\Delta T_{mb})$	$F_o+[a(+\Delta T_{po})+b(+T_{mb})]$	32
5	po sc	Rabbit	$(+\Delta T_{po}); (+\Delta T_{sc})$	$F_o+[a(+\Delta T_{po})+c(+\Delta T_{sc})]$	12
6	po s	Cat	$(+\Delta T_{po}); (+\Delta T_s)$	$F_o+[a(+\Delta T_{po})+d(+\Delta T_s)]$	23,42
7	po sc	Rabbit	$(+\Delta T_{po}); (+T_{sc})$	$F_o+[a(+\Delta T_{po})-c(+\Delta T_{sc})]$	12
8	po mb	Rabbit	$(+\Delta T_{po}); (-\Delta T_{mb})$	$F_o+[a(+\Delta T_{po})+(-b(-\Delta T_{mb}))]$	33
9	po mb	Rabbit	$T_{po}; (-\Delta T_{mb})$	$+(+aT_{po})+[-b(-\Delta T_{mb})]$	33
10	po	Cat, Rabbit Dog	$(-\Delta T_{po})$	$F_o-[+a(-\Delta T_{po})]$	9,12,23
11	po sc	Rabbit	$(-\Delta T_{po}); (\Delta-T_{sc})$	$F_o-[+a(-\Delta T_{po})+c(-\Delta T_{sc})]$	12
12	re	Rabbit	$T_{po}; (+\Delta T_{re}); (\Delta-T_{sc})$	$-e[+T_{re}(T_{po}+\Delta T_{sc})]$	12
13	po sc	Rabbit	$(-\Delta T_{po}); (+\Delta T_{sc})$	$F_o-[+a(-\Delta T_{po})+(-c(+T_{sc}))]$	12

TABLE 2 Preoptic-anterior hypothalamic units: Negative coefficients for preoptic temperature change

N	Temperature response	Species studied	Input temperature	Estimated output	Observer
14	po	Dog, Rabbit	$-T_{po}$	$-aT_{po}$	5,7
15	po	Dog, Rabbit Tilique, Cat	$+(-\Delta T_{po})$	$-a(-\Delta T_{po})$	4,5,7,8,22
16	po	Cat, Rabbit	$+(-\Delta T_{po})$	$F_o+[-a(-T_{po})]$	7,12
17	po sc	Rabbit	$+(-\Delta T_{po}); (-\Delta T_{sc})$	$F_o+[-a(-T_{po})-c(-T_{sc})]$	12
18	sc po	Rabbit	$(-\Delta T_{po}); (+\Delta T_{sc})$	$F_o+[-a(-\Delta T_{po})+c(+\Delta T_{sc})]$	12
19	po	Dog, Cat Rabbit	$(+\Delta T_{po})$	$F_o-[-a(+\Delta T_{po})]$	5,7,8,12,23,33
20	po sc	Rabbit	$(+\Delta T_{po}); (+\Delta T_{sc})$	$F_o-[-a(+\Delta T_{po})-c(+\Delta T_{sc})]$	12
21	po mb	Rabbit	$(\Delta+T_{po}); (+\Delta T_{mb})$	$F_o+[-a(+\Delta T_{po})-b(+\Delta T_{mb})]$	33
22	po mb	Rabbit	$(-\Delta T_{po}); +(-\Delta T_{mb})$	$F_o+[-a(-\Delta T_{po})-b(-\Delta T_{mb})]$	33

$+a\ T_{po}$) and the inhibiting input from the temperature insensitive units, $-F_o$, or, $+a\ T_{po}\ -F_o$. It is possible to think of the cell as having a threshold for activity and in this case $-F_o$ would be some sort of temperature insensitive quality built into the cell and not the result of activity of insensitive unit discharges. Experimental evidence on this point is not available at this time but the answer should be possible through studies of the response of #2 type units to neural transmitters. The Murakami hypothesis requires that unit #2 respond in a specific way to two transmitters. Unit #8, reported in the rabbit by Guieu and Hardy [12] responds to preoptic temperature (above normal only, i.e. $+\varDelta T_{po}$) and to midbrain temperature (below normal only, i.e. $-\varDelta T_{mb}$). Consider now the "output" for the type 8 unit. In these experiments the unit was spontaneously active at some minimal level which was independent of low preoptic temperature ($-\varDelta T_{po}$) and high midbrain temperature ($+\varDelta T_{mb}$) thus requiring a term representing the temperature independent firing rate (F_o). To that is added the additional activity which is proportional to the elevated preoptic temperature (i.e. $+a(+\varDelta T_{po})$). Also, there is added to F_o an activity which increased in proportion to the amount of the decrease of midbrain temperature (i.e. $+(-b(-\varDelta T_{mb}))$. The $+$ sign in front of the bracket has special meaning in that it signifies a facilitation by the function $(-b(-\varDelta T_{po}))$. For some units an inhibition is indicated for example in the case of neuron #10, for which the function is $-[+a(-\varDelta T_{po})]$, the negative sign indicating the inhibitory effect of the function, $+a\ (-\varDelta T_{po})$. Units of type 8 group increase their activity with any displacement of body temperature from its normal range and thus they could serve a "setpoint" function of some sort rather than a temperature detecting or transmitting function since they could not distinguish warm from cold. A similar type of algebra is used to describe all the other units in Tables 1 and 2 using the convention that a negative sign for a coefficient means a negative slope to the response curve and a negative sign in front of a parenthesis signifies an inhibiting action. The letters a,b,c,d and e have been assigned as categorical coefficients for changes in preoptic (po), midbrain (mb), spinal cord (sc), skin (s) and rectal (re) temperature respectively.

In many of the studies which have been made on preoptic units in the last 10 years, reference has been made to "warm" units which increase firing rate with increasing preoptic temperature, that is positive temperature coefficient, $+a$, or "cold" units which increase firing rate with decreasing preoptic temperature, or negative coefficient, $-a$. On this basis, Table 1 contains "warm" units and Table 2 "cold" units, but, as the data in the tables indicate, this distinction is rather arbitrary and may not be generally useful. About 1,000 units in the preoptic-anterior hypothalamus have been reported from various laboratories with respect to the unit sensitivity to local temperature. Of these, about 22% have been classified as warm units, 5% as cold units and 73% of the cells were either insensitive to temperatures between 32°C and 42°C or were only so slightly sensitive that they have been classified as insensitive. As can be noted in the tables the units may be uniformly sensitive to temperature (units #1 and #14) or may have a non-linear response; that is, the units may be insensitive over a certain temperature range. The temperature levels at which the changes in sensitivity occurred were either in or just above or below the normal temperature range of the animal. The data from different laboratories support the following conclusions:

a)   Temperature signals from thermal receptors in the preoptic region, midbrain, spinal canal, skin and probably the abdominal viscera converge on preoptic units;

b)   Thermal and nonthermal stimuli from the peripheral regions evoke activity of units in the preoptic region;

c)   Most preoptic units which respond to such stimulation have non-linear responses to preoptic temperature.

As can be seen from the "output" columns of Tables 1 and 2, the pattern of activity of the convergence is a summation of the thermal input signals, for example, neurons #4, #5, #6, #11, #17, #20, #21 and #22 show this effect.   Neuron #12 appears to have a multiplying action between preoptic, spinal cord and rectal temperatures, but the response of this neuron is difficult to analyze.   Neurons #8, #9, #13 and #18 have changes in activity whenever the body temperature is displaced from normal and as noted above, these effects remind one of "setpoints."   Neuron #7 appears to change activity if there is a gradient of temperature between preoptic region and spinal canal.

Since the clarification of our understanding of the way in which the central nervous system processes the temperature information from the preoptic region and other body areas is in its beginning stages, many other types of responses of preoptic, hypothalamic and other brain stem neurons must be anticipated.   Also, the data reviewed above are limited by the particular methodology employed in their study. For example, the unit #9 and perhaps also #12, under conditions of stable normal temperature of the animal's body (except for the manipulated preoptic temperature) would have been reported as a unit #1.   Similarly, the other units in the tables have not been studied under a great variety of body temperature changes, and thus the data must be considered as providing indicative rather than definitive descriptions of the unit activity.   With new researches the data will become more and more complex and thus, it becomes a question of importance to the further study of unit activity related to temperature to ask whether any rational relationship can be visualized between the types of units that already have been identified?   Must the data be considered as descriptive only or can they be assembled into hypothetical neuronal networks which may have a conceptual relationship to the known facts regarding physiological and behavioral temperature regulation?   Even though such an exercise will result initially in incorrect concepts, it perhaps can furnish a point of attack for future developments of more correct ideas.   Thus, I have undertaken to use the observed unit responses in the construction of a conceptual network of interconnections of units that have been described.   It is realized that the numbers of units studied are few in comparison to the many which exist in the preoptic anterior hypothalamus subserving many vital regulatory functions, and that the data available on any unit are fragmentary at best.   Furthermore, only circumstantial evidence is presently available to link the activity of the temperature sensitive units to the functions of physiological and behavioral temperature regulation.   Nevertheless the many types of evidence which now exist are completely compatible with the idea that the nervous elements of the brain stem which are temperature sensitive do serve thermoregulatory functions and thus justify analysis of unit activity in this context.

All of the neuron responses of Tables 1 and 2 were considered, even though only a single unit of the type may have been reported.   The unit activity was related to the observed temperature changes locally and at some distant site, when data were available, in terms of equations of the form indicated in the "output" columns:

Unit firing rate = function of local temperature and distant temperature + an activity component insensitive to temperature.

The following assumptions were made regarding interneuronal relationships:

a) Units responding linearly to local temperature *only*, over a wide range of temperatures (32–42 °C) are temperature sensors and furnish the POA temperature input into the system;

b) All other temperature sensitive POA units are interneurons which may receive inputs from temperature changes locally and elsewhere as well as from temperature insensitive units;

c) Synaptic transmission can be either facilitating or inhibitory (both can operate on a single cell) [3, 10];

d) Unit response is proportional to the amounts of transmitter substances released (three are required); these amounts in turn are proportional to the firing rates of units having inputs to the cell;

e) Interneurons are not generally spontaneously active; that is, if there are no inputs, such as can be observed at low or elevated body temperatures, the unit may be silent; if the unit is not silent under these conditions (e.g. unit #3) a temperature insensitive unit input is assumed;

f) No unit response can be omitted if sufficient data are available to clearly relate its response to temperature;

g) Unit inputs are selected so as to provide the output which agrees with experimental data from unit recordings without regard to possible thermoregulatory function;

h) Circuits may be separated on basis of the response of the unit to preoptic temperature, i.e. $\pm$ $(+\Delta T_{po})$ and $\pm$ $(-\Delta T_{po})$ for "warm" and "cold" circuits respectively.

Using these limiting assumptions [21], which are compatible with available knowledge of these neurons, it quickly became evident that only two networks would be required, one for preoptic temperatures above normal and the other for temperatures below normal. In Fig. 7, is shown the diagram for the network applicable to temperatures above normal and noted as "warm." The term "warm" in this case refers to the physiological meaning of the word, that is to activity in hyperthermia, rather than to the designation of the increasing of activity of a unit with increasing temperature. For example, units #10, #11 and #13 increase activity with increasing preoptic temperature but only at hypothermic $(-\Delta T_{po})$ levels, and so would not be included in the warm circuit. The beginning of the network is the hypothalamic warm sensor shown to the left as unit #1; the response of the unit is shown immediately above. The hypothalamic warm sensor has been discussed by several authors as being a neuron with, 1) a large linear response to temperature over a wide range of temperature; 2) a minimal response to anesthetics; 3) a minimal response to temperature changes in other areas; and 4) a distribution restricted largely to the area of the brain stem which has maximum effectiveness in evoking physiological #11 and behavioral thermoregulation #1. It is visualized that these units synapse directly with interneurons #2 and #12. Interneuron #2 is facilitated by unit #1 and inhibited by a temperature insensitive unit firing at a fixed rate. As pointed out by Murakami *et al.* [32], unit #2 has characteristics appropriate for an error signal generator and forms the base for the warm network since it has response only at elevated temperatures. The sequence of units #2, #3, #4, #5 and #6 provides for the development of the hypothalamic error signal due to hyperthermia and the subsequent summation of this signal with warm error signals from the midbrain, spinal cord and skin. The outputs from this chain are noted as W_1, W_2 and W_3 all of which increase with temperatures above normal and have a low-level, unchanging output for hypothermic temperatures. Unit #12 is the single reported instance of three identified inputs and it has a great peculiarity because it seems to be a multiplying rather than a summing unit. That is, the hypothalamic and spinal cord temperatures seem to control the sensitivity of this unit to changes in the rectal temperature. The output W_4 is also increased with high body temperature but the unit is silent in hypothermia. The units #7 and #9 seem to have responses to temperature in other areas which cancel that in the preoptic region. Their thermal functions may be that of detecting temperature differences or gradients. Unit #8 appears to have minimal response at normal body temperature but increased activity at both high and low temperatures. Such a unit could serve an alerting function and be related perhaps to thermal discomfort.

Units #19, #20 and #21 have negative temperature coefficients but only for temperatures above normal for preoptic, spinal cord and midbrain temperatures. For this reason, they necessarily belong to the warm network even though they have negative temperature coefficients, a characteristic of "cold" units. Their outputs W_5, W_6 and W_7 decrease with elevated body temperature. The total output from the warm preoptic network can be written in the form of an equation as:

$$S_w = (F_0 + W_1 + W_2 + W_3 + W_4) + (F_0 - W_5 - W_6 - W_7) \pm U \text{ or}$$
$$S_w = [F_0 + a\varDelta T_{po} + b\,(\varDelta T_{mb}) + c\,(\varDelta T_{sc}) + d\,(\varDelta T_s) + e\,\varDelta T_{re}\,(T_{po} + T_{sc})]$$
$$+ [F_0 - a\varDelta T_{po} - b\,(\varDelta T_{mb}) - c\,(\varDelta T_{sc})] \pm U \tag{2}$$

These outputs would provide marked stimulation and some inhibition with elevated temperatures perhaps acting as a sort of push-pull system. The facilitating outputs may operate on the respiratory and salivary systems and the decreased outputs on the metabolic rate and the vasomotor system. Unit 12 recalls the multiplying system suggested by Stolwijk and Hardy [38] to account for the control of sweating in resting man. This concept of the neuronal network appears compatible with a thermoregulatory function employing continuous proportional control.

It is useful to compare equation (2) with the computer control equations for man to see if the demands of the physiological regulator bear resemblance to the outputs which can be visualized from the neuronal data. The computer equation for hyperthermia (38) is:

$$S_w = a\,(+\varDelta T_{po}) + d\,(+\varDelta T_s) + h\,(+\varDelta T_{po})\,(+\varDelta \bar{T}_s) \tag{3}$$

There are obviously common factors between equations (2) and (3) but also there are several differences. For example, equation (2) is more complex than equation (3). This situation is to be expected, however, since equation (3) was developed with the limitation that it should contain only the terms which certain human physiological data on temperature regulation demanded. Clearly, some of the actual inputs to the physiological regulator will always be lumped together or omitted entirely from the computer equation and the computer model will thus be limited. In Fig. 8 is outlined the "cold" network of interneurons.

This network is simpler but of the same general form as the warm network. There is some question as to whether the "cold" sensor neuron exists. Only a few clear-cut cold sensor units have been described which fill all the requirements that have been set down for a warm sensor. As an alternative a warm sensor is shown in Fig. 8, with an inhibiting synapse on unit #15 supplying both the negative coefficient and the response only for hypothermic temperatures. Unit #15 thus becomes the key element for the cold network. There are only two outputs C_1 and C_2 which increase activity in the cold as shown from units #17 and #22 which sum the effects of the spinal cord, midbrain and preoptic region. Two units #18 and #13 appear to alter activity for both heating and cooling. Output C_3 decreases activity in hypothermia in combination with low spinal cord temperatures. The quation for the cold circuit can be written as,

$$S_C = (F_0 + C_1 + C_2) + (F_0 - C_3) \pm U \text{ or}$$
$$S_C = [F_0 + (-a(-\Delta T_{po})) + (-c(-\Delta T_{sc}))] + [F_0 - (+a(-\Delta T_{po}) + c(-T_{sc}))] \quad (4)$$

The corresponding computer equation which has been developed from human physiological considerations (38) includes terms corresponding to C_1 and additional terms not yet identified by neuronal recordings and is as follows:

$$S_C = +a(-\Delta T_{po}) + d(-\Delta T_s) + c(-\Delta T_{po})(-\Delta T_s) \quad (5)$$

Again, there are obvious similarities and differences. Equation (4) is in some respects more complex than equation (5) but does not contain some terms appearing in equation (5). In the computer equations as with the interneuron model two circuits

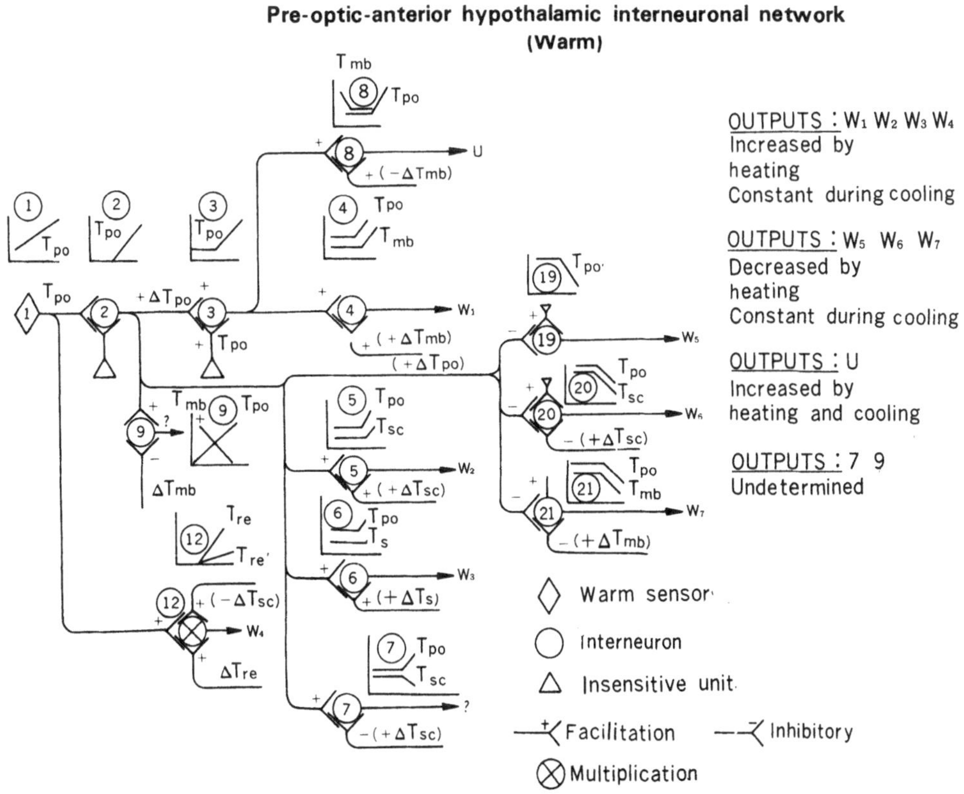

Fig. 7. Hypothetical interconnections among units of the preoptic-anterior-hypothalamic region responding to hyperthermic preoptic temperatures.

are required, one to operate in hyperthermia and another to function in hypothermia. It is instructive to consider in a qualitative manner how the neuronal networks should respond based on Tables 1 and 2 and Figs. 7 and 8 during an experiment in which the preoptic temperature is raised and clamped for a prolonged period. Assuming that the data apply to the monkey, an experiment of this sort is shown in Fig. 2b (top). It will be assumed also that before the preoptic heating begins, the animal is in thermally neutral conditions and the outputs from the warm circuit are minimal at the level of F_0. The same assumptions are made for the cold circuit. If the heating begins at time, t = o, then the following conditions will prevail:

Start of heating	Warm circuit		
Unit number	Effect on units	Effect on outputs	
1,2,3,4,5,6,7,8,9,12	↑	W_1, W_2, W_3, W_4, U	↑
19,20,21	↓	W_5, W_6, W_7	↓
	↔	———	↔

Start of heating —	Cold circuit		
1	↑	———	↑
14	↓	———	↓
10,11,13,15,16,17,22	↔	C_1, C_2, C_3, U_1, U_2	↔

The warm circuit is completely activated and thus the animal will demand cooling by both physiological and behavioral means. The cold circuit will be generally unactivated

Pre-optic-anterior hypothalamic interneuronal network
(Cold)

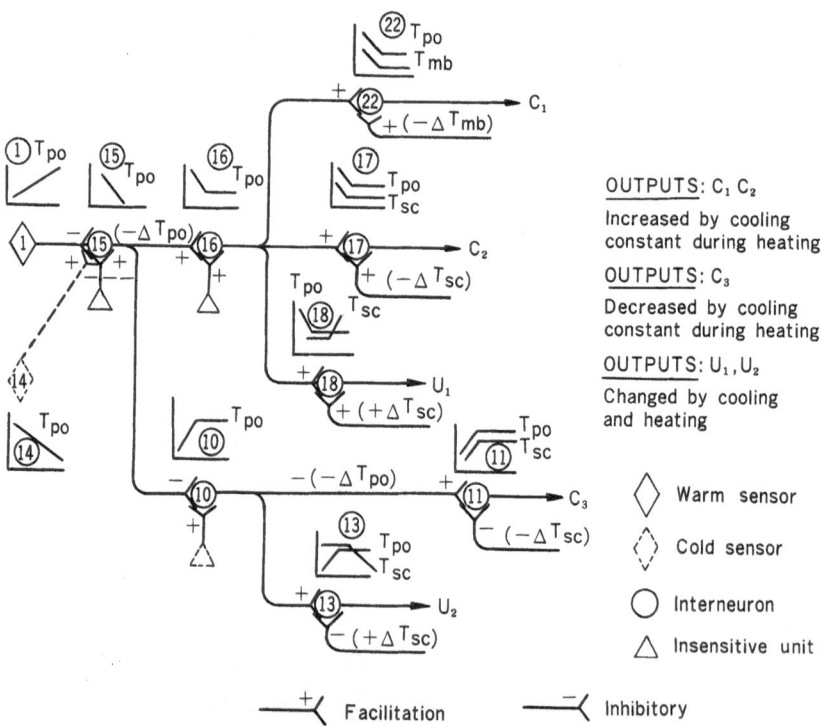

Fig. 8. Hypothetical interconnections among units of the preoptic-anterior-hypothalamic region responding to hypothermic preoptic temperatures.

because unit #15 will stop firing and the animal will not demand heating. These predictions are in complete accord with the actions seen in Fig. 2b (top).

After about an hour the animal comes into equilibrium and appears to regulate his core temperature about a level which is 3° lower than normal. The conditions of the warm and cold circuits will also have altered and can be visualized as follows:

After 90 minutes		Warm circuit		
Unit number	—	Effect on units	Effect on outputs	
8,9		↑↑	U	↑↑
1,2,3,4,5,6,7		↑	W_1, W_2, W_3	↑
12,19,20,21		↓	W_4, W_5, W_6, W_7	↓
——		↔	——	↔

After 90 minutes	—	Cold circuit		
		↑↑		↑↑
——			——	
1,17,22		↑	C_1, C_2	↑
11		↓	C_3	↓
10,13,14,15,16		↔	U	→

In this situation the drive for body cooling has been decreased somewhat by the decrease in W_4 and the cold circuit is activated by the effects of the peripheral inputs. These are very powerful since it is clear that high continuous heating of the preoptic region to 41–42 °C will be effectively balanced by the peripheral cold stimulation. Or:

$$C_1 + C_2 = W_1 + W_2 + W_3 \qquad (6)$$

This property of the physiological regulator was noted by Fusco et al. [11]. It might be noticed from the computer equation that the above experimental results for the squirrel monkey would not be predicted because there is no provision in the control equations for deep body temperatures other than the hypothalamic temperature or for the peripheral temperatures except for the skin. The "push-pull" outputs from the warm and cold networks form interesting points for speculation. The computer equations that have been developed contain two groups of output signals, one of which increases with hyperthermia and controls sweating and the other with hypothermia and controls shivering. Also, two sets of equations are developed by the model makers

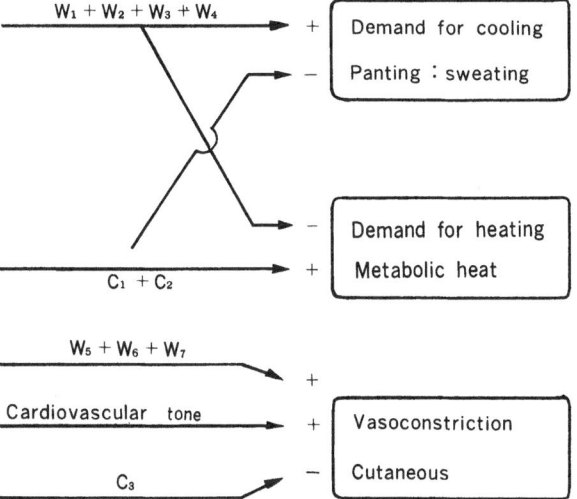

Fig. 9. Possible connections of warm and cold circuit outputs to thermoregulatory functions.

usually one for vasomotor response to heat and the other for vasomotor effects in the cold. On this basis one could suppose that $W_1 + W_2 + W_3 + W_4$ and $C_1 + C_2$ would combine to evoke sweating (or panting) and shivering respectively and that $W_5 + W_6 + W_7$ and C_3 would combine in some way to promote vasodilation or inhibition of vasoconstriction in hyperthermia and vasoconstriction in the cold. However, since W_5, W_6, W_7 and C_3 all are maximal at thermal neutrality these outputs would be respectively facilitory and inhibitory to vasoconstriction. Thus, the combined model of the outputs from the two circuits would have the form shown in Fig. 9. The preceding analysis does not *prove* anything and is not intended in this direction. The aim has been to look at the 22 observed unit responses and to relate them to each other to see if some rational scheme could be found. Having done this, the outputs of the networks could be examined in the light of already existing concepts of thermoregulation. However, the diagrams shown in Figs. 7 and 8 lack uniqueness and the important attributes of being necessary and sufficient. If the diagrams have any value it must lie in the direction of suggestions for further experimentation. As a beginning, naturally, all the assumptions upon which the models are based provide points of attack.

SUMMARY

1) Peripheral stimuli, both thermal and nonthermal, converge on temperature sensitive neurons of the preoptic-anterior hypothalamic area (POA) and provide important contributions to physiological and behavioral regulation of body temperature.

2) Heating and cooling of the POA stimulates both physiological and behavioral temperature responses which are limited by the development of opposing peripheral signals (probably thermal).

3) Thermal signals from the POA, midbrain reticular formation, spinal cord, viscera and skin converge on neurons of the POA in a summative and discrimitory manner so that internal thermal gradients and temperature displacements may be detected and evaluated.

4) The observed POA unit responses can be used as a basis for conceptualized interneuron networks, one for hypothermia and the other for hyperthermia. The unit activity suggests generally summative functions although differentiation and multiplication also are indicated.

5) Analysis of the outputs from conceptual models of the neuronal and computer thermoregulating systems indicates a compatibility of the two for proportional control and gain control although the neuronal model tends to be more complex.

REFERENCES

1. ADAIR, E.R., J.U. CASBY, and J.A.J. STOLWIJK (1970): *J. Comparative and Physiol. Psychology* **72**: 17.
2. BAZETT, H.C. (1941): Temperature, Its Measurement and Control in Science and Industry, Am. Institute of Physics Ed., Reinhold Publ. Corp., New York.
3. BLOOM, F.E., A.P. OLIVER, and G.C. SALMOIRAGHI. (1963): *Int. J. Neuropharmacology* **2**: 181.
4. CABANAC, M., T. HAMMEL, and J.D. HARDY (1967): *Science* **158**: 1050.
5. CABANAC, M., J.A.J. STOLWIJK, and J.D. HARDY. (1968): *J. Appl. Physiol.* **24**: 645.
6. CROSS, B.A., and J.D. GREEN (1959): *J. Physiol., London* **148**: 554.
7. CUNNINGHAM, D.J., J.A.J. STOLWIJK, N. MURAKAMI, and J.D. HARDY (1967): *Am. J. Physiol.* **213**: 1570–1581.

8. EISENMAN, J.S. (1969): *Am. J. Physiol.* **216:** 330.
9. EISENMAN, J.S., and D.C. JACKSON (1967): *Exp. Neurol.* **19:** 33.
10. FELDBERG, W., and R.D. MYERS (1964): *J. Physiol.* **175:** 303.
11. FUSCO, M.M., J.D. HARDY, and H.T. HAMMEL (1961): *Am. J. Physiol.* **200:** 572.
12. GUIEU, J.D., and J.D. HARDY (1970): *J. Appl. Physiol.* **29:** 675.
13. GUIEU, J.D., and J.D. HARDY (1971): Thermoregulation Comportementale, Lyon Symposium, M. Cabanac (ed.), *J. Physiol.* (Paris), pp 253–256.
14. HAMMEL, H.T. (1965): Physiological Controls and Regulation. W.S. YAMAMOTO and J.R. BROBECK, Eds., Saunders Co., Philadelphia, Pa.
15. HAMMEL, H.T. (1968): *Ann. Rev. Physiology* **30:** 641.
16. HAMMEL, H.T., D.C. JACKSON, J.A.J. STOLWIJK, J.D. HARDY, and S.B. STROMME (1963): *J. Appl. Physiol.* **18:** 1146.
17. HAMMOUDA, M. (1933): *J. Physiol.* **77:** 319.
18. HARDY, J.D. (1961): *Physiol. Reviews* **41:** 521.
19. HARDY, J.D. (1969): Brody Memorial Lecture VIII, Brain Sensors of Temperature, University of Missouri, Special Report 103.
20. HARDY, J.D. (1970): Physiological and Behavioral Temperature Regulation. Chas. C. Thomas Publ., Fort Lauderdale, Florida, U.S.A. P. 586.
21. HARDY, J.D., and J.D. GUIEU. (1971): Thermoregulation Comportementale, Lyon Symposium, M. Cabanac (ed.), *J. Physiol.* (Paris), pp 260–267.
22. HARDY, J.D., R.F. HELLON, and K. SUTHERLAND (1964): *J. Physiol.* (London) **175:** 242.
23. HELLON, R.F. (1969): *Experientia* **25:** 610.
24. HENRIQUES, F.C., JR. (1947): *Arch. Pathol.* **43:** 489.
25. HENSEL, H. (1952): *Ergeb. Physiol.* **47:** 166.
26. HENSEL, H. (1968): The Skin Senses, Dan Kenshalo, Ed., Chas. C. Thomas, Pub., Fort Lauderdale, Florida, USA, p. 398.
27. KELLER, A.D., and E.B. McCLASKEY (1964): *Am. J. Physiol.* **43:** 181.
28. KUNO, Yas. (1934): The Physiology of Human Perspiration, J. & A. Churchill, Ltd., London.
29. KUNO, Y. (1956): Human Perspiration, Chas. Thomas., Springfield, Ill., U.S.A.
30. LANDGREN, S. (1960): *Acta Physiol. Scand.* **48:** 255.
31. MARTIN, Charles J. (1930): *The Lancet*, Sept. 13, p. 561.
32. MURAKAMI, N., J.A.J. STOLWIJK, and J.D. HARDY (1967): *Am. J. Physiol.* **213:** 1015.
33. NAKAYAMA, T., and J.D. HARDY (1969): *J. Appl. Physiol.* **27:** 848.
34. OGATA, K. (1961): *Bull. Res. Inst. Diathetic Med.*, Kumamoto Univ., Kumamoto, Japan II, **1:** 58.
35. OGATA, K., T. SASAKI, and N. MURAKAMI (1966): *Bull. Inst. Constitutional Med.*, Kumamoto Univ., Japan **16:** 1.
36. RAWSON, R.O., K.P. QUICK, and R.F. COUGHLIN (1969): *Science* **169:** 919.
37. SMITH, L.W., and T. FAY (1939): *J. Am. Med. Assn.* **113:** 653.
38. STOLWIJK, J.A.J., and J.D. HARDY (1966): *Pflügers Archiv.* **291:** 129–162.
39. STUART, D.G., D.S. MAXWELL, J.N. HAYWARD, M.D. FAIRCHILD, W.R. ADEY, and R.W. PORTER (1963): *Biologica Inst. Estud. Med. Biol.*, Mexico **21:** 349.
40. TAKAGI, K. (1960): Essential Problems in Climatic Physiol., Kyoto, Nankodo.
41. THAUER, R. (1935): *Arch. Ges. Physiol.* **236:** 102.
42. WIT, A., and S.C. WANG. (1968): *Am. J. Physiol.* **215:** 1151.
43. WOOD, J.D. (1970): *Am. J. Physiol.* **219:** 159.
44. YOSHIMURA, H., K. OGATA, and S. ITOH. (1960): Essential Problems in Climatic Physiol. Kyoto, Nankodo.

Chapter 2

SPINAL CORD AND TEMPERATURE REGULATION

Rudolf THAUER and Eckhart SIMON

W. G. Kerckhoff-Institut der Max-Planck-Gesellschaft, Bad Nauheim
Physiologisches Institut der Universität Gießen, Germany

INTRODUCTION

Body temperature regulation in homeotherms is one of those biological phenomena which have given rise to numerous investigations aiming at the elucidation of general principles of central nervous control providing body homeostasis under varying external conditions. The discovery of hypothalamic thermosensitivity implied the question of whether control of the various thermoregulatory effectors is performed by a circumscribed hypothalamic center having developed as an unique structure, or by an integrated system of control loops evolved in various parts of the central nervous system, among which the hypothalamic area provides superior coordination.

This latter concept has, in part, been promoted by the fact that hypotheses built on the assumption of only one circumscribed hypothalamic thermoregulatory and thermosensitive region have failed to interpret satisfactorily the entire pattern of thermoregulatory responses. It has further been supported by considerations concerning the broad principles of central nervous performance. Central nervous control of somatomotor and autonomic effectors may be regarded as being achieved by hierarchic systems of control loops, in which every single element possesses, to a greater or lesser extent, its own limited regulatory abilities. These independent functions, however, are usually disclosed only, if the influences of higher parts of the control systems are excluded by pathological disturbances or by experimental interference.

With respect to temperature regulation, investigations of the last decade have largely confirmed the idea that integrated neuronal circuits involving ample parts of the central nervous system constitute the structural matrix of central nervous regulatory performance. The discovery of *spinal thermosensitivity*, and the disclosure of its physiological significance, not only involve consequences for the description of thermoregulatory performance in terms of systems analysis. These findings also offer a new experimental approach for the investigation of the neuronal mechanisms underlying central nervous thermosensitivity. With respect to the neuronal correlates of central nervous control, a new experimental access is likewise opened by the discovery of *basic thermoregulatory properties of spinal neuronal circuits*. These latter expectations based on the thermoregulatory functions of the spinal cord seem not to be entirely unjustified, if it is realized that many important principles of higher central nervous performance are grounded on elementary neuronal mechanisms as discovered in the spinal cord.

THERMOREGULATORY PERFORMANCE AND CENTRAL THERMO-
SENSITIVITY OF THE EXTRACEREBRAL BODY CORE

The idea of *extracerebral temperature regulation* in homeothermic organisms, which can be traced back to Goltz (Goltz and Ewald, 1896), was experimentally supported for the first time by ablation experiments (Popoff, 1934; Thauer, 1935; Thauer and Peters, 1938), in which a limited thermoregulatory function was found to persist after chronical spinal and midbrain transection. Proceeding from these findings and from clinical observations, and taking into account the variety of conflicting data on the hypo-thalamic heat regulating center, a conception of homeothermia was developed by Thauer in 1939 in which extracerebral thermoregulation was incorporated as an essential aspect. This implied the rejection of theories based on only one circumscribed thermoregulatory center in the hypothalamic region.

However, in spite of the above-mentioned observations on extracerebral thermoregulatory capabilities of spinalized or decerebrated animals and of patients with hypothalamic lesions, the concept of extracerebral thermoregulation was open to objections as long as the existence of *extracerebral central temperature detectors*, which had to be assumed for theoretical reasons, was not definitely established. Several investigations on this question were guided by the view that a "glomus caroticum of temperature regulation" (Thauer, 1962), i.e., central temperature sensors outside of the central nervous tissue, should exist. In fact, central thermosensitivity mediated by thermal sensors of this type seems to exist in various parts of the body core (Cort and McCance, 1953; Blatteis, 1960; Lippold, Nicholls, and Redfearn, 1960; Bligh, 1961). However, compared to the effects of peripheral or hypothalamic thermal stimulation, no consistent thermoregulatory responses were evoked by stimulation of these sensors.

The first evidence for a relevant extracerebral central thermosensitivity resulted, when an experimental design was chosen which enabled selective temperature changes of the whole extracerebral body core. Thus, all possible extracerebral central thermodetectors could be stimulated simultaneously. This was achieved by Hallwachs, Thauer, and Usinger (1961) in anesthetized dogs by means of heat exchangers interposed in the blood streams of the carotid arteries and the jugular veins and by a warm, stirred water bath in which the animals were submerged. The temperature of the extracerebral body core was lowered by cooling the blood of the jugular veins, while head and brain temperatures were kept at the normal level by heating the carotid blood. Under these conditions, cold shivering with a corresponding increase of oxygen consumption was evoked by extracerebral central cooling. Since cutaneous and hypothalamic temperature sensors were kept at normal or even elevated temperatures, this response could be explained only by stimulation of the hypothetical extracerebral deep thermoreceptors (Fig. 10). This observation was confirmed in a series of experiments in which an improved method of thermal isolation of the head from the trunk allowed more precise temperature changes (Rautenberg, Simon, and Thauer, 1963). It was further shown that the response to the extracerebral central cold stimulus could be modified by changes of brain temperature, indicating the specific nature of the extracerebral central thermosensitive structures (Simon, Rautenberg, and Thauer, 1963). Recently, similar experiments have been made with the crossed circulation technique, confirming the importance of extracerebral central thermosensitivity

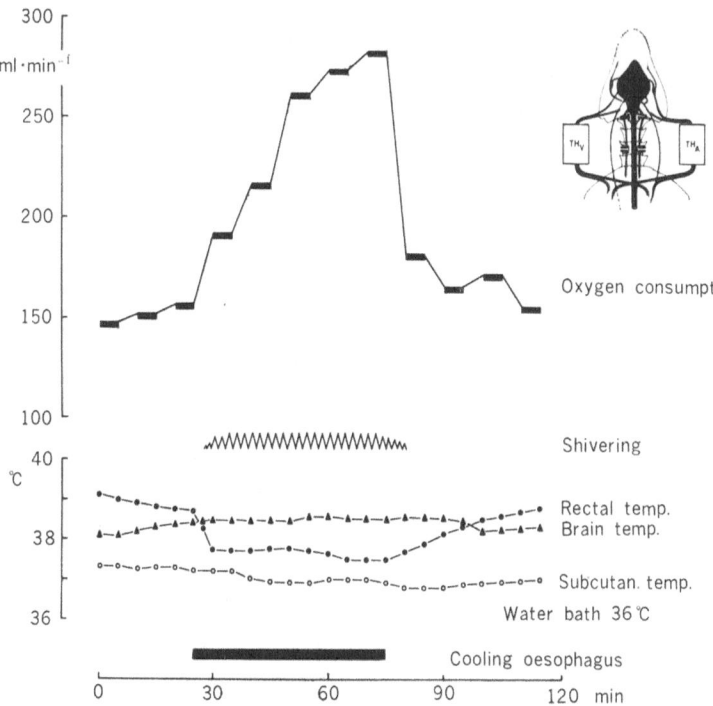

Fig. 10. Demonstration of extracerebral central thermosensitivity in an anesthetized dog. Head thermally isolated from trunk by heat exchangers interposed in the blood streams of the carotid arteries and the external jugular veins (TH$_A$ and TH$_V$ in the inset figure) and by ligation of the vertebral arteries and the tissues of the neck. Animal submerged in a warm, stirred water bath (36°C). Rise of oxygen consumption indicates increase of heat production by shivering during lowering of extracerebral central body temperature (see rectal temperature) which was performed by cooling of the venous heat exchanger and by cold water perfusion (black bar) of a metal thermode placed into the esophagus. Brain temperature slightly rising due to moderate warming of the arterial heat exchanger.
(From Rautenberg, Simon, and Thauer, 1963).

also for central heat stimulation (Hales, Kao, and Mei, personal communication).

SPINAL THERMOSENSITIVITY

After various experimental attempts, the vertebral canal was identified as the region where extracerebral central thermosensitive structures—or at least a considerable fraction of them—were localized. Among other considerations, reflections on hypothalamic thermosensitivity had led to the decision to search for thermosensitive elements in extracerebral central nervous tissues. As for extracerebral central thermosensitivity as a whole, initial evidence was furnished for thermosensitive structures in the vertebral canal by observing cold shivering and measuring oxygen consumption, when the structures of the vertebral canal were selectively cooled, either by perfusion of the spinal subarachnoidal space with cool artificial liquor or by cold water perfusion of a hairpin-like thermode of polyethylene tubing inserted into the spinal peridural space. In these experiments, which were carried out at first in anesthetized and later in unanestetized dogs (Simon, Rautenberg, Thauer, and Iriki, 1963, 1964; Simon,

Rautenberg, and Jessen, 1965), shivering was evoked by vertebral canal cooling usually within less than 2 min (Fig. 11). Due to the anatomical demarcation of the cooled area, vertebral canal cooling did not influence shell and core temperatures of thermoregulatory significance outside of the vertebral canal (skin temperature, central blood temperature, brain temperature). If ever, core temperatures changed in the opposite direction in consequence of increased heat production. Therefore, the responses to vertebral canal cooling had to be ascribed to the stimulation of cold sensitive structures localized within or close to the spinal cord. Experiments in dogs with chronic bilateral transection of the lumbo-sacral dorsal roots finally confirmed that the responses to vertebral canal cooling were evoked by stimulation of temperature sensible elements located in the spinal cord itself (Meurer, Jessen, and Iriki, 1967); shivering was produced in these animals by selective cooling of the deafferentated section of the spinal cord.

During these first investigations pointing to the existence of spinal thermosensitive structures, observations had already been made which revealed that these structures might exert a specific influence on the thermoregulatory system. For instance, cold

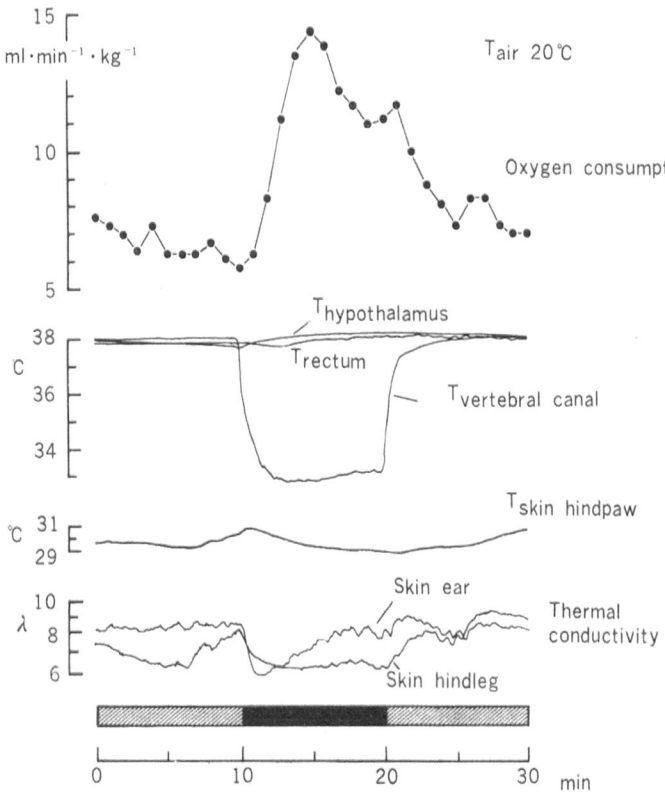

Fig. 11. Evocation of shivering as indicated by the rise of oxygen consumption during vertebral canal cooling at neutral ambient air temperature in an unanesthetized dog. Cooling performed by cold water perfusion (black bar) of a peridural vertebral canal thermode extending from C_2 to S_1. Decrease of thermal conductivity of ear and paw skin (heated thermocouple method) indicates reduction of cutaneous blood flow.—Notice rise of hypothalamic and rectal temperatures during vertebral canal cooling.
(Unpublished observation of Jessen, Simon, and Kullmann, 1968).

shivering elicited by peripheral or general body cooling was inhibited by heating and augmented by cooling of the vertebral canal (Rautenberg and Simon, 1964). Further, measurements of skin temperature and of cutaneous thermal conductivity had shown that skin blood flow was adequately influenced by thermal stimulation of the spinal cord (see Fig. 11).

> Additional experimental evidence for specific relations between temperature sensitivity within the vertebral canal and the temperature regulating system seemed, however, necessary, since thermal influences on spinal reflex mechanisms could have accounted for the responses described above. Effects of temperature on excitability and responsiveness of spinal neuronal circuits had been reported in the literature for warm-blooded as well as cold-blooded animals (for references see Klussmann, 1969 a, b; Pierau, Klee, and Klussmann, 1969). Therefore, several possibilities for the evocation of the observed responses had to be taken into consideration: These responses could have been elicited as unspecific temperature effects. Further, they could have been brought forth by a basically unspecific mechanism having, however, been incorporated into temperature regulation during the evolutionary development of homeothermia. Finally, these responses could have been mediated by specific thermosensitive structures. Discrimination between these possibilities on a neurophysiological basis, though necessary for final proof of specifity, seemed to be difficult and wearysome, especially, since criteria for a specific thermosensitivity of other neuronal structures—for instance of the hypothalamic thermosensitive elements—were not established. Therefore, another way of experimental approach to this problem was additionally assayed.

Evidence for the thermoregulatory specifity of spinal thermosensitivity could more likely be expected under a functional point of view from the systematic investigation of the responses of all known effectors of the temperature regulating system to thermal stimulation of the vertebral canal. Here, two aspects of thermal influences on thermoregulatory effectors had to be considered which, for methodological reasons, could not always be followed up in the same series of experiments. These were firstly the comparative analysis of the effector responses to spinal and to peripheral thermal stimulation to ascertain the identity of the responses evoked by these different stimuli, and secondly the determination of the threshold temperatures to find out whether the responses to spinal thermal stimulation could be evoked by temperature changes ranging within the natural limits of body temperature.

1. Thermoregulatory Responses to Thermal Stimulation of the Spinal Cord

Cold shivering: The type of tremor termed "shivering" is an adequate somatomotor response to cold stress and is the prevailing calorigenic thermoregulatory mechanism in many species. Analysis by electromyography and mechanography reveals several characteristic features of this cold induced tremor: Periodic "bursts" of activity often related to respiratory rhythm are frequently observed. Further, partial coordination of the discharges of different motor units brings forth, in the electromyogram, the pattern of "grouped discharges." Finally, species differences in average tremor frequency exist, which are closely correlated with body size. When these criteria were applied in the comparison of shivering evoked by external or by spinal cord cooling, no significant differences were found. Regardless of the way of evocation, cold shivering showed rhythmic bursts of shivering activity in anesthetized and awake dogs and rabbits, especially during weak shivering (Meurer, Iriki, Baumann, and Jessen, 1965; Kosaka and Simon, 1968 a). The average frequencies of the grouped discharges as well as the frequency ranges were the same for shivering induced by peripheral or spinal cord cooling (Fig. 12) (Kosaka and Simon, 1968 b). Consequently, cold induced tremor evoked by spinal cold stimulation followed the general relations between body size and average shivering frequency (Spaan and Klussmann, 1970). Finally, simultaneous thermal stimulation of spinal cord and hypothalamus by synergistic or antagonistic temperature changes revealed a complete functional identity, or interchangeability, of both thermosensitive sites with respect to activation or inhibition of cold shivering (Jessen, Simon, and Kullmann, 1968). Thus, all observations indicated that the same tremor-producing mechanism was activated by spinal, cutaneous or hypothalamic cold stimulation.

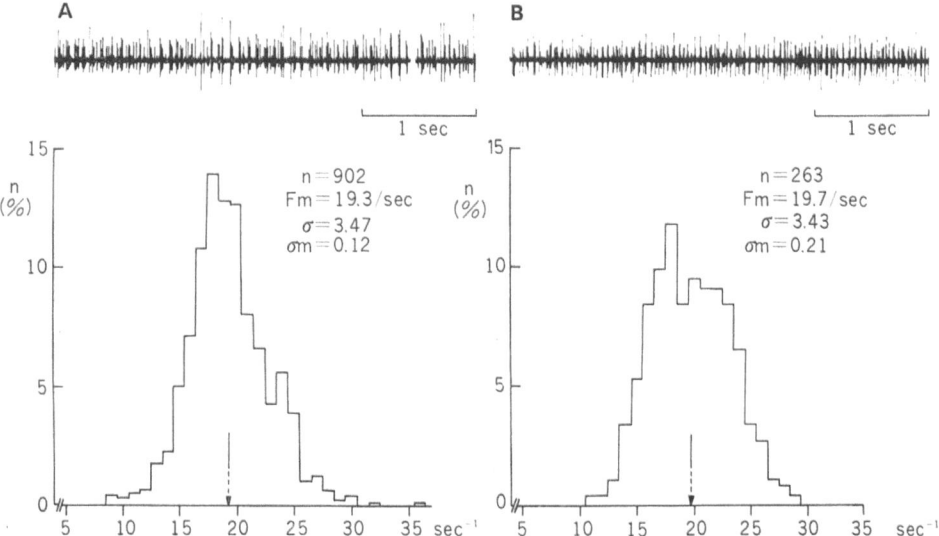

Fig. 12. Grouped discharges in the electromyograms of unanesthetized rabbits obtained from shivering under peripheral cooling (A) and spinal cord cooling (B). Original recordings (above) visualize the pattern of grouped discharges; histograms show the distribution of grouped discharge frequencies.
(From data of Kosaka and Simon, 1968 b).

Vasomotor responses: In awake and anesthetized animals of different species, skin temperature measurements at constant ambient temperatures, evaluation of cutaneous heat conductivity, and determination of cutaneous blood flow with electromagnetic flowmeters all showed a reduction of skin blood flow during cooling and an increase during heating of the spinal cord. As shown in Fig. 13, changes of conductive heat loss caused by these blood flow adjustments in the skin were often followed by changes of core temperature opposite to the direction of the spinal thermal stimulus (Jessen, Meurer, and Simon, 1967; Jessen, Simon, and Kullmann, 1968; Iriki, 1968). Analysis of the circulatory responses to spinal thermal stimulation showed that, in spite of the distinct regional adjustments of blood flow, only minor changes occurred in the systemic circulation as a whole during thermal stimulation of the spinal cord in the intact animal (Simon, 1969 a, b; Kullmann, Schönung, and Simon, 1970). This was apparently due to changes of blood flow in central (intestinal) vascular beds antagonistic to those in the skin (Kullmann, Schönung, and Simon, 1970). This regional antagonism, which was induced by likewise opposing changes of activity in sympathetic efferents supplying

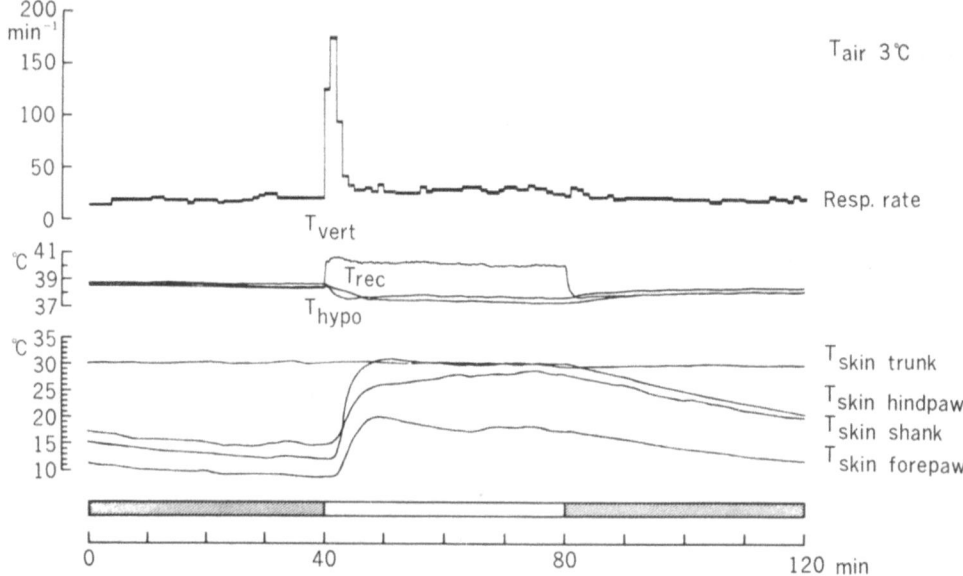

Fig. 13. Evocation of cutaneous vasodilatation as indicated by the rise of acral skin temperatures at low constant ambient air temperature during spinal cord heating in an unanesthetized dog. Heating performed by hot water perfusion (white bar) of a peridural vertebral canal thermode extending from C_2 to S_1. The rise of respiratory rate during the early stage of heating indicates thermal panting. Notice the fall of hypothalamic and rectal temperatures during spinal cord heating. (From Jessen, Meurer, and Simon, 1967).

cutaneous and visceral vascular areas (Walther, Iriki, and Simon, 1970), corresponds with observations on regional changes of blood flow under external or hypothalamic thermal stimulation (Rein, 1931; Schönung, Wagner, Jessen, and Simon, unpublished observations). Thus a complete conformity of the vasomotor responses to peripheral, hypothalamic, and spinal thermal stimulation may be stated.

Panting: This typical thermoregulatory response which provides evaporative heat loss in many species also could be activated by spinal heat stimuli (Fig. 14). All aspects of thermal panting were apparent in the awake dog, when the spinal cord was selectively heated; besides tachypnoea, especially the opened mouth, the protruded tongue with the typical to-and-fro movements, and increased salivation (Jessen, 1967). Intensity and duration of panting proved to be dependent not only on the intensity of the spinal heat stimulus but were also influenced by the ambient temperature conditions. At low ambient temperatures panting lasted, as a rule, only for a short time, during which core temperature fell significantly (see Fig. 13). At warm conditions, panting could persist for a much longer time. A similar influence of ambient temperature on panting evoked by spinal cord heating was observed also in pigeons (Rautenberg, 1967; 1969). In this species it was further shown that panting evoked by elevating ambient temperature could be suppressed completely by a sufficiently strong spinal cold stimulus. In anesthetized rabbits, respiratory frequency could be elevated by spinal cord heating, and, conversely, an elevated—but not a normal—respiratory frequency could be lowered by spinal cord cooling. Ablation experiments in this species showed that the influences of spinal thermal stimulation on respiration were mediated by diencephalic, probably hypothalamic structures (Kosaka, Simon, Thauer, and Walther, 1969). This fits well

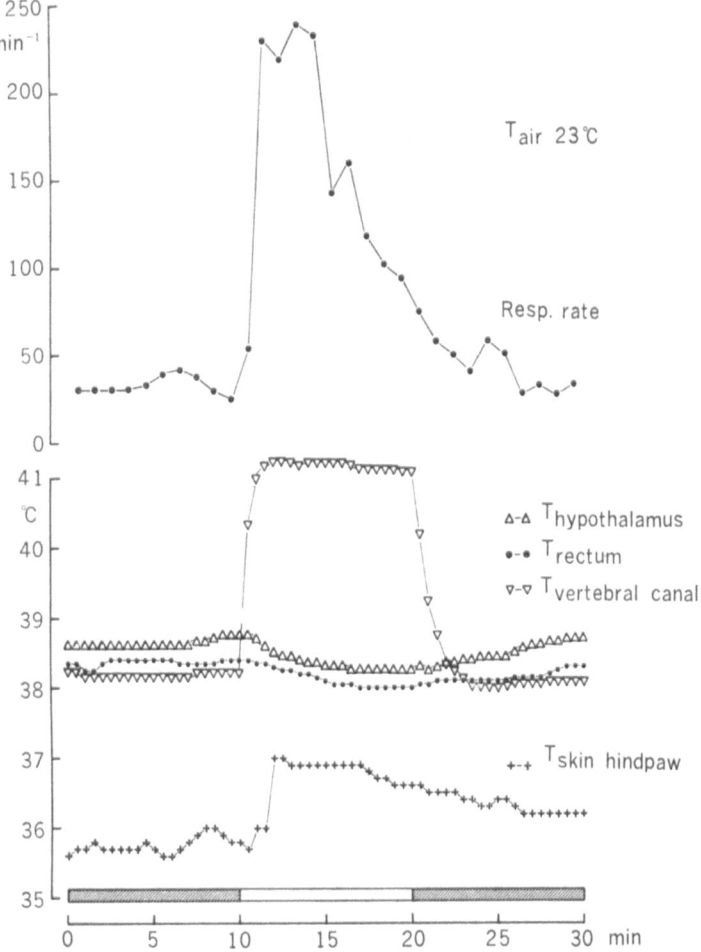

Fig. 14. Evocation of panting as indicated by the rise of respiratory rate at neutral ambient air temperature during spinal cord heating in an unanesthetized dog. Heating performed by hot water perfusion (white bar) of a peridural vertebral canal thermode extending from C_2 to S_1. The rise of paw skin temperature indicates cutaneous vasodilatation.—Notice the fall of hypothalamic and rectal temperatures during spinal cord heating.
(From Jessen, 1967).

in the conception that spinal thermosensitive structures are closely connected with the thermoregulatory system.

Sweating: The influence of spinal thermosensitive structures on this second mechanism providing evaporative heat loss can be studied only in a few species, which—like man—produce sweat in significant amounts. In the ox (bos taurus) sweating can account for about 2/3 of total evaporative heat loss. Investigations carried out by Hales and Jessen (1969) in this species showed that, besides thermal panting, increase of water vapor loss from the skin was evoked by spinal cord heating. The amount of sweating depended on the intensity of the spinal heat stimulus and on the ambient temperature conditions. This interdependence of spinal and other thermosensitive structures in determining sweat rate confirmed that spinal thermosensitivity is integrated in the thermoregulatory system.

Piloerection: While it is difficult to detect changes of pilomotor activity in furred experimental animals, significant changes in the arrangement of the plumage could be observed in pigeons during thermal stimulation of the spinal cord (Rautenberg, 1967). As ascertained by photographic recording (Fig. 15), fluffing induced by low ambient temperature was reduced by spinal cord heating. Conversely, at warm ambient conditions the animals fluffed their plumage when the spinal cord was cooled. Additionally, a distinct change of *behaviour* became manifest during spinal cooling, as the animals squatted down and covered their legs with their feathers.

2. *Spinal Temperature Thresholds for Thermoregulatory Effector Activation*

Direct evaluation of threshold temperatures for the various thermoregulatory responses evoked by thermal stimulation of the spinal cord was carried out in samples of awake rabbits and pigeons. Some of the results are summarized in the Table 3. Estimations of threshold temperatures for heat production and evaporative heat loss in dogs by linear extrapolation of stimulus-response curves are considered in a following chapter.

Comparison of the threshold temperatures in Table 3 with core temperature variations occurring in the same species under various other conditions can be made on the basis of data available from the literature and from own observations. In awake rabbits exposed to low ambient temperatures (−3 to +10°C) the onset of shivering occurred, on the average, at a rectal temperature of 38.4°C, while in single cases core

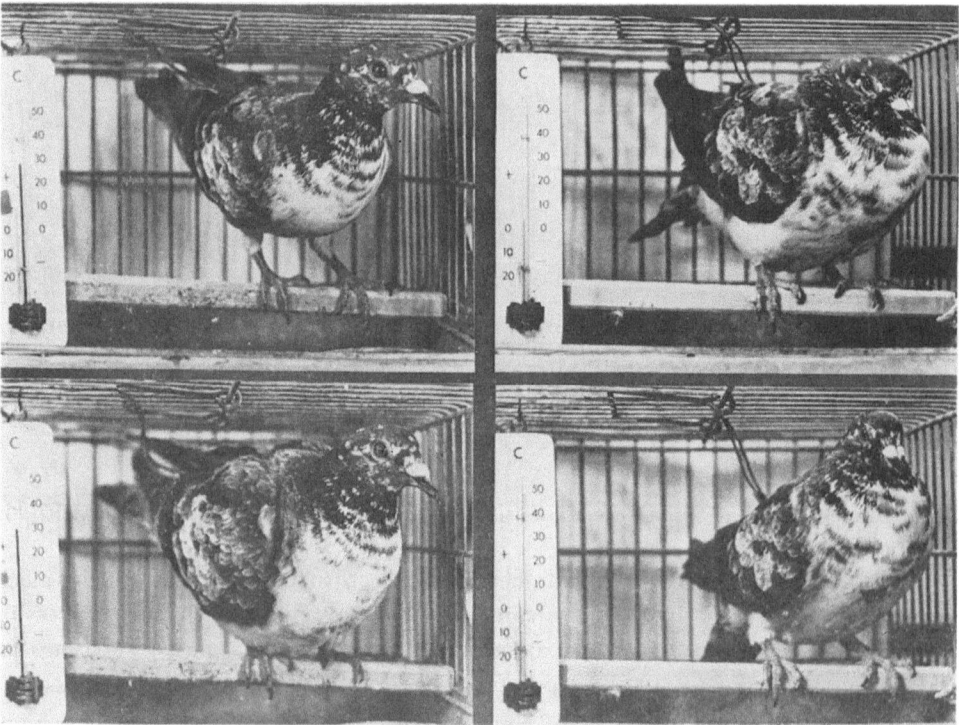

Fig. 15. Changes in the state of piloerection induced by thermal stimulation of the spinal cord in an unanesthetized pigeon. Thermal stimulation performed by cold or hot water perfusion of a peridural vertebral canal thermode extending from Th$_3$ to C$_2$. Left side: Pigeon at warm ambient air temperature before (above) and during (below) spinal cord cooling. Right side: Pigeon at cold ambient air temperature before (above) and during (below) spinal cord heating. (From Rautenberg, 1967).

TABLE 3 Vertebral canal temperatures at the onset and at the end of various thermoregulatory responses during periods of spinal cord cooling and heating

Awake animals Thermoregulatory response	Ambient air temp. °C	Vertebral canal temp. At onset at end of response °C °C		Core temp.
Shivering				
Pigeon	25	38.6	39.0	40.6
(Rautenberg, 1967, 1969)	30	37.4	37.8	40.3
Rabbit	28–33	37.1	37.8	38.8
(Kosaka and Simon, 1968 a)				
Panting				
Pigeon	25	43.2	42.8	40.0
(Rautenberg, 1967, 1969)	30	42.5	42.4	40.2
Cutaneous vasoconstriction				
Pigeon	30	39.8	—	40.3
(Rautenberg, 1967, 1969)				
Cutaneous vasodilatation				
Pigeon	25	41.1	—	40.6
(Rautenberg, 1967, 1969)				
Rabbit	25	39.8	—	39.2
(Iriki, 1968)	17	41.3	—	39.0

temperatures below 38 °C were observed (Kosaka and Simon, 1968 a). On the other hand, elevations of rectal temperatures up to 42 °C were reported for rabbits in fever (Grant, 1949). In awake, resting pigeons exposed to ambient temperatures at the lower limit of thermoneutrality (25 °C), core temperatures varied to values as low as 39 °C, while during flight and excitement temperatures as high as 43–44 °C were measured (Hart and Roy, 1967; Rautenberg, 1967).

If the data of the table are compared against these observations, threshold temperatures for spinal thermosensitivity are found to be partly outside, but partly, however, inside the range of core temperature variations which is delineated by the above-mentioned data obtained under not too severe conditions. It must further be considered that the "true" thresholds were probably closer to the normal body temperature; for it can be assumed that the methods used for the control of effector activation, e.g. electromyographical recording from a circumscribed muscle area, only exceptionally detected the very first onset of activation. In any case, spinal threshold temperatures ranging, at least partially, within the limits of natural core temperature variations indicate that a basic precondition for physiological significance of spinal thermosensitivity is fulfilled, and thus support the view that spinal thermosensitive structures may have a specific sensory function.

In considering some other aspects of spinal threshold temperatures for effector activation it must be taken into account that their levels may be considerably influenced by other factors impinging on the thermoregulatory control system. In the case of temperature regulation, hypothalamic, peripheral and possibly other temperature sensors in addition to spinal thermosensitive structures transmit error signals to the controller. If it is assumed that transmission of a fixed load error to the controller is required for activation of a thermoregulatory effector, then stimulus intensity in one sensor necessary to evoke a response must depend on what error signals arrive from the remaining sensors. Consequently, spinal threshold temperatures must depend on peripheral and central temperature conditions and vice versa. It must be further taken into consideration that only indirect conclusions can be drawn about the sensitivity of a temperature sensor from its threshold temperatures, sensitivity being determined rather by the slope of the stimulus-response curve. However, provided that the temperature conditions of the other sensors remain the same, the degree of deviation from neutral temperature of threshold temperature for effector activation will be the smaller, the more sensitive is the investigated sensor. Additional information about the sensitivity of a sensor can further be obtained from the effect of its subliminal stimulation on the thresholds of the remaining sensors.

In conformity with these considerations, the level of spinal temperature thresholds was definitely influenced—as shown in the table—by external temperature conditions, a phenomenon which corresponds to the influence of ambient temperature on hypothalamic temperature threshold. Conversely, skin and core temperature thresholds, e.g. for panting, were dependent on spinal cord temperature. If, for example, in pigeons ambient temperature was gradually elevated, panting occurred, on the average, at an ambient temperature of 35.9 °C, when rectal and vertebral canal temperatures had risen to 41.9 °C and thoracic skin temperature to 41.4 °C. If, under the same conditions, vertebral canal temperature was "clamped" at the normal level of 40 °C, panting occurred only after a rise of ambient temperature to 37.3 °C, of rectal temperature to 42.8 °C, and of thoracic skin temperature to 42.2 °C (Rautenberg, 1967). It is worth mentioning that this core temperature was higher than the spinal threshold temperature for panting during selective spinal cord heating at 30 °C air temperature. Not least, the inclusion of spinal thermosensitivity into the temperature regulating system is underlined by the observations of Brück and Wünnenberg (1967 a, b) in guinea pigs. In this species the threshold conditions for cold shivering could be described by an equation in which subcutaneous and spinal cord temperatures were the relevant variables. The common reference value for these parameters was found to be shifted by cold acclimatization without any change of their interdependence.

NEURONAL CORRELATES OF SPINAL THERMOSENSITIVITY

The specific nature of spinal thermosensitivity, which seems to be well established by the reported findings (Thauer, 1968), provokes the further question of its structural basis. No evidence has been obtained, so far, for conduction of signals over the dorsal roots arising from thermoreceptor-like structures at the surface of or in close proximity to the spinal cord (Klussmann, 1964; 1969 a; Meurer, Jessen, and Iriki, 1967). Therefore, it is assumed that—as in the hypothalamus—thermosensitivity is based on temperature sensitive neurons.

1. Temperature Effects on the Activity of Ascending Spinal Neurons

The close involvement of spinal thermosensitivity in temperature regulation rises the question of interconnections between the spinal and the supraspinal parts of the thermoregulatory system. While the influence of spinal thermal stimuli on pathways descending from supraspinal thermoregulatory centers may be explained by temperature effects on spinal neurons constituting the spinal sections of these pathways, influence of spinal cord temperature on the activity of ascending spinal neurons is additionally required, if it is also assumed that connections in the opposite direction, i.e. from spinal thermosensitive structures to—e.g.—the hypothalamus, do exist.

Afferent conduction of signals arising from thermal stimulation of the spinal cord was discussed by Thauer in 1964 and was confirmed by indirect evidence, when evocation of panting during spinal cord heating was observed (Jessen, 1967). Investigation of responses to spinal cord heating after partial transection of the spinal cord in guinea pigs (Wünnenberg and Brück, 1968 a) and in rabbits (Kosaka, Simon, Walther, and Thauer, 1969) indicated that these signals were conducted in the ventrolateral tracts. It was further shown that the influences on respiratory rate of spinal heat and cold stimuli were mediated by diencephalic, probably hypothalamic structures (Kosaka, Simon, Thauer, and Walther, 1969). In this latter investigation indirect evidence for the existence of cold activated as well as heat activated ascending spinal neurons was suggested by the arousal responses following both kinds of thermal stimulation, which implied that the ascending reticular activating system was influenced in the same manner by heating and cooling.

Direct evidence for heat-sensitive ascending units was obtained in guinea pigs from extracellular micro-recording in the rhombencephalic part of the medial lemniscal pathway or, respectively, in the spinothalamic tract during heating of the cervical spinal cord (Wünnenberg and Brück, 1968 b; Wünnenberg, 1969). The existence of heat-sensitive ascending spinal units was confirmed in cats by micro-recording at the cervical level of the spinal cord during heating of the thoracic and lumbosacral portions (Fig. 16) (Simon and Iriki, 1970 a, b). Additionally, though less frequently,

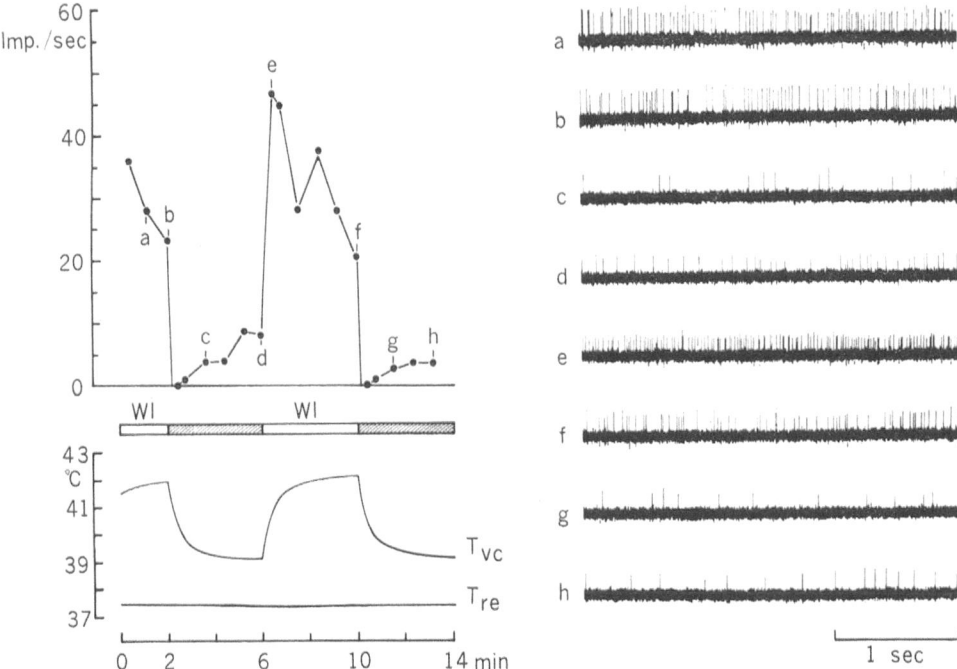

Fig. 16. Discharge of a spinal neuron recorded at C_3 in the spinothalamic tract showing a combined dynamic and static activation by spinal cord heating. Anesthetized, artificially ventilated cat. Left side: Courses of discharge rate and of vertebral canal (T_{vc}) and rectal (T_{re}) temperatures during periods of neutral (hatched bars) and hot (white bars) water perfusion of a peridural vertebral canal thermode extending from Th_1 to S_1. Right side: Original recordings at the points of the response curve indicated by the letters.
(From Simon and Iriki, 1970 b).

ascending units were detected which were activated by spinal cord cooling (Fig. 17).
High spinal transection at C_1/C_2 ensured that only afferent activity was recorded.
Activation of ascending units by spinal cord cooling under neuromuscular blockage
by succinyl choline or curare indicated that cold-sensitive ascending units were stimulated
by temperature effects on intraspinal neurons rather than by way of muscle spindles
driven by changes of efferent motoneuron discharge.   This assumption is also congruent
with the results of histological control of the recording sites as determined by micro-
marking.   Both heat- and cold-sensitive units were located outside of the spinocerebellar
tracts in the spinothalamic pathway of the anterolateral funiculi.

The neurophysiological observations on ascending units activated by spinal cord cooling
and heating do not, by themselves, allow a definite conclusion concerning a possible
specific thermoregulatory function.   A very distinct PD-sensitivity of some of the heat-
and cold-sensitive units closely resembling that of peripheral thermoreceptors may be
considered as an argument for a specific sensory function of these neurons.   This is
further suggested by the observation of hypothalamic units which were simultaneously
influenced by hypothalamic and by spinal thermal stimulation (Guieu and Hardy, 1970,
and personal communication).

2.   Local Temperature Effects on Spinal Neurons

From a more general point of view, susceptibility of spinal neurons to temperature
changes is indicated by the influence of local spinal temperature on the "dorsal root

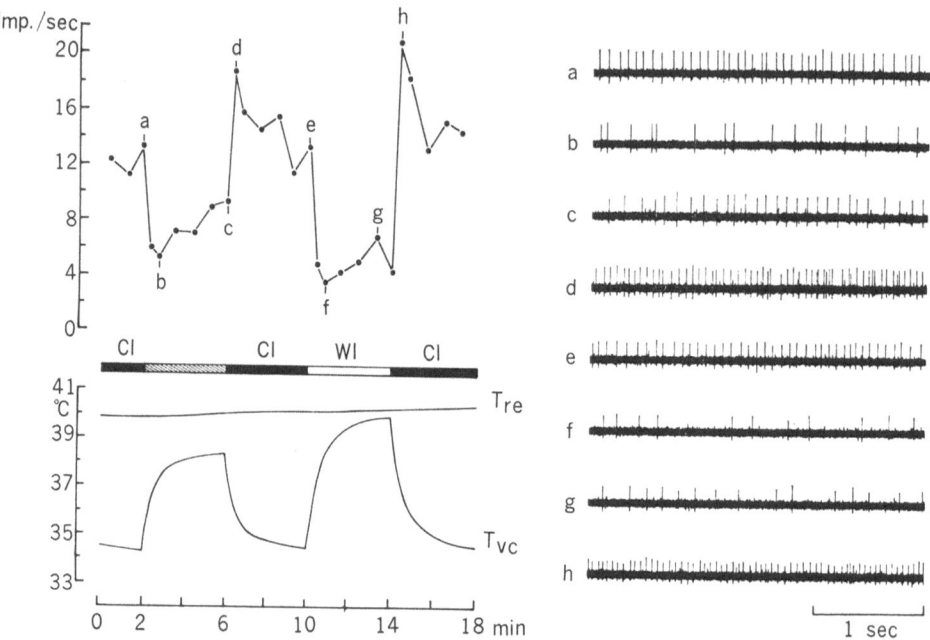

Fig. 17.   Discharge of a spinal neuron recorded at C_3 in the spinothalamic tract showing a combined dynamic and static activation by spinal cord cooling.   Anesthetized, artificially ventilated
cat.   Left side: Courses of discharge rate and of vertebral canal (T_{vc}) and rectal (T_{re}) temperatures
during periods of neutral (hatched bars), cold (black bars), and hot (white bar) water perfusion
of a peridural vertebral canal thermode extending from Th_1 to S_1.   Right side: Original recordings
at the points of the response curve indicated by the letters.
(From Simon and Iriki, 1970 a).

reflex" (Barron and Matthews, 1938 a, b; Tönnies, 1938, 1939), and by the "hyper-responsiveness" of spinal motoneurons following spinal cord hypothermia (Brooks, Koizumi, and Malcolm, 1955; Koizumi, 1955).   These phenomena by themselves do not suggest a direct connection with the variety of thermoregulatory responses to thermal stimulation of the spinal cord.   However, it may be inferred that the cellular mechanisms underlying this temperature dependence of spinal neuronal activity might basically be identical with or similar to those which constitute specific spinal thermosensitivity.   Quantitative differences of the temperature coefficients and/or special interconnections might then account for the specific influences on the thermoregulatory system.   Proceeding from this hypothesis, the phenomenon of hyperresponsiveness of motoneurons was chosen by a research group in our institute as a starting point for investigations on the mechanisms underlying neuronal thermosensitivity.   With respect to the experimental techniques established and to the amount of data already accumulated, the motoneuron appeared as the most suitable type of neurons for this purpose.   Recordings from ventral root filaments showed that the discharge rates of motoneurons were definitely influenced by variations of spinal cord temperature. Maximum discharge rates were observed in the hypothermic range which, however, differed for the various types of motoneurons.   For instance, maximum activity of

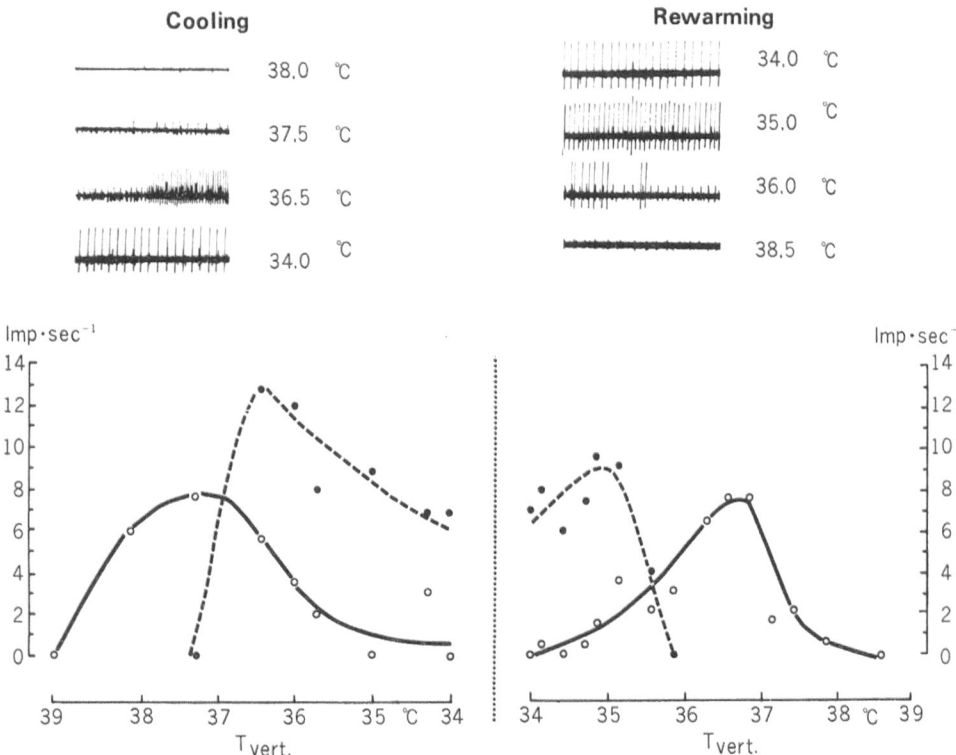

Fig. 18. Discharges of motoneuron fibers in a ventral root filament during spinal cord cooling and rewarming in an anesthetized cat. Above: Original recordings show the discharges of a small γ-motoneuron and of a big α-motoneuron at various spinal cord temperatures. Below: Discharge rates of the γ-motoneuron (solid lines) and of the α-motoneuron (broken lines) plotted as a function of spinal cord temperature.
(From data of Klussmann, 1969 a).

γ-motoneurons was reached at temperatures within or slightly below the normal range of body temperature, while the big α-motoneurons had maximum discharge rates at definitely lower spinal cord temperatures (Fig. 18) (Klussmann, 1964, 1969 a; Klussmann, Stelter, and Spaan, 1969). The different maxima may be considered as analogous to those of the peripheral thermoreceptors, at least with respect to static sensitivity. As a rule, however, the maximum discharges of all types of motoneurons were found in the normo- and hypothermic ranges but not in the definitely hyperthermic range.

These observations suggested that direct investigation of the motoneuronal properties would give further information about the cellular events underlying neuronal thermosensitivity, at least for cold sensitivity. It could be assumed that indirect temperature effects on the motoneurons, for instance those mediated by suprasegmental structures involved in temperature regulation, might become insignificant, if the temperature of only one spinal segment was selectively changed. Intracellular recordings from α-motoneurons in a locally cooled area of the spinal cord showed that duration and amplitude of evoked mono- and polysynaptic excitatory postsynaptic

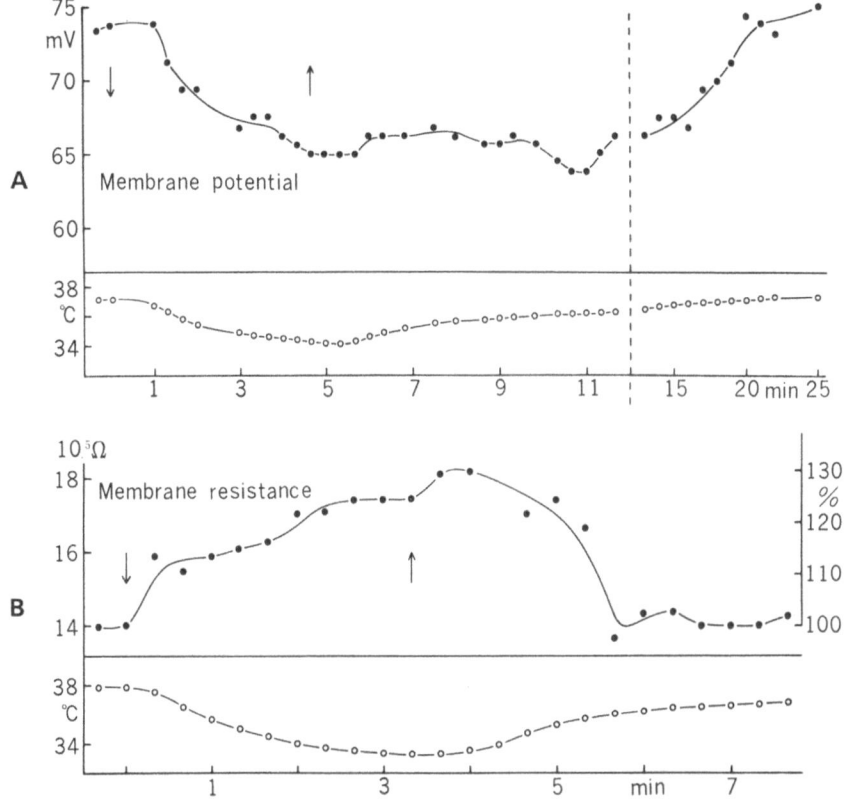

Fig. 19. Membrane properties of a lumbar motoneuron as influenced by local spinal cord cooling. Data obtained by intracellular micro-recording technique in an anesthetized cat. The upper diagram (A) shows the courses of the resting membrane potential and of local spinal cord temperature, the lower diagram (B) shows the courses of membrane resistance and of local spinal cord temperature, both during periods of local cooling and rewarming.
(From Pierau, Klee, and Klussmann, 1969).

potentials increased with falling temperature and more frequently exceeded the excitatory threshold of the neuron (Pierau, Klee, and Klussmann, 1969). This cold-induced increase of excitability developed in spite of a cold-induced increase of evoked inhibitory postsynaptic potentials (Pierau, Wurster, and Spaan, 1969). However, as demonstrated for recurrent inhibition, this latter effect probably did not result from an increased firing rate of experimentally stimulated inhibiting interneurons (Pierau, Spaan, and Golda, 1970). Therefore, the simultaneous increase of excitatory and inhibitory postsynaptic potentials rather seemed to indicate a cold induced change of the electric properties of the motoneuron membrane as the underlying event. In fact, the slight depolarisation of the membrane and the simultaneous increase of electrical membrane resistance observed during cooling (Fig. 19) could explain the cold-induced changes of both excitatory and inhibitory postsynaptic potentials (Pierau, Klee, and Klussmann, 1969). The observation that also after-hyperpolarisation of the motoneuron is enlarged during hypothermia (Pierau and Klussmann, 1970) likewise fits in this interpretation. These membrane effects, which apparently account for the increased excitability of the motoneuron in a certain range of spinal hypothermia (Pierau and Spaan, 1970), are regarded as the electrophysiological correlates of temperature dependent changes of membrane function, which might also constitute the cellular basis for specific spinal thermosensitivity (Fig. 20).

The question of whether cellular mechanisms similar to those observed in motoneurons do account also for the described thermosensitivity of ascending units needs further investigation, particularly, since the existence of some sort of spinal "thermoreceptors" is not yet definitely excluded. At present, changes of membrane properties observed

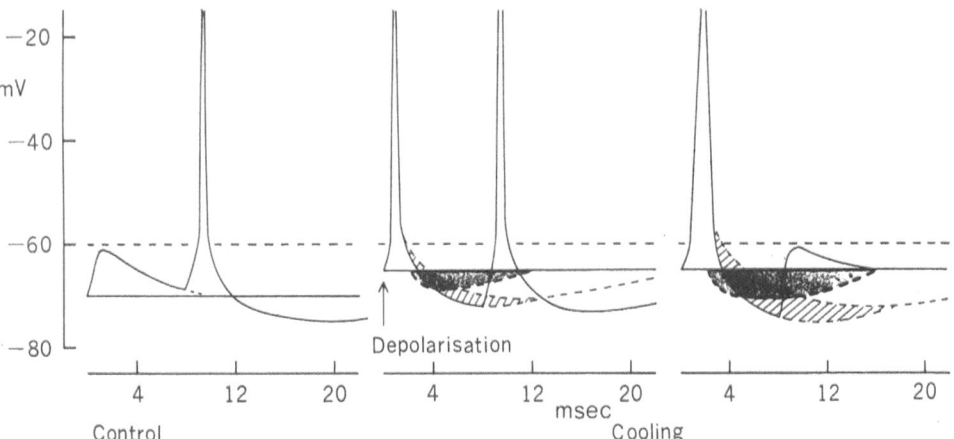

Fig. 20. Schematic survey of the changes of EPSP, IPSP, and after-hyperpolarisation occurring in a spinal (moto-) neuron during spinal cord hypothermia. At normal temperature (left figure), only the second out of two EPSPs following each other in a certain time distance reaches the threshold of excitation. During moderate hypothermia (middle figure), membrane depolarisation and enlargement of EPSP already make the first EPSP surpass the threshold of excitation, i.e., the discharge rate is increased; at this state of hypothermia, the slight increase of (recurrent) IPSP (shaded area) and of after-hyperpolarisation (hatched area) following the first spike is not sufficient to cause suppression of the second spike. During stronger hypothermia (right figure), IPSP and after-hyperpolarisation become more pronounced so that the second discharge is suppressed, i.e., discharge rate is reduced again.
(From Pierau and Klussmann, 1970).

in motoneurons during spinal cord cooling can explain the static responses of cold-sensitive ascending neurons, while findings corresponding to the dynamic component of response are equivocal. Though no correlate for heat activation could as yet be established in investigations on motoneurons, it may be assumed that in certain other spinal neurons the minimum values of membrane potential and of electrical membrane conductivity are attained in the hyperthermic range.

THERMOREGULATORY PERFORMANCE AT THE SPINAL LEVEL

Discussion on the first observations of the role of spinal cord in temperature regulation (Thauer, 1964) was not restricted solely to "afferent function." With regard to earlier observations in chronically spinalized animals it was suggested that "synapses concerned with the mediation of thermoregulatory reflexes or formations of cells exerting control functions might exist outside of the hypothalamus;" those elements of the central nervous system preferably concerned with efferent functions were included in this speculation. These considerations implied that spinal central nervous structures might account for the extracerebral thermoregulatory performance claimed by Thauer in 1939.

Experimental support for the concept of spinal control functions in temperature regulation could, as a matter of fact, only be expected for those responses which were mediated by spinal efferent neurons. Attempts were made to obtain evidence in spinalized animals. In most cases, thermal stimuli were applied directly to the spinal cord, since this kind of stimulation acted quickly and did not alter the thermal state of the animal as a whole. However, the effects of peripheral thermal stimulation were also regarded.

Spinal thermoregulatory performance, i.e. transformation of a thermal stimulus into an adequate activation of thermoregulatory effectors by spinal structures, was first confirmed for cold shivering (Klussmann, Simon, Halbfass, Rautenberg, and Kosaka, 1966). In anesthetized dogs spinalized at the level of C_2, spinal cord cooling elicited visible tremor which—apart from having lower intensity and being predominantly confined to the trunk muscles—could not be discriminated from regular cold shivering. Electromyographical controls in anesthetized spinalized dogs further revealed that during general body cooling at low ambient temperatures increase of motor activity, though no visible shivering, occurred (Simon, Klussmann, Rautenberg, and Kosaka, 1966). Increase of motor activity during external cold stimulation in chronically spinalized, awake rabbits was found to appear after the same slight fall of core temperature as in intact rabbits; hence, activation of peripheral cold receptors seemed to contribute to stimulation of motor activity in the spinal animal (Kosaka and Simon, 1968 a). Comparative analysis of the electromyograms (Fig. 21) further revealed that cold-induced motor activity in spinal rabbits showed the same patterns of tremor bursts and of grouped discharges as noted in cold shivering in intact animals, implicating the same tremor-producing system in both cases (Kosaka and Simon, 1968 b). This finding confirmed the spinal genesis of cold shivering which had been suggested before by several authors (Jung, 1941; Birzis and Hemingway, 1957 a, b; Stuart, Kenneth, Ishikawa, and Eldred, 1966 b).

In contrast to shivering, definite effects on cutaneous blood flow of thermal stimuli could not be observed immediately after spinal transection in the experimental animals.

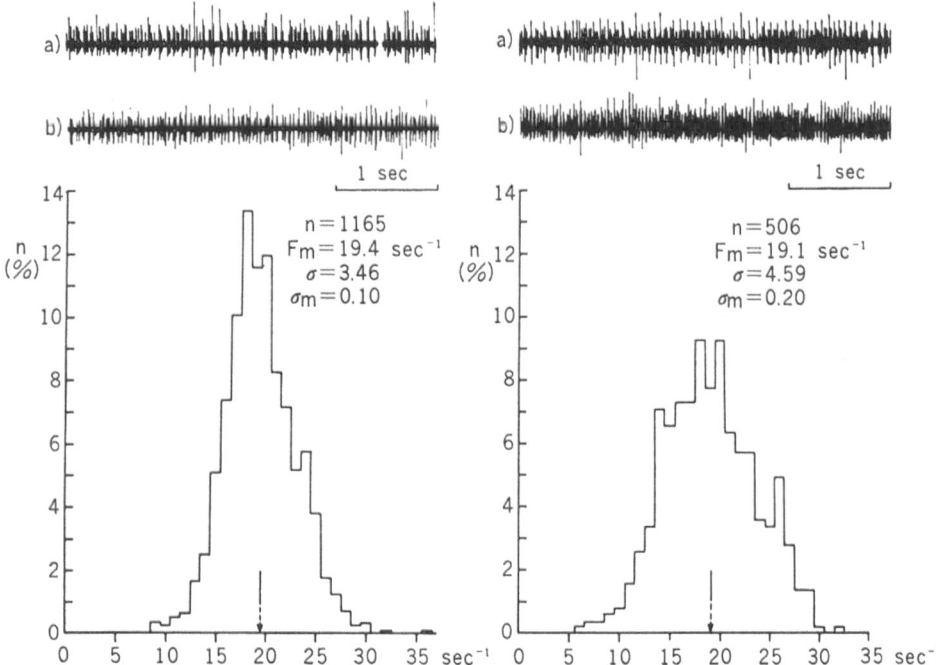

Fig. 21. Grouped discharges in the electromyograms of unanesthetized intact (left side) and chronically spinalized (right side) rabbits. Original recordings obtained under either peripheral (a) or spinal cord (b) cooling visualize the pattern of grouped discharges; histograms show the distribution of grouped discharge frequencies observed in intact and spinalized animals. (From data of Kosaka and Simon, 1968 b).

This corresponded to the general experience that vegetative spinal reflexes remain depressed for a longer time. However, in the chronically spinalized dog, cutaneous vasoconstriction at the hindpaws could be evoked by selective cooling of the isolated section of the spinal cord (Walther, Simon, and Jessen, 1969). A similar observation had already been made in spinal rabbits under external cooling (Thauer, 1935).

Evidence for thermoregulatory functions of spinal structures can also be derived from observations of Randall, Wurster, and Lewin (1966) on thermal sweating in the spinal man. Subjects with high spinal cord lesions showed a weak but significant increase of sweating when exposed to hot ambient conditions. The authors concluded "that the spinal cord, isolated from hypothalamic and brain-stem influences, is capable of independent mediation of thermally induced sweating." Further, observations were made indicating that the vasomotor system also participates in the thermoregulatory adjustments of the spinal man.

The knowledge added by these findings to earlier statements on the thermoregulatory functions of spinal central nervous structures enables the expression of a consistent hypothesis on the spinal cord as the site of extracerebral temperature regulation (Simon, 1968): Efferent neurons of the spinal cord mediate the activation of several thermoregulatory effectors, such as shivering, sweating, piloerection, and skin blood flow. The spinal cord contains thermosensitive structures with specific importance for core temperature reception. Basic control functions are established in spinal structures transforming thermal stimuli into adequate responses of the thermoregulatory effectors. Thus, regulatory functions are accomplished by spinal structures which can be termed as functions of controllers, of central sensors providing feedback signals, and of elements transmitting controller output to the effectors. Cutaneous thermoreceptors may be adjoined as peripheral sensors providing anticipatory control against external disturbances. The spinal cord may be regarded, therefore, as a comparatively simple model for the intricate complete nervous control system accomplishing temperature homeostasis in homeothermic organisms (Simon, 1967).

Experimental approach to problems of temperature regulation by investigating this "spinal model" seemed especially promising for the elucidation of the shivering mechanism. In the case of shivering induced by spinal cord cooling, it could be suggested from the experiments described in a previous chapter that tremor was initiated by direct temperature effects on the α-motoneurons. As further shown by recordings from muscle spindle afferents (Klussmann, 1969 b), the concomitant reduction of γ-motor activity often resulted in a diminution of the "dynamic index" (Matthews, 1962) of muscle spindle responses to muscle distention. Since this effect may facilitate oscillations in the muscle spindle loop, it could support the development of a coordinated, rhythmic activity of motor units, i.e. of a tremor, during spinal cord cooling (Klussmann, Stelter, and Spaan, 1969).

Other investigations, however, revealed that not only the muscle spindle loop but also intraspinal neuronal connections contributed to the rhythmicity of the motoneuronal output constituting shivering activity. As shown by experiments with dorsal root transection (Stuart, Kenneth, Ishikawa, and Eldred, 1966 a; Meurer, Jessen, and Iriki, 1967), the function of the proprioceptive control system of the muscles consisted in the coordination of tremor activity rather than in generation of the tremor rhythm itself. Tremor more likely was produced by an intraspinal mechanism (Klussmann, Spaan, Stelter, and Rau, 1969), which was probably activated not only by spinal thermal stimulation but also by signals arising from peripheral thermoreceptors or from supraspinal thermoregulatory centers (Kosaka and Simon, 1968 b). This was confirmed by the observation that the close correlation between body size and shivering frequency was apparently not based on parameters exerting their influences through the muscle spindles, for instance not on the resonance frequency of the oscillating system (Spaan and Klussmann, 1970).

THERMOREGULATORY SIGNIFICANCE OF SPINAL THERMOSENSITIVITY

While new insights into the problems of evolution of homeothermia can be expected from the discovery of thermoregulatory performance at the spinal level (Thauer, 1967), spinal thermosensitivity is placed into the foreground, if the physiological significance of spinal contributions to temperature regulation is discussed (Bligh, 1966; Benzinger, 1969). Investigations with special reference to this question have only recently been brought to a provisional close (Rautenberg, 1969; Jessen, 1970).

The contributions of spinal cord and hypothalamus to total central thermosensitivity were studied by Jessen in conscious dogs with a method introduced by Hammel for investigations on the hypothalamic temperature sensors (Hammel, Jackson, Stolwijk, Hardy, and Strömme, 1963; Hammel, 1965): The relation between thermal stimulus and effector activity (heat production, respiratory evaporative heat loss) was described by calculating linear regressions from the experimental data. By this method the threshold temperature of activation is determined as the point of intersection between the regression line and the resting effector activity (resting heat production, resting respiratory heat loss), while sensitivity of the investigated thermosensitive area is given by the slope of the regression line (Fig. 22).

Owing to the excentric position and to the comparatively small diameter of the peridural thermode, considerable transversal temperature gradients are established in the spinal cord of larger animals, e.g. the dog, during spinal thermal stimulation. The effective thermal stimulus, therefore, could not be evaluated directly from temperature measurements. Calculations of regression lines were, therefore, based on "mean spinal cord temperatures" which were determined as the mean values of numerous temperature measurements at the same stimulus intensity (perfusion temperature) in arbitrary points of the vertebral canal.

In conscious dogs, the relation between heat production and mean spinal cord temperature could be described by linear regression equations (Jessen and Mayer, 1971). At indifferent ambient temperatures between 18 and 24 °C, temperature thresholds for activation of heat production ranged between 37 and 38 °C. Slopes of the regression lines between -0.3 and -0.7 kcal/(kg.hr. °C) were determined in four animals (Jessen, 1970). Maximum heat production evoked by spinal cord cooling amounted to three times the resting value. Under warm external conditions (30 °C) the thresholds for increase of heat production were shifted to lower mean spinal cord temperatures. For activation of respiratory evaporative heat loss by spinal cord heating at indifferent ambient conditions (18–24 °C) spinal temperature thresholds between 40 and 41.5 °C were determined, while the regression lines had slopes of 1.2 kcal/(kg.hr. °C). At warm ambient temperatures (30 °C), the threshold was shifted to lower spinal cord temperatures, while the slope did not change significantly (For example, see Fig. 22).

Results obtained from related investigations on hypothalamic thermosensitivity in the same group of animals provided a reliable basis for conclusions on the significance of spinal thermosensitivity. Hypothalamic threshold temperatures for activation of heat production at indifferent ambient temperatures (18–24 °C) ranged between 36.5 and 38.8 °C. The highest value calculated for the slope of regression lines was -0.7 kcal/ (kg.hr. °C) and thus did not differ significantly from the corresponding figures found for spinal cold stimulation. In conformity with the results of Hammel and coworkers (Hammel, Jackson, Stolwijk, Hardy, and Strömme, 1963; Hellström and Hammel, 1967) and with our own observations on spinal temperature thresholds, hypothalamic threshold temperatures were shifted by several degrees to lower values at warm ambient conditions (30 °C). The relation between hypothalamic temperature and respiratory evaporative heat loss at warm ambient air temperature (30 °C) was investigated in one animal. Here, a threshold temperature of 39 °C was found. The slope of the regression line was determined as 0.9 kcal/(kg.hr. °C) and thus did not differ significantly from the corresponding value for spinal heat stimulation. At indifferent ambient conditions, the threshold was shifted to temperatures between 41 and 42.5 °C. In the narrow temperature range above these high hypothalamic temperatures, heat loss increased steeply. Therefore, reliable slopes could not be calculated.

Comparison of the total of data obtained from thermal stimulation of the hypothalamus and of the spinal cord does not reveal major differences with regard to thresholds and sensitivities between both central thermosensitive sites. Consequently, spinal cord and hypothalamus may be regarded in the dog as functionally equivalent temperature sensors. The data of Hellström and Hammel (1967) indicating a higher hypothalamic thermosensitivity in the dog (heat production: -0.7 to -1.2 kcal/(kg.hr.°C); respiratory evaporative heat loss: 0.8 to 3.2 kcal/(kg.hr.°C)) can be explained by their experimental conditions which did not exclude the participation of spinal thermosensitive structures.

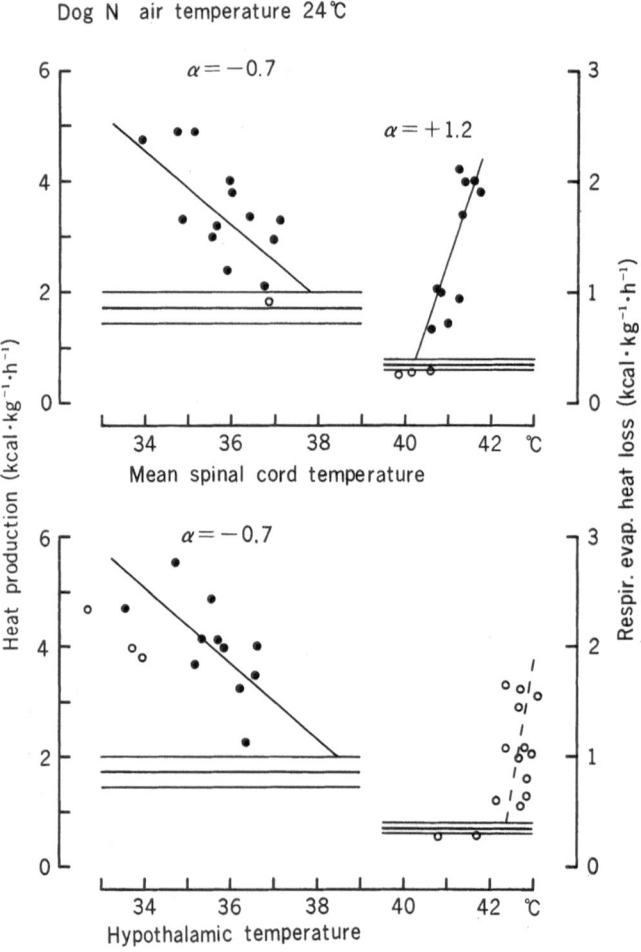

Fig. 22. Heat production (left diagrams) and respiratory evaporative heat loss (right diagrams) in an unanesthetized dog observed during periods of spinal cord (above) or hypothalamic (below) heating and cooling at indifferent ambient air temperature. Thermal stimulation was performed by cold or hot water perfusion of a peridural vertebral canal thermode extending from C_2 to S_1 and, respectively, by perfusion of a set of six stainless steel thermodes inserted stereotaxically into the preoptic region.—Every circle in the diagrams shows the response obtained during one five-min-period of heat or cold stimulation plotted as a function of the corresponding "mean spinal cord temperature" or, respectively, hypothalamic temperature. The lines paralleling the abscissae represent the resting levels with standard deviations of heat production and, respectively, respiratory evaporative heat loss. The regression lines were calculated from the filled circles; responses to hypothalamic heating were obtained only in a narrow temperature range which did not allow reliable calculation of a regression line.
(From Jessen and Mayer, 1971).

The physiological significance of spinal thermosensitivity was further confirmed by experimental data obtained with a different method in awake pigeons (Fig. 23) (Rautenberg, 1969). Heat production elevated by external cold conditions (10°C) was definitely influenced by small variations of spinal cord temperature ranging within 1°C above and below normal core temperature. The relation between heat production and spinal cord temperature within this range was described by a regression line with a slope of −1.8 kcal/(kg.hr.°C). This value indicates a sensitivity of spinal temperature sensors considerably higher than in the dog. This may be explained by the fact that a relevant hypothalamic thermosensitivity could, as yet, not be discovered in this species (Rautenberg, 1970). The suggestion that the spinal cord represents the predominant central thermosensitive site in pigeons is underlined by the changes in body heat content under the above-mentioned conditions. Lowering of spinal cord temperature by 1°C induced a rise of extraspinal core temperature (rectal tem-

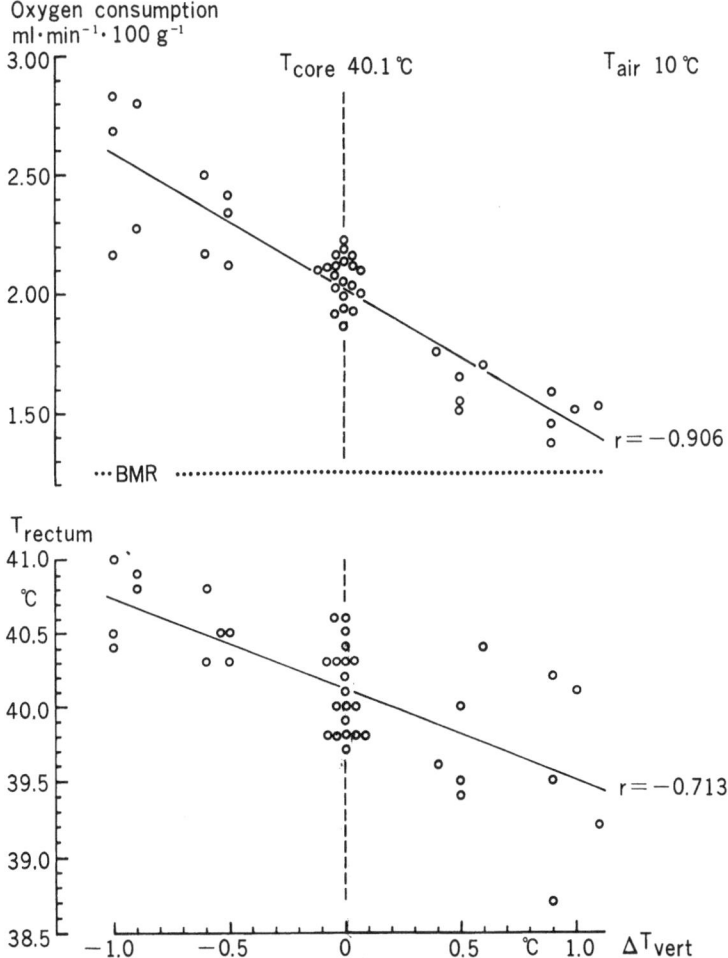

Fig. 23. Influence of small variations of spinal cord temperature ($T_{vert.}$) on oxygen consumption (upper diagram) and on rectal temperature (lower diagram) in five unanesthetized pigeons exposed to constant low ambient air temperature.
(From data of Rautenberg, 1967).

perature) by 0.6 °C. Core temperature was lowered by the same amount when spinal cord temperature was increased by 1 °C.

Finally, spinal and hypothalamic thermosensitivity may be compared on the basis of results obtained from hypothalamic and ascending spinal temperature-sensitive neurons by micro-recording. Spinal heat-sensitive ascending units recorded in the guinea pig had an average static sensitivity of 2(Imp./sec)/°C (Wünnenberg, 1969). In cats average static sensitivities of eight heat- and eight cold-activated units were determined (Fig. 24) (Simon and Iriki, 1970 b). If derived from the regression lines calculated for each of both groups of neurons over a temperature range from 26 to 42 °C in cold-sensitive units and over a range from 35 to 45 °C in heat-sensitive units, average static sensitivities of −1.3(Imp./sec)/°C and of 3.7(Imp./sec)/°C were obtained. If calculated from the steepest parts of the single response curves, average maximum static sensitivities of −2.8(Imp./sec)/°C for cold-sensitive neurons and of 5.6(Imp./sec)/°C for heat-sensitive neurons were found.

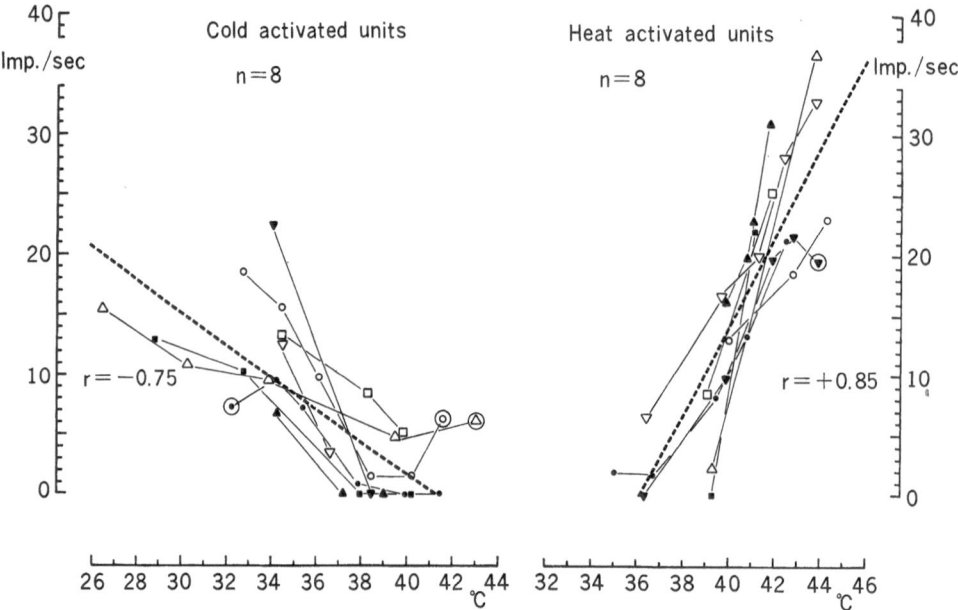

Fig. 24. Steady discharge rates of eight cold sensitive (left side) and eight heat sensitive (right side) ascending spinal neurons activated by thermal stimulation of the spinal cord. Every symbol represents the steady discharge rate obtained at the end of a stimulation period of four min duration plotted as a function of the corresponding vertebral canal temperature. Regression lines were calculated from the total of data except the encircled symbols. Data obtained from experiments in cats. (From data of Simon and Iriki, 1970 b).

Hypothalamic heat-sensitive neurons recorded in cats had a mean static sensitivity of 4.2 (Imp./sec)/ °C (Nakayama, Hammel, Hardy and Eisenman, 1963), while cold-sensitive units were not detected. For heat-sensitive hypothalamic neurons in the dog, average static sensitivities of 7(Imp./sec)/°C (Hardy, Hellon, and Sutherland, 1964) and 3.5 (Imp./sec)/°C (Cunningham, Stolwijk, Murakami, and Hardy, 1967) were reported. The corresponding values for cold-sensitive units, being observed less frequently were −1(Imp./sec)/°C and −3.3(Imp./sec)/°C. Among the thermosensitive hypothalamic neurons recorded in rabbits (Hellon, 1967), heat-sensitive type A units showed sensitivities between 4.9 and 1.2(Imp./ sec)/°C, while the sensitivity of one cold-sensitive type A unit was determined as −0.8(Imp./sec)/°C.

Comparison of the data obtained from hypothalamic and from ascending spinal
thermosensitive units clearly shows that the neuronal susceptibilities for temperature
changes are of the same order of magnitude in both regions.   If, for present purposes,
the fact is left out of account that the specific function of the thermosensitive
neurons of neither hypothalamus nor spinal cord is, as yet, definitely established, no

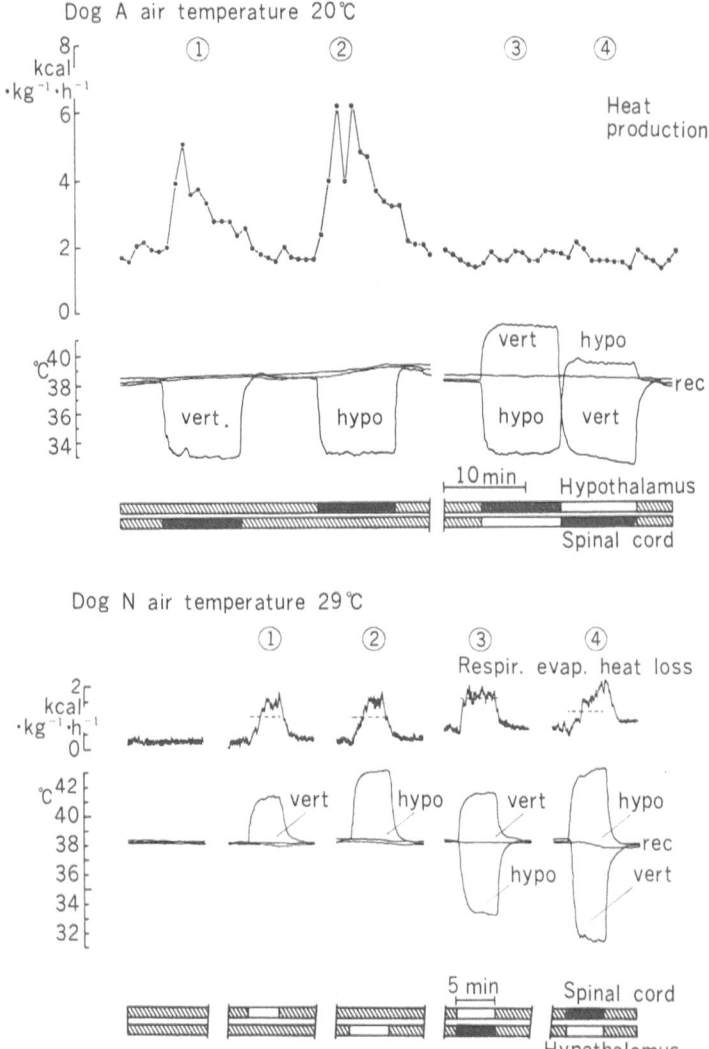

Fig. 25. Single experiments in unanesthetized dogs demonstrating the functional identity and interchangeability of spinal and hypothalamic temperature sensors under the conditions of simultaneous antagonistic thermal stimulation.   Experimental design as described in Fig. 22; core temperatures measured: vertebral canal (vert), hypothalamic (hypo), and rectal (rec) temperatures.   Upper
diagram: Effects on heat production.   Response to selective spinal cord cooling (1) is canceled by
simultaneous hypothalamic heating (4); response to selective hypothalamic cooling (2) is suppressed
by simultaneous spinal cord heating (3).   Lower diagram: Effects on respiratory evaporative heat
loss.   Response to selective spinal cord heating (1) cannot be canceled by simultaneous hypothalamic
cooling (3); likewise, the response to selective hypothalamic heating (2) is not suppressed by simultaneous spinal cord cooling (4).
(From Jessen and Simon, 1971).

difference between the spinal and hypothalamic thermosensitive structures seems to exist with respect to sensitivity. It also seems to be common for both thermosensitive areas that the heat-activated units are more sensitive and greater in number than the cold-sensitive neurons.

Functional identity of spinal and hypothalamic temperature sensors is especially indicated by the fact that their signals proved to be completely interchangeable with respect to their effects on the temperature regulating system (Jessen, 1970). This is most clearly demonstrated by the effects of selective thermal stimulation of either temperature sensitive area on the stimulus-response relation for the other area. For example, the regression line describing the relation between heat production and spinal cord temperature was shifted by hypothalamic heating to lower and by cooling to higher threshold temperatures. The relation between heat production and hypothalamic temperature was influenced by variations of spinal cord temperature in exactly the same manner.

An even more impressive demonstration of functional identity and interchangeability of spinal and hypothalamic temperature sensors is afforded by the effects of simultaneous antagonistic changes of spinal and hypothalamic temperatures (Fig. 25) (Jessen and Simon, 1971). Stimulation of heat production, for instance, evoked by spinal

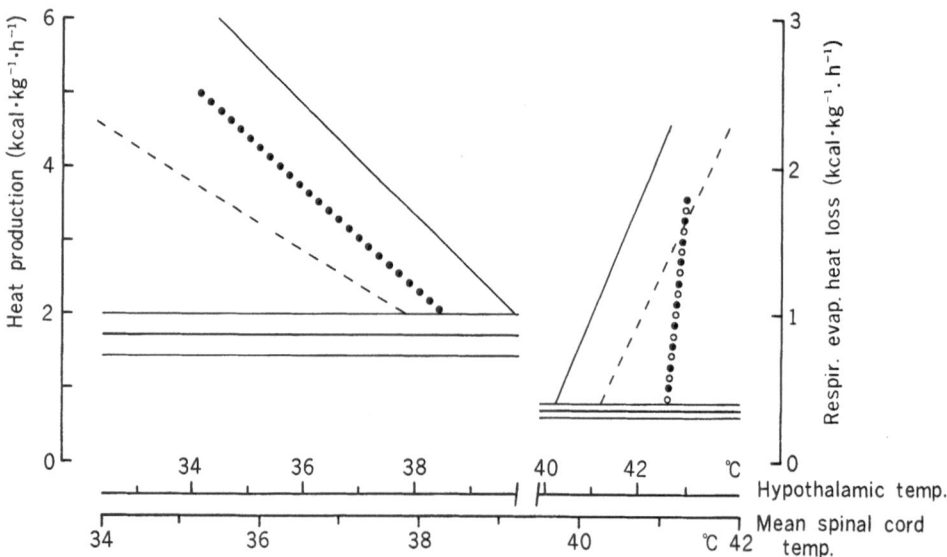

Fig. 26. Influence of simultaneous synergistic thermal stimulation of spinal cord and hypothalamus on heat production and respiratory evaporative heat loss (solid regression lines) as compared with selective stimulation of either spinal cord (broken regression lines) or hypothalamus (dotted regression lines). The diagram was constructed according to Fig. 22, and broken and dotted regression lines are identical with those in that figure. Two abscissae had to be drawn for comparison of selective and simultaneous stimulations, because somewhat different values of mean spinal cord temperature and hypothalamic temperature were obtained, when hypothalamic and peridural vertebral canal thermodes were perfused with water of the same temperature.—Comparison of the regression lines shows the narrowing of the distance between the threshold temperatures for increase of heat production and those for respiratory evaporative heat loss under the conditions of simultaneous thermal stimulation of spinal cord and hypothalamus.

(From Jessen and Ludwig, 1971).

cord cooling, could be canceled by simultaneous hypothalamic heating, and vice versa. On the other hand, activation of heat loss induced by strong heat stimulation in one area could not be suppressed by simultaneous cooling of the other area, and it made no difference, whether spinal cord or hypothalamus were heated or cooled, respectively. Apart from the interesting observation that strong central heat stimulation has a preponderant influence with respect to evaporative heat dissipation, these findings imply a common final pathway or integrating system, which does not discern between signals arising from spinal or hypothalamic temperature sensors.

Finally, concerning central thermosensitivity as a whole, another gap has been narrowed by the discovery of spinal temperature sensors. While in intact animals and in human beings under natural conditions the "central thermostat" works with remarkable accuracy, hypotheses on the underlying control system which are based on the hypothalamus as the sole central temperature detector have always been faced with the temperature differences between the thresholds of, e.g., heat production and evaporative heat loss becoming evident under the conditions of selective thermal stimulation of the hypothalamus. As demonstrated by Jessen and Ludwig (1971) in dogs, this threshold distance, which amounted to 2–4 °C for selective thermal stimulation of hypothalamus or spinal cord, was considerably reduced by simultaneous and synergistic stimulation of both areas, sometimes to immeasurable values (Fig. 26). It may thus be concluded that the combined sensitivities of hypothalamus and spinal cord are great enough to account for a precise control of core temperature within the limits of physiological core temperature variations.

SUMMARY

The spinal cord has been established as a central nervous region, where central temperature sensors of physiological significance are localized. All investigated thermoregulatory effectors are adequately influenced by thermal stimuli applied to the spinal cord. Spinal threshold temperatures for effector activation are dependent in an adequate manner from the external and hypothalamic thermal states and are ranging, under appropriate conditions, within the limits of natural core temperature variations. Heat- and cold-sensitive neurons are conducted in the spinothalamic tracts which show dynamic and static responses to variations of spinal cord temperature. Their static sensitivities are of the same order of magnitude as those of hypothalamic temperature sensors.

Spinal structures not only fulfill sensory functions in temperature regulation. Basic thermoregulatory control mechanisms are also localized at the spinal level of the central nervous system. Therefore, the spinal cord is regarded as a suitable experimental model for investigations of the neuronal mechanisms which constitute central thermosensitivity and central nervous thermoregulatory effector control. Corresponding model experiments in spinal motoneurons have suggested the hypothesis that temperature dependent changes of the soma membrane properties might account for the thermosensitivity of spinal neurons.

The spinal temperature sensors are functionally identical with the hypothalamic temperature sensors. Signals from both central thermosensitive regions are combined to one common sensory input for the central nervous control system providing body temperature regulation. The combined sensitivities of the hypothalamic and spinal temperature sensors seem to be sufficient to account for a central sensory input great enough to allow a precise control of body temperature within the limits of physiological core temperature variations.

REFERENCES

1. BARRON, D.H., and B.H.C. MATTHEWS (1938 a): *J. Physiol. (Lond.)* **94**: 26 p.
2. BARRON, D.H., and B.H.C. MATTHEWS (1938 b): *J. Physiol. (Lond.)* **94**: 27 p.
3. BENZINGER, H.T. (1969): *Physiol. Rev.* **49**: 671.
4. BIRZIS, L., and A. HEMINGWAY (1957 a): *J. Neurophysiol.* **20**: 91.
5. BIRZIS, L., and A. HEMINGWAY (1957 b): *J. Neurophysiol.* **20**: 156.
6. BLATTEIS, C.M. (1960): *Amer. J. Physiol.* **199**: 697.
7. BLIGH, J. (1961): *J. Physiol. (Lond.)* **159**: 85 p.
8. BLIGH, J. (1966): *Biol. Rev.* **41**: 317.
9. BROOKS, C. McC., K. KOIZUMI, and J.M. MALCOLM (1955): *J. Neurophysiol.* **18**: 205.
10. BRÜCK, K., and W. WÜNNENBERG (1967 a): *Pflügers Arch.* **293**: 215.
11. BRÜCK, K., and W. WÜNNENBERG (1967 b): *Pflügers Arch.* **293**: 226.
12. CORT, J.H., and R.S. McCANCE (1953): *J. Physiol. (Lond.)* **120**: 115.
13. CUNNINGHAM, D.J., J.A.J. STOLWIJK, N. MURAKAMI, and J.D. HARDY (1967): *Amer. J. Physiol.* **213**: 1570.
14. GOLTZ, F., and I.R. EWALD (1896): *Pflügers Arch.* **63**: 362.
15. GRANT, R. (1949): *Amer. J. Physiol.* **159**: 511.
16. GUIEU, J.D., and J.D. HARDY (1970): *J. Appl. Physiol.* **29**: 675.
17. HALES, J.R.S., and C. JESSEN (1969): *J. Physiol. (Lond.)* **204**: 40 p.
18. HALLWACHS, O., R. THAUER, and W. USINGER (1961): *Pflügers Arch.* **274**: 115.
19. HAMMEL, H.T. (1965): Neurons and Temperature Regulation. In: W.S. Yamamoto and J.R. Brobeck (edi.), Physiological Controls and Regulations. Saunders, Philadelphia, 1965.
20. HAMMEL, H.T., D.C. JACKSON, J.A.J. STOLWIJK, J.D. HARDY, and S. STRÖMME (1963): *J. Appl. Physiol.* **18**: 1146.
21. HARDY, J.D., R.F. HELLON, and K. SUTHERLAND (1964): *J. Physiol. (Lond.)* **175**: 242.
22. HART, J.S., and O.Z. ROY (1967): *Amer. J. Physiol.* **213**: 1311.
23. HELLON, R.F. (1967): *J. Physiol. (Lond.)* **193**: 381.
24. HELLSTRÖM, B., and H.T. HAMMEL (1967): *Amer. J. Physiol.* **213**: 547.
25. IRIKI, M. (1968): *Pflügers Arch.* **299**: 295.
26. JESSEN, C. (1967): *Pflügers Arch.* **297**: 53.
27. JESSEN, C. (1970): Rückenmark und Hypothalamus: gleichartige und gleichwertige Temperaturfühler des Körperkerns. Habilitationsschrift, Gießen.
28. JESSEN, C., and O. LUDWIG (1971): *Pflügers Arch.*, **324**: 205.
29. JESSEN, C., and E. Th. MAYER (1971): *Pflügers Arch.*, **324**: 189.
30. JESSEN, C., K.A. MEURER, and E. SIMON (1967): *Pflügers Arch.* **297**: 35.
31. JESSEN, C., and E. SIMON (1971): *Pflügers Arch.*, **324**: 217.
32. JESSEN, C., E. SIMON, and R. KULLMANN (1968): *Experientia (Basel)* **24**: 694.
33. JUNG, R. (1941): *Z. ges. Neurol. Psychiat.* **173**: 263.
34. KLUSSMANN, F.W. (1964): *Experientia (Basel)* **20**: 450.
35. KLUSSMANN, F.W. (1969 a): *Pflügers Arch.* **305**: 295.
36. KLUSSMANN, F.W. (1969 b): *Pflügers Arch.* **305**: 316.
37. KLUSSMANN, F.W., E. SIMON, H.J. HALBFASS, W. RAUTENBERG, and M. KOSAKA (1966): *Pflügers Arch.* **289**: R 23.
38. KLUSSMANN, F.W., G. SPAAN, W.J. STELTER, and B. RAU (1969): *Pflügers Arch.* **312**: R 108.
39. KLUSSMANN, F.W., W.J. STELTER, and G. SPAAN (1969): *Fed. Proc.* **28**: 992.
40. KOIZUMI, K. (1955): *Amer. J. Physiol.* **183**: 35.
41. KOSAKA, M., and E. SIMON (1968 a): *Pflügers Arch.* **302**: 333.
42. KOSAKA, M., and E. SIMON (1968 b): *Pflügers Arch.* **302**: 357.
43. KOSAKA, M., E. SIMON, R. THAUER, and O.E. WALTHER (1969): *Amer. J. Pysiol.* **217**: 858.
44. KOSAKA, M., E. SIMON, O.E. WALTHER, and R. THAUER (1969): *Experientia (Basel)* **25**: 36.
45. KULLMANN, R., W. SCHÖNUNG, and E. SIMON (1970): *Pflügers Arch.* **319**: 146.
46. LIPPOLD, O.C.J., J.G. NICHOLLS, and J.W.T. REDFEARN (1960): *J. Physiol. (Lond.)* **153**: 218.
47. MATTHEWS, P.B.C. (1962): *Quart. J. exp. Physiol.* **47**: 324.
48. MEURER, K.A., M. IRIKI, Ch. BAUMANN, and C. JESSEN (1965): *Pflügers Arch.* **285**: 63.
49. MEURER, K.A., C. JESSEN, and M. IRIKI (1967): *Pflügers Arch.* **293**: 236.
50. NAKAYAMA, T., H.T. HAMMEL, J.D. HARDY, and J.E. EISENMAN (1963): *Amer. J. Physiol.* **204**: 1122.

51. Pierau, F.K., M.R. Klee, and F.W. Klussmann (1969): *Fed. Proc.* **28:** 1006.
52. Pierau, F.K., and F.W. Klussmann (1971): Internat. Symposium of Comparative Thermoregulation, Lyon. *J. Physiol. (Paris)*, **63:** 380.
53. Pierau, F.K., and G. Spaan (1970): *Experientia (Basel)* **26:** 978.
54. Pierau, F.K., G. Spaan, and V. Golda (1970): *Pflügers Arch.* **316:** R 61.
55. Pierau, F.K., R.D. Wurster, and G. Spaan (1969): *Pflügers Arch.* **307:** R 100.
56. Popoff N.F. (1934): *Pflugers Arch.* **234:** 137.
57. Randall, W.C., R.D. Wurster, and R.J. Lewin (1966): *J. Appl. Physiol.* **21:** 985.
58. Rautenberg, W. (1967): Die Bedeutung der peripheren und zentralen Thermosensitivität für die Temperaturregulation der Taube. Habilitationsschrift, Bochum.
59. Rautenberg, W. (1969): *Z. vergl. Physiol.* **62:** 235.
60. Rautenberg, W. (1971): Internat. Symposium of Comparative Thermoregulation, Lyon. *J. Physiol. (Paris)*, **63:** 396.
61. Rautenberg, W., and E. Simon (1964): *Pflügers Arch.* **281:** 332.
62. Rautenberg, W., E. Simon, and R. Thauer (1963): *Pflügers Arch.* **278:** 337.
63. Rein, H. (1931): *Ergebn. Physiol.* **32:** 28.
64. Simon, E. (1967): *Arch. Sci. physiol. (Paris)* **21:** 215.
65. Simon, E. (1968): Spinal Mechanisms of Temperature Regulation. *24th internat. Congr. Physiol. Sci.*, Washington D.C., Vol. **VI** p. 289–290.
66. Simon, E. (1969 a): *J. Neuro-Viscer. Relat.* **31:** 223.
67. Simon, E. (1969 b): *J. Neuro-Viscer-Relat.* **31:** 260.
68. Simon, E., and M. Iriki (1970 a): *Experientia (Basel)* **26:** 620.
69. Simon, E., and M. Iriki (1971 b): Internat. Symposium of Comparative Thermoregulation, Lyon. *J. Physiol. (Paris)*, **63:** 415.
70. Simon, E., F.W. Klussmann, W. Rautenberg, and M. Kosaka (1966): *Pflügers Arch.* **291:** 187.
71. Simon, E., W. Rautenberb, and C. Jessen (1965): *Experientia (Basel)* **21:** 476.
72. Simon, E., W. Rautenberg, and R. Thauer (1963): *Pflügers Arch.* **278:** 361.
73. Simon, E., W. Rautenberg, R. Thauer, and M. Iriki (1963): *Naturwissenschaften* **50:** 337.
74. Simon, E., W. Rautenberg, R. Thauer, and M. Iriki (1964): *Pflügers Arch.* **281:** 309.
75. Spaan, G., and F.W. Klussmann (1970): *Pflügers Arch.* **320:** 318.
76. Stuart, D.G., O. Kenneth, K. Ishikawa, and E. Eldred (1966 a): *Amer. J. phys. Med.* **45:** 74.
77. Stuart, D.G., O. Kenneth, K. Ishikawa, and E. Eldred (1966 b): *Amer. J. phys. Med.* **45:** 91.
78. Thauer, R. (1935): *Pflügers Arch.* **236:** 102.
79. Thauer, R. (1939): *Ergebn. Physiol.* **41:** 607.
80. Thauer, R. (1962): Die Auslösungsmechanismen der chemischen Temperaturregulation. *22nd inter. Congr. physiol. Sci.*, Leiden Vol. **II,** p. 390–397.
81. Thauer, R. (1964): *Naturwissenschaften* **51:** 73.
82. Thauer, R. (1967): Homoiothermie als Fortschritt und Schicksal des Menschen. Jahrb. 1967 der Max-Planck-Gesellschaft, München, pp. 39–75.
83. Thauer, R. (1968): Temperature reception in the spinal cord. Symp. about Physiological and Behavioral Temperature Regulation, New Haven. In: Physiological and Behavioral Temperature Reguration. J.O. Hardy, A. Ph. Eagge, and J.A.J. Stolwijk (eds.). Thomas, Springfield, 1970, pp. 472–492.
84. Thauer, R., and G. Peters (1938): *Pflügers Arch.* **239:** 483.
85. Tönnies, J.F. (1938): *J. Neurophysiol.* **1:** 378.
86. Tönnies, J.F. (1939): *J. Neurophysiol.* **2:** 515.
87. Walther, O.E., M. Iriki, and E. Simon (1970): *Pflügers Arch.* **319:** 162.
88. Walther, O.E., E. Simon, and C. Jessen (1969): *Pflügers Arch.* **307:** R 98.
89. Wünnenberg, W. (1969): *Pflügers Arch.* **312:** R 118.
90. Wünnenberg, W., and K. Brück (1968 a): *Pflügers Arch.* **299:** 1.
91. Wünnenberg, W., and K. Brück (1968 b): *Nature* **218:** 1268.

CHAPTER 3

NEURAL FACTORS AFFECTING THE REGULATORY RESPONSES OF BODY TEMPERATURE

Korehiro OGATA and Naotoshi MURAKAMI

Department of Physiology, Institute of Constitutional Medicine, Kumamoto University, Kumamoto, Japan

WORKING HYPOTHESIS OF BODY TEMPERATURE REGULATION

First, the authors would like to propose a working hypothesis regarding the central nervous mechanism of body temperature regulation. This working hypothesis was first presented in 1966 [31], but it became necessary to make some revision owing to recent advances in our research.

Fig. 27 shows our whole concept of body temperature regulation based on the observations available at the present stage of our research. This is simplified and summarized from the viewpoint of control theory. A continuous line stands for the pathway of cold stress, and a broken line, heat stress. The diagram does not represent the anatomical neuronal connection.

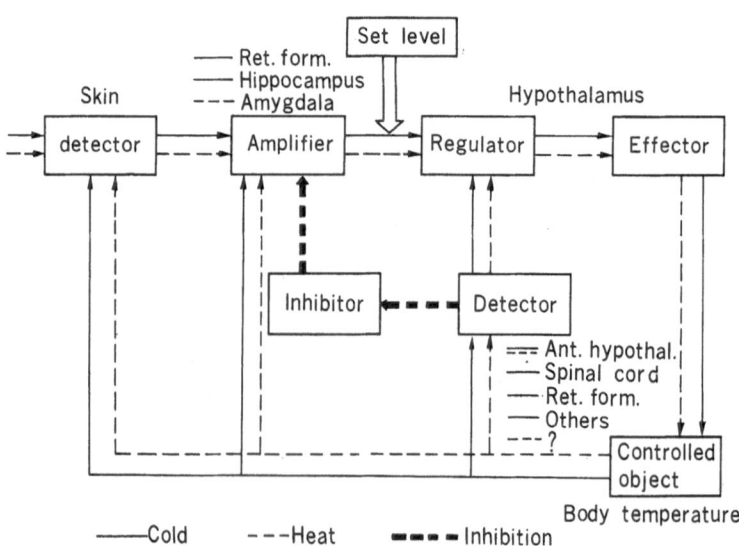

Fig. 27. Diagram of body temperature regulation.

An external thermal stress is detected by thermal receptors in the skin. Thermal information from the skin sensors is transmitted to an amplifier. Cold sensation may be amplified mainly by the mesencephalic reticular activating system. The hippo-campus will also take some part in amplifying the sensation. In the case of a warm sensation the amygdaloid nuclei would serve as an amplifier.

The activated sensation induces the activity of the regulator and, in turn, the effector. Here the hypothalamus might be seen as a kind of regulator. Between the amplifier and the regulator, a "set level" exists which determines the level or rhythmic variation in body temperature.

Through these lines of control the controlled object, in other words the body tem-perature, is maintained. Deviation or load error may occur, which is corrected through feedback to the skin sensor and also to the amplifier.

Another line of feedback goes through the detector in the anterior hypothalamus, and this may operate in the case of local heating and cooling. While we accepted the existence of a central warm receptor in our previous working hypothesis, we could not admit the existence of a central cold-sensitive structure. However, cold-sensitive cells in the anterior hypothalamus were found recently. Thus, both cold and warm information from the skin and the hypothalamus are transmitted to the regulator and a high level of precision may be maintained.

Besides the thermosensitive structures in the skin and the anterior hypothalamus, recent observations suggested that thermosensing elements may also exist in deep tissues outside the hypothalamus, i.e. in the spinal cord (Thauer et al. [33, 10]), in the re-ticular formation (Nakayama [24]), and in some others. Thermal information from these elements may also be transmitted to the regulator. On this subject Bligh [3] pointed out that "the evidence related only to cold sensitivity. Detection has depended upon gross thermal changes and it could not be assumed that this sensitivity to cold is concerned in normal thermoregulation, although this is possible." The results obtained in our laboratory are generally in line with his opinion.

The inhibitory system in the hypothalamus also has ascending and descending influence on various kinds of physiological functions. The inhibitory effect seems to increase during local heating of the heat detector in the hypothalamus, and is followed by remarkable inhibition in cold responses. On the contrary, local cooling of the detector may reduce the inhibitory effect on cold responses. Therefore, responses to cold may occur more easily.

In the following chapters this hypothesis will be discussed on the basis of experimental findings which were mainly observed in our laboratory. Among them our attention in this paper is especially devoted to some findings which were obtained after the latest review published in 1966.

THE RELATIVE IMPORTANCE OF PERIPHERAL AND CENTRAL DETECTION OF THERMAL STRESS

With regard to the activation of the regulatory mechanism of body temperature, several well-established and inconsistent views of its central vs. peripheral origin prevail. Recent studies have revealed that the regulatory mechanism is not purely central or peripheral in origin, but rather more complicated than was assumed by previous investigators.

Many experiments were also performed in our laboratory on this problem, and we pointed out that the high dependence of the regulatory mechanism upon temperature perceptions from the skin sensor may be responsible [31, 28, 29].

Our research then naturally expanded to include the question of whether or not there exist such cells in the hypothalamus which respond sensitively to direct heating and cooling. The results observed in our laboratory suggest that elevating the temperature of the anterior hypothalamus might activate thermoregulatory responses to heat, but lowering the temperature rarely resulted in activating responses to cold in neutral or hot environment [21]. Hereupon we must recall Thauer's interpretation [34]: Regulation in a hot environment is achieved both by reflexes originating in warm receptors in the skin and the effect of increased blood temperature on a central heat sensitive mechanism, while in a cold environment the regulation depends exclusively on the stimulation of the cold receptors of the skin. (Recently his conception was extended to include not only the skin receptors but also those in the spinal cord [10, 33].) Benzinger [1] concluded that central receptors play the greatest part in the control of responses to heat while responses to cold may depend more upon peripheral receptors. In 1961, Nakayama et al. [24] obtained single unit activity of the anterior hypothalamus in the anesthetized cat which responded with an increase of discharge frequency to a rise in hypothalamic temperature of less than 1 °C. So the initiation of responses to heat due to heating of central receptors became definite.

However, recent evidence in some species indicates that there are central structures which respond to quite small falls in temperature by initiating a rise in oxygen consumption. Hardy et al. [8] found temperature sensitive cells which increased their firing rate with local cooling of the anterior hypothalamus. It became clear that the relative importance of peripheral and central detection of thermal stress in control of body temperature must be examined more precisely.

Under these circumstances, Murakami et al. [22] studied the same subject at the J.B. Pierce Foundation Laboratory. The earlier experiments were conducted on animals maintained under chloralose-urethan anesthesia and the question arises as to the possible direct effect of the anesthetics on the activity level of the temperature-sensitive neurons. The question is especially important since peripheral stimulation by heat and cold produced no effect on these neurons in the anesthetized animal and marked effects would be anticipated according to some current theories of temperature regulation. It was felt essential, therfore, to obtain data from the unanesthetized animal. Thus the following experiments were conducted to study the influence of anesthetic agents and immobilizing drug upon temperature-sensitive units in the unanesthetized dog. An encephale isole preparation was utilized in these studies and the animal was considered to be in an unanesthetized state following a sufficiently long period of time to allow full recovery from the inhalation anesthetic (ether) administered prior to the surgical procedure. The area explored was bounded by the anterior commissure and the optic chiasm, extending from the midline to about 5 mm laterally. Sixty-five temperature-sensitive units were observed in a total of 55 dogs, in both the unanesthetized and anesthetized states. These units demonstrated changes in firing rate in response to induced changes in hypothalamic temperature (35–41 °C) and each could be classified basically as either warm- or cold-sensitive.

In Table 4 the frequency of the appearance of each type of unit is shown. "Warm-sensitive" means the temperature-sensitive unit which is characterized by an increased

TABLE 4 Pattern of firing rate of temperature-sensitive units in relation to hypothalamic temperature

Temperature-sensitive units	Total		Unanesthetized		Anesthetized	
	Number of cases	%	Number of cases	%	Number of cases	%
Warm-sensitive units	47	72.3	17	77.3	30	69.8
Cold-sensitive units	6	9.2	1	4.5	5	11.6
Phasic units	12	18.5	4	18.2	8	18.6

firing rate with rising hypothalamic temperature within the temperature range of 35–41 °C. "Cold-sensitive" means the temperature-sensitive unit characterized by a negative relationship between the firing rate and the hypothalamic temperature. "Phasic" units in this table means those units which increase the firing rate during the rising stage of hypothalamic temperature, and do not mean the so-called temperature-sensitive units in which the firing rate depends not only upon the hypothamic temperature level but also upon the rate of temperature change. The frequency of the appearance of all types of temperature-sensitive units as well as the nature of their thermal response did not significantly differ between the unanesthetized and the chloralose-urethanized dog. Further efforts were made to determine the effect of anesthetics

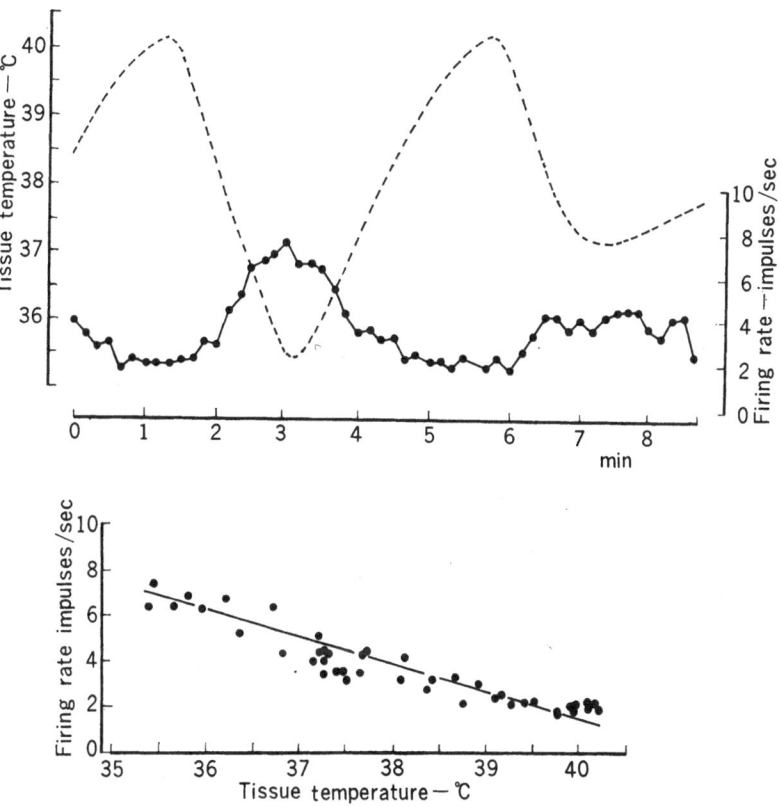

Fig. 28. Firing rate of a primary cold-sensitive unit plotted against the tissue temperature.

upon the level of activity of both the temperature-sensitive and temperature-insensitive neurons. Murakami *et al.* [22] reported that anesthetics in small amounts reduced the spontaneous firing rate of neurons having high activity (5 impulses/sec) but did not affect the spontaneous activity of neurons with low firing rates (0.5–1 impulses/sec). Moreover, the thermal sensitivity of warm-sensitive neurons was slightly decreased. It could be speculated that the former neuron must have been a secondary polysynaptic one, while the latter neurons were the primary sensors. An anesthetic in larger amounts (chloralose (6.5 mg/kg)-urethan (65 mg/kg) or thiopental sodium (70 mg/kg)), decreased and often suppressed the response of warm-sensitive units to temperature change. Gallamine triethiodide reduced both the spontaneous firing rate and thermal sensitivity of warm-sensitive neurons but did not affect the spontaneous firing rate of the temperature-sensitive units. The hypothermia induced by anesthetics and immobilizing drugs may thus result from a thermoregulatory response to the decreased level of activity of temperature-sensitive units.

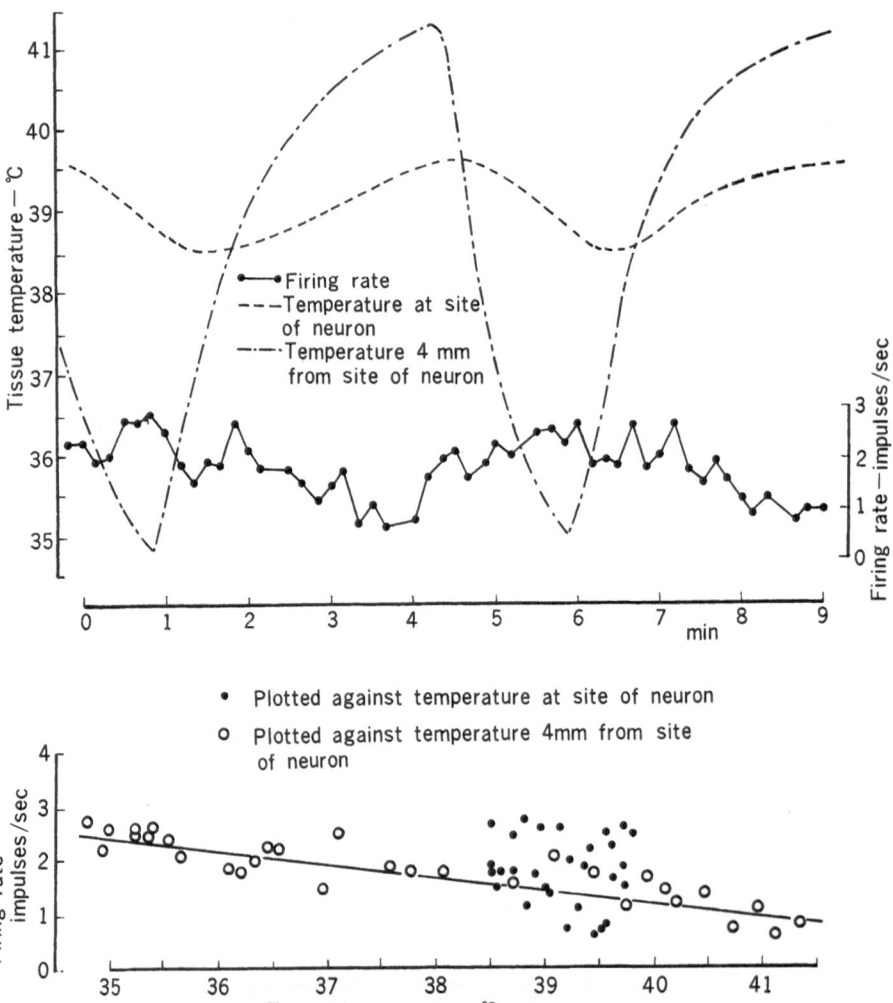

Fig. 29. Changes in firing rate of a secondary cold-sensitive unit as related to the calculated tissue temperature near the neuron.

Now the authors would like to make a few remarks as to the presence of the cold-sensitive units which demonstrate an increase in discharge frequency upon lowering of the local temperature. Recently it has been suggested that those neurons are regarded as interneurons which are driven by the cold receptors lying in the caudal part of the brain. By making corrections in neuron temperature, Murakami (unpublished) demonstrated two kinds of cold-sensitive units in the anterior hypothalamus. Fig. 28 shows one of the primary cold-sensitive units having a good linear relationship between impulse frequency and local temperature. In Fig. 29, where other neurons were observed to undergo changes in firing rate which followed variations in brain temperature at a site other than the actual location of the unit, these are regarded as secondary neurons. From these results we might speculate the existence of these two kinds of cells which respond sensitively to cooling in the anterior hypothalamus. Next, pharmacological research on the nature of the temperature-sensitive neuron is necessary in order to determine the transmitter substance at the synapse with which the temperature-sensitive neuron activates the thermoregulatory system. It was found that carbacol injected intracarotically reduced the spontaneous firing rate of all units as well as the temperature sensitivity of the warm-sensitive units in the dog, while strychnine did not affect the spontaneous activity of neurons (unpublished). Studies on the effects of not only these drugs but catecholamine and 5-HT on the activity of temperature sensitive neurons are carried out iontophoretically now by the use of a five barrel microelectrode.

The next question is whether there exists a cold sensitive neuron in the posterior hypothalamus. A moderate cooling and heating of the posterior hypothalamus caused no thermoregulatory responses, while an intensive cooling even inhibited shivering which had been observed previously; on the contrary the animal shivered vigorously with an intensive warming if he had already started to shiver. From these results it could be inferred that there is no thermoreceptor in the posterior hypothalamus which drives the heat production system (S. Takata, and N. Murakami—unpublished).

ACTIVATING AND INHIBITORY MECHANISM OF THERMAL SENSATION

In our laboratory, reaction with regard to heat production when exposed to cold was observed in leprosy patients with seriously impaired skin sensation [27, 36]. Resting heat production and body temperature were determined on a leprosy patient along with a healthy control. Then they were unclothed and exposed to cold at the same time. As was expected, the healthy man suffered a chill at once and after a few minutes he started to shiver markedly, while the patient scarcely complained of a chill at all at that time. In the healthy control, oxygen consumption during this stage increased, but not all in the patient. The body temperature in the healthy man did not show any decrease, while in the patient it fell progressively. After about 15 minutes when the fall of body temperature exceeded 1 °C, the patient began to suffer a chill for the first time and showed a marked increase in oxygen consumption. Here we would like to postulate a regulatory mechanism as follows.

A fall in core temperature will in the first place make the skin more sensitive to cold, and through this increased sensitivity cold is felt in the same environment in which it was not felt before, and other reactions to cold will develop. This suggests a close association of core temperature with thermal sensibility. Thus we studied the relationship between the rectal temperature level and the threshold of thermal sensation in the skin experimentally [13, 31]. The subject took a cold water bath of 23 °C for 50 minutes, which resulted in a lowering of rectal temperature from 37.2 °C to 35 °C; the threshold of warmth and pain were observed before and after the bath. The determination of the latent period was made by applying a heat ray to a skin area on the flexor surface of the forearm, the temperature of which was kept same in both cases by making use of a thermostat box. The threshold of warmth and pain with low rectal temperature became distinctly higher. We also observed the effect of a hot water bath at 43 °C for 40 minutes, which raised the rectal temperature up to 38.9 °C. The threshold of warmth and pain became lower significantly. The threshold of cold pain sensation was elevated at high rectal temperature, while the threshold became lower at temperatures low enough to cause a feeling of chill.

In the next stage of our research the site of the activation of these thermal sensation was investigated. Since it was proved that the ascending sensory system gives off collaterals to the reticular substance, through which consciousness as well as sensation is maintained (Magoun *et al.* [15]), the activity of the mesencephalic reticular formation in the unanesthetized rabbit was observed during progressive stages of cold exposure. The highest activity was found in a rectal temperature range between 34 °C and 33 °C [18, 31].

Besides these experiments, the behavior of the unanesthetized rabbit in consecutive stages of exposure to extreme cold was observed [31, 35]. The heat production rose to a maximum at a rectal temperature level of 35 °C in the course of the experiment, which was twice as high as the initial level. The range of body temperature in which maximum heat production was observed coincided well with the range of body temperature in which maximum electrical activity of mesencephalic reticular formation appeared.

Based on the assumption that a possible influence of autonomic activity on the sensibility of temperature senses could be expected, patterns of electrical activity of mesencephalic reticular formation were observed by giving repeated stimuli to the hypothalamic sympathetic zone or ventromedial nucleus in an unanesthetized rabbit [19, 31]. On stimulation of the sympathetic zone electrical activity of the reticular formation developed a pattern with high-voltage fast waves, which resembled after-discharge, along with systemic sympatheticotonic reactions suggesting sham rage. Seventy to 80 seconds after stimulation the pattern was replaced by electrical high frequency activity of a different nature. The results of electrical stimulation were confirmed also by an injection of epinephrine [19, 31], which produced a transitory rise in the evoked potential of the mesencephalic reticular formation. These findings may prove the possibility of influence of the sympathetic center upon activity of the mesencephalic reticular formation. Finally, it is inferred that the reticular ascending activating system is one of the major factors controlling cold sensation, which is the generator of somatic reaction to cold.

Besides the reticular formation, another type of ascending activating system for cold sensation was observed in our laboratory [16, 31]. The electrical activity of the hippocampus in unanesthetized rabbits during progressive cooling was studied. As the body was cooled down hippocampal rhythmic slow waves were distinctly observed.

But below the rectal temperature level of 28 °C these waves disappeared and small fast waves remained. This result suggests that the hippocampus also takes part in the regulation of body temperature against cold. Here a question is asked as to whether the hippocampus acts by itself as a regulatory center for cold or if the pattern is developed by way of the hypothalamic activity system. We gave electrical stimulation to the hippocampus of an unanesthetized rabbit under neutral temperature environment and no shivering could be induced on the electromyogram. On the contrary, when the rabbit was exposed to cold and was shivering slightly, electrical stimulation of the hippocampus induced more shivering. It seemed reasonable to infer that the hippocampus acts as a subsidiary activating system for cold sensation.

With a rise in rectal temperature due to heat exposure, the sensibility to warmth, as is mentioned above, is increased. Consequently continuing from the preceding case of cold exposure one might assume the presence of an activating system for warm sensation to be located in the mesencephalic reticular formation, too. The height and pattern of the evoked potential in the mesencephalic reticular formation of an unanesthetized rabbit induced by a single electrical shock to the sciatic nerve in succeeding stages of heat exposure were observed [20, 31]. But no essential changes were seen throughout the experiment.

Repeated stimulation to the hypothalamic parasympathetic zone or lateral hypothalamic nucleus was given. This procedure naturally induced vagotonia but it did not affect the electrical pattern of the mesencephalic reticular formation [19, 31]. One point to be remembered, however, is that the mesencephalic reticular formation was represented only by the medial part of the reticular formation on the frontal plane of P8, according to Sawyer's atlas. Therefore, some other parts in the reticular formation should be investigated as well.

Our next target was the amygdala. Electrical stimulation by square pulses was given to the lateral part of the basal amygdaloid nucleus or nucleus T' Völsch [11, 31]. The fibers from the parasympathetic zone of the hypothalamus proceed to this nucleus. The results showed that under a cool ambient temperature up to

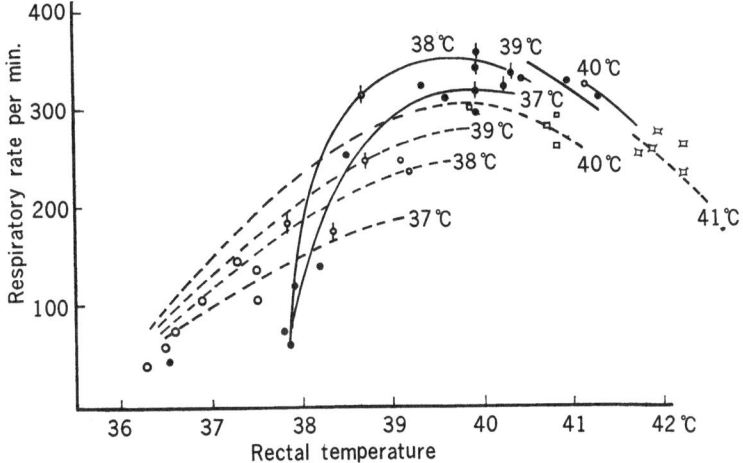

Fig. 30. The effect of different skin temperatures on respiratory rate and rectal temperatures following destruction of the amygdaloid nuclei.

11 °C no effect of stimulation was observed on rectal temperature, but when the ambient temperature was as high as 30 °C, the stimulation always resulted in a significant fall in rectal temperature. These findings suggest that the afferent impulses from the peripheral thermoreceptors deal with these phenomena. Furthermore, responses to heat in an unanesthetized rabbit on destruction of the limbic system were observed. In Fig. 30 the amygdaloid nuclei were bilaterally destroyed one week prior to the experiment [11, 31]. The solid line represents the result of a rabbit with bilateral destruction and the broken line stands for the control experiment, in which there was no destruction. As one of the responses to heat, respiratory rate is plotted against rectal temperature and is grouped according to respective levels of skin temperature. In the control experiment, a gradual increase in the respiratory rate with a rise in rectal temperature following exposure to heat is closely associated with the level of skin temperature; that is, at the same rectal temperature level, the higher the skin temperature is the more increased the rate of respiration. The curves representing this relationship at respective skin temperature levels are parabola-like with a peak at the rectal temperature of 40 °C and convergence at a point of 36 °C. In the case of cerebral lesion, three characteristic points are noted: A remarkable shift in the set point to a higher rectal temperature level, a sudden rise in respiratory rate with an increasing rectal temperature, and a smaller dependence of respiratory rate on the level of skin temperature, that is the respiratory curve at various skin temperature levels come close together. These results suggest that the decreased effect of skin temperature level after the destruction of amygdala is proof of the smaller dependence

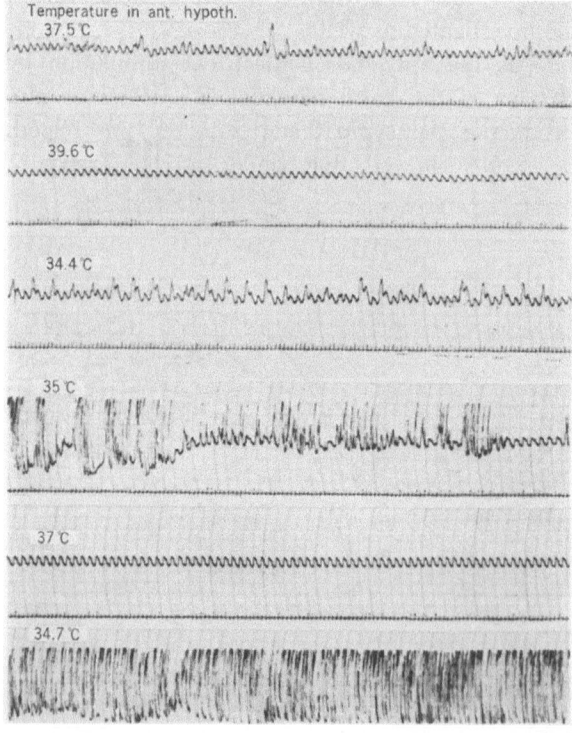

Fig. 31. Respiratory movement at different temperature levels of the anterior hypothalamus.

of heat responses on thermal sensation through the skin. An elevated set point with a sharp rise in the response suggests the participation of direct heating of the center in the regulatory mechanism. Therefore, it is reasonable to assume that the amygdaloid nucleus acts as one of the activating systems of warm sensation.

In the next stage of our researches, influences of local warming and cooling of the anterior hypothalamus upon somatic activity were observed [21, 31]. In Fig. 31 the respiratory movement, which was indicative of the degree of restlessness of the body, was traced during the cooling and heating period of the anterior hypothalamus of the rabbit. The local heating induced a remarkable depression in the restlessness of the body, while the local cooling resulted in an increased restlessness; this would be due to suppression of the inhibitory effect of the anterior hypothalamus. From these results, it is inferred that warming of the thermosensitive structure in the anterior hypothalamus would influence the physiological functions of cold responses and remarkable inhibition of cold responses would be induced. On the contrary, local cooling of this detector may reduce the inhibitory effect on cold responses.

ACTIVITY OF THE REGULATOR AND THE EFFECTOR

Maintenance of relatively constant body temperature requires control through both the somatic and autonomic nervous systems, so it is obvious that several different levels of the central nervous system may work together. It is beyond question that collection of thermal information from various parts of the body is the first step in body temperature regulation. The thermal information must be processed in the CNS, especially in the hypothalamus, and in turn thermoregulatory responses must be activated. Thus the body temperature will be well regulated within a narrow range. In any case, it is obvious that body temperature regulation is accomplished in the hypothalamus. But neuronal connections in the center where integration of thermoregulatory function is achieved are still not so clear-cut, and many investigators have differing opinions regarding it. Observations of changes in the activity of the hypothalamus were performed in our laboratory during exposure to cold [19, 31]. We demonstrated that during cold exposure activity of the parasympathetic center does increase, along with activity of the sympathetic center. The activity of the autonomic center with the progress of cold exposure was observed by introducing bipolar needle electrodes into the ventromedial hypothalamic nucleus (b-sympathetic zone) and into the lateral hypothalamic nucleus (c-parasympathetic zone) [14]. The frequency of the EEG from the sympathetic zone began to increase below the rectal temperature level of 37–36°C. A maximum which was reached at 34–33°C was followed by a notable decrease in frequency with the progress of cooling. The parasympathetic pattern also showed a slight increase in frequency on exposure to cold. When the rectal temperature fell down to 33–31°C the tendency was noticeably strengthened. A peak of increased frequency at 29–27°C was followed by a progressive decrease. In a certain stage below 20°C, concurrent with the excitation before death, a transient increase in frequency was observed on both EEG's. The excitation of the parasympathetic nervous system during cold exposure seems strange and unreasonable. But Gelhorn [7] proved in the dog that at a rectal temperature of 25–29°C a reduction of the adrenergic responses resulted from hypothalamic stimulation, whereas at the same body temperature the action of acetylcholine and histamine were increased. Another proof supporting our findings was furnished by Hirasawa [9] who demonstrated that the excitation of either system makes the other system unstable, and the disappearance of such excitation yields increased irritability of the other. The balance between excitation levels of both centers was recognized as an important factor in thermoregulatory functions.

Based on such assumptions, it seems very reasonable to presume that the activity of center of body temperature regulation is related closely to the activity of the sympathetic and parasympathetic zones in hypothalamus and that the balance between excitation levels of both zones play the most important role in producing regulatory responses.

Recently the concept of "neurochemical system of thermoregulation" which was proposed by Feldberg and Myers [5, 6] in 1963 has attracted special interest. In studies using amines concentrated highly in the hypothalamus, they noted their implication in the control of body temperature and proposed the new concept of temperature regulation.

In connection with this new problem a series of experiments were also undertaken in our laboratory to determine what kinds of mechanism are activated in thermoregulation [17, 23]. In the first place, following intraventricular injection of catecholamine, 5-HT and acetylcholine, the activity level in the hypothalamic autonomic center and the hippocampus, which are responsible for the central mechanism in thermoregulation, and the rectal temperature were observed in unanesthetized rabbits. With the injection of noradrenaline (10 μg), the activity level of b-sympathetic zone in the hypothalamus was elevated prior to a rise in rectal temperature, and θ waves, α waves and β waves became significantly more dominant. In the hippocampus EEG, α waves and θ waves also appeared dominantly in hyperthermia following intraventricular injection of noradrenaline. An elevation of activity level in the hippocampus returned to an initial level before the rectal temperature reached the maxmum value. When hypothermia was produced by intraventricular injection of 5-HT (200 μg) the activity level of the b-sympathetic zone in the hypothalamus was lowered markedly with a fall in rectal temperature. In the c-parasympathetic zone in the hypothalamus the alteration of activity level, which is dominant in θ waves, α waves and β waves and poor in δ waves, was followed by a fall of rectal temperature. These alterations implied a remarkable elevation of activity level in the c-parasympathetic zone of the hypothalamus. Acetylcholine in doses of 20–50 μg caused a dose-dependent hyperthermia which showed the shortest latent period.

In the second case, in hyperthermia and hypothermia following intraventricular injection of catecholamine, 5-HT and acetylcholine, rectal, average skin temperature and metabolic rate were measured and then heat balance was made for each 5-min period. On injection of noradrenaline (10 μg) heat production increased about 110–200% as much as before the injection. The larger the increment of heat production, the greater the rise in rectal temperature. There was no detectable change in heat loss in three out of five cases, and heat loss was inhibited slightly in two out of five cases. Intraventricular injection of 5-HT (200 μg) caused no detectable change in heat production in most of the cases. In only a few instances a slight decrement in heat production during hypothermia was seen. But, a remarkable increment of heat loss coincided well with hypothermia. Acetylcholine (20–50 μg) injected intraventricularly had no effect on heat production with the only exception being a slight decrement occurring during the peak stage of hyperthermia. Nevertheless, a remarkable increment of heat loss was caused simultaneously during hyperthermia.

From these findings it could be concluded that hyperthermia with noradrenaline or adrenaline was produced as a result of activation of the heat production system and slight inhibition of the cooling system in thermoregulation. Hypothermia due to 5-HT injection was caused mainly by activation of the cooling system and not by heat production. Hyperthermia caused by acetylcholine resulted exclusively from an inhibition of the cooling system and had no relation to the heat production system. Furthermore, it could be inferred that the loss of temperature sensitivity in warm sensitive cells in the preoptic region yield an intense depression of the cooling system, as is usually observed during fever. From these results a simple neuronal model was proposed in Fig. 32 following the neuronal model proposed by Bligh and Cottle [4]. Our model is slightly different from theirs in the acting site of noradrenaline and acetylcholine. It could be inferred that these drugs, noradrenaline and 5-HT, participate to process thermal information at the first synapse in either the pathways from cold receptors to heat production effectors, or from warm receptors to heat loss effectors. Anyhow input of the central thermal information to the regulator would be mediated by such a neurochemical system.

In thermoregulation, the shivering system and vasomotor system will be available as effectors in the heat production system. In addition, the effectors of the cooling system might be the vasomotor and sweating systems. Among these three systems, sweating can be investigated only in the human being. The posterior hypothalamus has recently been considered to be merely the site of synapse for the transmission of driving cold impulses from the skin, rather than the heat maintenance center which it was assumed to be in the dual center theory. In our laboratory, it was found by the electrical stimulation experiments carried out by Takata and Murakami (unpublished) that the posterior hypothalamus includes the shivering center, the discending pathway of which controls development of shivering, the shivering inhibition center which reduces the intensity of shivering on electrical stimulation, and another area which has nothing

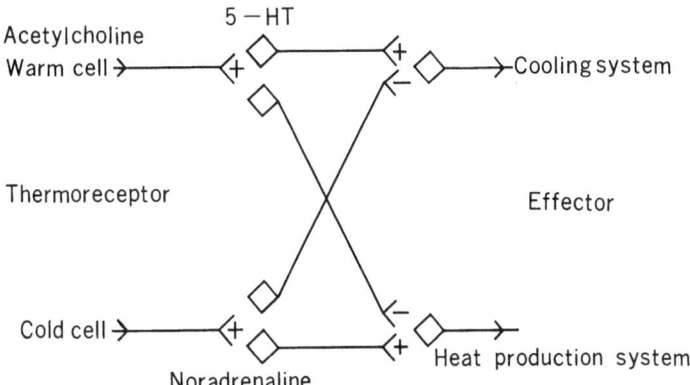

Fig. 32. Schema showing an acting site of noradrenaline, 5-HT and acethycholine in the anterior hypothalamus.

to do with shivering. The shivering center localized in the dorsomedial posterior hypothalamus is equivalent with what was described by Birzis *et al.* [2] in the cat. Influences of ambient temperature on the electrical activity of shivering center were shown schematically in Fig. 33. On frequency analysis of EEG's in the shivering center, θ waves and α waves essential in posterior hypothalamus increased at lower ambient temperature and decreased at higher ambient temperature when each wave was compared with the value in ambient temperature 20 °C. However, δ waves behaved conversely in relation to ambient temperature. From these results it would be inferred that the activity in the shivering center is activated by thermoreceptors in the skin, especially cold receptors, or is inhibited by warm receptors. If so, the activity in the shivering center should also be affected significantly by changes in deep body temperature, through a thermoreceptive structure in the anterior hypothalamus particularly. In Fig. 34 it was shown that the activity level in the shivering center is changed considerably by local temperature changes in the anterior hypothalamus even if ambient temperature is maintained constant. Based on these results we must conclude that the integration of shivering, the activity of the shivering center, is a function of preoptic temperature as well as ambient temperature and that it is likely that the activity of the shivering center is proportional to the product of skin temperature and preoptic temperature. This thermoregulatory trend is observed not only in the shiver-

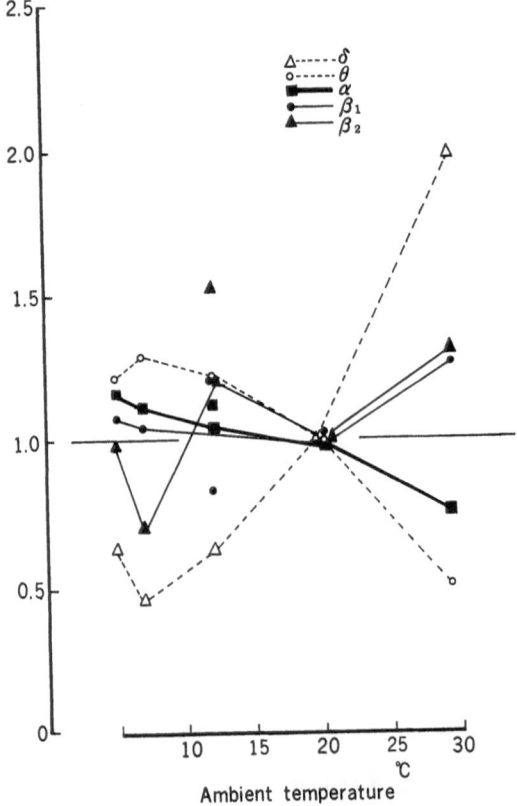

Fig. 33. Frequency analysis of EEG in the shivering center during exposure to various ambient temperature, when each wave was compared with the value in ambient temperature 20 °C.

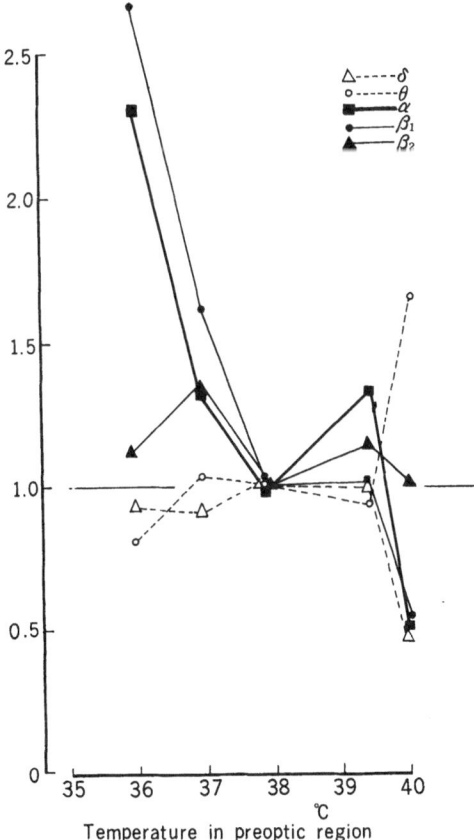

Fig. 34. Frequency analysis of EEG in the shivering center during a local temperature change in anterior hypothalamus, when each wave was compared with the value in preoptic temperature 37.9°C.

ing system, but in the vasomotor system as well, and could be a common characteristic of the thermoregulatory effector system. Murakami (unpublished) studied quantitatively reflex change of blood flow occurring in one pinna when thermal stress is applied to the other pinna. The reflex change of blood flow depended on preoptic temperature as well as the intensity of thermal stress. Even if the same thermal stress is given, the higher temperature in preoptic area caused a more marked change of blood flow, the lower a smaller change or none at all.

From all the results mentioned above it could be speculated that thermoregulatory responses must be triggered by a thermal signal from the skin at first and that the trigger action activating thermoregulatory responses should also be a function of deep body temperature, detected through the hypothalamic thermosensor and the extra-hypothalamic thermosensor in the midbrain, spinal cord and so on. That is to say, thermoregulatory responses exist as hierarchical system. Vasomotor reaction is the first thermoregulatory response met, and consequently, after the skin temperature reached above or below a limited temperature, other responses develop to maintain a constant body temperature.

A POSSIBLE FACTOR FOR SETTING THE LEVEL AND RHYTHMIC VARIATION IN BODY TEMPERATURE

In Fig. 27, a "set level" is installed. "Set level" here means the structure which determines the level or rhythmic variation in body temperature. Causes of the level and the fluctuation in body temperature have long been studied in many ways from the last century on by a number of investigators. But every one of the theories failed to give a clear-cut interpretation of the mechanism. In this chapter we would like to propose vestibular function as one of possible factors in the phenomena. In the present stage of our research we can not decide where the "set level" should be installed in Fig. 27. We put it temporarily between the amplifier and the regulator.

The primary point of discussion is what serves as a pace maker to circadian rhythm of body temperature. An opportunity to make a few comments on this problem was given to us by the voyage from Hamburg to Kobe [30]. Ogata left Hamburg on November 29, 1961, aboard a boat for Japan, passing through the North Sea, the Mediterranean Sea and Indian Ocean, and arrived in Kobe on January 16, 1962. The east-bound voyage resulted in a shorter periodicity of daily routine of 23 hours and 40 minutes, oral temperature was taken every two hours as a rule, but in some critical cases frequent determination was made.

In Fig. 35, SS stands for seasickness and $(-)$ denotes being unaware of seasickness; $(+)$ slight seasickness; $(++)$ moderate seasickness with poor appetite; and $(+++)$ seasickness severe enough to cause him to be confined to bed. Dizzy here means having a sensation of dizziness even after the ships' pitching and rolling had subsided.

The curve on November 28, taken while at anchor showed a typical diurnal pattern with a morning rise, a plateau during the daytime and a evening fall. The boat set sail from Hamburg on the following day and was overtaken by a storm in the North Sea with an instantaneous wind velocity of 30 meters per second. The subject suffered from severe seasickness. Body temperature on the storm-tossed day developed

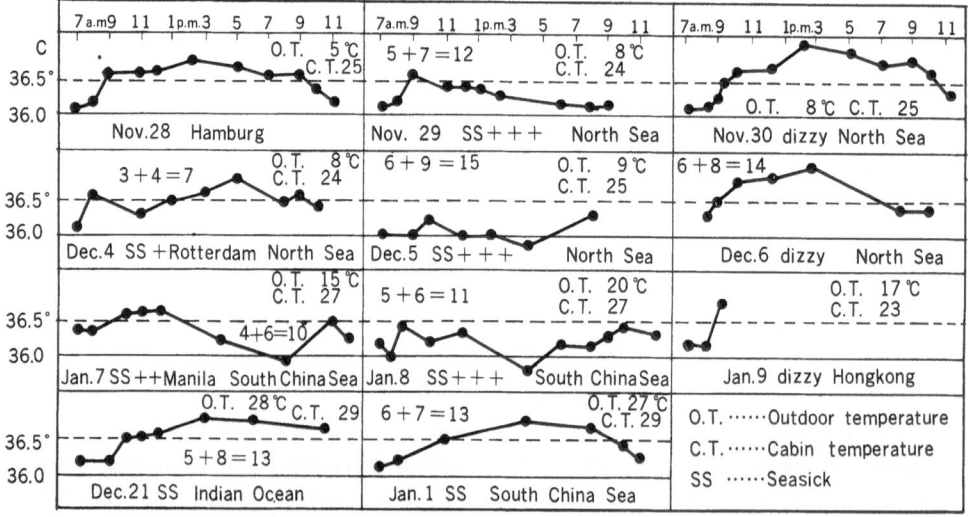

Fig. 35. Diurnal variation in body temperature on particular days during voyage.

a morning rise at 9 a.m. which was followed by a gradual fall throughout the day. Such a low level of body temperature always accompanied severe seasickness as in the curves of December 5, January 7 and 8 and the like. On December 21 and January 1, pitching and rolling was evaluated as 13. This number represents the grades of swell and wave as an index of the sea and 13 means an instantaneous wind velocity of 30 meters per second. But at that point the subject developed neither seasickness nor the lowering of body temperature. Therefore, the lowering of body temperature is not absolutely attributable to the pitching and rolling themselves but rather to seasickness as a natural consequence of the former.

Body temperature rhythm during vertigo caused by a mechanism other than motion sickness is shown in Fig. 36. A pulmonary tuberculosis patient was treated with streptomycin and when the total amount of streptomycin exceeded 35 g the patient complained of a feeling of vertigo, one of the side effects on the VIIIth nerve. Showing scarcely any diurnal fluctuation, the curves of body temperature during daytime remained practically at the same level as in the early morning. The basal metabolism fell down progressively to 29.6 kcal/m²/hr. But on administration of an antihistaminic agent vertigo was alleviated considerably, basal metabolism took an upward turn and body temperature regained diurnal fluctuation.

As an important factor in diurnal variation of body temperature, further evidence is furnished by the case of children in favor of a probable relationship with the vestibular functions. Kleitman and others [12] gave statistical evidence as to establishment of the adult type of diurnal temperature curve during the second year of a child's life, when the nervous system develops greatly and a child learns to walk. Consequently we observed the diurnal temperature rhythm on 127 deaf-mutes, aged 8 to 13, whose condition is often complicated by some defect in the vestibular functions. Nothing remarkable was noticed in the temperature pattern of any case [31, 32]. However, special consideration should be paid to the fact that the subjects observed were all in the

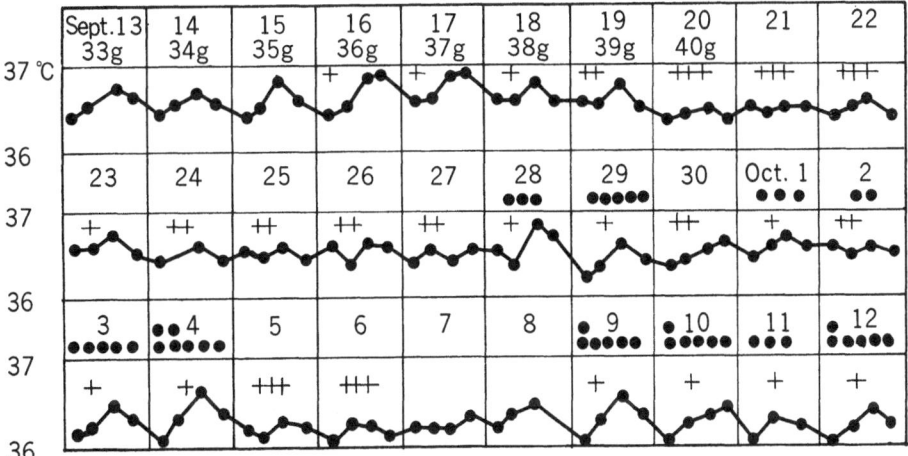

Fig. 36. Effect of vertigo on body temperature rhythm. Development of vertigo due to streptomycin and alleviation by antihistaminic administration.

+ ++ +++: Degree of vertigo.

· · · · · : Number of 10 mg tablets of an antihistaminic drug.

33–40 g: Total amount of streptomycin injected.

chronic stage and they might have established some sort of compensation for the accompanying functions. Similarly in the previous case of adaptation to conditions causing seasickness the body temperature was not lowered. Elevation of temperature rhythm during prolonged sensation of dizziness after a storm is compatible with our observations that vertigo caused by visual distortion is entirely different from the case of streptomycin treatment, and has no inhibitory effect on oxygen consumption in the least, but there is a trace of a tendency at work to bring about an elevation in metabolism [26, 31].

Based on these findings it may be reasonable to presume that vestibular functions act as a factor in setting the level and rhythmic variation in body temperature.

SUMMARY

1) A working hypothesis regarding the central nervous mechanism of body temperature regulation is proposed from the view point of control theory, and the hypothesis is discussed on the basis of experimental findings which were mainly observed in our laboratory.

2) The exact proportions for the effects of peripheral and central thermal receptors cannot be evaluated at this time. It has been made clear that there exist two types of temperature sensitive neurons in the anterior hypothalamus, and that one is primary and the other secondary. Then, these temperature sensitive neurons show different effects of anesthetics and immobilizing agents respectively. In connection with thermoreception in the posterior hypothalamus, it could be inferred that there is no thermoreceptor in the posterior hypothalamus which drives the heat production system.

3) Information from the thermal detectors may be affected through activating or inhibitory structures. Cold sensation would be amplified mainly by the mesencephalic reticular activating system. The hippocampus may also take some part in amplifying cold sensation. As for warm sensation, the amygdaloid nuclei would serve as an amplifier. Remarkable inhibition of cold responses is induced by local heating of the heat detector in the hypothalamus. On the contrary, local cooling of the detector may reduce the inhibitory effect on cold responses.

4) The balance between excitation levels of the sympathetic and parasympathetic zones in hypothalamus plays an important role in producing regulatory responses.

5) A neurochemical system of thermoregulation was studied with attention to heat balance. Consequently, it was shown that input of the central thermal information to the regulator would be mediated by this system.

6) There exists a shivering center and a shivering inhibition center in the posterior hypothalamus. The activity of the shivering center localized in the dorsomedial posterior hypothalamus is a function of deep body temperature as well as ambient temperature and it is likely that the activity is proportional to the product of skin temperature and preoptic temperature.

7) Based on a finding that there exists a close relationship between the circadian variation of body temperature and vestibular functions, an assumption was proposed that vestibular functions may act as a factor for setting the level and rhythmic fluctuation in body temperature.

REFERENCES

1. BENZINGER, T.H. (1969): *Physiol. Rev.* **49**: 671.

2. BIRZIS, L., and A. HEMINGWAY (1957): *J. Neurophysiol.* **20:** 91.
3. BLIGH, J. (1966): *Biol. Rev.* **41:** 317.
4. BLIGH, J., and W.H. COTTLE (1966): *Experientia* **25:** 608.
5. FELDBERG, W., and R.D. MYERS (1963): *Nature (Lond.)* **200:** 1325.
6. FELDBERG, W., and R.D. MYERS (1964): *J. Physiol.* **173:** 226.
7. GELHORN, E. (1955): *Acta Neurovegetativa* **11:** 90, cited from *Ann. Rev. Physiol.* (1957) **19:** 93.
8. HARDY, J.D., R.F. HELLON, and K. SUTHERLAND (1964): *J. Physiol.* **175:** 242.
9. HIRASAWA, K. (1949): *Nagai-Shoten* **270:** (in Japanese).
10. IRIKI, M. (1968): *Pflüg. Arch.* **299:** 295.
11. KATAYAMA, J. (1965): *Bull. Inst. Constit. Med.* **16:** 51 (in Japanese).
12. KLEITMAN, N., S. TITELBAM, and H. HOFFMANN (1937): *Am. J. Physiol.* **119:** 48.
13. KORI, N. (1955): *Bull. Res. Inst. Diath. Med.* **6:** 143 (in Japanese).
14. KUROTSU, T. (1949): *No-Kenkyu* **3:** 39 (in Japanese).
15. MAGOUN, H.W., and G. MORZZI (1949): *Clin. Neurophysiol.* **1:** 455.
16. MINAKAMI, M. (1967): *Bull. Inst. Constit. Med.* **17:** 256 (in Japanese).
17. MIYAMOTO, Y. (1970): *Bull. Inst. Constit. Med.* **20:** 347 (in Japanese).
18. MURAKAMI, N. (1959): *Bull. Res. Inst. Diath. Med.* **10:** 235 (in Japanese).
19. MURAKAMI, N. (1959): *Bull. Res. Inst. Diath. Med.* **10:** 243 (in Japanese).
20. MURAKAMI, N. (1966): *Bull. Constit. Med.* **16:** 218 (in Japanese).
21. MURAKAMI, N. (1966): *Bull. Inst. Constit. Med.* **17:** 23 (in Japanese.)
22. MURAKAMI, N., J.A.J. STOLWIJK, and J.D. HARDY (1967): *Am. J. Physiol.* **213,** 1015.
23. MURAKAMI, N., Y. MIYAMOTO, and K. OGATA (1970): *J. Physiol. Soc. Japan* **32:** 443.
24. NAKAYAMA, T., J.S. EISENMAN, and J.D. HARDY (1961): *Science* **134:** 560.
25. NAKAYAMA, T. (1968): *Proc. Int. Nat. Union Physiol. Sci.* 4. Abstracts of Lect. and Symp. Washington. D.C.: 287.
26. OGATA, T. (1954): *Bull. Res. Inst. Diath. Med.* **5:** 39 (in Japanese).
27. OGATA, K. (1957): *Bull. Res. Inst. Diath. Med.* **7:** Suppl.: 1.
28. OGATA, K. (1960): Essential Problem in Climatic Physiology, Nankodo, Tokyo, 26.
29. OGATA, K. (1961): *Bull. Inst. Constit. Med. Kumamoto Univ.* **11:** Suppl.: 1.
30. OGATA, K., and T. SASAKI (1963): *Jap. J. Physiol.* **13:** 84.
31. OGATA, K., T. SASAKI, and N. MURAKAMI (1966): *Bull. Inst. Constit. Med. Kumamoto Univ.* **16:** Suppl.: 1.
32. SASAKI, T. (1953): *Bull. Res. Inst. Diath. Med.* **3:** 262 (in Japanese).
33. THAUER, R., and G. PETER (1937): *Pflüg. Arch. ges. Physiol.* **239:** 483.
34. THAUER, R. (1961): *Arch. Sc. Physiol.* **15:** 95.
35. WATANABE, S. (1957): *Bull. Res. Inst. Diath. Med.* **7:** 197 (in Japanese).
36. YAGI, I. (1961): *Bull. Res. Inst. Diath. Med.* **11:** 423 (in Japanese).

CHAPTER 4

THERMOSENSITIVE NEURONS IN THE BRAIN

Teruo NAKAYAMA

Department of Physiology, Nagoya University School of Medicine, Nagoya, Japan

The methods utilized by physiologists in an analysis of brain function have been principally sectioning of the brainstem, production of localized lesions, physical, chemical or electrical stimulation of a specific area and the recording of electrical activity. In the history of the research on temperature regulation, each of these experimental approaches has been followed. Ablation of the cerebral cortex and the thalamus did not impair the maintenance of normal body temperature while lesions limited to the hypothalamus caused definite disturbances in temperature regulatory function. Thermal stimulation of the hypothalamus has been known to initiate appropriate thermoregulatory responses. In 1961 the unit activity of the temperature sensitive neuron was first recorded in the hypothalamus [11], although some d. c. potential changes associated with changes in brain temperature were reported by C von Euler [6] in 1950.

In this paper, the following four topics will be considered. 1. The warm sensitive neuron, 2. The cold sensitive neuron, 3. The effect of skin temperature on neuron activity in the brainstem, 4. The effect of pyrogen on the thermally sensitive neuron. Although most of the experiments to be discussed were performed in anesthetized animals, the data does not significantly differ from the results obtained in unanesthetized animals. In early studies, diathermic heating was used to raise the hypothalamic temperature. To control the brain temperature more precisely, however, conductive warming and cooling was more commonly used in later studies. It must be pointed out that the brain temperature was not measured at the location of the recording electrode because of technical difficulties. This matter will be referred to later.

THE WARM SENSITIVE NEURON

In the cat, anesthetized by urethane, unit discharges which increased their firing rate during local heating were recorded in the preoptic area [12]. In Fig. 37 the spike discharges of the preoptic neuron at various brain temperatures are shown. The firing rate increased from 11.6 to 25.1 impulses per sec with an elevation of the local temperature from 38 to 39.8 °C. The respiratory rate nearly doubled. The temperature characteristic of these warm sensitive neurons is that the discharge frequency increases and decreases in proportion to the rise and fall in local temperature between 35 and 40 °C with a high Q_{10} coefficient of five or' more and very little adaptation in the steady state, this being regarded as a most suitable feature in a biological thermostat. These warm sensitive neurons were localized histologically to

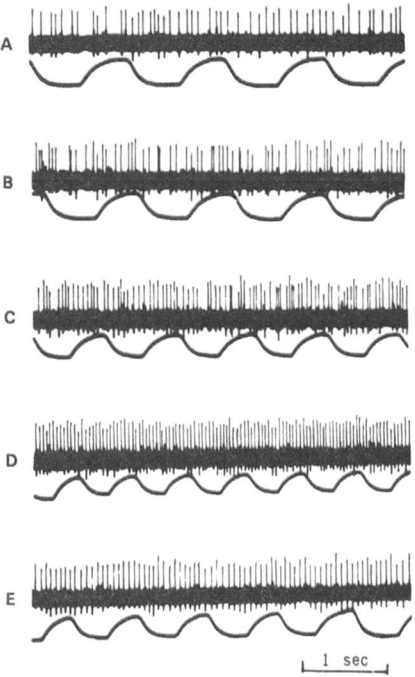

Fig. 37. Unit discharge of the preoptic neuron and respiratory rate during heating of the preoptic area. **A**: Control (38 °C). **B, C, D**: During heating (max. temp. 39.8 °C). **E**: 20 sec after cessation of heating.

the midline region immediately rostroventral to the anterior commissure. There are many neurons which respond to a rise in local temperature with a small positive coefficient. Such an increase in firing rate, however, is regarded as a non-specific reaction to temperature. In some warm sensitive neurons, the number of discharges per sec increases in proportion to local temperature only within a limited temperature range [4, 9]. These neurons are reported to be sensitive to barbiturates. Cunningham *et al.* [3] analyzed the non-linear relationship between impulse frequency and local temperature and found that the measured brain temperature does not always show the actual neuron temperature from which the unit activity is being recorded. When the discharge frequency was replotted against the tissue temperature at the location of the neuron, a linear relationship was obtained. However, in some cases, a non-linear relationship could not be eliminated by the correction of temperature. Replotting of the discharge frequency against calculated neuron temperature resulted simply in a shift in the hysteresis curve. Further analysis has shown that in this case firing rate has a linear relationship with the tissue temperature 2 mm from the thermode and 6 mm away from the location of the unit whose activity is being recorded. This means that the neuron under observation is driven by the true thermoreceptors lying in another area of the brain tissue.

In Fig. 38, unit 1 increased the firing rate at preoptic temperatures of above 37.5 °C but maintained a constant firing level below this temperature, thus showing a non-linear relationship to changes in local tissue temperature. This preoptic neuron, however, was influenced also by changes in the midbrain temperature concurrent

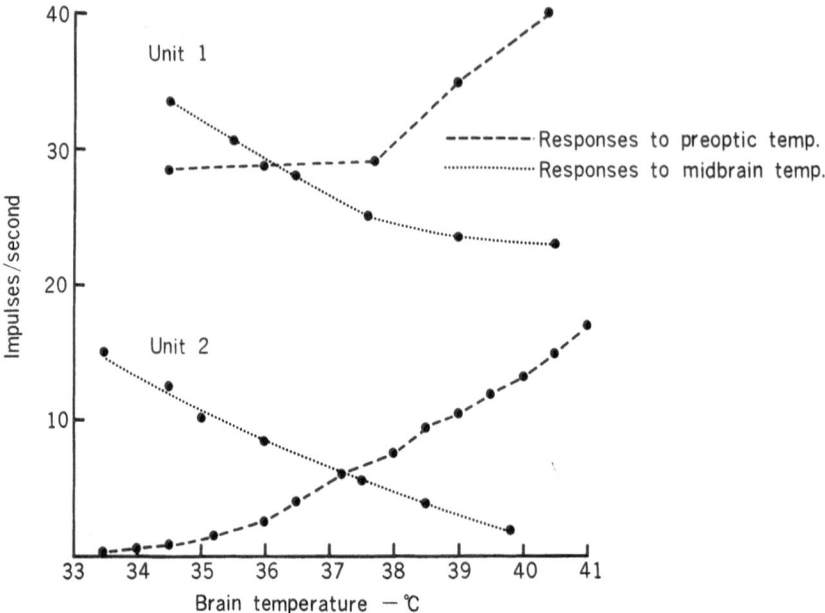

Fig. 38. Steady-state response of preoptic neurons to changes in preoptic and midbrain temperature. While recording the response to temperature changes in the preoptic area, the midbrain temperature was kept constant and vice versa.

with a constant local temperature. Unit 2 demonstrates a linear relationship between discharge frequency and the local temperature, which does not necessarily mean, however, that the unit is a warm receptor. As is seen, the firing rate of this unit was increased by a fall in the midbrain temperature. These findings indicate that both units 1 and 2 are interneurons. Can units such as this, driven by both midbrain cold receptors and preoptic warm receptors, ever play any significant role in temperature regulation?

For the time being, the criteria for judging whether a unit is a true thermodetector or not may be stated as follows: If a unit in the preoptic area has a very high Q_{10}, shows a linear relationship between firing rate and temperature, is insensitive to anesthetic depression and is not influenced by changes in midbrain temperature, it may then be identified as a warm sensor.

THE COLD SENSITIVE NEURON

The existence of units which demonstrate an increase in discharge frequency upon lowering of the local temperature has been reported in the septal area, but only over a limited range of temperature. These neurons are sensitive to anesthetics and are generally regarded as interneurons [4]. Hardy *et al.* [8] have shown the presence of units which have a negative coefficient to temperature in the preoptic area of the dog, but the temperature sensitivity of these units is generally low. The average ratio of the number of warm-sensitive units to cold-sensitive units encountered in the preoptic and septal area was reported to be about 5:1. Murakami's histological data indicate that most cold-sensitive neurons were in the septal area [10].

These findings suggest that the septal or preoptic interneurons are driven by the cold receptors which may lie in the caudal part of the brain, because it is known that under certain circumstances the temperature of the tissue 1 cm away from the thermode is modified by conductive cooling. Accordingly, an experiment was designed in which the preoptic and midbrain temperatures of a rabbit were controlled independently [13]. It was found that only one unit out of 51 in the preoptic-septal area decreased the discharge frequency during local warming while the midbrain temperature was kept constant.

On the other hand, a number of units were found in the mesencephalic reticular formation to be very sensitive to a reduction in the local temperature while the preoptic temperature was locked at a constant level (Fig. 39). Twelve neurons out of 146 units recorded from the reticular formation did not respond to a change in the preoptic temperature, were not influenced by mechanical stimulation to the body surface and demonstrated an inverse relationship between local temperature and discharge frequency. In the steady state, little adaptation was observed in these neurons and the negative temperature coefficients were higher than Q_{10} −2. The histological localization of these neurons showed a wide distribution within the mesencephalic reticular formation, dorsal to the red nucleus.

Other cold sensitive neurons were driven by mechanical stimulation applied to the body surface. Generally, neurons which showed a higher rate of discharge were depressed to a certain extent by a rise in local temperature but the discharges did not disappear, indicating that the spontaneous firing of these neurons is maintained by two mechanisms, i.e. local temperature and non-specific sensory influences. At first, only those neurons which were cold sensitive but were not influenced by non-thermal stimuli were considered to be cold receptors. Later studies (unpublished), however,

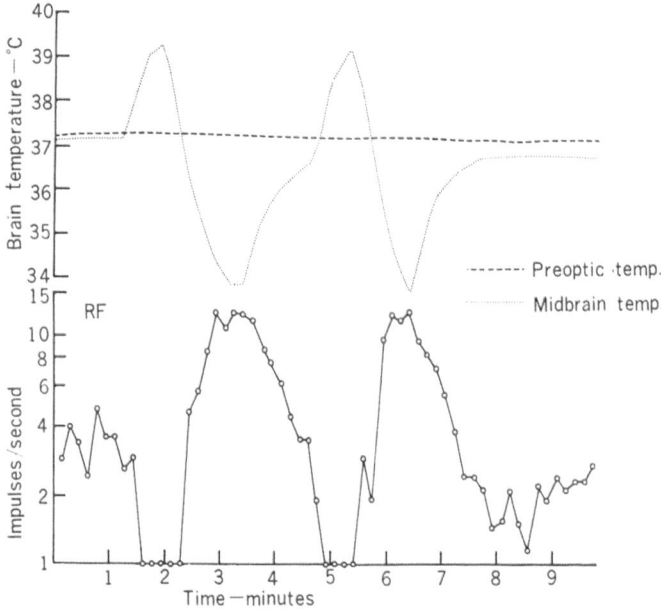

Fig. 39. Response of a unit within the reticular formation to changes in local temperature.

revealed that the spontaneous firing rate was inhibited by systemic administration of small amounts of anesthetic, while the thermosensitivity of the neuron was not impaired. This finding may suggest that the neuron driven by a non-thermal stimulus is itself sensitive to a change in local temperature.

THE EFFECT OF SKIN TEMPERATURE UPON UNIT ACTIVITY WITHIN THE BRAINSTEM

One of the main problems in thermophysiology and a matter of much discussion is whether the heat loss response is driven by an elevation in skin temperature, in brain temperature or both. Murakami *et al.* [10] observed the effect of peripheral thermostimulation applied to a limited area upon unit activity in the preoptic area in both the anesthetized and unanesthetized dog, but could not find a significant change in the firing rate of either warm sensitive or insensitive neurons. According to Wit and Wang [15], the firing rate of some preoptic neurons of the cat was increased upon a rise in ambient temperature with a further increase in discharge with elevation in the brain temperature. These results may indicate the convergence of both the central and peripheral input of temperature information.

To see the effect of skin temperature upon activity within the brainstem reticular formation, shaved rabbits were immersed in water and the water temperature was changed rapidly, maintaining a constant flow of water. As was already pointed out, there are cold sensitive neurons in the midbrain reticular formation; therefore, the brain temperature must be kept constant in order to evaluate the effect of peripheral thermal stimulation in the overall level of activity.

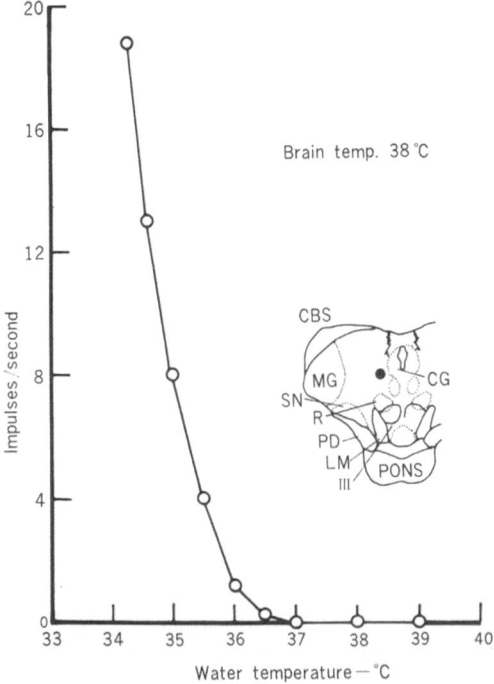

Fig. 40. Steady-state response of a reticular unit to various skin (water bath) temperatures.

Some reticular units were not influenced by changes in preoptic or local temperature. Elevation of the water temperature to 40 °C also had no effect upon local activity. The firing rate was increased significantly, however, with a fall in the water temperature. The increased firing rate was maintained as long as the water temperature remained low, and very little adaptation was observed.

In Fig. 40, the steady state discharge of a reticular unit was plotted against water temperature while the brain temperature was maintained at 38 °C. At a water temperature of 37 °C or higher, no discharge was recorded. This is not because the neuron is inhibited but simply due to the lack of afferent impulses from the skin. The unit could be activated by mechanical stimulation to the skin, giving phasic discharges up to 20 impulses per sec at a water temperature of 37.4 °C, a temperature at which no spontaneous firing would normally be observed.

It is interesting to see that the temperature of the water in which an animal is immersed and the local brain temperature may both influence neurons within the reticular formation. Some units increased and decreased their discharge frequency upon the fall and rise of either the brain temperature or of the water temperature, respectively. If either one of the temperatures is kept low, the rise of the other temperature did not reduce the firing rate.

EFFECT OF PYROGEN ON THE THERMALLY SENSITIVE NEURON

Following intravenous injection of typhoid vaccine in rabbits, the warm unit of the hypothalamus was inhibited with a latency of 7–13 min. A reverse effect was observed in the cold unit [2]. According to Eisenman [5], the thermosensitivity of the central warm detectors was depressed by administration of Piromen, but the firing rate of high Q_{10} unit was unchanged at 38 °C. In other words, the thermal-response curve rotated around the normal core temperature. This means that the resetting of the thermoregulatory set point cannot be attributed to a change in the activity of central warm detectors. As was mentioned, there are ample cold units in the brainstem reticular formation. A local injection of leucocyte pyrogen into the midbrain produced fever in the conscious rabbit [14]. The effect of typhoid vaccine was observed on the unit activity of the reticular formation. The discharge frequency of cold units driven by mechanical stimulation to the body surface was increased by the intravenous injection of typhoid vaccine with a variable latency ranging from a few minutes to 35 minutes. In Fig. 41, A, B and C show control discharges at brain temperatures of 38 °, 36 ° and 34 °C, respectively. D is the record taken 33–36 min. after the intravenous injection of vaccine. While the brain temperature was kept constant at 36 °C, the firing rate increased to the level it would normally be if the local temperature were about 34 °C. Thus, the results add further support to the idea that the reticular formation may be involved in the regulatory mechanism of body temperature.

Wit and Wang [16] studied the effect of sodium salicylate on the firing rate of preoptic neurons following the injection of pyrogen. When the brain temperature had been elevated by 1 °C due to exposure of the animal to a high ambient temperature for more than one hour, both firing rate of the preoptic unit and the respiratory rate were increased. Intracarotid injection of pyrogen depressed the neuron activity as well as the respiratory rate within 15–30 min. after the injection. Subsequent injection

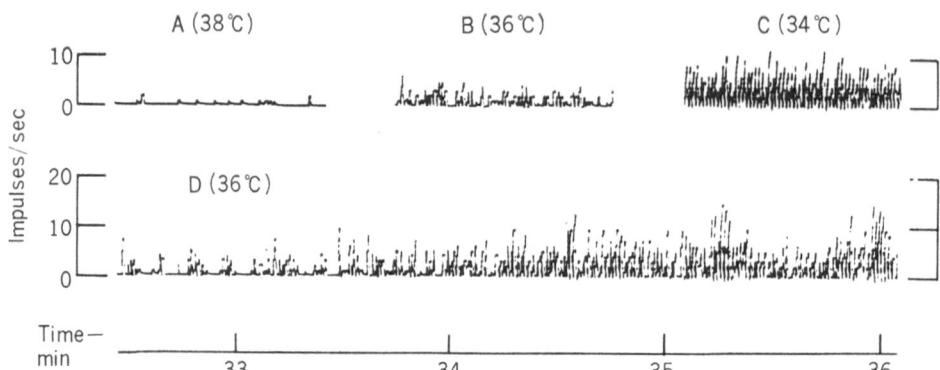

Fig. 41. Effect of pyrogen on a cold unit of the reticular formation. **A, B, C**: Control discharge. **D**: Record taken 33–36 min after systemic injection of typhoid vaccine.

of salicylate resulted in a return to the pre-pyrogen level of neural discharge within 30 min. When ambient and body temperature declined, neuronal activity and respiratory rate decreased. Based on these results, it was concluded that pyrogen induced fever is due to a depression in the thermal sensitivity of the preoptic neuron and that the antipyretic effect of salicylate is the result of the reversal of this pyrogen depression.

CONCLUSION

Thus the major findings from studies of single unit activity were presented in relation to temperature regulation. Some of these units may function as true thermoreceptors. Others appear to be interneurons in an afferent or efferent thermoregulatory pathway. More neurophysiological data must be accumulated, however, to evaluate the role of each class of neurons in the complex neural network involved in temperature regulation. Although there remains a big gap between our knowledge of unit activity within the nervous system and that of thermoregulatory responses, it will not be useless speculating as to the possible mechanism of temperature regulation.

Benzinger [1] has postulated that the preoptic warm sensors and the cutaneous cold receptors play a major role in heat loss and heat producing responses, respectively. The effect of cutaneous warm receptors may not be significant, but the afferent activities stemming from them are known to influence the central warm receptors. On the other hand, cutaneous cold receptors activate the brainstem reticular formation, which itself is very sensitive to a fall in local brain temperature. It seems that the reticular formation is as important as the hypothalamus in the regulation of body temperature. A rise or fall in body temperature with or without thermal stress was explained as a shift of a set point which is formed by combination of hypothalamic high Q_{10} thermal activity and low Q_{10} non-thermal activity of the reticular formation [7]. Using an electrical model of temperature regulation as an analogy, non-thermal activity of the reticular formation or of the hypothalamus was often regarded as a reference level and the difference between the firing rates of thermally sensitive and insensitive neurons would make an error signal.

At the time when Hammel *et al.* [7] proposed the adjustable set point theory, the effect of peripheral and central cold stimuli had not been observed on the unit activity of the reticular formation. Since then, it has been found that the reticular neuron is very sensitive to a fall in skin temperature just as the preoptic neuron is to a rise in brain temperature. The effect of pyrogen has been found to be inhibitory to the preoptic warm unit and facilitatory to the reticular cold unit. For the time being, therefore, it might be appropriate to suppose a simple model composed of warm sensitive activity of the preoptic area and cold sensitive activity of the reticular formation (see Fig. 42). The latter is influenced also by non-thermal factors. There is no need to assume an indifferent or a reference activity within the central nervous system. The warm- and cold-sensitive activities may function reciprocally, as is the case in the spinal extensor and flexor activities.

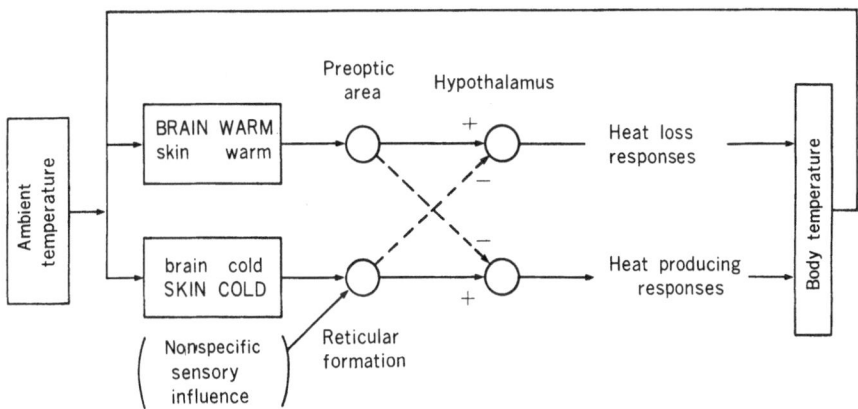

Fig. 42. A simplified model for temperature regulation.

SUMMARY

The studies of various investigators into the nature of thermally sensitive neuron are summarized as follows.

1) Neurons were found which increased their steady state discharge frequency, proportional to the change in temperature with a thermal sensitivity of $Q_{10} > 5$. These neurons were localized in the most rostral aspect of the hypothalamus, mainly ventral to the anterior commissure near the midline.

2) The relationship between firing rate and temperature was not linear over the entire temperature range for all warm-sensitive neurons, but was characterized in some neurons by a sharp deflection in their steady state response curve. Neurons of this type were also characterized by their sensitivity to barbiturates and wider anatomical distribution. They were functioning as interneurons which received impulses from the primary thermoreceptors.

3) The presence of cold-sensitive neurons in the preoptic area has been reported. However, the number of such neurons was very limited and their temperature sensitivity rather low. In the brainstem reticular formation, a number of neurons were found to be very sensitive to a fall in local temperature and demonstrated little adaptation in the steady state. Most of them were influenced by mechanical stimulation given to the body surface.

4) More than half of the neurons studied in the reticular formation were activated by peripheral cooling. Some neurons were driven by local cooling, peripheral cooling and by mechanical stimulation to the body surface.

5) Following systemic administration of pyrogen the warm-sensitive neurons in the preoptic area and in the reticular formation showed a reduced activity, while the cold-sensitive neurons increased their level of spontaneous discharge. A thermally insensitive neuron was not affected by the pyrogen.

6) It is suggested that the brainstem reticular formation, where thermal and non-thermal information are integrated, may play an important role in the neuronal network of body tempertaure regulation.

REFERENCES

1. BENZINGER, T.H. (1969): *Physiol. Rev.* **49**: 671.
2. CABANAC, M., J.A.J. STOLWIJK, and J.D. HARDY (1968): *J. Appl. Physiol.* **24**: 645.
3. CUNNINGHAM, D.J., J.A.J. STOLWIJK, N. MURAKAMI, and J.D. HARDY (1967): *Am. J. Physiol.* **213**: 1570.
4. EISENMAN, J.S., and D.C. JACKSON (1967): *Exp. Neurol.* **19**: 33.
5. EISENMAN, J.S. (1969): *Am. J. Physiol.* **216**: 330.
6. EULER, C. VON (1950): *J. Cell. Comp. Physiol.* **36**: 333.
7. HAMMEL, H.T., D.C. JACKSON, J.A.J. STOLWIJK, J.D. HARDY, and S.B. STRØMME (1963): *J. Appl. Physiol.* **18**: 1146.
8. HARDY, J.D., R.F. HELLON, and K. SUTHERLAND (1964): *J. Physiol.* **175**: 242.
9. HELLON, R.F. (1967): *J. Physiol.* **193**: 381.
10. MURAKAMI, N., J.A.J. STOLWIJK, and J.D. HARDY (1967): *Am. J. Physiol.* **213**: 1015.
11. NAKAYAMA, T., J.S. EISENMAN, and J.D. HARDY (1961): *Science* **134**: 560.
12. NAKAYAMA, T., H.T. HAMMEL, J.D. HARDY, and J.S. EISENMAN (1963): *Am. J. Physiol.* **204**: 1122.
13. NAKAYAMA, T. and J.D. HARDY (1969): *J. Appl. Physiol.* **27**: 848.
14. ROSENDORFF, C., J.J. MOONEY, and C.N.H. LONG (1970): *Fed. Proc.* **29**: 523.
15. WIT, A., and S.C. WANG (1968): *Am. J. Physiol.* **215**: 1151.
16. WIT, A., and S.C. WANG (1968): *Am. J. Physiol.* **215**: 1160.

PART II

SWEATING AND HEAT ADAPTABILITY

MORPHOLOGICAL ATTEMPTS TO SOLVE SOME UNSETTLED PROBLEMS ON THE HUMAN ECCRINE SWEAT GLANDS

JUNZO OCHI and YUTAKA SANO

Department of Anatomy, Kyoto Prefectural University of Medicine, Kyoto, Japan

Up to the present a considerable number of morphological and physiological investigations on the human eccrine sweat glands have been carried out to clarify the mechanism of sweating. Many normal and pathological findings on the eccrine glands at the level of fine structure have been also reported. Nevertheless, morphological bases for some important physiological phenomena of the eccrine gland have not yet been determined. For example, the existence of the "transitional portion" with a special structure between the secretory and ductal portions, the relation of this special portion or proximal duct to the reabsorption of sweat in reference to the effect of desoxycorticosterone acetate (DCA), and the difference in autonomic innervation between mentally stimulated eccrine glands and thermally stimulated ones have yet to be investigated. In order to settle these problems, it is necessary for us to conduct human, not animal, experiments, but these inevitably involve serious limitations. In the present article we tried morphologically to solve these important but difficult problems, using biopsied materials from the authors themselves and from volunteers.

WHETHER THE "TRANSITIONAL PORTION" WITH THE SPECIAL STRUCTURES EXISTS IN THE HUMAN ECCRINE SWEAT GLAND OR NOT

It may be of interest to briefly survey the literature on the so-called transitional portion of the eccrine sweat gland. More than two decades ago Ito and Enjo (1949) found microscopically a short intercalated portion with special structures between the secretory and the ductal portion and referred to it as the "transitional portion" (in German: "Übergangsteil"). It consisted of a layer of tall columnar epithelial cells in which no secretory granules were observed. The Golgi apparatus of these cells formed a simple network in the supranuclear region and the mitochondria were rod-shaped or filamentous. Several years later Montagna, Chase and Lobitz (1953) discerned a gradual transition between the secretory and the coiled ductal portion, and they regarded this initial piece of the duct as the "transitional region." It had two layers of epithelial cells, of which the basal layer is composed of cuboidal cells and the superficial one of flat cells with a fine cuticular border to the lumen. After Loewenthal (1960, 1961) it was found that there existed, however, a dilated ampulla at the junction of the secretory and ductal portions of the eccrine sweat gland. It showed specialized morphological features in contrast to the transitional portion (or region) reported by Ito and Enjo and by Montagna, Chase and Lobitz. The ampulla opens into the just distally located sphincter with large myoepithelial cells and possesses a single row of parietal cuboidal cells on an occasional myoepithelial cell. The extreme delicacy of the cuticula in the epithelial cells and the presence of canaliculi among the cells is also apparent. Loewenthal speculated that the ampulla functions in the reabsorption of sweat constituents and that the sphincter indicates a contractile structure. In his book Montagna (1962) thereafter described that the transition between the secretory and the ductal segment is abrupt and denied the special structures maintained by Loewental, because of the poor quality of the illustrations in the papers. After his work it was thought that the transitional region was essentially not different from the initial part of the duct.

Electron microscopically Hibbs (1958), using the biopsied materials from volar skin and subcutis, demonstrated that the eccrine sweat gland is composed of the following four portions: The coiled secretory portion, the transitional zone, the coiled portion of the duct with two layers of cells, and the straight ascending portion of the duct. Among them the transitional region encountered in some sections has one layer of epithelial cells, some of which is occasionally observed to extend all the way from the basement membrane to the lumen. In this zone myoepithelial cells are sparse. Notwithstanding the above description, it is strange that Hibbs does not show the electron micrographs which explain these findings. Recently Shibasaki and Ito (1967) reported that between the secretory and the coiled ductal portion of the human axillar eccrine sweat gland the presence of the short transitional portion (Ito and Enjo, 1949) was electron microscop-

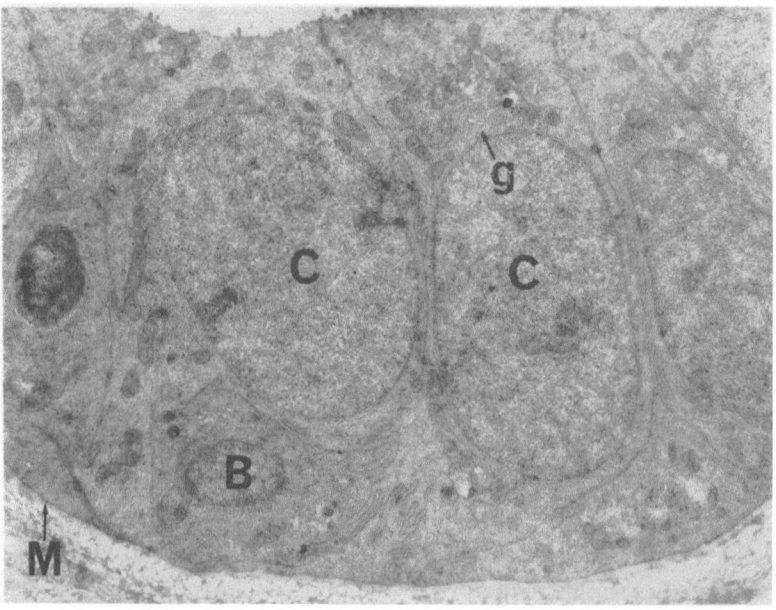

Fig. 43. Transitional portion. Tall columnar cells (C) extend from the basement membrane to the lumen. Between the basal regions of two columnar cells a small basal cuboidal cell (B) is located on the basement membrane. A process of a myoepithelial cell (M) can be observed at the left bottom of the figure. g: Golgi apparatus. × 5,000.

ically confirmed. The authors, however, have doubts about their observations and will now comment on them, in connection with their own observations.

During electron microscopic observation of the eccrine sweat gland in the skin of the human arm, the authors have sometimes found a short area at the junction of the secretory and the ductal portion which seems to be structurally a mixture of these two. In an occasional thin section this area is located within a group of coiled secretory and ductal cells. This short section is considered to be part of a gradual transition between the other two. As can be seen in Fig. 43, the transitional portion is fundamentally composed of one layer of tall columnar cells extending from the basement membrane to the lumen. Sometimes the small basal cuboidal cell as observed in the secretory portion was situated on the basement membrane. In the columnar cells no or few small vacuoles could be found near the lumen. The Golgi complex is mostly found in the supranuclear region, the rough-surfaced endoplasmic reticulum in the infranuclear region and mitocondria in both regions. Desmosomes between the neighboring cells are developed in the apical side and interdigitations formed by the lateral membrane of the cells are not as complicated as those found in the secretory portion. There was neither basal infolding in the basal part of the cells nor secretory canaliculi among the cells. Less frequently, small processes of a myoepithelial cell extend into this transitional region. These characteristic findings correspond well to those of Hibbs (1958). The authors could not, however, detect the presence of the special transitional portion, the existence of which had been asserted by Shibasaki and Ito (1967).

In the course of further observations the authors found by chance structures very similar to the "transitional portion," which are nothing other than small blood vessels in the vicinity of the sweat glands (Fig. 44a, b). The wall of the vessel is composed of a layer of cuboidal endothelial cells attached by an interrupted row of flattened pericytes. The cuboidal endothelial cell possesses apical cytoplasmic processes of various sizes but neither a characteristic cuticular border nor distinguished intercellular interdigitations. It often contains fine perinuclear filaments, small clusters of free ribosomes, multivesicular bodies and some stick-like dense bodies with longitudinal filaments. The pericyte is located outside of the endothelial cell and has characteristics of the smooth muscle. On and near the lateral and the basal cell membranes of the endothelial cells and the inner and outer walls of the pericyte a large number of pinocytotic or reverse pinocytotic vesicles can be observed. The most important finding is the interposition of a fairly wide irregular extracellular space with basement membrane between the endothelium and pericyte. These findings were quite different from those obtained in other part of the eccrine sweat gland, but very similar to those describing the "transitional portion" of the eccrine gland as reported by Shibasaki and Ito (1967). In the lumen of the blood vessel an erythrocyte can be frequently seen, strongly suggesting that this tubule is a blood vessel, not a sweat gland. On the other hand, it was already reported by Hibbs, Burch and Phillips (1958) that the blood vessels of human skin possess a special structure different from the blood vessels seen in other organs. Their report states that blood vessels of this type are found predominantly in the vicinity of sweat glands, and are lined by endothelial cells with the following characteristics: (1) small dense rod-shaped granules in the cytoplasm; (2) large bundle of very fine filaments in the perinuclear cytoplasm; (3) groups of small vesicles in the cytoplasm, each group enclosed by a membrane; (4) thicker endothelium, the cells in contracted vessels being pyramidal or columnar in

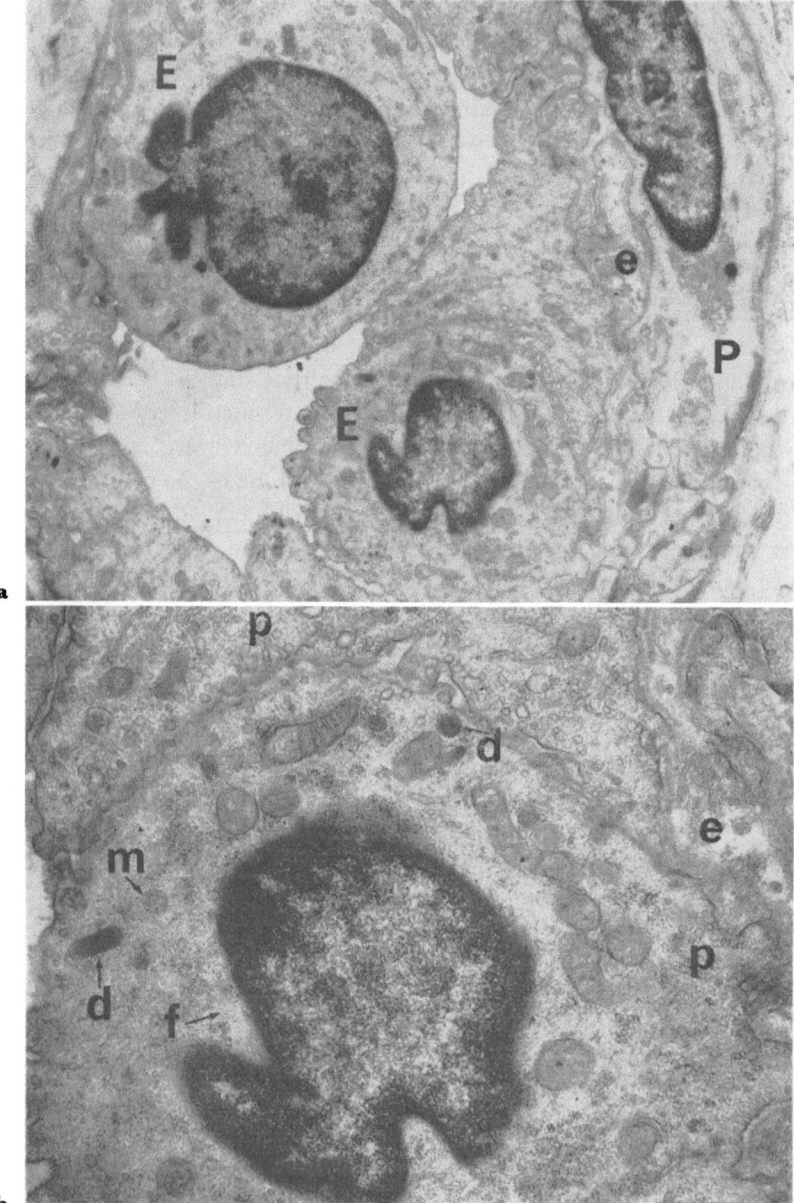

Fig. 44. A small vessel in the vicinity of the eccrine sweat gland.

   a, Lower magnification of the vessel. The wall is composed of a row of cuboidal endothelial cells (E), outside of which the flattend pericyte (P) is attached. e: Extracellular space interposed between the endothelial cell and the pericyte. × 3,600.

   b, Larger magnification of a cutting-out of **a**. The endothelial cell contains fine perinuclear filaments (f), free ribosomes, multivesicular bodies (m) and dense bodies (d). To the left of the figure a longitudinally sectioned dense body is seen and on the top of the figure a transversely sectioned dense body. e: Extracellular space. p: Pinocytotic or reverse pinocytotic vesicles. × 15,500.

shape. They attribute the transport of fluid to the secretory portion of the sweat gland to this type of vessels.

Based on the authors' own observations and those of Hibbs, Burch and Phillips, it is concluded that the transitional portion found by light microscopy (Ito and Enjo, 1949) would not correspond to that found later electron microscopically (Shibasaki and Ito, 1967), but rather to the part detected by the authors, and that the transitional portion with electron microscopically special structures whose presence is maintained by Shibasaki and Ito is nothing but of a special type of blood vessel near the sweat gland.

ON THE DUCTAL REABSORPTION OF SWEAT AND THE EFFECT OF DCA

The most important constituent of sweat except for water is sodium chloride. It is physiologically well known that the sweat from human eccrine glands is hypotonic and that the concentration of sodium chloride in the sweat is lower than that of blood plasma, becoming lower and lower as sweating decreases. The hypotonicity of eccrine sweat is explained as the result of selective ductal reabsorption of sodium chloride from the precursor sweat with isotonicity to blood plasma secreted by epithelial cells of the secretory coiled portion (Kuno, 1956; Schwartz and Thaysen, 1956; Lloyd, 1962; Schulz et al., 1965). When sweating is weak or less profuse, the ductal reabsorption is effective because of the slow flow of the precursor sweat in the duct. On the contrary, when sweating is very profuse, the reabsorption becomes less effective due to the accelerated flow of the precursor fluid in the duct, resulting in an increased concentration of sodium chloride in the sweat (Kuno, 1956; Cage and Dobson, 1965). It is also widely known that mineralocorticoid from the adrenal cortex plays a significant role in the reabsorption of sodium chloride in the renal tubuli, and that this hormone lowers also the content of sodium chloride in the sweat (Conn et al., 1948; Lobeck and McSherry, 1963). In fact, patients with a hypofunction of the adrenal cortex secrete sweat with an increased concentration of sodium chloride. The salt-conserving action of the eccrine sweat gland after treatment with desoxycorticosterone acetate (DCA) may result from a promotion of the ductal reabsorption of sodium chloride or from a decrease in the amount of precursor sweat secreted by the secretory portion which had been metabolically altered, or from both of these factors. This is not yet fully established.

Based on the chemical reaction of potassium pyroantimonate to sodium ions, Komnick and Komnick (1963) have devised a histochemical method for the electron microscopic detection of sodium ions in the tissues. This method and its modifications were applied to several tissues with some success (salt gland—Komnick and Komnick, 1963; Lennep, 1968: sweat gland—Grand and Spicer, 1967; Ochi, 1968; kidney—Bulger, 1969; Mizuhira and Amakawa, 1966; Nolte, 1966; intestine—Yamada, 1967; choroidal epithelium—Torack and LaValle, 1970; cornea—Kaye, Cole and Donn, 1965; muscle—Shiina et al., 1970; Zadunaisky, 1966; gall bladder—Kaye, et al. 1966, and so on). We therefore used a modification of this method to examine the transport of sodium ions in the human eccrine sweat gland, in reference to the ductal reabsorption of sodium ions and the effect of DCA.

As a control, a 3 mm punch biopsy of the skin of a volunteer, a normal 25-year-old male Japanese, was taken from the radial side of the left fore-arm, where sweating was locally induced by the iontophoresis of 0.5% pilocarpine (3 mA, 50 V, 5 min) and the tissue was treated as described just below.　On the third day after administration of DCA for two days (20 mg/day, intramuscular inj.) to the subject (Lobeck and McSherry, 1963), a punch biopsy of the same size as the control was taken from the same region just after iontophoresis under the same conditions.　Each specimen was fixed for two hours in (1) 3% glutaraldehyde containing 2% potassium pyroantimonate and (2) after rinsing with an s-collidine buffer, postfixed for one hour in 2% OsO_4 buffered with the same solution containing pyroantimonate in the same concentration (Ochi, 1968).　Following fixation the materials were routinely embedded in Epon.　Thin sections were lightly stained with uranyl acetate and lead citrate.

Parallel to the morphological investigation, the amount of sweat and the contents of sodium and potassium ions in the sweat were also determined.　The results are presented in Table 5.　The sweating rate and the Na/K ratio fell to about a third after administration of DCA.

TABLE 5　Effects of DCA upon the sweating rate and the content of sodium and potassium ions in sweat

	Sweating rate (mg/cm²-20 min)	Na (mEq/l)	K (mEq/l)	$\dfrac{Na}{K}$
H. A., man, aged 25				
Control	23.5	42.5	7.4	5.7
DCA	8.7	22.8	13.6	1.7
(20 mg × 2 days)				

Note:　1.　Radial side of upper fore-arm.
　　　　2.　Induction of sweating: Pilocarpine iontophoresis (0.5%, 3 mA, 50 V, 5 min).
　　　　3.　Sweat collection: 12.56 cm², 20 min.

In thin sections prepared for detection of sodium ions with the pyroantimonate method, the dark (mucoid) and clear cells (as defined light microscopically by Montagna, Chase and Lobitz, 1953 and confirmed electron microscopically by Munger, 1961) could be observed.　The dark cell was filled with an indefinite number of secretory vacuoles of various sizes containing mucopolysaccharide in the apical cytoplasm, and the prominent Golgi complex in the supranuclear region.　The cytoplasm is rich in free ribosomes but rough-surfaced endoplasmic reticulum is sparse.　Among the secretory vacuoles there are lipid droplets of various sizes and densities.　The clear cells possess electron opaque cytoplasm, in contrast with the light microscopic finding as stained by basic dyes.　On the lateral wall of this cell numerous intercellular interdigitations were found which often formed an intercellular canaliculus with adjacent cells.　This type of cell contained a number of glycogen granules and small vesicles of various sizes and densities. Inconspicuous Golgi apparatus was present, but neither rough-surfaced endoplasmic reticulum nor lipid droplets were seen.

Contrary to the observations of Munger (1961), the intercellular canaliculi were sometimes seen also between adjacent clear and dark cells and between the clear and myoepithelial cells, and further between dark cells.　In the resting eccrine sweat gland precipitates of sodium pyroantimonate were observed mostly along the plasma membrane of dark and clear cells composing the secretory portion, and occasionally between

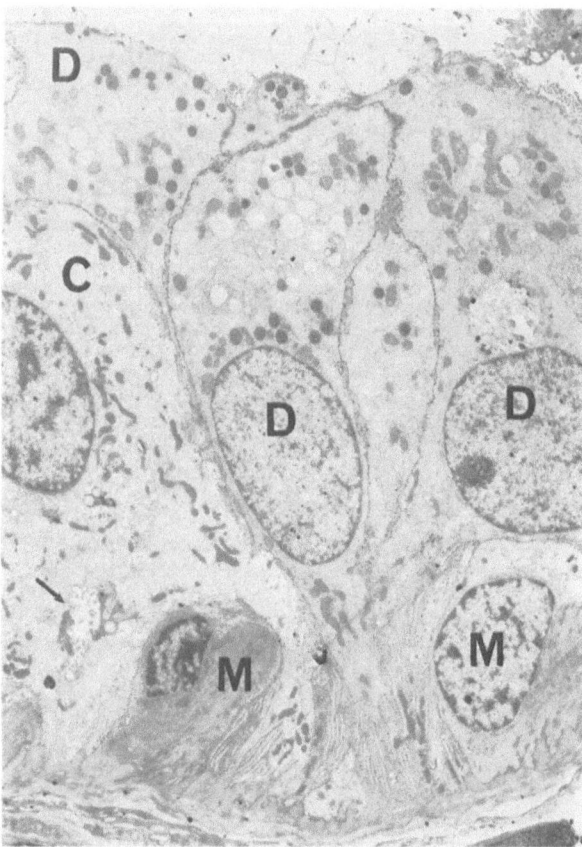

Fig. 45. Secretory portion after sweating by pilocarpine iontophoresis. Deposits of sodium pyro-antimonate are observed in large numbers on membranes of the dark (D) and clear cells (C) and on the inner membrane of myoepithelial cells (M). In the dark cell there are a small number of secretory vacuoles and lipid droplets. A prominent Golgi complex is located in the supranuclear region. In the clear cell with the cytoplasm of a decreased density, glycogen granules were largely disappeared. The lower left arrow in the figure shows an intercellular canaliculus which is formed by a clear cell and a myoepithelial cell. × 3,400.

the membranes of these cells. Cell organells were lacking in such deposits.

When sweating was induced by pilocarpine iontophoresis, apical secretory vacuoles and lipid droplets were depleted to a great extent and Golgi apparatus became more prominent, as shown in Fig. 45. As described by Munger (1961), the cytoplasmic density of clear cells decreased, and glycogen granules largely disappeared, although the degree of these changes varied from cell to cell. A striking change is the condensation of mitochondria. These mitochondria became slender and had matrices of greater opacity than normal. Deposits of sodium pyroantimonate were observed in large numbers on membranes forming basal infoldings and on the apical and complicated lateral membrane of dark and clear cells, and also on the inner membrane of myoepithelial cells (Fig. 46a). In larger magnification, these deposits were seen to be spindle or ovoid in shape on the inner surface of the plasma membrane. Occasionally the precipitations were found to be free between the membranes of adjacent cells. On the lateral membrane of dark cells the deposits seemed to align more closely than on the wall of clear

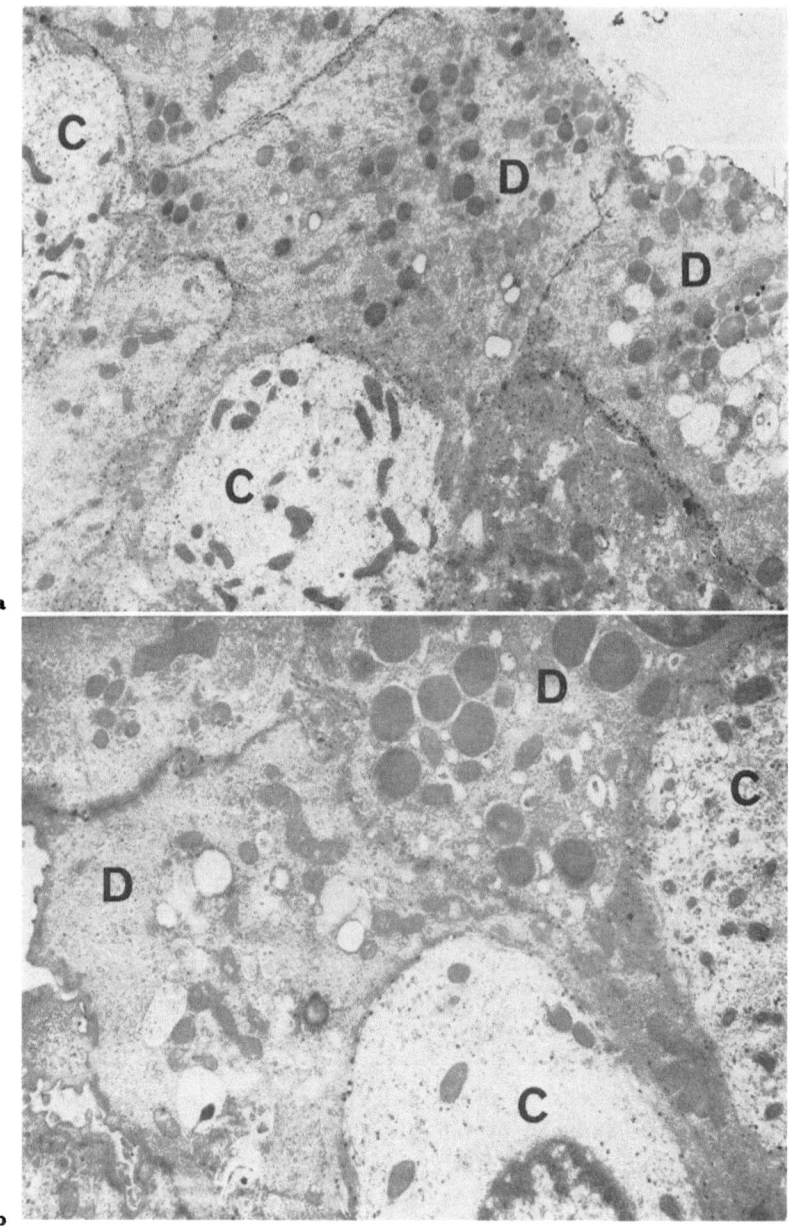

Fig. 46. DCA effects on the secretory portion.

  a, The secretory portion stimulated pilocarpine iontophoretically. The deposits of sodium pyroanti-monate are observed more closely on the lateral membrane of the dark cell (D) than on that of the clear cell (C). × 4,200.

  b, The secretory portion stimulated in the same way after DCA. The deposits appear somewhat in decreased numbers. In a clear cell (right) glycogen granules are increased in number while in a clear cell (below) those are decreased. × 87,00.

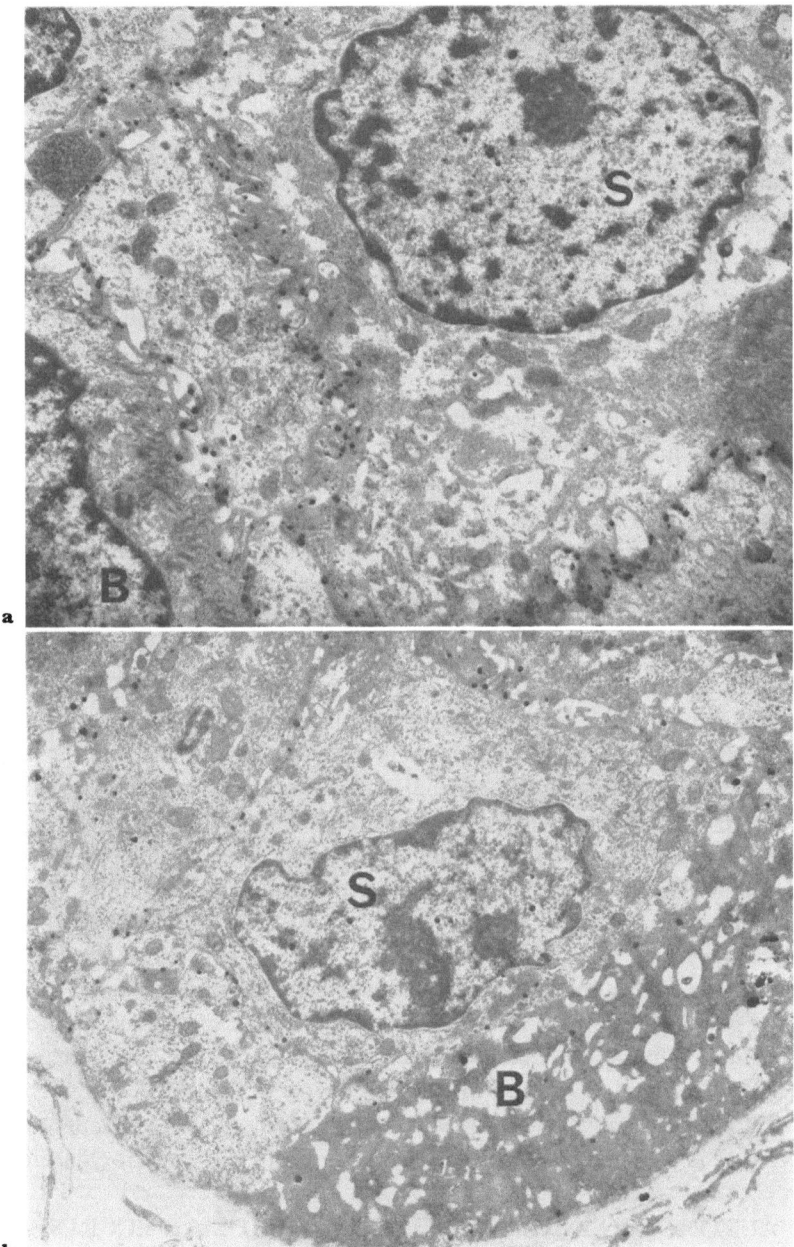

Fig. 47. DCA effects on the ductal portion.

a, The duct which belongs to the secretory portion showed in Fig. 46a. Somewhat larger precipitates are less closely found on the membranes of the superficial (S) and the basal cell (B). × 8,000.

b, The duct which belongs to the secretory portion showed in Fig. 46b. The deposits are more sparsely observed on the membranes of the superficial (S) and the basal cell (B). Note the vacuolization and the darkening of the remnant cytoplasm. × 4,000.

cells, suggesting that the dark cell plays a role in the transport of sodium ions. It had already been reported that Na$^+$ and K$^+$-activated ATPase are abundant in the basal infolding and between the cell walls of the sweat glands in the rat foot pads (Matsuzawa and Kurosumi, 1963).

In the DCA-pretreated sweat gland the dark cells of the secretory segment contained a decreased number of secretory vacuoles with irregular sizes and forms. Occasionally the secretory vacuoles became larger and fused with each other into large vacuoles occupying the regions around the nucleus. The number of glycogen granules in the clear cells are generally increased. However, in some clear cells glycogen granules largely disappeared. Most mitochondria seen in these cells had a normal conformation. The distribution of the reaction products on a unit length of the cell membrane seemed somewhat sporadic as compared with that of the DCA-untreated gland. On the lateral membranes in some regions composed of dark cells the deposits of sodium pyroantimonate were distributed almost in the same manner as the control (Fig. 46b). Also, in this case no precipitations were observed in the cytoplasma, as though a few larger precipitations were occasionally found in the nucleus (Spicer, Hardin and Greene, 1968).

In the proximal duct some larger precipitates of sodium pyroantimonate were found either in the membrane of the superficial and the basal cells, or between these cell membranes. The distribution of the precipitates was sparse in comparison with that in the secretory portion (Fig. 47a). This finding corresponds to that observed in the sweat gland of the rat foot pad (Ochi, 1968). But Grand and Spicer (1967) reported that the membranes of cells in the sweat duct lack precipitates like those seen in the dark cells of the coiled secretory portion. The presence of the precipitates on the membranes of cells in the proximal duct indicates that a membrane associated active transport of sodium exists in this area. After treatment with DCA the number of precipitates seen in the duct seemed to be somewhat smaller. The most conspicuous results seen were irregular vacuolization of the cytoplasm of basal cells and darkening of the remaining cytoplasm (Fig. 47b). These may suggest a sort of cell alteration elicited by DCA.

Considered together with the physiological observations of Robinson *et al.* (1955) and of McConahay, Robinson and Newton (1964), these findings indicate that in the human eccrine sweat gland DCA affects metabolically the secretion of sodium chloride from the secretory portion, refuting the claim that DCA accelerates the ductal reabsorption of sodium chloride in the same way as in the tubular part of the nephron. The decrease in sodium chloride secretion in the DCA treated eccrine sweat gland might be thought of as a saving of energy necessary for the reabsorption of the sodium chloride.

AUTONOMIC INNERVATION OF THE HUMAN ECCRINE SWEAT GLAND

It is widely known that the human eccrine sweat gland is innervated by postganglionic sympathetic *cholinergic* fibers from the paravertebral ganglia. However, an adrenergic mechanism of sweating is also proposed in man (Chalmers and Keele, 1951; Evans, 1957; Haimovici, 1950; Ikai *et al.* 1969; etc.). Nowadays a considerable number of observations on cholinergic and adrenergic double innervation have been reported from both physiological and pharmacological viewpoints (Sonnenschein *et al.*, 1951; cf. Kuno, 1956). The activity of cholinesterase (Hurley, Shelley and Koelle, 1953; Hellman, 1955; Beckett, Bourne and Montagna, 1956; Montagna and Ellis, 1958; Miyake, 1966) and monoamine oxidase (Hellmann, 1955; Yasuda and Montagna, 1960; Miyake, 1966) were light microscopic histochemically demonstrated in the human eccrine sweat glands. But convincing direct evidence for the innervation of this gland is still lacking, because of the difficulty in demonstrating the presence of the neurotransmitter itself. For showing the adrenergic fibers to the sweat gland, we used the light microscopic formaldehyde-induced fluorescence method for catecholamines of Falck and Hillarp, and the potassium permanganate method for the electron microscopic detection of granular vesicles in the sympathetic nerves (Ochi, 1969), in addition to the routine fixation with glutaraldehyde and OsO_4. The specimens were taken from both the radial side of upper fore-arm and the hypothenar on the same side, in order to compare the innervation of the sweat glands in these regions in which sweating is induced thermally and psychically, respectively.

Fluorescence microscopy: No distinct adrenaline-specific fluorescent nerve fibers or terminals were detected around either the secretory or the ductal portions of the sweat gland from the fore-arm or from the hypothenar, contrary to expectation (especially in

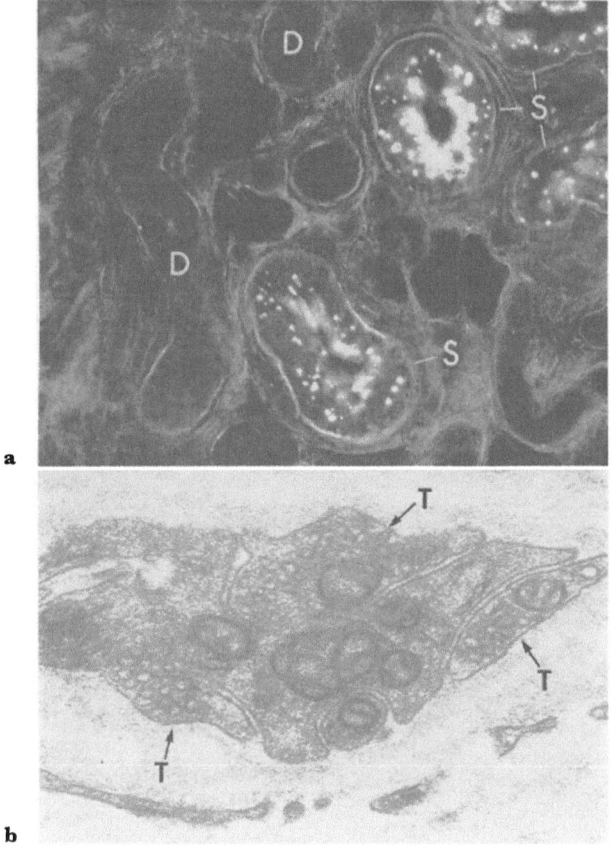

Fig. 48. Human hypothenar eccrine sweat gland.

a, Fluorescence microscopic finding. No distinct noradrenaline-specific fluorescent nerve terminals are found. Surrounding the sweat gland, elastic fibers with faint unspecific green fluorescence are frequently observed. D: Duct, S: Secretory portion. × 380.

b, Electron microscopic finding ($KMnO_4$-fixation). Nerve terminals (T) near the sweat gland which are partly covered with the cytoplasm of a Schwann cell contain no small granular vesicles. × 38,000.

the case of psychically-induced hypothenar sweating). In the secretory portion the apical region of cells were filled with a number of yellow, intensely fluorescent droplets which may correspond to lipid droplets on the fine structural level (Fig. 48a).

Electron microscopy: On the sections of glutaraldehyde-OsO$_4$ fixed materials, nerve terminals or preterminals with a large number of clear synaptic vesicles (500 Å diameter) and occasionally a few large granular vesicles (about 1200 Å diameter) were found surrounding the gland, mostly near to a myoepithelial cell of the secretory portion, incompletely covered by the cytoplasma of a Schwann cell. The myoepithelial cell and the terminals were separated by a distance over ca. 1 μ, and a bundle of collagen fibers and processes of a fibrocyte were interposed more frequently in the case of the fore-arm sweat gland than in the hypothenar one. These nerve terminals formed no synaptic direct

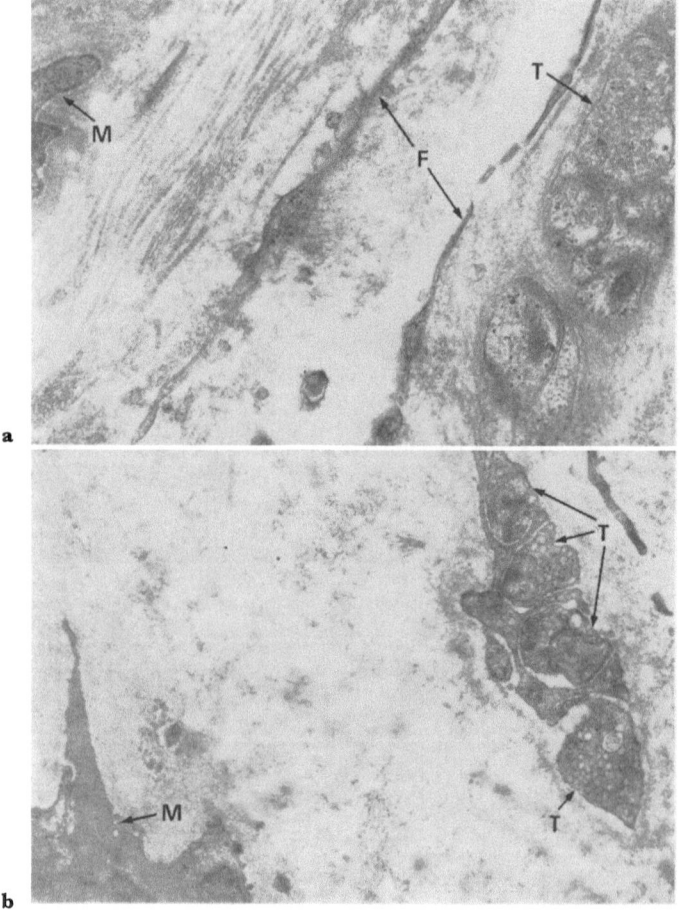

Fig. 49. Difference of the innervation between the fore-arm and the hypothenar eccrine sweat gland (glutaraldehyde-OsO$_4$ fixation).

a, Fore-arm eccrine sweat gland. The myoepithelial cell (M) and the nerve terminal (T) are frequently separated by thin processes of fibrocytes (F). A large granular vesicle is found among a number of agranular (synaptic) vesicles within the terminal. × 17,000.

b, Hypothenar eccrine sweat gland. Note no interposition of processes of the fibrocyte. Besides agranular vesicles a few number of large granular vesicles are also found in the nerve terminals (T). M: Myoepithelial cell. × 22,000.

contacts with the myoepithelial cell or the secretory cells (Fig. 49a, b).   Nerve terminals seemed to appear more frequently in the hypothenar than in the fore-arm sweat gland. Less frequently, near the proximal duct, there were a few small nerve terminals partly covered by a Schwann cell.   Using the $KMnO_4$ fixation, it was also confirmed that the nerve terminals or preterminals possess no small granular vesicles which could be considered noradrenaline-storing structures on the electron microscopic level (Fig. 48b).

These morphological findings indicate that the hypothenar (psychically stimulated) sweat glands are more intimately innervated by autonomic nerves than those of the fore-arm (thermally stimulated) and that the autonomic nerves to the sweat gland were probably cholinergic, not adrenergic.   The response of the human eccrine sweat glands to adrenaline may, therefore, be caused humorally, not by adrenergic fibers.

SUMMARY

1)   It is found electron microscopically that there is a short portion between the secretory and the coiled ductal cells composed of a layer of tall columnar cells with an occasional basal and myoepithelial cell.   This portion is considered to correspond to the transitional portion as found by light microscopy (Ito and Enjo, 1949).   A similar area with such special structures detected electron microscopically by Shibasaki and Ito (1967) represents only a contracted small blood vessel in the vicinity of the human eccrine sweat glands.

2)   By using the potassium pyroantimonate method for electron microscopic detection of sodium ions, the transport of sodium ions in the eccrine sweat gland was observed. In the secretory portion, numbers of the precipitates of the resulting sodium pyroantimonate were detected, aligned mainly along the lateral plasma membranes of the dark and clear cells, especially the former.   A few deposits of a somewhat larger size appeared among the ductal cells.   Treatment with DCA caused a considerable decrease in the number of deposits on the lateral wall of the cells of the secretory portion, while it caused a minimal decrease in the number of deposits among the ductal cells.   These facts suggest that DCA alters the sodium secreting activity of the epithelial cells in the secretory portion, rather than accelerating the ductal reabsorption of sodium.

3)   By means of the formaldehyde-induced fluorescence method for light microscopical demonstration of catecholamines and the potassium permanganate fixation for electron microscopic detection of noradrenaline containing granular vesicles in the sympathetic nerve endings, it was established that autonomic nerves to the eccrine sweat gland are cholinergic and mostly terminate near the myoepithelial cell.   On the level of fine structure there are no synaptic direct terminals at the secretory or myoepithelial cells. No pronounced difference in innervation between the fore-arm and the hypothenar eccrine sweat glands were found, except in that the myoepithelial cell and the nerve endings were often separated by slender processes of the fibrocyte in the former gland, though this is not the case in the latter gland.

ACKNOWLEDGEMENTS

The authors would like to thank Dr. T. Morimoto, Dept. of Physiology, for the use of his physiological data, seen in the present paper.   They also thank Mr. T. Matsuura, B. Sci. for his assistance in a part of this work, and Miss S. Sugino for typing the manuscript.

REFERENCES

1. BECKETT, E.B., G.H. BOURNE, and W. MONTAGNA (1956): *J. Physiol (Lond.)*, **134**: 202.
2. BULGER, R.E. (1969): *J. Cell Biol.* **40**: 79.
3. CAGE, G.W., and R.L. DOBSON (1965): *J. clin. Invest.* **44**: 1270.
4. CHALMERS, T.M., and C.A. KEELE (1951): *J. Physiol. (Lond.)* **114**: 510.
5. CONN, J.W., L.H. LOUIS, M.W. JOHNSTON, and B.J. JOHNSON (1948): *J. clin. Invest.* **27**: 529.
6. EVANS, C.L. (1957): *Brit. Med. Bull.* **13**: 197.
7. GRAND, R.J., and S.S. SPICER (1967): *Mod. Probl. Pediat.* **10**: 100.
8. HAIMOVICI, H. (1950): *J. Appl. Physiol.* **2**: 512.
9. HELLMANN, K. (1955): *J. Physiol. (Lond.)* **129**: 454.
10. HIBBS, R.G. (1958): *Amer. J. Anat.* **103**: 201.
11. HIBBS, R.G., G.E. BURCH, and J.H. PHILLIPS (1958): *Amer. Heart J.* **56**: 662.
12. HURLEY, H.J., W.B. SHELLEY, and G.B. KOELLE (1953): *J. invest. Dermatol.* **21**: 139.
13. IKAI, K., K. SATO, K. SUGIYAMA, Y. OTSUKA, and H. NITTA (1969): *Nagoya Med. J.* **15**: 47.
14. ITO, T., and K. ENJO (1949): *Seitai no Kagaku (Tokyo)* **1**: 69 (in Japanese).
15. KAYE, G.I., J.D. COLE, and A. DONN (1965): *Science* **150**: 1167.
16. KAYE, G.I., H.O. WHEELER, R.T. WHITLOCK, and N. LANE (1966): *J. Cell Biol.* **30**: 237.
17. KOMNICK, H. u. U. KOMNICK (1963): *Z. Zellforsch.* **60**: 163.
18. KUNO, Y. (1956): Human Perspiration. Charles C. Thomas Publ., Springfield, Illinois.
19. LENNEP, E.W. v. (1968): *J. Ultrastruct. Res.* **25**: 94.
20. LLOYD, D.P. (1962): In: Eccrine Sweat Glands and Eccrine Sweating. Advances in Biology of Skin. Vol. 3. p. 127. W. Montagna, R.A. Ellis and A.F. Silver (eds.). Pergamon Press, New York.
21. LOBECK, C.C., and N.R. MCSHERRY (1963): *J. Pediat.* **62**: 393.
22. LOEWENTHAL, L.J.A. (1960): *J. invest. Dermatol.* **34**: 233.
23. LOEWENTHAL, L.J.A. (1961): *J. invest. Dermatol.* **36**: 171.
24. MATSUZAWA, T., and K. KUROSUMI (1963). *J. Electronmicr.* **12**: 175.
25. MCCONAHAY, T.P., S. ROBINSON, and J.L. NEWTON (1964): *J. Appl. Physiol.* **19**: 575.
26. MIYAKE, K. (1966): *Okajimas Fol. anat. jap.* **42**: 219.
27. MIZUHIRA, V., and T. AMAKAWA (1966): *J. Histochem. Cytochem.* **14**: 770.
28. MONTAGNA, W. (1962): The Structure and Function of Skin. 2nd Ed., Academic Press, New York and London.
29. MONTAGNA, W., H.B. CHASE, and W.C. LOBITZ, JR. (1953): *J. invest. Dermatol.* **20**: 415.
30. MONTAGNA, W., and R.A. ELLIS (1958): *Ann. histochem.* **3**: 1.
31. MUNGER, B.L. (1961): *J. biophys. biochem. Cytol.* **11**: 385.
32. NOLTE, A. (1966): *Z. Zellforsch.* **72**: 562.
33. OCHI, J. (1968): *Histochemie* **14**: 300.
34. OCHI, J. (1969): *Acta histochem. cytochem.* **2**: 13.
35. ROBINSON, S., J.R. NICHOLAS, J.H. SMITH, W.J. DALY, and M. PEARCHY (1955): *J. Appl. Physiol.* **8**: 159.
36. SCHULZ, K., K.J. ULLRICH, E. FRÖMTER, H. HOLZGREVE, A. FRICK, u. U. HEGEL (1965): *Pflügers Archiv ges. Physiol.* **284**: 360.
37. SCHWARTZ, I.L., and J.H. THAYSEN (1956): *J. clin. Invest.* **35**: 114.
38. SHIBASAKI, S., and T. ITO (1967): *Arch. histol. jap.* **28**: 285.
39. SHIINA, S., V. MIZUHIRA, T. AMAKAWA, and Y. FUTAESAKU (1970): *J. Histochem. Cytochem.* **18**: 644.
40. SONNENSCHEIN, R.R., H. KOBRIN, H.D. JANOWITZ, and M.I. GROSSMAN (1951): *J. Appl. Physiol.* **3**: 573.
41. SPICER, S.S., J.H. HARDIN, and W.B. GREENE (1968): *J. Cell Biol.* **39**: 216.
42. TORACK, R.M., and M. LaVALLE (1970): *J. Histochem. Cytochem.* **18**: 635.
43. YAMADA, E. (1967): *Arch. histol. jap.* **28**: 419.
44. YASUDA, K., and W. MONTAGNA (1960): *J. Histochem. Cytochem.* **8**: 356.
45. ZADUNAISKY, J.A. (1966): *J. Cell Biol.* **31**: C 11.

CHAPTER 6

LOCAL DETERMINANTS OF SWEAT GLAND ACTIVITY

Tokuo OGAWA

Department of Physiology, Niigata University School of Medicine, Niigata, Japan

The human eccrine sweat glands are innervated by cholinergic sympathetic nerves and their activity is under the nervous control of the central thermoregulatory mechanism, with a possible minor role played by adrenergic mechanisms [37, 41]. However, the magnitude of responses of the sweat glands to centrally-derived sudomotor impulses may not be consistent, i.e., conditions at the sweat gland, or conditions in the micro-environment of the glands exert considerable influence upon their activity and responsiveness. Wada and his colleague [80–83] performed extensive studies on mechanisms of local sweating and factors influencing on them. In this article, factors affecting local sweating will be discussed with special reference to generalized sweating.

Local factors discussed in the present article include the following conditions which have been recognized to affect locally the activity of sweat glands: 1) Local temperature; 2) local blood flow; 3) hydration of the epidermis and possibly the dermis; and 4) local training. Furthermore, the possibility of adaptive responses in the gland to prolonged or repeated heat exposures is to be considered.

LOCAL TEMPERATURE

It has been widely recognized that skin temperature affects the rate of generalized sweating through activation of peripheral thermoreceptors and the central thermoregulatory mechanism [3, 16, 74, 85]. The present article, however, is concerned with only the local influence of skin temperature on the secretory activity of the sweat glands.

Local heating of a skin area may cause sweat production by the regional sweat glands or increase locally the rate of sweating.

In the absence of generalized sweating, local heating to a skin temperature above 38 °C may sometimes cause activation of the regional sweat glands, whereas heating to 42 °C or above always does [5, 38, 41, 49, 63]. Sweating thus elicited is strictly confined to the heated area and is not abolished after denervation, atropinization, or procainization, and this effect of local heating is attributed to a direct glandular activation, possibly by facilitation of the metabolic process of the secretory cells. A weakened sweat response by atropinization or procainization at a relatively high ambient temperature [38, 63] and a decrease in skin temperature threshold for sweat production with an elevation of ambient temperature [5] suggest participation of subthreshold sudomotor impulses, which will be discussed later. Such intense heating, however, generally brings the skin temperature to an apparently unphysiological range and therefore is not considered to be of physiological significance.

A local increase or decrease in the rate of sweating has been noted during local heating or cooling, respectively, within a physiological range of skin temperature in the presence of generalized sweating [16, 41, 78] (Fig. 50). Quick or delayed appearance of sweating

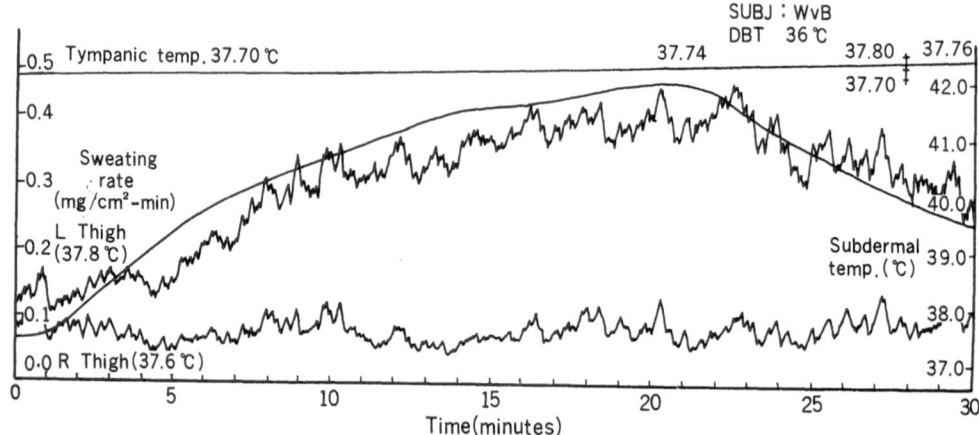

Fig. 50. Effect of local heating on the rate of spontaneous sweating. Sweat rate on a left thigh area varies with changes in the local subdermal temperature (From Bullard *et al.* [16]).

at the heated or cooled area, respectively, has also been noted following a rise in room temperature or the start of physical exercise [78]. Lloyd [46] observed on the footpad of the cat that the latency for sweat emergence following direct stimulation of the regional nerve was shortened with increase in local temperature, and noted that it took place in the face of an increased rate of ductal reabsorption with the increased temperature. If less than 1/1500 of the total skin surface or an area of 10 cm² is heated by 10 °C, the mean weighted skin temperature will increase by less than 1/150 °C, or 0.007 °C. Thus, it may be assumed that the heating does not affect the central thermoregulatory mechanism. No responses occur at the contralateral site, nor at the adjacent area, and the effect is considered to be strictly local.

The rate of regional sweating is not a linear function of the local skin temperature, but the effect of the local temperature increases as the temperature rises [16, 51] (Fig. 51). A similar pattern derived from the effect of local temperature has been observed in sweating from the footpad of the squirrel monkey, which has been shown to exhibit thermal sweating [52].

Several possible mechanisms may be thought to be responsible for the local effect of changes in skin temperature on sweat gland activity: 1) The physical environment may be altered so that the gradients driving evaporation may be changed; 2) there may be a temperature coefficient or Q_{10} effect of the secretory process; 3) changes in sweat rate may be secondary to vascular changes; 4) the release of the transmitter substance, acetylcholine, at the neuroglandular junction may be temperature-dependent; 5) sensitivity of the receptor mechanism of the secretory cells to the transmitter substance may be affected by skin temperature; and 6) an axon reflex may be evoked by local heating.

Huheey and Adams [36] assert, on the basis of their observations on evaporative water loss from the cat footpad, that the increase in evaporative rate with elevation of skin

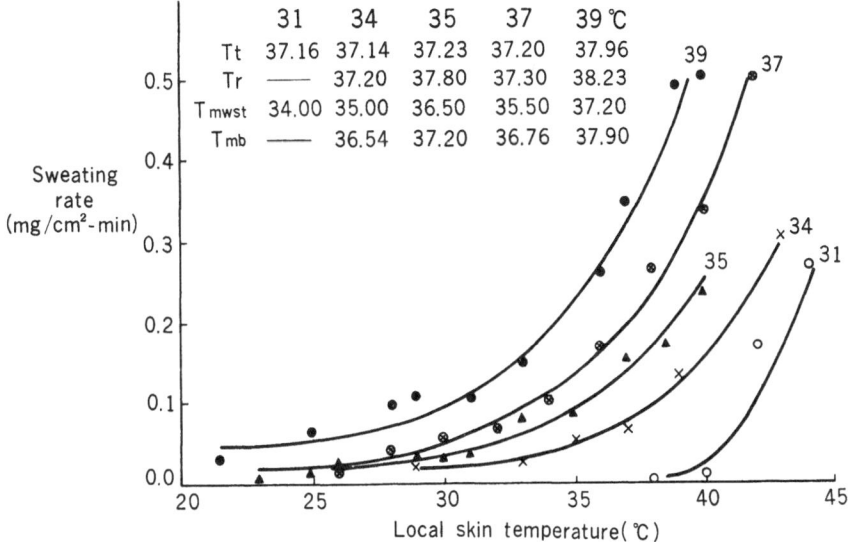

Fig. 51. Regional sweat rate versus local skin temperature. Five experiments at different ambient temperatures (shown at the top of each curve) on two subjects. T_t = tympanic temperature, T_r = rectal temperature, T_{mwst} = mean weighted skin temperature, T_{mb} = calculated body temperature (From Bullard et al. [16]).

temperature in maximal sweating condition (made by direct neural stimulation) is caused by the increase in water vapor pressure gradient between skin surface and air. Their study does not exclude the concept that the increased water vapor pressure in the heated skin area is due to an increased activity of the sweat glands, and therefore the rate-limiting factor determining maximal sweating has been left unsolved. The ratio of the increase in evaporation rate to the elevation of skin temperature has been found much higher in studies on human sweating [16, 51] than in their study on the footpad sweating. Increased insensible perspiration with elevated skin temperature has also been attributed largely to changes in physical environment such as the water vapor pressure gradient and hydraulic conductance [12, 36], while variations in sweat gland activity have also been thought to participate in the increase [31, 32, 62]. At any rate, such changes in evaporative water loss with temperature changes are extremely small compared with those in the rate of local sweating. In various modern methods of sweat rate recording, very dry air is circulated at a fairly high flow rate through a circumscribed test skin area and water excreted onto the skin surface is evaporated immediately. In this situation, therefore, the activity of the sweat glands is the limiting factor of the evaporation rate.

The cellular metabolism is considered to be temperature-dependent and the Q_{10} values are thought to be around two to three. On the other hand, an increase in sweat rate with elevation of skin temperature possesses higher Q_{10} values, especially at a relatively high level of skin temperature. Therefore the increase in cellular metabolism cannot fully account for an increase in the regional rate of sweating with elevation of skin temperature.

The effect of changes in local blood circulation on sweat secretion generally appears very slowly [41], whereas the effect of changes in local temperature is much more rapid. Furthermore, full cutaneous vasodilatation is expected at an ambient temperature above

32–33 °C, and changes in the local temperature are even more effective on sweat rate [16] (Fig. 51). These observations exclude the possibility that facilitation of sweating by local heating may be secondary to local vascular changes.

MacIntyre *et al.* [48] noted that the increased sweating by local heating was closely associated with the sudomotor neural activity and postulated that the local elevation of temperature increased the amount of transmitter substance released for each neural impulse arriving at the neuroglandular junction. A temperature dependence of acetylcholine release and of its resynthesis has been demonstrated in sympathetic ganglia, atria and brain tissue [10, 17, 50, 73], and their hypothesis is to postulate that these phenomena are applicable to the neuroglandular junction of the sweat gland.

Recently, Ogawa [55] observed that the threshold concentration of various cholinergic sudorific agents for inducing local sweating by intradermal injection was reduced at the heated skin area. This effect of local heating was apparent even at a very low room temperature, below 18 °C, where subthreshold sudomotor neural impulses were absent or negligible [56, 58]; the effect also persisted after regional nerve block or procainization. These observations indicate that the sensitivity of the sweat glands to cholinergic stimuli, inclusive of transmitter substance released at the neuroglandular junction, increases with the elevation of local temperature. On the other hand, the threshold concentration of adrenaline for local sweating was found not to be affected by local heating [55]. Similarly, local heating increased distinctly the rate of local sweating induced by intradermal administration of a cholinergic agent, but not significantly that of an adrenergic agent (not more than the increase in evaporative rate attributable to changes in physical environment by heating) [57]. These observations suggest that the effect of local heating on glandular activity is not the result of a simple elevation of cellular metabolic rate, and further that the secretory cells of sweat glands possess a receptor mechanism specific for cholinergic and adrenergic stimuli, respectively, and that cutaneous heating is likely to increase the sensitivity of specific receptor sites of glandular cells.

In the case of generalized sweating, an increase in the sweat rate at the heated skin area is explained by an increase in the release of transmitter substance at the neuroglandular junction and/or by an increase in sensitivity of the glandular cells to transmitter substance. The localized increase in the rate of spontaneous sweating caused by local heating is comparable to the increase in drug-induced sweating caused by local heating to the same degree under regional nerve block [57], indicating the predominant effect of changes in glandular sensitivity to the transmitter substance. On the other hand, Bullard [14] noted that local sweating induced by electrical stimulation of the regional nerve was more effectively facilitated by local heating than drug-induced sweating, and attributes this to the increased release of transmitter substance at the neuroglandular junction in addition to the increased sensitivity of the glandular cells to transmitter substance at the heated skin area. With either explanation, enhanced receptor sensitivity or transmitter release, the quantitative effect of local temperature alterations on sweating activity would be the same.

It has been demonstrated by many authors [41, 68, 80] that axon reflex sweating can be produced by faradic stimulation to the skin and by intradermal injection of agents with nicotinic action and various sodium salts, and its mechanism has been thoroughly investigated by Wada and his colleague [80—82]. Possible participation of an axon reflex in the increased sweat rate accompanying local heating has been suggested [9]. However, this possibility has been disputed on the basis of the observations that the increase in sweat rate is sharply limited to the heated area [16], and that the threshold concentration of a nicotinic agent required to induce axon reflex sweating is not affected by local heating [55].

The significance of localized response of the sweat glands to skin temperature in the overall regulation of human sweating has not been fully evaluated. Obviously, this local modulation of sweat gland activity affects the central thermoregulatory process through interaction with the neural feed back influence on skin temperature [16, 51]. Practically, the subject rarely show a wide range of skin temperatures at various regions in a steady laboratory thermal condition. However, with transient changes of ambient temperature, the effect of skin temperature can be evidenced. Furthermore, in daily life considerable regional differences in skin temperature may be expected on a variety of occasions, such as variously clothed conditions, radiant heating (sun-bath, bonfire, etc.), warm bath, physical exercise in a cold weather, etc.

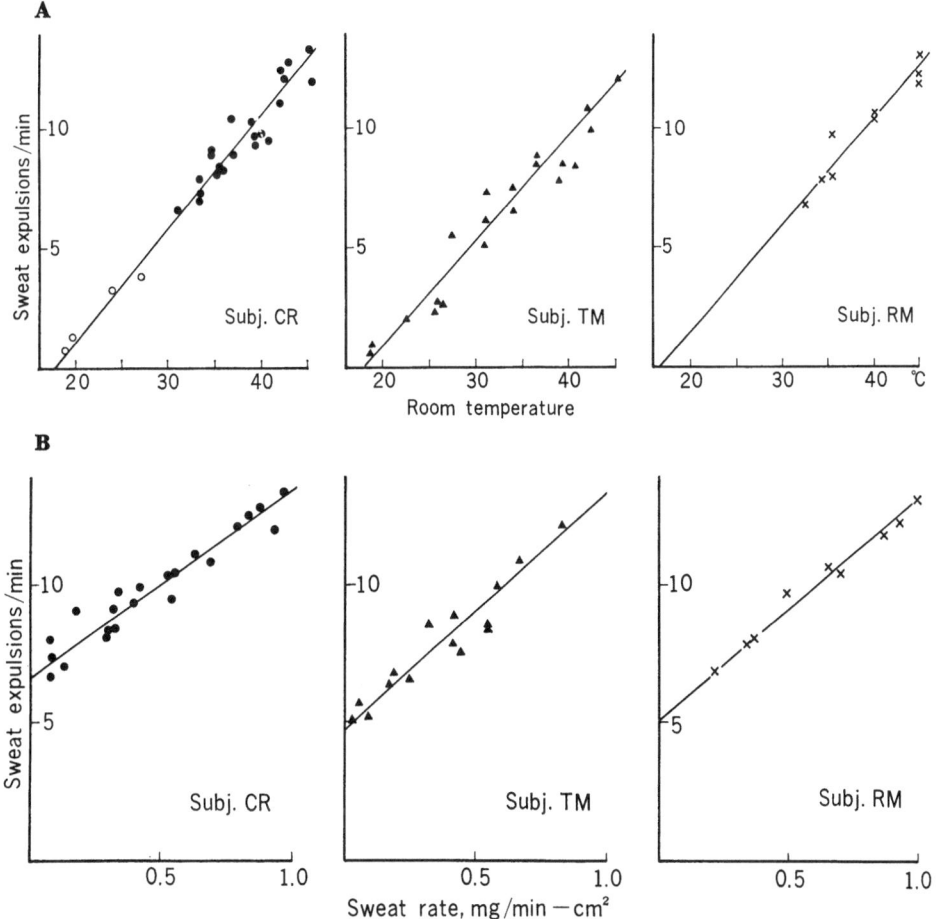

Fig. 52. Plots of frequency of pulsatile sweat expulsions synchronous at different sites, versus room temperature (A), and versus forearm sweat rate (B). ○, ▲ in A = drug-induced sweating, other symbols = spontaneous sweating.

In conventional theories about the human temperature control system, skin temperature is considered to act as a multiplier [74, 85]. The effect of local skin temperature appears also to be multiplicative [51]. The earlier initiation of sweating at the heated area with exercise or elevation of room temperature must then be explained by assuming that sudomotor neural impulses are arriving at the neuroglandular junction in the absence of generalized sweating. Indirect evidence for such subthreshold impulses and their dependence upon environmental temperature has been presented by several investigators [5, 37, 40, 49, 62, 76, 83]. Recently Ogawa [56] and Ogawa and Bullard [58] reported the direct evidence: Small expulsions of sweat were observed in the continuous recording of local sweating produced by an intradermal administration of a sudorific agent in the absence of generalized sweating and they occurred simultaneously at different test areas as sweat expulsions in generalized sweating. Frequency of sweat expulsions is linearly related to ambient temperature regardless of the presence or absence of generalized sweating [59] (Fig. 52A).

LOCAL BLOOD FLOW

It has been widely recognized that vasomotor and sudomotor impulses are largely independent of each other. While the activation of both sympathetic pathways can be simultaneously seen in mental sweating (cold sweating) and in shock, thermal sweating is not associated with vasoconstriction [68]. Instead, the activation of the sweat glands is usually accompanied by vasodilatation.

Evidence that the vasodilatation is not simply due to the release of vasoconstrictor tone, but involves an active vasodilator mechanism has been presented by Fox and Hilton [29]: the bradykinin-forming enzyme is released from the activated sweat glands and bradykinin is formed in the immediate vicinity of the gland and affects the network of blood vessels surrounding the gland and also nearby vessels. Obviously the vasodilatation favors the production of copious sweat, but the significance of its role has not been assessed. Sweating accompanied by vasoconstriction such as cold sweating, sweating in shock and local sweating induced by intradermal administration of adrenaline or noradrenaline, is either short-lasting or relatively low in rate, suggesting that ample water reservoir is prerequisite at least to copious sweat secretion.

Another important aspect of blood flow in sweat gland activity is oxygen supply. Arterial occlusion has been shown to reduce sweating rather gradually [41, 64, 79]. The diminution of sweating develops only after five to 15 min. of occlusion and sweating eventually ceases, but with profuse sweating this process appears to be accelerated [20, 41]. The sweat glands persist in responding to direct radiant heat [64] and to locally administered pilocarpine during occlusion [48]. Consequently, the sweat-inhibitory effect of arterial occlusion has been attributed to anoxia of sudomotor nerve endings, causing the reduction in the amount of transmitter substance released at the neuroglandular junction for each neural impulse.

On the other hand, occlusion also reduces response of the secretory cells to a sudorific agent. Sweat rate as well as the number of active glands in drug-induced local sweating in a cool environment or under regional nerve block is reduced during occlusion in a pattern similar to natural sweating in a warm environment and to reflex sweating induced by indirect heating [4, 20] (Fig. 53). Response to acetylcholine injected during occlusion is greatly reduced, compared with the response in the unoccluded area [20],

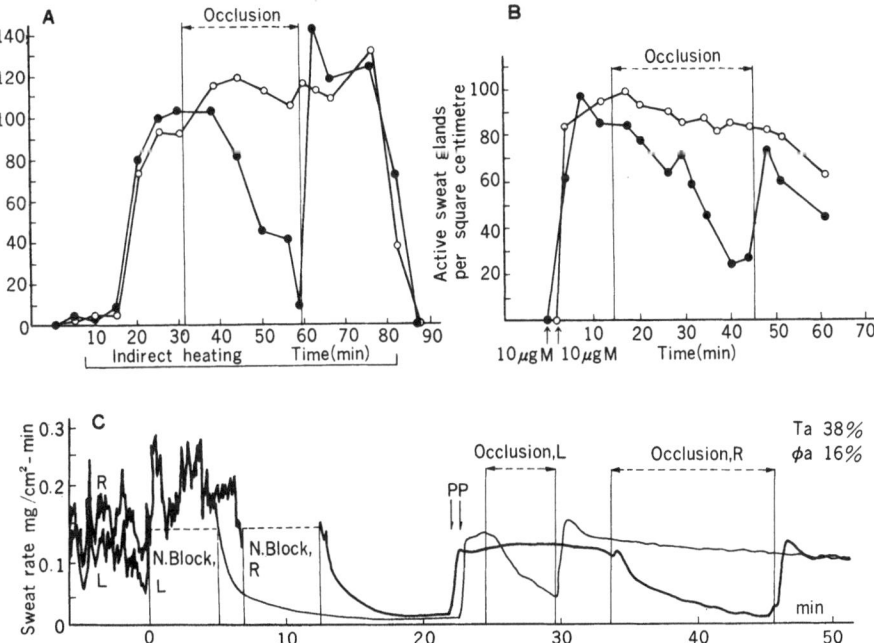

Fig. 53. Effect of arterial occlusion on: (A) the number of sweat glands activated reflexly by indirect heating, (B) that by an intradermale injection of metacholine (from Collins *et al.* [20]), and (C) the rate of sweating induced by an intradermal injection of pilocarpine (P, 1 μg in 0.1 ml) under nerve block. In A and B, ●—● = occluded arm, ○—○ = unoccluded arm; in C, R and L denote right and left forearm areas, respectively; note that spontaneous sweating on the volar aspect of forearms has been checked by injections of 2% xylocaine around the radial and ulnar antebrachial cutaneous nerves.

but the magnitude of sweating response to the drug injection at different times in the course of occlusion hardly varies [4]. There may be two mechanisms involved in ischemic suppression: one is 'fatigue' at the neuroglandular junction and the other is changes in the secretory mechanism itself.

Changes in the composition of sweat also occur during occlusion; especially consistent are increases in lactate and urea concentrations [79]. This fact may suggest reduced activity of the ischemic secretory cells.

On the other hand, it has been suggested that some chemical substance may be produced by ischemic tissues and, upon release of occlusion, act centrally to depress sweating [41, 64]. This hypothesis is based on the observation that, upon release of the occlusion, sweating is depressed for some time not only at the site previously occluded but also at the control site. However, this can be alternatively explained by a sudden heat loss from the core by rewarming of cooled blood and tissues in the occluded region, since a definite drop of tympanic temperature is noted upon release of occlusion, although a drop can still be observed with a very warm area of occlusion [2]. Contrarily, gradual increases in sweat rate at an unoccluded site as well as increases in tympanic temperature are seen during occlusion of a limb and are attributed to the decreased heat loss from the core [3].

In short, anoxia of sudomotor nerve endings and/or of the secretory cells appears to play a primary role in the depression of sweating at the site deprived of blood supply, while production of unknown humoral substance and/or local cooling may play an additional role.

HYDRATION STATUS OF THE SKIN

Enough evidence has been presented to establish that reabsorption of water takes place through the sweat duct as sweat produced by the secretory cells travels towards the skin surface [23, 41, 45, 47, 53, 71, 77]. Reabsorbed water diffuses into the epidermis and the dermis, and it is conceivable that the hydration status of the skin may affect the rate of water reabsorption and consequently the appearance of sweat on the skin surface. If a skin area is artificially hydrated by keeping it wet for a length of time and then the rate of evaporation from the area is recorded at a room temperature slightly below the critical level for spontaneous sweating, small sweat expulsions can be observed on the otherwise smooth exponential curve [58] (Fig. 54).

The sweat duct must be filled with sweat produced by the secretory cells before sweat appears on the skin surface. This filling will be counteracted by reabsorption, and if the rate of reabsorption exceeds the filling rate, sweat will not be excreted out of the sweat pore. As shown in Fig. 52B, spontaneous sweating appears on the forearm with a frequency of five sweat expulsions per min. or more [59]. With expulsive sweat gland activity below this frequency, the rate of sweat production is considered to be paralleled

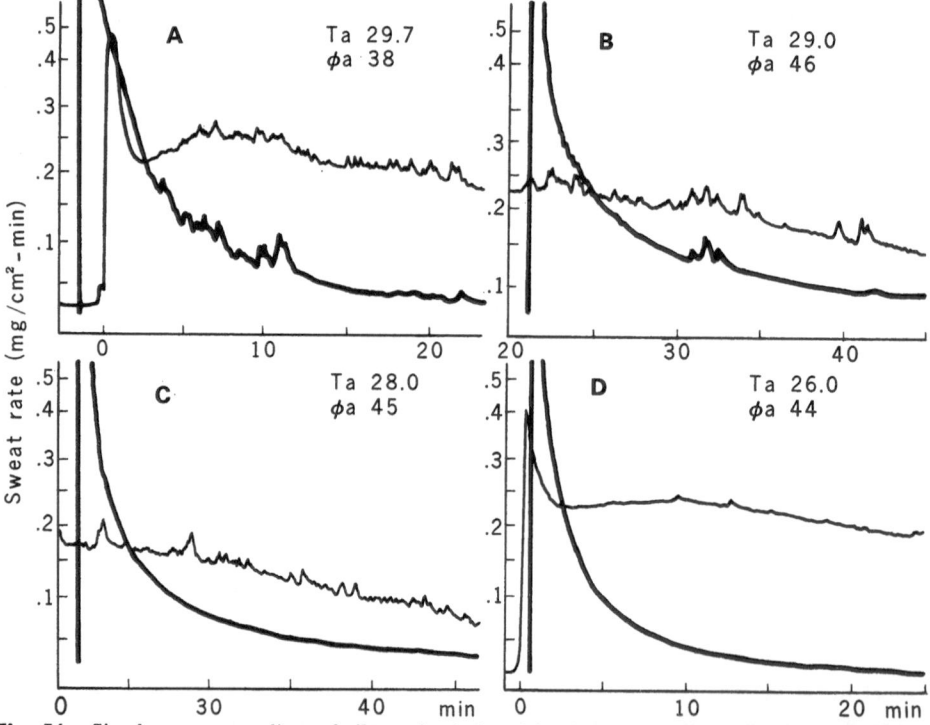

Fig. 54. Simultaneous recordings of pilocarpine-induced local sweating (thin line) and evaporation rate from a moistened, otherwise untreated skin area (thick line) at four different room temperatures (T_a) in a single subject. ϕa = relative humidity. Two curves are taken from skin areas of different forearms. Small fluctuations of the exponential evaporation curve indicate sweat expulsions which appear synchronously with those of the pilocarpine sweating curve (From Ogawa and Bullard [58]).

by reabsorption rate. This relation has been well demonstrated by Lloyd [45] on sweating from the hind footpad of the cat induced by electrical stimulation of the centrally severed plantar nerve. In Fig. 55, the latency for sweat emergence is plotted against the frequency of stimulation which reflects the rate of sweat formation. The lower the frequency, the longer is the latency and also the lower the sweat rate, and at very low frequencies of stimulation, sweat never appears, indicating that the rate of sweat formation is exceeded by the capacity of reabsorption.

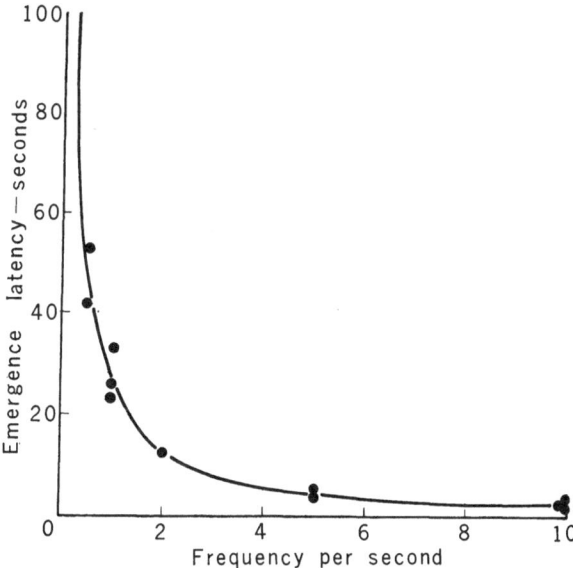

Fig. 55. Latency for sweat emergence at the footpad surface of the cat as a function of frequency of plantar nerve stimulation, the sweat ducts having been filled by an precedent maximal stimulation (From Lloyd [45]).

Adams [1], who conducted the same type of experiments as Lloyd's but used a method of continuously recording the evaporation rate, made similar observations and further stated that the hydration of the stratum corneum is affected by low-level sweat gland activity. He proposed a microcirculation of water diffusing from the sweat ducts through the upper epidermis back to the capillaries. Since hydration of the epidermis affects the rate of insensible perspiration, a low level of sweat gland activity is considered to contribute to insensible perspiration as has been suggested by many investigators [31, 32, 62, 68, 76].

On the other hand, Lloyd [45] demonstrated on the cat footpad that the latency of sweat emergence following a maximally effective neural stimulation was a linear function of the duration of the rest period between stimulations up to 60 min. at which point the increase in latency ceased. This indicates that reabsorption of the fluid in the sweat duct takes place at a constant rate, and Lloyd suggests that water reabsorption may likely occur near the base of gland, presumably at the initial thin segment of the duct near its junction with the secretory portion, rather than along the length of duct; the levelling off of the latent period may indicate that the fluid in the duct has been reabsorbed completely by that time. Thompson [77] has also suggested that the reabsorptive mechanisms may reside mainly in a deep dermal portion of the sweat duct. This assumption is based on a histochemical demonstration of the survival of apparently functional sweat glands in autogenous skin grafts devoid of the epidermis and of a papillar portion of the dermis implanted subcutaneously.

Bullard [15] measured following percutaneous electrical stimulation of the lateral antebrachial cutaneous nerve in man the latency for sweat emergence from a forearm area and the latency for reaching a steady level of the sweat rate in relation to the stimulation interval. The results were somewhat different from those reported by Lloyd on the cat footpad [45]: the latency for sweat emergence was hardly altered for 20 min. or more of the stimulation interval, then showed a sigmoidal pattern of increase, while the latency for reaching a steady state began to increase immediately after the preceding stimulation stopped. These observations may reveal that water is continuously removed from the epidermis, but that it takes some time before an effective diffusion gradient develops for water reabsorption through the duct to exceed slow sweat production by the unstimulated secretory cells, although more information is needed for accurate evaluation.

The hydration status of the skin may not be relevant in steady sweating conditions, because the epidermis at this time is considered to be practically saturated with water, whereas in transitory conditions and in states of low-level sweat gland activity, the degree of epidermal hydration may participate in determining sweat emergence, stabilization of sweat rate and the rate of insensible perspiration.

The case of overhydration or prolonged hydration of the skin, however, is quite different. It has been demonstrated by Hertig et al. [33, 34] that immersion of the body in warm water (36 °C and above) produces sweating which declines markedly after reaching a peak within one hour (Fig. 56). Such progressive decrement of sweat rate

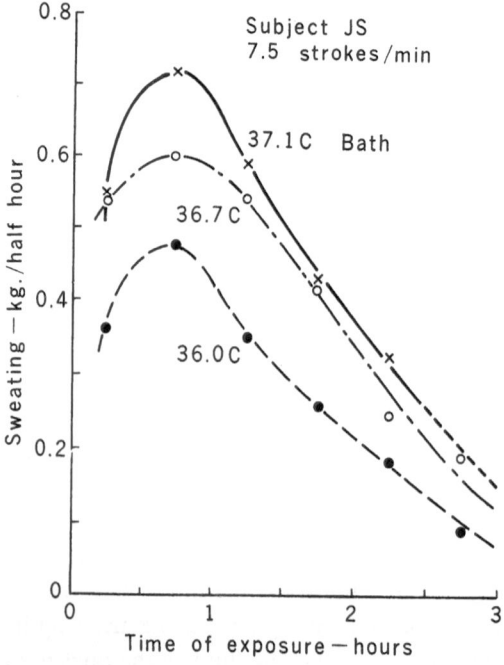

Fig. 56. Time course of sweat rate in warm water at three levels of temperature and at a constant physical activity (From Hertig et al. [34]).

has been called 'hidromeiosis.' The decline begins within 15 min. of immersion if the body has been preheated, and proceeds exponentially for at least five hours towards a zero sweat rate [7]. Presoaking in water of neutral temperature (30–32 °C) also causes a depression in sweat rate in the subsequent heat exposure or warm bath [8, 33]. Hidromeiosis can be reproduced locally by wetting or immersing a localized area [21, 65], and the decline in sweat rate with total body immersion has also been attributed to peripheral changes caused by hydration of the skin [21, 33]. The decline is reduced with immersion in dilute saline and abolished in 15% [7, 33], or even 10% NaCl solution [21]. These observations clearly indicate that diffusion of water into the skin is prerequisite to the hidromeiotic effect of immersion and is responsible for the degree of sweat depression, since the rate of water diffusion is a function of salinity of the solution wetting the skin [13]. More precisely, the hidromeiosis associated with wetting the skin depends on hydration of the stratum corneum, since it is prevented or reversed by epidermal stripping [11].

The most readily conceivable explanation for the hidromeiotic effect of skin soaking would be that swelling of the horny layer might occlude mechanically the sweat duct orifice [65, 70, 72]. This may most effectively occur on the palm and sole, where the horny layer is by far thicker than in other regions, and swelling of the layer as can be noted by characteristic whitening and wrinkles of the skin surface may narrow the sweat ducts, causing increased resistance to sweat secretion, or even occlude the ducts. However, Brebner and Kerslake [8] noted that the presence of sweating during presoaking (warm bath or exercise) accelerated markedly the depression of sweat rate in the subsequent heat exposure, compared with the sweat depression following soaking without sweating (by rest in a bath of neutral temperature), whereas the rate of sweating during presoaking was unimportant. Accordingly, they concluded that the rate of decrement of sweating was increased if sweat ducts were perfused, and suggested that the closure of the sweat ducts might be produced by swelling of the cells of duct walls along the epidermis, rather than by swelling of the stratum corneum. Laminated condensation of keratin in this part of the sweat duct [54] supports this view.

The decrement of sweating has also been demonstrated during prolonged heat exposure and has often been referred to as 'sweat gland fatigue' [69]. It is provoked more readily and more rapidly in humid heat than in dry heat [66] (Fig. 57). Although its picture may be complicated by systemic factors such as dehydration [44], elevated body temperature [44], etc., 'sweat gland fatigue' is considered to be essentially of the same nature as hidromeiosis in the warm bath, being primarily attributed to peripheral defects. The key phenomenon apparently is swelling of the stratum corneum (especially of the highly keratinized sweat duct walls), since suppression of sweating is promoted by factors which accelerated cutaneous hydration, such as high humidity, high skin temperature and full activation of the sweat glands [21].

A question arises as to whether exhaustion of the secretory cells takes place and participate in hidromeiosis [30, 43, 61, 75]. One basis for this possibility is the alteration in salt content of sweat with prolonged sweating. The decline in sweating is accompanied by a progressive rise in the salt concentration of sweat, which may indicate failure of the sweat glands to produce hypotonic secretion [43]. However, this explanation is contradicted by the fact that a sudden reduction in skin temperature during 'sweat gland fatigue' produces an immediate decrease in sweat chloride concentration [84]. Consequently, the increase in salt content of sweat during 'sweat gland fatigue' may be at-

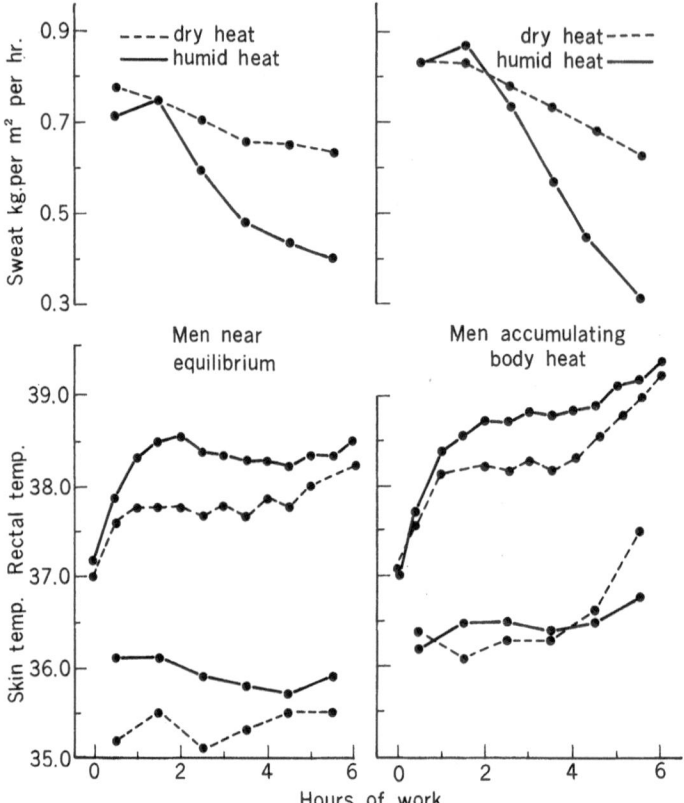

Fig. 57. Time course of total sweat rate during physical exercise in hot-dry and hot-wet environment among men maintaining thermal eqilibrium (left) and men not maintaining thermal equilibrium (right). (From Robinson and Gerking [66]; redrawn by Sargent [69]).

tributed to an increase in water reabsorption with an increased skin temperature. Besides, the concentration of sweat chloride does not invariably increase during hidromeiosis [67].

Reduction in sweat production in response to locally acting drugs during hidromeiosis is another ground for attributing hidromeiosis to exhaustion of the secretory cells [75]. Furthermore, during heat exposure, the sweat glands pretreated with atropine produce more sweat when released from atropine effect than the unatropinized glands [75]. However, a reduced response to local administration of acetylcholine is observed in a hot humid environment, but not in dry heat; pretreatment with atropine also prevents this reduction [21]. Moreover, the sweat glands which had been 'fatigued' in an arm bag showed a recovery in the activity after removal of the bag in a hot dry environment [21]. These observations indicate that even the highly activated sweat glands will not go into 'fatigue' peripherally without skin wetting, and the 'fatigued' sweat glands will regain their activity as soon as the skin is dried. Nevertheless, more evidence is required to rule out the possible development of exhaustion of the secretory cells during hidromeiosis.

The concept of mechanical occlusion of the sweat ducts may also need further evaluation. In histological observations of the ducts in hidromeiosis, Dobson et al. [24] failed to detect any changes in the keratin rings at the duct orifice. Furthermore, Peter and

Wyndham [61] showed that the decrease in activity of the sweat glands developed more rapidly on the back than on the chest in their unacclimatized subjects in spite of supposedly similar degrees of hydration in the two skin areas, and that the hypoactivity was not reversed even after the back skin became virtually dry due to the diminished glandular activity.

PERIPHERAL CHANGES ASSOCIATED WITH HEAT ACCLIMATIZATION AND SWEAT GLAND TRAINING

It has been generally recognized that repeated daily exposures to heat lead to an increase in the capacity to secrete sweat. The increased sweat output may be due to a combination of central and peripheral factors, but recent evidence suggests that the increased sweat rate with heat acclimatization is, at least in a large part, peripheral in origin, i.e., due to increased sweat gland activity. There is some evidence that changes in the central thermoregulatory mechanism occur during heat acclimatization [28, 40, 86]. This problem however is beyond the scope of this article.

The effect of training of the sweat glands by repeated local heating has been shown to encourage their activity [18, 19, 27, 39]. The sweat glands can also be trained by repeated daily intradermal injections of a sudorific drug [18].

If the skin temperature of a local area is controlled during daily exposures to heat, sweat gland activity of this area is markedly modified from that of other areas: local cooling prevented the local increase in sweating capacity, while local heating augmented the latter [27] (Fig. 58). However, the results shown in Fig. 58 indicate that hyperthermia is a more effective stimulus than local heating, suggesting that local temperature itself is not the predominant factor. Results of similar experiments all support the concept that the increase in sweating capacity during heat acclimatization is largely dependent upon sweat gland activity during heat exposure [6, 19].

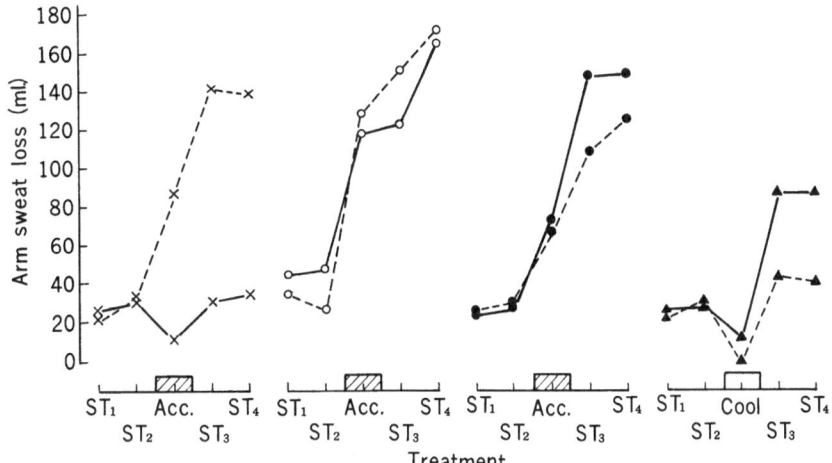

Fig. 58. Total arm sweat losses for four different treatment groups before ($ST_{1,2}$) during (Acc.) and after ($ST_{3,4}$) the 15-day treatment period. Acc. = acclimatization by control hyperthermia of Fox, during which one arm is immersed in water at temperatures of 13°C (×), 37°C (○), 43°C (●); subjects of the last group are not acclimatized (Cool), one arm being immersed in water at 43°C (▲). —— = treated arm, - - - - = control arm. ST = standard hyperthermia test (From Fox et al. [27]).

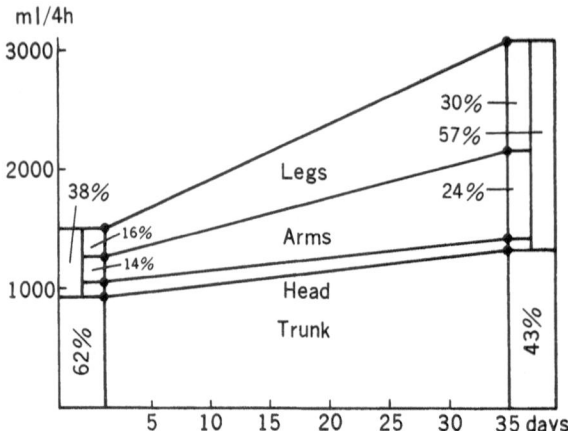

Fig. 59. Changes of total sweat rate and of percentage contribution of different surface areas during the 35-day acclimatization period (From Höfler [35]).

Changes in the regional distribution of sweating have been noted during heat acclimatization: the increment in activity of the sweat glands in the extremities is greater than that on the trunk [35] (Fig. 59); that on the back is more than that on the chest [61]. These observations may indicate regional differences in adaptive functioning of the sweat glands.

The peripheral mechanism of the increase in sweat gland activity with heat acclimatization has not been established. Collins *et al.* [18] have shown that the threshold concentration of acetylcholine for inducing local sweating is not changed with acclimatization. Similarly, Craig *et al.* [22] have reported that the same doses of atropine given intravenously cause the same amount of depression in sweat rate before and after acclimatization. These observations indicate that increased sweat gland activity with heat acclimatization does not involve changes in sensitivity of the glands to the transmitter substance. It may be that each sudomotor impulse releases a greater amount of acetylcholine.

Recently, Elizondo *et al.* [25] observed that the magnitude of increase in sweat rate in response to local heating was significantly reduced after heat acclimatization, both in spontaneous sweating and in acetylcholine-induced sweating, and suggested that sweat gland activity was less dependent upon local skin temperature, and might be more directly controlled by the central thermoregulatory processes after acclimatization. It may be conceivable that the increased sweat gland activity caused by acclimatization and that caused by local training may be different in nature. In other words, adaptive responses in the sweat glands to repeated heat exposures may not involve the same mechanism as the local training effect. This assumption awaits further evaluation.

Heat acclimatization not only increases but also prolongs glandular activity, i.e., it delays 'sweat gland fatigue' [61]. This reduction in the rate of sweat suppression is more distinct in an arm exposed to a hot-wet condition than in an arm exposed to a hot-dry condition [26]. These phenomena further complicate the understanding of the mechanism, since they involve the still-controversial mechanism of 'sweat gland fatigue.'

SUMMARY

Various changes in conditions at the sweat gland or in the microenvironment of the sweat glands may affect sweat gland activity and modify the magnitude of centrally controlled thermoregulatory responses. Local temperature appears to exert a multiplicative effect on sweat secretion. Local increase in skin temperature is considered to enhance sweating by increasing sensitivity of the glandular receptor mechanism and possibly by increasing release of the transmitter substance at the neuroglandular junction. Significance of vasomotor tone has not been assessed, although vasodilatation favors copious sweat secretion. Mechanisms of ischemic suppression of sweating are controversial: ischemia may cause 'fatigue' at the neuroglandular junction and/or it may affect the secretory mechanism per se. The status of cutaneous hydration appears to affect the rate of water reabsorption through the sweat ducts and thus the emergence of sweat and stabilization of sweat rate. Overhydration or prolonged hydration causes progressive decrement of sweat rate, 'hidromeiosis.' This effect has been explained by mechanical occlusion of the sweat duct orifices by swelling of the horny layer or by exhaustion of the secretory cells; neither explanation is yet convincing.

Increased sweat secretion in association with heat acclimatization appears in a larger part to be peripheral in origin, although its mechanism has not been established. The sweat glands can be trained by repeated local heating or repeated intradermal administration of a sudorific drug, but increased sweat gland activity by training may not be of the same nature as that associated with heat acclimatization.

REFERENCES

1. ADAMS, T. (1966): *J. Appl. Physiol.* **21:** 1004.
2. BANERJEE, M., and R.W. BULLARD: Personal communication.
3. BANERJEE, M.R., R. ELIZONDO, and R.W. BULLARD (1969): *J. Appl. Physiol.* **26:** 787.
4. BANERJEE, M., and T. OGAWA: Unpublished data.
5. BENJAMIN, F.B. (1953): *J. Appl. Physiol.* **5:** 594.
6. BREBNER, D.F., and D. McK. KERSLAKE (1963): *J. Physiol.* **166:** 13P.
7. BREBNER, D.F., and D. McK. KERSLAKE (1964): *J. Physiol.* **175:** 295.
8. BREBNER, D.F., and D. McK. KERSLAKE (1968): *J. Physiol.* **194:** 1.
9. BRONOW, R.S., D.T. DESILETS, and R.R. SONNENSCHEIN (1958): *Proc. Soc. Exp. Biol. Med.* **97:** 272.
10. BROWN, G.L. (1954): *J. Physiol.* **124:** 26P.
11. BROWN, W.K., and F. SARGENT, II. (1965): *Arch. Environ. Health* **11:** 442.
12. BUETTNER, K. (1953): *J. Appl. Physiol.* **6:** 229.
13. BUETTNER, K.J.K. (1959): *J. Appl. Physiol.* **14:** 261.
14. BULLARD, R.W. (1970): *Physiologist* **13:** 158.
15. BULLARD, R.W. (1971): *J. Physiol. (Paris)* **63:** 218.
16. BULLARD, R.W., M.R. BANERJEE, and B.A., MacINTYRE (1967): *Int. J. Biometeor.* **11:** 93.
17. BURN, J.H., and A.S. MILTON (1959): *Brit. J. Pharmacol.* **14:** 493.
18. COLLINS, K.J., G.W. CROCKFORD, and J.S. WEINER (1965): *Arch. Environ. Health* **11:** 407.
19. COLLINS, K.J., G.W. CROCKFORD, and J.S. WEINER (1966): *J. Physiol.* **184:** 203.
20. COLLINS, K.J., F. SARGENT, and J.S. WEINER (1959): *J. Physiol.* **148:** 615.
21. COLLINS, K.J., and J.S. WEINER (1962): *J. Physiol.* **161:** 538.
22. CRAIG, F.N., E.G. CUMMINGS, H.L. FROEHLICH, and P.F. ROBINSON (1969): *J. Appl. Physiol.* **27:** 498.
23. DOBSON, R.L. (1962): In: Advances in Biology of Skin, Vol. 3, W. Montagna, R.A. Ellis and A.F. Silver (eds.). Pergamon Press, Oxford—London—New York—Paris, p. 54.
24. DOBSON, R.L., V. FORMISANO, W.C. LOBITZ, JR. and D. BROPHY (1958): *J. Invest. Dermat.* **31:** 147.
25. ELIZONDO, R.S., M.R. BANERJEE, T. OGAWA, and R.W. BULLARD (1970): *Physiologist* **13:** 189.
26. FOX, R.H., R. GOLDSMITH, I.F.G. HAMPTON, and T.J. HUNT (1967): *J. Appl. Physiol.* **22:** 39.
27. FOX, R.H., R. GOLDSMITH, I.F.G. HAMPTON, and H.E. LEWIS (1964): *J. Physiol.* **171:** 368.
28. FOX, R.H., R. GOLDSMITH, D.J. KIDD, and H.E. LEWIS (1963): *J. Physiol.* **166:** 548.
29. FOX, R.H., and S.M. HILTON (1958): *J. Physiol.* **142:** 219.
30. GERKING, S.D., and S. ROBINSON (1946): *Am. J. Physiol.* **147:** 370.
31. GOODMAN, A.B., and A.V. WOLF (1969): *J. Appl. Physiol.* **26:** 203.
32. HEERD, E., and K. OHARA (1962): *Pflügers Arch. ges. Physiol.* **276:** 32.
33. HERTIG, B.A., M.L. RIEDESEL, and H.S. BELDING (1961): *J. Appl. Physiol.* **16:** 647.

34. HERTIG, B.A., M.L. RIEDESEL, and H.S. BELDING (1962): In: Advances in Biology of Skin, Vol. 3, W. Montagna, R.A. Ellis and A.F. Silver (eds.). Pergamon Press, Oxford—London—New York—Paris, p. 213.
35. HÖFLER, W. (1968): *J. Appl. Physiol.* **25:** 503.
36. HUHEEY, M.J., and T. ADAMS (1967): *J. Appl. Physiol.* **22:** 939.
37. IKAI, K., K. SUGIYAMA, Y. OTSUKA, and H. NITTA (1970): *Jap. J. Physiol.* **20:** 250.
38. ISSEKUTZ, B., JR., G. HETENYI, and A. DIOSY (1950): *Arch. Int. Pharmacodyn.* **83:** 133.
39. ITO, S., and J. ADACHI (1934): *J. Orient. Med.* **21:** 93.
40. JANOWITZ, H.D., and M.I. GROSSMAN (1950): *J. Invest. Dermat.* **14:** 453.
41. KUNO, Y. (1956): Human Perspiration. Thomas, Springfield.
42. KUNO, Y. (1965): Proc. 23rd Int. Congr. Physiol. Sci., Excerpta Medica Intern. Congr. Series No. 87, p. 3.
43. LADELL, W.S.S. (1945): *Brit. Med. Bull.* **3:** 175.
44. LADELL, W.S.S. (1955): *J. Physiol.* **129:** 8P.
45. LLOYD, D.P.C. (1959): *Proc. Nat. Acad. Sci.* **45:** 405.
46. LLOYD, D.P.C. (1961): *Proc. Nat. Acad. Sci.* **47:** 358.
47. LOBITZ, W.C., and H.L. MASON (1948): *Arch. Dermat. Syphilol.* **57:** 907.
48. MacINTYRE, B.A., R.W. BULLARD, M. BANERJEE, and R. ELIZONDO (1968): *J. Appl. Physiol.* **25:** 255.
49. McLAUGHLIN, J.T., and R.R. SONNENSCHEIN (1963): *J. Invest. Dermat.* **41:** 27.
50. MILTON, A.S. (1958): *J. Physiol.* **142:** 25P.
51. NADEL, E.R., R.W. BULLARD, and J.A.J. STOLWIJK (1971): *J. Appl. Physiol.* **31:** 80.
52. NADEL, E.R., and J.T. STITT (1970): *Physiologist* **13:** 267.
53. NITTA, H. (1953): *Nagoya Med. J.* **1:** 59.
54. O'BRIEN, J.P. (1947): *Brit. J. Dermat.* **59:** 125.
55. OGAWA, T. (1970): *J. Appl. Physiol.* **28:** 18.
56. OGAWA, T. (1970): *Tohoku J. Exp. Med.* **100:** 255.
57. OGAWA, T., and R.W. BULLARD (1970): *Physiologist* **13:** 275.
58. OGAWA, T., and R.W. BULLARD (1971): *J. Appl. Physiol.* In press.
59. OGAWA, T., and R.W. BULLARD (1971): *J. Physiol. (Paris).* **63:** 371.
60. PEARCY, M., S. ROBINSON, D.I. MILLER, J.T. THOMAS, and J. DeBROTA (1956): *J. Appl. Physiol.* **8:** 621.
61. PETER, J., and C.H. WYNDHAM (1966): *J. Physiol.* **187:** 583.
62. RANDALL, W.C. (1946): *Am. J. Physiol.* **147:** 391.
63. RANDALL, W.C. (1947): *Am. J. Physiol.* **150:** 365.
64. RANDALL, W.C., R. DEERING, and I. DOUGHERTY (1948): *J. Appl. Physiol.* **1:** 53.
65. RANDALL, W.C., and C.N. REISS (1957): *J. Invest. Dermat.* **28:** 435.
66. ROBINSON, S., and S.D. GERKING (1947): *Am. J. Physiol.* **149:** 476.
67. ROBINSON, S., S.D. GERKING, E.S. TURRELL, and R.K. KINCAID (1950): *J. Appl. Physiol.* **2:** 654.
68. ROTHMAN, S. (1954): Physiology and Biochemistry of the Skin. Univ. of Chicago Press, Chicago.
69. SARGENT, F., II. (1962): In: Advances in Biology of Skin, Vol. 3, W. Montagna, R.A. Ellis and A.F. Silver (eds.). Pergamon Press, Oxford—London—New York—Paris, p. 163.
70. SARKANY, I., S. SHUSTER, and M.C. STAMMERS (1965): *Brit. J. Dermat.* **77:** 101.
71. SCHWARTZ, I.L., J.H. THAYSEN, and V.P. DOLE (1953): *J. Exp. Med.* **97:** 429.
72. SHELLEY, W.B., and P.N. HORVATH (1950): *J. Invest. Dermat.* **14:** 193.
73. SLAT, B., K. KOSTIAL, and H. LORKOVIC (1965): *Arch. Intern. Physiol.* **73:** 627.
74. STOLWIJK, J.KJ., and J.D. HARDY (1966): *J. Appl. Physiol.* **21:** 967.
75. THAYSEN, J.H., and I.L. SCHWARTZ (1955): *J. Clin. Invest.* **34:** 1719.
76. THOMAS, P.E., and A. KAWAHATA (1962): *J. Appl. Physiol.* **17:** 999.
77. THOMPSON, N. (1960): *Clin. Sci.* **19:** 95.
78. VAN BEAUMONT, W., and R.W. BULLARD (1965): *Science* **147:** 1465.
79. VAN HEYNINGEN, R., and J.S. WEINER (1952): *J. Physiol.* **116:** 404.
80. WADA, M. (1960): In: Essential Problems in Climatic Physiology, H. Yoshimura, K. Ogata and S. Itoh (eds.). Nankodo, Tokyo, p. 185.
81. WADA, M. (1954): *J. Invest. Dermat.* **23:** 63.
82. WADA, M., T. ARAI, T. TAKAGAKI, and T. NAKAGAWA (1952): *J. Appl. Physiol.* **4:** 745.
83. WADA, M., S. SATO, W. KOYAMA, H. HAYASHI, and J. HANAWOKA (1968): *Tohoku J. Exp. Med.* **95:** 297.
84. WEINER, J.S., and R.E. VAN HEYNINGEN (1952): *J. Appl. Physiol.* **4:** 725.
85. WYNDHAM, C.H. (1965): *J. Appl. Physiol.* **20:** 31.
86. YOSHIMURA, H. (1964): In: Handbook of Physiology, Section 4: Adaptation to the Environment, D.B. Dill, E.F. Adolph and C.G. Wilber (eds.). Am. Physiol. Soc., Washington, D.C., p. 109.

CHAPTER 7

ADRENALINE SWEATING

KIMIO IKAI and YASUHIRO HASEGAWA

Department of Physiology, Nagoya City University Medical School, Nagoya, Japan

ADRENALINE SWEATING IN ECCRINE GLANDS

1. Survey of Past Works

Since Dale and Feldberg (1934) demonstrated the release of acetylcholine in sweat from the cat's paw on stimulation of the sudomotor nerve, the mechanism causing sweating in the footpad of the cat has been recognized to be cholinergic. In man, cholinergic drugs such as pilocarpine, acetylcholine and methacholine have been shown to stimulate the sweat gland when administered locally, while atropine, locally or systemically, can counteract this effect. Moreover, the intradermal administration of atropine abolished spontaneous sweating in the palm as well as on the general body surface. This stimulation and inhibition of sweating is considered to be based on cholinergic innervation at present. With this concept in mind, we will review past works concerning adrenaline-induced sweating in man and animals.

Haimovici (1948, 1950) reported that systemic administration of neosynephrine and adrenaline caused an increase in sweating in the palm and that systemically administered dibenamine, an adrenergic blocking agent, inhibited spontaneous palmar sweating. He further showed the positive effect of adrenaline, noradrenaline and isopropylnoradrenaline and the blocking action of systemically administered dibenamine against these catecholamines, suggesting that in man the sweat gland may receive adrenergic as well as cholinergic innervation. Around the same time, Kisin (1948) and Wada (1950) observed that the sweat glands are stimulated by systemically and locally administered adrenaline.

Sonnenschein et al. (1949, 1951) also observed that locally administered adrenaline, noradrenaline, isopropylnoradrenaline and neosynephrine caused sweating which was inhibited by dibenamine, but not by atropine. However, since the local sudorific effect of these catecholamines was difficult to demonstrate in the palm, and the spontaneous sweating of the forearm was not inhibited by dibenamine iontophoresis, they concluded that the existence of an adrenergic innervation of the sweat gland was not proven. Sonnenschein et al's. and Haimovici's observations were confirmed by Chalmers and Keele (1951, 1952). However, Chalmers and Keele showed that the palmar sweating induced by both acetylcholine and adrenaline given locally was blocked by atropine, while Sonnenschein et al. did not find this inhibitory effect of atropine; they also found that spontaneous palmar sweating was not blocked by a locally administered adrenergic blocking agent, while Haimovici reported inhibition by a systemically administered adrenergic blocking agent.

Nakamura and Hatanaka (1958) observed the effects of denervation of the cat's sweat glands on their responsiveness to adrenaline and some other drugs, and reported that adrenaline elicited a sweat response which was abolished by dihydroergotamine, but not by atropine. Lloyd (1959) also observed that the sweat gland of the cat footpad responded to locally administered adrenaline and noradrenaline, and that atropine had no blocking effect on it. He considered that this result was due to direct activation of the secretory cells by adrenaline and noradrenaline, and that the gland is essentially innervated cholinergically. After further observation, however, Lloyd (1963, 1964, 1968) claimed that high doses of anti-adrenergic substances such as guanethidine, bretylium and dibenamine inhibited the response of the cat's foot pad sweat gland to plantar nerve stimulation, and presented this as evidence for an adrenergic component.

Foster and Weiner (1970) reported recently that the blocking effect of guanethidine and phentolamine on sweat response in the cat's foot pad gland to plantar nerve stimulation was so feeble that the extremely high doses which cause anti-cholinergic action could not reveal any significant measure of inhibition, and that small doses of atropine were as effective as these large doses of guanethidine or phentolamine. The results obtained in the human forearm sweat gland were reported to confirm those obtained in the cat concerning the relative ineffectiveness of anti-adrenergic substances when compared with atropine. Thus, it was concluded that there are only cholinergic fibers innervating the sweat gland in the cat footpad as well as in the human forearm.

Sakurai and Montagna (1964) observed that the eccrine gland of the mongoose lemur or green monkey responded to intradermally administered adrenaline, although the sweat amount was small and the response was not as constant as that obtained with mecholyl stimulation. Spontaneous sweating was suppressed by atropine in every case, but not by dihydroergotamine. Thus, both functional activity and neuroglandular transmission in the palmar eccrine sweat gland of the monkey seemed to be similar to that in man.

Takahashi (1964) reported that spontaneous sweating of central origin in the toe-pads of dogs was easily blocked by local administration of atropine, but not by dihydroergotamine. This indicates a cholinergic nerve supply to the sweat gland, although locally induced adrenergic agents were as effective as cholinergic agents in eliciting sweat responses in the toe-pad gland of the dog whose spontaneous sweating had been eliminated.

Hayashi and Nakagawa (1963) observed in the rat in which spontaneous sweating had been carefully abolished by blocking or cutting the sciatic nerve, that local sweating induced by acetylcholine and mecholyl was abolished by atropine, and that induced by adrenaline was abolished by dihydroergotamine as well as by atropine.

Sivadjian et al. (1959, 1965) blocked spontaneous sweating in the footpad of mouse by intraperitoneal injection of atropine. Hayashi (1968) observed in the mouse that adrenergic agents also elicit sweat secretion, although they were less potent than cholinergic agents, and that the spontaneous sweating was eliminated with relatively low concentrations of atropine, but not with relatively high concentrations of dihydroergotamine. He suggested that the sweat glands of the plantar surface of the mouse receive a cholinergic nerve supply.

From the above listed investigations in the cat, monkey, dog, rat and mouse, it seems likely that the eccrine sweat glands in the toe-pad of these animals are cholinergically innervated as they are in the eccrine sweat gland of the human general body surface.

2. *Author's Diagrammatic Representation of Adrenaline Sweating*

Results concerning the sudorific effect of adrenaline on the human general body surface are contradictory in some of their details. While Kuno (1962, 1965) observed an augmentation with a smaller amount of adrenaline (0.1–0.3 mg) and a depression with a larger amount (0.6 1.0 mg), Foster *et al.* (1967) postulated that circulating adrenaline may not potentiate sweat gland activity unless the concentration is high, since intravenous infusion of adrenaline in doses between 2–20 μg/min produced no sweating, while intraarterial infusion of it in doses between 2–10 μg/min produced a distinct sweat response in the forearm (Barcroft and Swan, 1953).

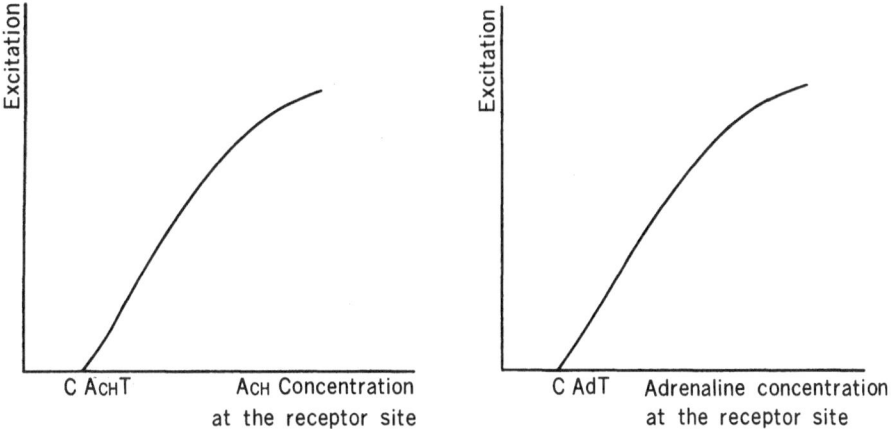

Figs. 60 a and b. Diagrammatic representation of the correlation between the excitation of the sweat gland and the concentrations of acetylcholine and adrenaline at the receptor site.

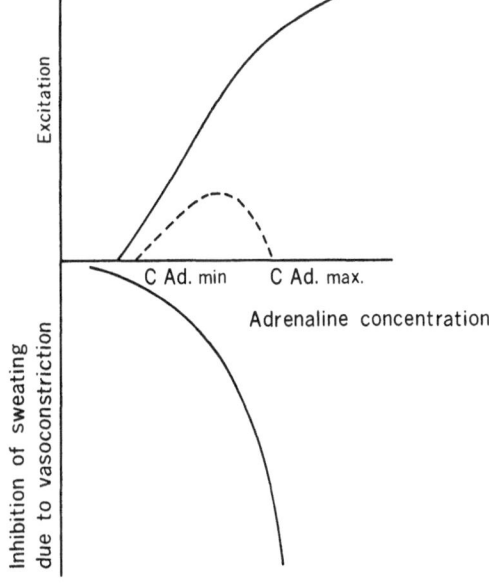

Fig. 60 b′. Diagrammatic representation of correlation between actual sweating activity and the concentration of adrenaline. Fig. 60b′ is composed of excitation at the receptor site and inhibition of actual sweating due to vasoconstriction by adrenaline, and indicates the effective or optimal concentrations of adrenaline between C Ad. Min, and C Ad. Max., eligible to cause sweating activity.

These conflicting results may be interpreted according to the authors' diagrammatic representation of adrenaline sweating, correlating the actual sweating response with the excitatory response of the sweat gland to adrenaline and acetylcholine, as follows:

As shown in Fig. 60, the sweat gland is sensitive to both acetylcholine and adrenaline, and *excitation of the sweat gland* is seen whenever the concentration of acetylcholine or adrenaline is above C AchT, or C AdT, respectively. When the concentration of adrenaline is high in the gland, the volume of blood supply to the sweat gland decreases due to vasoconstriction, and consequently the volume of primary sweat decreases despite the excitation of the sweat gland. Adrenaline sweating combined with histamine-induced vasodilatation was shown to produce a large amount of sweat in the human forearm (Authors' unpublished data).

Fig. 60b′ shows *excitation of the sweat gland* and inhibition of sweating by adrenaline, and indicates the effective or optimal concentrations of adrenaline C Ad.Min and C Ad.Max., able to cause actual sweating. A dotted line indicates actual sweating activity. While adrenaline sweating occurs, vasoconstriction around the sweat duct also occurs. Therefore, inhibited ductal sodium reabsorption results in the production of sweat with a high sodium concentration, as observed in adrenaline-induced sweat (Ikai *et al.*, 1968, 1970).

Acetylcholine or adrenaline seems to rarely exist alone in the gland, and probably both act in the gland together. If the concentrations of acetylcholine and adrenaline are both below C AchT and C AdT, the sweat gland is thought to be activated by combination of both their actions. In the case reported by Kuno (1962, 1965) adrenaline in low concentrations potentiates a sweat response, whereas pilocarpine in low concentrations cannot produced sweating.

Combining Fig. 60a and 60b′ on a graph, with acetylcholine concentration on the X axis, and adrenaline concentration on the Y axis, results in another graph (Fig. 61) on which border lines are plotted between the occurance and non-occurance of sweating

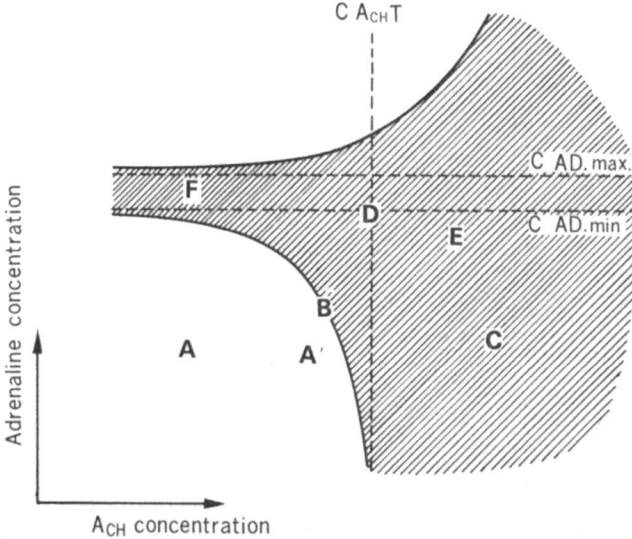

Fig. 61. Concentrations of acetylcholine and adrenaline at the secretory coil in various kind of sweating.

response. Sweating response caused by adrenaline and acetylcholine concentrations is indicated by a dark area in the Figure.

At rest: No sweating response occurs on the general body surface when there is no thermal nor emotional stress, since both acetylcholine and adrenaline concentrations are low (indicated on Fig. 61 as Area A).

Intermittent sweating in the palm: While the subjects are awake, however, the palmar sweat glands receive impulses from the cerebral cortex (but not from the thermoregulatory center), and the amount of released acetylcholine increases. Therefore, the palm reveals an intermittent sweat response when the subjects are awake (Area B). Area B may repeat changing position from the sweating to the non-sweating zone and from the non-sweating to the sweating zone.

Cholinergic sweating: Sweating on the human general body surface due to exogenously administered acetylcholine, or spontaneous sweating on the cat's paw caused by stimulation of the plantar nerve, is based on the status change from A to C, as is the case in the thermal sweating. This change could be reversed by a cholinergic blocking agent, and not by an adrenergic blocking agent, as observed by many investigators.

Thermal sweating: When thermal stress is given, a greater amount of acetylcholine is released from the postganglionic sympathetic nerve fibers at a signal from the thermoregulatory center, and the concentration of acetylcholine at the gland is increased. Except when thermal stress is especially severe, the amount of adrenaline released from the adrenal medulla does not increase. Therefore, the concentrations of acetylcholine and adrenaline causing thermal sweating may be plotted around C in Fig. 61, as in the case of cholinergic sweating.

Emotional palmar sweating: When emotional stress is given, the amount of adrenaline released from the adrenal medulla increases, as does the concentration of adrenaline in the gland. Acetylcholine concentration at the gland also increases, due to an increased stimulation from the cerebral cortex. Therefore, the concentrations of acetylcholine and adrenaline in emotional sweating are presumed to be around D in Fig. 61. That the emotional palmar sweating may be, or may not be blocked by cholinergic blocking agent, could be assumed from the position of D.

Emotional body sweating: When the environmental temperature is high, the concentration of acetylcholine in the gland is high (A'), and hence, whenever emotional stress is given at this high environmental temperature, A' is shifted upward to D. Emotional sweating may also occur in the general body surface at a high environmental temperature. Emotional body sweating has been reported by Kuno (1956) to occur at environmental temperatures above 30 °C. Kennard (1963) also observed emotional body sweating at temperatures above 32 °C, but not below 26 °C.

Exercise sweating: Sweating caused by strenous physical exercise has been noted to have a shorter latency than thermal sweating, and was described by Kuno (1956) as being located between emotional sweating and thermal sweating with characteristics of both. It is also known that adrenaline and noradrenaline are released from the adrenal medulla through physical exercise, as is the case in sweating in the horse, reported by Evans *et al.* (1956). The position of the concentrations of acetylcholine and adrenaline concerning this sweating is presumed to be E, because the concentration of acetylcholine must be increased by excitation of the thermoregulatory center.

Adrenaline sweating: Exogenous adrenaline can cause sweating whenever the concen-

TABLE 6 Electrolyte concentration in the human body sweat induced by cholinergic and adrenergic receptor mechanisms

Data of the noradrenaline sweating and adrenaline sweating indicate that they were obtained on the different days from one of the two subjects, unless encircled with the frame.

Data encircled with the frame indicate that the noradrenaline sweating or adrenaline sweating were compared with the control (pilocarpine) sweating on the same days on the same subjects (noradrenaline sweating or adrenaline sweating performed successively after the control (pilocarpine) sweating were compared with control sweating on the same space lines, respectively).

	Noradrenaline sweating					Control (pilocarpine) sweating					Adrenaline sweating				
	Sweat rate G/100 cm² 30 min.	NA mEq/L	CL mEq/L	K mEq/L	NA/K	Sweat rate G/100 cm² 30 min.	NA mEq/L	CL mEq/L	K mEq/L	NA/K	Sweat rate G/100 cm² 30 min.	NA mEq/L	CL mEq/L	K mEq/L	NA/K
	2.8	66.0	62.0	4.3	15.35	1.4	46.8	54.0	3.5	13.37	1.8	51.8	58.6	3.9	13.26
	3.0	49.6	46.9	3.5	14.17	1.9	36.0	37.2	3.8	9.47	4.7	56.8	58.6	3.0	18.93
	0.8	40.4	32.7	3.4	11.88	4.1	54.0	42.9	3.0	18.00	1.1	29.6	31.0	6.2	4.77
	3.0	48.0	44.0	4.4	10.91	1.9	37.6	32.7	3.9	9.64	0.6	44.0	42.4	6.3	7.00
	1.6	47.2	48.5	3.8	12.42	2.8	46.8	43.3	4.0	11.90	3.0	55.6	45.1	2.9	19.28
	3.4	58.0	54.1	4.2	13.81	1.8	29.2	32.1	4.6	6.35	2.1	49.6	49.0	4.2	11.81
	1.5	48.0	52.4	4.2	11.43	3.5	42.0	41.6	4.0	10.50	1.7	40.0	50.0	4.0	10.00
	2.5	40.4	40.6	3.0	13.47	1.0	14.5	19.7	4.9	2.96	1.0	20.8	18.6	3.9	5.08
	2.0	64.8	58.7	4.2	15.43	0.6	14.0	22.6	4.0	3.60	2.1	34.4	35.0	4.3	8.00
	2.5	57.6	57.4	4.2	13.95	1.5	24.2	27.6	3.5	6.91	1.6	34.8	33.3	4.6	7.57
	1.4	52.8	50.8	3.2	15.88	1.2	21.0	20.5	4.0	5.25	2.0	38.0	38.8	4.0	9.50
	1.7	46.4	45.2	5.6	8.29	1.3	27.0	31.4	4.1	6.59	4.1	45.4	39.6	4.4	10.32
	—	—	—	—	—	4.5	58.0	47.2	6.8	8.53	3.1	56.8	51.9	5.8	9.80
Mean	2.2	51.6	49.4	4.0	13.08	2.1	34.7	34.8	4.2	5.77	2.2	42.9	42.5	4.4	10.41
SD	0.8	8.1	7.9	0.7		1.2	13.8	10.3	0.9		1.2	10.8	11.0	1.0	
Difference Percent-change	+4.8%	+48.7%	+41.9%	−2.4%	+125.0%						+4.8%	+23.7%	+21.3%	+4.8%	+80.4%
		S_1	S_2	NS_1	S_3							S_4	S_5	NS_2	S_6

Note: S_1: Significant ($0.001<P<0.005$), S_2: Significant ($P<0.005$), S_3: Significant ($P<0.001$), NS_1: Not significant ($P>0.1$), S_4: Significant ($P<0.001$), NS_2: Non-significant ($0.05<P<0.1$), S_5: Nonsignificant ($0.05<P<0.1$), NS_2: Not significant ($P>0.1$), S_6: Significant ($0.01<P<0.05$).

tration in the gland reaches C Ad.Min., or by status changes from A to F, even if the concentration of acetylcholine is too low to cause sweating. The range of the optimal concentration of adrenaline to cause sweating is very narrow, and thus the reason why sweating does not occur when the concentration of adrenaline is too low or too high, may be easily interpreted. The reason why adrenaline-induced sweating cannot be blocked by atropine, as was reported by many investigators, is that Area F is never off the sweating zone (zone of the concentrations of acetylcholine and adrenaline, able to cause sweating), even if much shifted toward the left on Fig. 61. By blockage with adrenergic blocking agents, on the other hand, Area F will be off the sweating zone when shifted downward on Fig. 61.

3. High Sodium Sweat in Adrenaline Sweating

The chloride concentration in sweat, as reported by Houstek and Jirka (1967), was higher in sweat induced by adrenaline than in that by pilocarpine. Ikai et al. (1968, 1970) confirmed this, and observed a higher sodium concentration as well (Table 6). The results were interpreted to be due to (1) decreased ductal sodium reabsorption due to the rapid expulsion of sweat by the contraction of myoepithelium which is under adrenergic control, and (2) an adrenergic innervation of the dark cells, a primitive component in the eccrine gland, secreting so-called sodium reabsorption inhibiting factor which acts on cholinergically secreted primary sweat from the clear cells. However, the second possibility is now rather questionable, since Foster and Weiner (1970) clearly demonstrated in the cat and man that the blocking effect of guanethidine and phentolamine on sweat response is due to their anti-cholinergic action, and that there are only cholinergic fibers innervating sweat glands in the cat footpad as well as in the human forearm. It should be added to the first interpretation that the vasoconstriction around the duct also results in reduced ductal sodium reabsorption. Some elevated sodium concentrations observed in sweat induced emotionally or by strenuous physical exercise, as reported by Ikai et al. (1968, 1969, 1970) could be interpreted similarly.

ADRENALINE SWEATING IN APOCRINE GLANDS

1. Apocrine Sweat Gland in Man

Rothman (1954) deduced that the human apocrine sweat gland has a dual innervation from his observation that there are two kinds of apocrine sweat, different in appearance: (1) One secretion, a viscid, milky or turbid white droplet by a semiholocrine mechanism appears at hair follicle orifices following pharmacological (adrenaline) as well as emotional or sensory stimuli, and is probably due to the adrenergic contraction of myoepithelium. This secretion does not appear in response to heat, and cannot be inhibited by atropine. (2) A second secretion, a clear, colorless, watery fluid, also appears to emanate from the same hair follicle orifices in response to heat, cholinergic and emotional stresses, and is probably cholinergic in function.

Shelley and Hurley (1951, 1952, 1953, 1960), on the other hand, believed that the human apocrine glands are exclusively adrenergic based on their finding that the human apocrine sweat gland produced only one secretion, the viscid, turbid white or milky sweat. The clear, aqueous "follicular fluid," which Rothman believed to be a product of cholinergic secretion, is in reality eccrine sweat which arises from adjacent eccrine sweat duct pores and collects at the follicular orifices, giving a false impression of its

TABLE 7   Comparison of eccrine and apocrine sweat glands in man and animals with respect to cholinergic and adrenergic innervation

	Cholinergic innervation	Adrenergic innervation
Eccrine glands in man, cat, dog, rat and mouse	+	—
Apocrine gland in man	—, (+ ?)	—
Apocrine gland in monkey	—, (+ ?)	—, (+ ?)
Apocrine gland in dog	—	+
Apocrine gland in horse and donkey	—	+
Apocrine gland in cattle, sheep and goat	—	+

origin: Turbid, true apocrine secretion is nerver seen on cholinergic stimulation.

Shelley and Hurley have differentiated between "apocrine sweating" and "apocrine secretion;" that is, the former term represents the expulsion of pooled apocrine fluid by the contraction of myoepithelium under adrenergic innervation, while the latter represents a slow, more or less continuous production of apocrine fluid, not under the adrenergic innervation but humorally controlled by adrenaline in the blood stream. It has been reported by these authors that the "apocrine sweating" could not be blocked by sympathectomy, as is the case in eccrine sweating. This suggests that the existence of adrenergic innervation in apocrine sweating also is doubtful.

Moreover, Aoki (1962) observed that the human apocrine sweat gland discharged a viscous sweat, regardless of whether stimulation was adrenergic or cholinergic, only at the site of injection, thus eliminating the possiblity that emotional, sensory or mechanical stimulations might elicit sweat response. The selective inhibition of the effect of acetylcholine as well as of mecholyl by atropine, seems to leave almost no doubt that this apocrine sweat was due to direct cholinergic stimulation.

In conclusion, there is no evidence so far that the human apocrine glands are supplied with secretory nerves of any kind, and it is doubtful that they have either adrenergic or cholinergic innervation even if some cholinesterases have been observed around the human sweat gland by Aaviak, 1955; Montagna and Ellis, 1960; Yasuda, Machida and Suzuki, 1963; Montagna, 1964; they may, however, be controlled humorally with catecholamines in the blood flow, or with exogenously induced cholinergic and adrenergic agents.

2. *Apocrine Sweat Gland in the Monkey*

Sakurai and Montagna (1964) observed in the mongoose lemur a spontaneous sweating as well as adrenaline and mecholyl sweating only in the lower belly and not in the rest of the hairy skin regions. Although they concluded that the apocrine sweat glands in the hairy skin of the mongoose lemur are probably not sensitive to sudorific agents at all, there is little doubt that the glands which revealed the sweat response might be the eccrine glands. This of course is against their concept that this kind of monkey has eccrine glands only on the volar surface of the hands and feet; elsewhere on the body only apocrine glands are present. We have observed, in the hairy skin regions of the Japanese monkey (Macaca fuscata), spontaneous sweating at high environmental temperatures as well as sweating caused by locally administered pilocarpine and adrenaline. This sweating has been identified as "eccrine," from their physicochemical properties and their independent emergence from the hair follicle orifices, and has been confirmed to be blocked by atropine. The apocrine sweat gland in the hairy skin of the Japanese monkey has not so far been observed to respond to any kind of stimulation (our unpublished data).

On the other hand, Aoki (1962) has reported that the apocrine glands in the hairy skin of the Nycticebus coucang revealed not only a response to adrenaline and acetylcholine but also axon reflex sweating, thus suggesting autonomic innervation in the apocrine sweat gland. However, since the differentiation between "apocine sweating" and "apocrine secretion" was not made, whether the axon reflex sweating was due to an excitation of the myoepithel or of the apocrine gland itself is questionable.

3. *Apocrine Sweat Glands in the Horse and Donkey*

Copious sweating in the horse is a familiar phenomenon, and hence ample observations have been reported, as reviewed by Evans and Smith (1956). Evans *et al.* (1956) demonstrated that intradermal or intravenous administration of adrenaline to the horse caused sweating which could not be blocked by adrenergic blocking agents, and that cholinergic agents given intradermally and intravenously caused sweating which could be inhibited by atropine and augmented by an anticholinesterase such as prostigmine. Noradrenaline was ineffective in causing sweating in the horse, although it caused hair erection which was blocked by dibenamine. Isopropylnoradrenaline produced responses similar to those elicited by adrenaline. From the negative effect of noradrenaline in causing sweating, Evans and Smith concluded that the sweat gland of the horse is directly stimulated by adrenaline in the blood circulation, but not by a nerve mechanism. Aoki, Kimura and Wada (1959), on the other hand, have reported that the sweat gland of the horse is reactive to noradrenaline as well.

Robertshaw and Taylor (1968), however, demonstrated in the donkey that (1) the donkey perspired on exposure to heat and in response to intravenous infusion of adrenaline, (2) thermal sweating was abolished by bethanidine, an adrenergic-neuron blocking agent, but not by atropine, (3) sympathetic decentralization by preganglionic sympathectomy abolished thermal sweating but adreno-medullary denervation had no effect, (4) exercise resulted in sweating in both sympathetically innervated and decentralized skin and in the innervated skin of animals which had previously undergone adreno-medullary denervation, (5) insulin-induced hypoglycemia produced sweating in sympathetically decentralized skin and in innervated skin in two out of four animals. Adreno-medullary denervation abolished the sweat gland response to insulin administration. They further showed that (6) cold exposure inhibited the response of innervated sweat glands but not that of decentralized glands to adrenaline infusion. From these results they concluded that heat-induced and exercise-induced sweating in the donkey is controlled by adrenergic nerves, and that adreno-medullary secretion may contribute to sweating during exercise. Cutaneous blood flow was considered to be important in the response of the glands to humoral stimulation. From the view-point of the adrenergic innervation of the sweat gland, observations that heat-induced sweating could not be blocked by atropine, as reported by Muto (1916), Evans and Smith (1956) and Usenik (1958) would be easily understood. Although the mechanism controlling sweating in the horse seems to be further complicated by the fact that their sweat glands respond to intradermal injection of cholinergic agents and that the nerve fibers around the sweat glands are reactive for specific cholinesterase (Jenkinson, 1968), Usenik (1958) interpreted the action of acetylcholine releasing adrenaline from the adrenal medulla, based on his experiment in which acetylcholine, unlike adrenaline, did not induce sweating in an adrenalectomized horse. Aoki *et al.* (1959) on the contrary concluded that acetylcholine can have a direct action on horse sweat glands since the glands in vitro preparations responded to it.

4.   Apocrine Sweat Gland in the Dog

Experiments by Aoki and Wada (1951) and Aoki (1955) revealed that the apocrine gland in the hairy skin of the dog responded to local application of both adrenergic and cholinergic agents, while spontaneous sweating of nervous mechanism scarcely occurred. The sudorific effect of adrenaline was selectively inhibited by dihydroergotamine and that of acetylcholine and mecholyl by atropine, but was not affected by sympathectomy.

Iwabuchi (1967) observed that an infusion of adrenaline and noradrenaline into the non-anesthetized dog caused general sweating, suggesting that circulating catecholamines act directly on the gland.   General sweating which could be induced by asphyxiation was easily inhibited at the site of intradermal injection of dihydroergotamine in relatively low concentrations as well as at that of atropine in relatively high concentrations, but was not abolished by bilateral adrenal medullectomy.   From these results he concluded that the inhibitory effect of atropine on sweating produced by asphyxiation does not imply the presence of a cholinergic component in the nervous mechanism, and presumed that the glands of the hairy skin of the dog are innervated by adrenergic sympathetic nerve fibers.   He also showed that sweating on asphyxiation did not occur in sympathetically denervated skin, especially in animals which had been deprived of adrenal medullary secretion, suggesting that a nervous mechanism is involved in this form of sweating.

Aoki and Wada (1951), however, could induce sweating with radiant heat in localized areas of skin, even when the nerve supply had been removed by sympathectomy either with or without excision of the dorsal roots including their ganglia.   This evidence suggests that heat-induced sweating may have a different controlling mechanism from sweating induced by asphyxiation.

5.   Apocrine Sweat Gland in the Cattle

Muto (1916) reported that intravenous administration of pilocarpine produced marked sweating in the calf, concluding that the sweat gland of the ox is cholinergic.   Ferguson and Dowling (1955) observed the formation of sweat in response to an intradermal injection of adrenaline, and Taneja (1959) showed that dibenamine inhibited this response and reduced the moisture loss from the skin in a hot environment.

Findlay and Robertshaw (1965) reported that the sudorific effect of locally administered drugs was most potent with adrenaline, less potent with noradrenaline and isopropyl-noradrenaline, and that the sweating was partially inhibited by tolazoline (priscol), an adrenaline inhibitor, but not by atropine.   None of the cholinergic agents showed any sudomotor activity.   Sympathetic denervation considerably reduced thermal sweating, but did not abolish the response to intravenous or intradermal adrenaline.   Adrenomedullary denervation did not reduce the moisture loss from normal skin at environmental temperatures up to 40 °C.   Thermal sweating was abolished by adrenergic blocking agents such as bethanidine and dibenamine, but not by propranalol.   Adrenaline-induced sweating was blocked by dibenamine but not by bethanidine or propranalol.   From these observations, Findlay and Robertshaw concluded that sweating in cattle is controlled by an adrenergic mechanism requiring intact sympathetic nerves, and that under mild heat stress adreno-medullary secretion does not stimulate the sweat gland. Sweating is mediated by alpha receptors, there being no beta receptor component.

Joshi *et al.* (1968) have reported that in Haiana cattle under both cool and hot conditions, adrenaline, pilocarpine and acetylcholine stimulated sweat secretion, but atropine did not inhibit either drug-induced or thermally-induced sweating, concluding that the sweat gland in Haiana cattle is adrenergic in nature.

6. *Apocrine Sweat Gland in the Sheep and Goat*

The apocrine sweat gland of the sheep was demonstrated to respond to heat stimulation by Bligh (1961). Waites and Voglmayr (1963) showed that the scrotum of the sheep responded to heat stimulation as well as to intravenous administration of adrenaline, and that the response to heat stimulus was markedly reduced by sympathetic denervation. They claimed that sweating in this species is controlled by an adrenergic mechanism. Hayashi (1968) demonstrated that the sweat glands in the hairy skin of the sheep respond to intradermal or intravenous adrenaline, but not to pilocarpine, carbaminoylcholine or mecholyl. Intradermal noradrenaline was less potent and isopropylnoradrenaline was ineffective. By partial sympathectomy alone or combined with bilateral adrenal medullectomy, he showed that thermoregulatory sweating was produced primarily by excitation of the sympathetic adrenergic sweat nerves when heating was mild, and additionally by catecholamines from the adrenal medulla when their secretion was increased in association with heating.

Apocrine sweat gland in the hairy skin of the goat was investigated by Nakayama and Arimura (1955), Marzulli and Callahan (1957), Kimura and Aoki (1962), and Robertshaw (1968). While local administration of adrenaline was observed to be effective in inducing sweating in all experiments, pilocarpine was reported to be effective only by Nakayama and Arimura. The exposure of the animal's whole body to heat was revealed to be ineffective in causing sweat response in Nakayama and Arimura's experiment, but was demonstrated to cause sweating on the general hairy skin surfaced by other investigators. Kimura and Aoki also indicated that noradrenaline was effective in eliciting local sweating, but that neither isopropylnoradrenaline nor any of cholinergic agents were effective. They stated that dihydroergotamine, atropine and sympathetic denervation inhibited thermal sweating, but not the localized sweating induced by directly applied radiation. Robertshaw, besides confirming most of the above observations by Kimura and Aoki, demonstrated further that bilateral denervation of the adrenal medulla had no effect on the sweating pattern in either the sheep or the goat. He stated that sweating in the sheep and goat is controlled by an adrenergic mechanism, that the secretion of the adrenal medulla under conditions of mild heat stress does not stimulate the gland, and that the sweating is mediated by adrenergic alpha receptor, since thermal sweating was inhibited by alpha adrenergic blocking agents such as bethanedine or dibenamine but not by beta adrenergic blocking agents such as propranolol; further, he stated that sweating induced by intravenous adrenaline was blocked by dibenamine but not by propranolol.

From these observations it seems that sweating in the sheep and goat is similar to that in the ox, except in that isopropylnoradrenaline can cause mild sweating in the ox but not in the sheep and goat. Unilateral sympathectomy, thoracic in the calf (Findley and Robertshaw, 1965) and lumbar in the sheep (Waites and Voglmayr, 1963) and goat (Kimura and Aoki, 1962), considerably reduced sweating activity in response to heat on the denervated areas of the animals, but did not reduce the response of the gland to injected adrenaline.

SUMMARY

In surveying the sweating responses of the apocrine sweat glands in man and animals to cholinergic and adrenergic administrations and to their blocking agents, although many of the observations, especially those in animals, lack the differentiation of the excitability of the glands from the actual sweating response to the stimulation and inhibition, it was concluded that the apocrine sweat glands in the hairy skin surface of the cattle, sheep and goat seem to show adrenergic innervation. The apocrine glands of the horse and donkey also seem to show adrenergic innervation but they respond more intensely to locally administered cholinergic agents, compared with the apocrine glands in cattle, sheep and goats. Supposing Kuno's hypothesis concerning the evolutional development of the sweat glands from the apocrine to eccrine type to be true, it is therefore assumed that the apocrine sweat glands in the cattle, sheep and goat are more primitive than the human eccrine sweat gland, which has lost adrenergic innervation and is only controlled cholinergically. The adrenergic innervation in the apocrine sweat glands in man and monkey also seems to have degenerated and only remains in the myoepithelium. Accordingly, whether the actual sweating response is caused by adrenergic or cholinergic agents, the apocrine secretion may be only humorally potentiated with locally induced adrenaline or acetylcholine or with circulating catecholamines released from the adrenal medulla during emotional stress. The innervation of the apocrine sweat glands in the dog and horse would rank between the man-monkey group and cattle-sheep-goat group, although the dog is rather close to the former and the horse close to the latter.

REFERENCES

1. AAVIAK, O.R. (1955): *J. Invest. Dermat.* **24**: 103.
2. AOKI, T. (1962): *J. Invest. Dermat.* **39**: 115.
3. AOKI, T. (1962): *J. Invest. Dermat.* **38**: 41.
4. AOKI, T. (1955): *J. Invest. Dermat.* **24**: 545.
5. AOKI, T., and M. WADA (1951): *Science* **114**: 123.
6. AOKI, T., S. KIMURA, and M. WADA (1959): *J. Invest. Dermat.* **33**: 441.
7. BARCROFT, H., and H.J.C. SWAN (1953): Sympathetic Control of Human Blood Vessels. p. 118, Edward Arnold, London.
8. BARNET, A.J. (1951): *Nature* **167**: 482.
9. BENJAMIN, F.B. (1963): *J. Appl. Physiol.* **5**: 594.
10. BLIGH, J. (1961): *Nature Lond.* **189**: 582.
11. BLOZOVSKI, M., and J. SIVADJIAN (1959): *Arch. int. Pharmacodyn.* **123**: 58.
12. CHALMERS, T.M., and C.A. KEELE (1951): *J. Physiol.* **114**: 510.
13. CHALMERS, T.M., and C.A. KEELE (1952): *Brit. J. Dermat.* **64**: 43.
14. DALE, H.H., and W. FELDBERG (1934): *J. Physiol.* **82**: 121.
15. DARROW, C.W. (1937): *Arch. Neurol. Psyph.* **37**: 641.
16. ELLIOTT, T.R. (1905): *J. Physiol.* **32**: 401.
17. EVANS, C. LOVATT, D.F.G. SMITH, and H. WEIL-MALHERBE (1956): *J. Physiol.* **132**: 542.
18. EVANS, C., LOVATT, and D.F.G. SMITH (1956): *Proc. Roy. Soc. Lond.* B **145**: 61.
19. FERGUSON, K.A., and D.F. DOWLING (1955): *Aust. J. agric. Res.* **6**: 641.
20. FINDLAY, J.D., and D. ROBERTSHAW (1965): *J. Physiol.* **179**: 285.
21. FOSTER, K.G., J. GINSBURG, and J.S. WEINER (1967): *J. Physiol.* **191**: 131 P.
22. FOSTER, K.G., and J.S. WEINER (1970): *J. Physiol.* **210**: 883.
23. GORDON, B.I., and H.I. MAIBACH (1965): *A.M.A. Arch. Dermat.* **92**: 192.

24. HAIMOVICI, H. (1948): *Proc. Soc. exp. Biol. and Med.* **68:** 40.
25. HAIMOVICI, H. (1950): *J. Appl. Physiol.* **2:** 512.
26. HARRISON, J., and P.C.B. MACKINNON (1963): *Am. J. Physiol.* **204:** 785.
27. HAYASHI, H., and T. NAKAGAWA (1963): *J. Invest. Dermat.* **41:** 365.
28. HAYASHI, H. (1968): *Tohoku J. exp. Med.* **94:** 361.
29. HAYASHI, H. (1968): *Tohoku J. exp. Med.* **95:** 289.
30. VAN HEYNINGEN, R. and J.S. WEINER (1952): *J. Physiol.* **116:** 404.
31. HOUSTEK, J., and M. JIRKA (1968): *Vnitr. Lek.* **13:** 713, 1967.
32. HURLEY, H.J., and W.B. SHELLEY (1960): The Human Apocrine Sweat Gland in Health and Disease. Charles C Thomas, Springfield, Ill.
33. IKAI, K., K. SUGIYAMA, Y. OTSUKA, and H. NITTA (1970): *Jap. J. Physiol.* **20:** 250.
34. IKAI, K., K. SATO, H. KOZAWA, and H. NITTA (1970): *Proc. Japan Acad.* **46:** 203.
35. IKAI, K. (1968): *Cystic Fibrosis Club Abstracts* **9:** 9.
36. IKAI, K. (1968): *J. Invest. Dermat.* **50:** 272.
37. IKAI, K. (1968): *Proc. Int'l Union Physiol. Sci.* **7:** 207.
38. IKAI, K., K. SATO, K. SUGIYAMA, Y. OTSUKA, and H. NITTA (1969): *Nagoya Med. J.* **15:** 47.
39. ISSEKUTZ, B. JR., G. HETENYI, JR., and A. DIOSY (1950): *Arch. int. Pharmacodyn.* **83:** 133.
40. IWABUCHI, T. (1967): *J. Invest. Dermat.* **49:** 61.
41. JENKINSON, D.M., and P.S. BLACKBURN (1968): *Res. Vet. Sci.* **9:** 165.
42. JOSHI, B.C., R.E. MCDOWELL, and D.P. SADHU (1968): *J. Dairy Sci.* **51:** 905.
43. KENNARD, D.W. (1963): *J. Physiol.* **165:** 457.
44. KIMURA, S., and T. AOKI (1962): *Tohoku J. exp. Med.* **76:** 8.
45. KISIN, E.E. (1949): *Vestnik venerol. i. dermat.* **5:** 27, 1948. Quoted in *Chem. Abstr.* **43:** 2323.
46. KUNO, Y., T. YAMADA, and K. OHARA (1962): *Proc. Japan Acad.* **38:** 227.
47. KUNO, Y. (1965): Proc. 23rd Int'l Congr. Physiol. Sci., Excerpta Medica International Congress Series No. 87, page 3.
48. KUNO, Y. (1956): Human Perspiration. Charles C Thomas, Springfield, Ill.
49. LLOYD, D.P.C. (1959): *Nature* **184:** 277.
50. LLOYD, D.P.C. (1963): *J. Physiol.* **169:** 116 P.
51. LLOYD, D.P.C. (1964): *J. Physiol.* **175:** 74 P.
52. LLOYD, D.P.C. (1968): *Proc. natn. Acad. Sci. U.S.A.* **59:** 816.
53. MACINTYRE, B.A., R.W. BULLARD, M.R. BANERJEE, and R. ELIZONDO (1968): *J. Appl. Physiol.* **25:** 255.
54. MARZULLI, F.N., and J.F. CALLAHAN (1957): *J. Am. Veter. Med. Assoc.* **131:** 80.
55. MONTAGNA, W., and R.A. ELLIS (1960): *Am. J. Phys. Anthrop.* **18:** 69.
56. MONTAGNA, W. (1964): *J. Invest. Dermat.* **42:** 119.
57. MUTO, K. (1916): *Mitt. med. Fak. Tokio* **15**(2): 365.
58. NAKAMURA, Y., and K. HATANAKA (1958): *Tohoku J. exp. Med.* **68:** 225.
59. NAKAYAMA, T., and A. ARIMURA (1955): *J. Physiol. Soc. Jap.* **17:** 774.
60. OGAWA, T. (1970): *J. Appl. Physiol.* **28:** 18.
61. OGAWA, T. (1970): *Tohoku J. exp. Med.* **100:** 255.
62. RANDALL, W.C. (1947): *Am. J. Physiol.* **15:** 365.
63. ROBERTSHAW, D., and C.R. TAYLOR (1968): *J. Physiol.* **197:** 81 P.
64. ROBERTSHAW, D. (1968): *J. Physiol.* **198:** 53.
65. ROTHMAN, S. (1954): Physiology and Biochemistry of the Skin. The University of Chicago Press, Chicago.
66. SAKURAI, M., and W. MONTAGNA (1964): *J. Invest. Dermat.* **42:** 411.
67. SAKURAI, M., and W. MONTAGNA (1964): *J. Invest. Dermat.* **43:** 279.
68. SIVADJIAN, J., M. VAURIN, and H. MATGE (1965): *Arch. int. Pharmacodyn.* **153:** 359.
69. SONNENSCHEIN, R.R. (1949): *Proc. Soc. exp. Biol. and Med.* **71:** 654.
70. SONNENSCHEIN, R.R., H. KOBRIN, and M.I. GROSSMAN (1949): *Am. J. Physiol.* **3:** 573.
71. SONNENSCHEIN, R.R., H. KOBRIN, H.D. JANOWITZ, and M.I. GROSSMAN (1951): *J. Appl. Physiol.* **3:** 573.
72. SHELLEY, W.B. (1951): *J. Invest. Dermat.* **17:** 255.
73. SHELLEY, W.B., and H.J. HURLEY (1952): *Arch. Dermat and Syph.* **66:** 156.
74. SHELLEY, W.B., and H.J. HURLEY (1953): *J. Invest. Dermat.* **20:** 285.
75. TAKAHASHI, Y. (1964): *Tohoku J. exp. Med.* **83:** 205.
76. TANEJA, G.C. (1959): *J. agric. Sci.* **52:** 66.
77. USENIK, E.A. (1958): *Diss. Abstr.* **18:** 255.
78. WADA, M., and T. TAKAGAKI (1948): *Tohoku J. exp. Med.* **49:** 284.
79. WADA, M. (1950): *Science* **111:** 376.
80. WAITES, G.M.H., and J.K. VOGLMAYR (1962): *Nature (Lon.)* **196:** 965.
81. WAITES, G.M.H., and J.K. VOGLMAYR (1963): *Aust. J. agric. Res.* **14:** 839.
82. YASUDA, K., H. MACHIDA, and T. SUZUKI (1963): *Folia Anat. Jap.* **39:** 135.

CHAPTER 8

SALT CONCENTRATION IN SWEAT AND HEAT ADAPTABILITY

Kōkichi OHARA

2nd Department of Physiology, Nagoya City University Medical School, Nagoya, Japan

Sweat volume as well as the salt concentration in sweat (expressed usually as NaCl concentration in sweat) shows adaptation to differing amounts of heat, this adaptation due either to artificial training in resistance to heat or to living in a hot climate. Sweating is thus a good source of information about heat adaptability. Therefore it has been widely used as a guide in studies relating to this problem.

Various parameters have been used in investigating sweating, such as sweat volume, salt concentration in sweat, numbers of active sweat glands, threshold core temperature for initiation of sweating, changes in sweat volume per unit change in core temperature, rate of sweat suppression and others. Among the factors mentioned above, salt concentration in sweat is considered, as pointed out by Kuno [2], to be the most reliable index of heat tolerance. The lowering of salt concentration in sweat after heat exposure was demonstrated by a large number of investigators [3–13]. However, no definite conclusion have been drawn about the extent to which salt concentration in sweat represents heat adaptability, either quantitatively or qualitatively. At the present stage of investigation the problem seems to be answered not theoretically but by empirical explanation drawn from accumulated experimental data covering a large number of subjects, all demonstrating varying adaptability to heat.

THE STANDARD VALUE OF SALT CONCENTRATION IN SWEAT IN INDIVIDUALS

Since salt concentration in sweat is influenced by various factors, physiological and/or experimental, it is difficult to give it any standard value. To solve this problem sweat sampling should be performed under controlled experimental conditions. To determine the salt concentration in sweat, fluctuation due to the following factors should be taken into account.

1. Fluctuation due to Body Region

Sweating in the palm, sole and axilla differ generally from that of the general body surface due to thermoregulation (Kuno [2]). A higher salt content than in other areas was reported in palm sweat by Dill *et al.* [10], Ikai *et al.* [14], Lobitz and Osterberg [15] and Van Heyninger and Weiner [16]. Even in the case of the general body surface, volume and composition of sweat fluctuate according to the region. Since salt content in sweat is also related to sweat rate the issue is even further complicated.

It is therefore difficult to choose any one body region as the standard one for sweat sampling, and using of mixed sweat from the general body surface seems to be the best solution.   However, there are technical difficulties involved in the collection of mixed sweat such as avoiding contamination, evaporation and condensation.   Because of the difficulties in collecting mixed sweat due to variation in standardized sweat rate, the situation may better be met by collecting sweat in different body areas and obtaining mean values.

2.   Fluctuation due to Sweat Rate

There are many reports which deal with variations in sweat composition according to sweat rate.   Because of this variation, any measurement of salt concentration in sweat which was taken without regard to sweat rate is less meaningful.   Salt concentration in sweat is correctly expressed when it is relative to a given rate of sweating, and the rate of its increase to that of sweat rate.   For practical purpose Kuno [2] proposed using maximal salt concentration as a standard.   Salt concentration in sweat increases as sweating become profuse in response to any sudorific stimulus, as demonstrated in Fig.

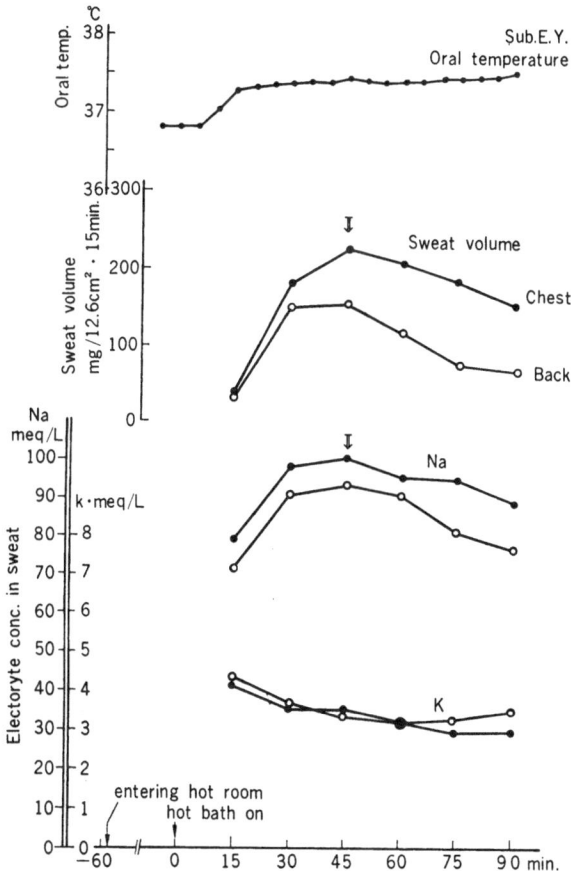

Fig. 62. Sweat volume, sweat sodium concentration and body tempeature during heat exposure. Maximal sweat rate and maximal sodium concentration in sweat were given by those indicated by arrows. Kalium content in sweat is also given in the figure.

62, reaching a maximal concentration and remaining unchanged for a considerable period of time, as long as sweating is at its maximum. As sweating is suppressed after a maximum period, salt concentration usually declines with decreasing sweat rate, however the parallel relationship between the two is less pronounced than when sweat rate is increasing. Occasionally sweat salt concentration continues to increase during the suppression period to reach a very high level, approaching that of blood plasma (Kyutoku [3] and Ohara [17]). The mechanism of this sudden increase in salt content has not yet been fully elucidated. Some investigators consider it to be a demonstration of fatigue in the sweat glands (Collins and Weiner [18] and Sibinga and Barbero [19]). In any case, the values obtained in this period should not be used as a standard.

3. *Fluctuation due to Salt or Water Intake*

The effect of salt intake on salt concentration in sweat was studied by Robinson *et al.* [5] who demonstrated that the salt content in sweat decreased with a daily intake of 3 gr NaCl and increased with a 11.8 gr daily intake. The onset of an adjustment by the regulating mechanism for salt discharge in sweat was about three days later than that of the kidney, where increased salt intake was followed by an increased excretion of salt within one to two hours (Robinson *et al.* [20]). According to Sigal and Dobson [21] subjects with a low salt intake (0.5 gr NaCl per day) had a consistently lower rate of sodium excretion in sweat than those with a high salt intake (16–28 gr NaCl per day). The sweat rate was said not to be affected by salt intake. On the other hand, Schwartz and Thaysen [22] and Kyutoku [3] found no effect of salt intake upon salt content in sweat. As for the effect of water intake, Pearcy *et al.* [23] reported that sweat rate during work in heat in deliberately dehydrated men was consistently about 15% below the rate observed when they were fully hydrated. Cage *et al.* [24] found that drinking one to three liters of water caused an increase in sweat rate but no changes in sweat composition (Na, K, Cl and lactate). It may be said that, though standardized dietary intake of salt and water is recommended, there is no significant deviation in salt concentration in sweat due to these factors, as long as no artificial deficiency or surfeit is created.

4. *Fluctuation due to Cutaneous Blood Flow (Local Skin Temperature)*

A higher salt concentration in sweat was reported by Robinson *et al.* [25] in the arm where skin temperature had been warmed to about 36–37 °C than that in the arm where skin temperature was lower by about 10 °C than the former. A lower chloride content was observed by Ladell [26] in sweat from the arm after arterial occlusion. Van Heyninger and Weiner [27] also reported that chloride content in sweat decreased after arterial occlusion but that this was not due to changes in skin temperature. No direct effect of skin temperature upon salt concentration in sweat was observed by Dill *et al.* [10] and Cage and Dobson [28] when observing sweating during exercise. From these findings it may be concluded that the effect of skin temperature, though it can influence sweat volume locally as well as centrally through the thermoregulatory reflex, does not greatly affect salt concentration in sweat, as long as salt concentration is measured in relation to sweat rate and as long as no great thermal or circulatory change is induced artificially in the area of skin tested.

5. *Fluctuation due to Thermal and Exercise Sweating*

It was pointed out by Kuno [2] that the general features of sweating vary according to whether the sweating is caused thermally or by muscular exercise. Kuno [29] said that thermal sweating is induced essentially by nervous action while during exercise sweat secretion is caused largely by a humoral process due to adrenaline discharge. Differences in sweat composition were also reported by Ikai *et al.* [14], sodium concentration being higher in exercise sweat than in thermal sweat taken at the same sweat rate. Sweat composition in the case of adrenergic sweating will be discussed in detail in Ikai's report in this monograph. It thus seems necessary to standardize the causal agencies of sweating to determine standard values in sweat composition.

METHOD FOR THE DETERMINATION OF STANDARD VALUES
FOR SWEATING IN INDIVIDUALS

Considering the factors discussed above which influence the volume of sweat and salt concentration in sweat, sampling of sweat was made by the following standardized procedures. Sweat was collected from the chest and back of subjects wearing only swimming trunks with the filter paper method using a sweatc up (Ohara [17]) made of acrylate plaster covering a skin area of 12.6 cm^2. Sweating was induced in a room with a controlled temperature of 30 °C and a relative humidity of 60–70% with immersion of both legs to just below the knee in a stirred water bath of 43 °C. Sweat samples were collected at intervals of 15 minutes for 90 minutes following the immersion. Sweat volume and sodium concentration in sweat was measured by gravimetric and flame-photometric methods, respectively. Maximum sweat rate as well as maximum sodium concentration in sweat was estimated as demonstrated in Fig. 62. Averages obtained from the two sampled areas were used as the standard value for individuals. Oral temperature was measured with a thermistor thermometer at intervals corresponding to the period of maximal sweat rate.

SWEATING FUNCTION EXPRESSED AS A COMBINATION OF SWEAT
VOLUME AND SALT CONCENTRATION IN SWEAT

Sweating ability can be expressed in terms of various factors, among which sweat volume and salt concentration in sweat are most significant in relation to heat adaptability. Adaptable changes in both of these areas has been widely studied, and it was found that their respective adaptative development differs. Upon application of heat whether it is intermittent, transitory or perpetual, salt concentration in sweat declines. On the other hand, sweat volume increases at first, but decreases as heat exposure is prolonged, as is evidenced in the case of inhabitant of the tropics (Kosuge and Kawahata [30]). Habituation processes (Hensel [31] and Glaser and Whittow [32]) may be responsible for this. We lack direct evidence about the relationship between heat tolerance and the physiological loss of salt and water in sweat. However, it may be that loss of these materials in sweat causes not only heat loss through evaporation but also disturbances in volume and composition of body fluid through which various thermoregulatory functions are secondarily affected. Sweating ability must be represented in its relation to heat adaptability, as an index involving sweat volume and salt concentration together. "Sweating type," as it is expressed, is a combined evaluation of sweat volume and salt concentration in the sweat of individuals.

SWEATING TYPE AS AN INDICATOR FOR SWEATING
ABILITY

Values of sweat volume and sodium concentration in sweat are plotted in Fig. 63, with
sweat volume as abscissa and sodium concentration as ordinate, for 109 Japanese subjects studied in the same season (summer).   There is very wide individual variation in
both variables, but individuals can be assigned to one of the four types of sweating ability
when the values of the two parameters investigated are evaluated as high or low as compared with respective mean values obtained for the population.   The determination
of the sweating type of individuals is simply made according to the location of individuals
in four sections bounded by vertical and horizontal lines through the population mean,
as demonstrated in the figure.   Four types were named as follows: type 1 (high sweat
volume, high salt concentration), type 2 (high sweat volume, low salt concentration),
type 3 (low sweat volume, high salt concentration) and type 4 (low sweat volume, low
salt concentration).   The characteristics of sweating types thus determined are as follows:

1. *Individuality of Sweating Type*
It was demonstrated by Ohara [11] and Sargent *et al.* [33] that sweat volume and salt
concentration in sweat show reproducible patterns though they vary very much indi-

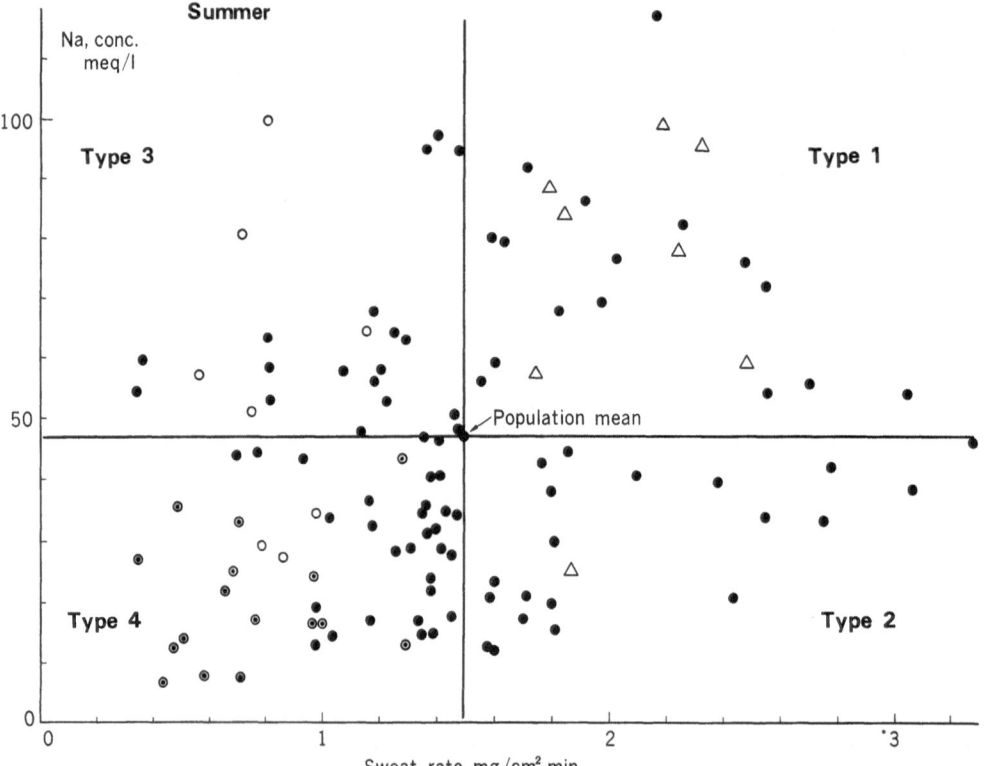

Fig. 63. Distribution of sweat volume and sodium concentration in sweat in Japanese subjects.
Determination of sweating type, see text. ●: Non-Ainu Japanese males, ⊙: Non-Ainu Japanese
females, △: Ainu males, ○: Ainu females.

vidually.   The same thing can be confirmed in various other reports made on sweating. This fact results in an individual ranking order refering to these two parameters.   The ranking order is, as shown in Fig. 64, unchanged with the season.   Since sweating type is to be determined based upon evaluation of the two parameters relative to the respective population mean (in other words, due to their ranking order in the population), it necessarily shows a pattern which persists regardless of changes in season.   The following findings confirm the individuality of sweating type.   The absolute values of sweat volume and salt concentration in sweat vary in individuals with the season, resulting in changes in the population mean.   Fig. 65 demonstrates the distribution pattern of the measures in 214 Japanese subjects.   In spite of seasonal changes, sweating type of individuals was found to be not influenced by season when the assessment was made with reference to the

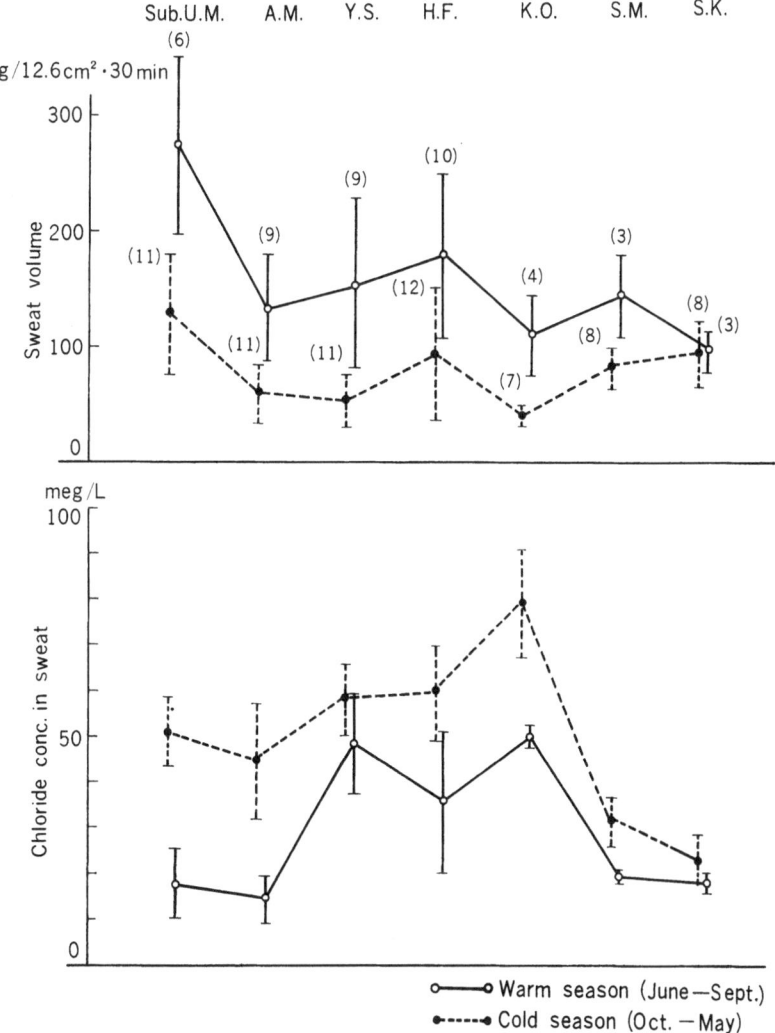

Fig. 64.   Season independet individual ranking order of sweat volume and salt concentration in sweat.   Numbers given in the upper figure are numbers of estimation made in the respective season. Vertical bars are standard deviation of the measures.   The figure was made using data from Ohara's report [11].

population mean in the respective season.   Fig. 66 shows the sweating type of 35 persons subjected to experiments both in summer and winter.   In the figure, population means in two seasons are plotted so as to overlap one another.   Eighteen out of 35 persons stayed in the same section irrespective of the season.   When individual variations due to technical and/or physiological factors are taken into account, very few individuals of the total 35 were considered to show an essentially different sweating type according to season.   The reproducibility of sweating type independent of season was also confirmed by Osada et al. [13].   It is therefore conceivable that the sweating type represents some permanent constitutional condition not influenced by short term exposure to heat such as changes in season, which cause only transitory adaptation.

2. Relationships with Other Thermoregulatory Functions

A close relationship was observed between sweating type and increase in body temperature as well as body temperature level after heat exposure.   As demonstrated in Fig. 67 with Japanese males in summer and winter, larger increase in body temperature and higher levels of body temperature were observed in types 1 and 3 as compared with

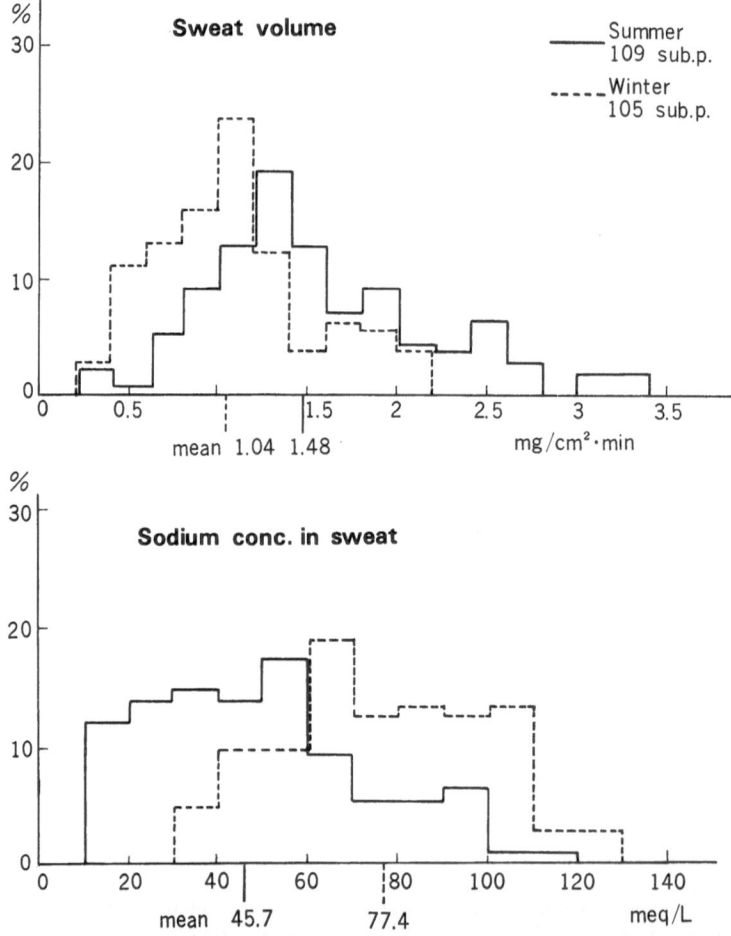

Fig. 65. Seasonal changes in frequency distribution of sweat volume as well as sodium concentration in sweat for 214 Japanese subjects.   Respective sample means are given downward.

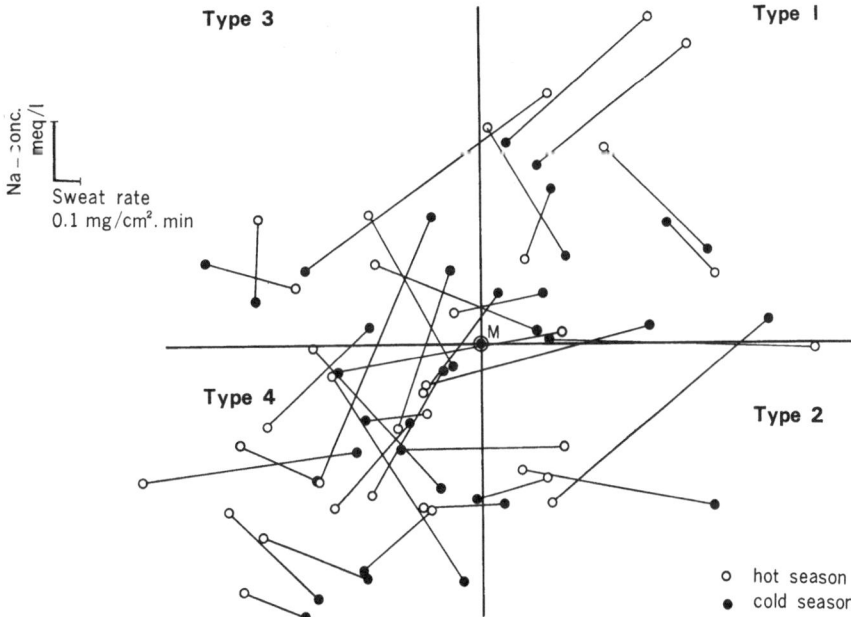

Fig. 66. Reproducibility of sweating type, unrelated to season.

types 2 and 4. The between-types differences in the increase as well as in the elevated levels of body temperature following the heat exposure were found statistically significant in summer experiments, while they were less significant in winter. In the figure, the latent time with which the sweating tended to decline during heat exposure is also demonstrated. Type 1 showed the longest latency period. This means that in type 1, as a high sweat volume and high salt content type, the loss of water and salt in sweat is facilitated more by prolonged profuse sweating. In addition, it was observed that all the subjects (three out of 214 cases) who fainted during heat exposure or could not accomplish the experiment were those designated as type 1. From all these findings it may be concluded that type 1 is the least tolerant of heat, type 3 resembling type 1, and that types 2 and 4 can tolerate heat best.

3. Frequency Distribution of Sweating Types in Groups Differently Adapted to Heat

While it is assumed that heat adaptability in individuals is indicated by sweating type, adaptability of any group may better be represented by the frequency distribution of the sweating types of its members. The frequency distribution of sweating types are summarized in Fig. 68 for various groups which differ from each other ecologically or racially. For non-Ainu Japanese males types 2 and 4, especially type 4, are frequently observed in a group living in the Nagoya district (mild climate), while types 1 and 3 are frequent in a group born and living in Hokkaido, a northern island of Japan (colder climate). The distribution pattern for each group is essentially the same in summer and winter. The difference in distribution pattern is considered to be caused by the ecological situation of the groups. The observation shows that types 2 and 4 occurred more frequently in the group more adapted to heat and, to the contrary, types 1 and 3 were more frequent in the group less adapted to heat.

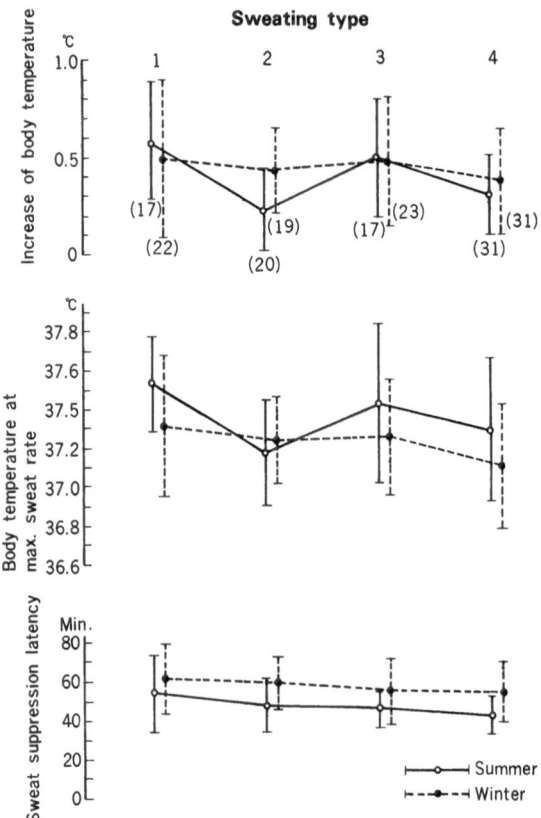

Fig. 67. Relationship between sweating type and increase in body temperature, level of increased body temperature and latency period of sweating suppression during heat exposure. Numbers given in parenthesis are numbers of subjects assigned to each respective type. Vertical bars are standard deviation.

A remarkable racial difference was found between Ainu males and non-Ainu Japanese males born and living in the same district in Hokkaido island. Though no great difference was observed between the two groups in living habits and food intake, Ainu males showed a high percentage of type 1 when compared with non-Ainu Japanese males, especially in summer. This indicates that Ainu males discharge large amounts of sweat of high salt concentration in summer. This finding contradicts that by Kawahata and Sakamoto [34] who could not find any detectable difference in sweat volume and salt content in sweat between the two races, except for smaller numbers of active sweat glands in the Ainu. A significantly narrower distribution was also demonstrated by calculation of F-values for sweat volume in the Ainu in summer as compared with non-Ainu Japanese (Fig. 63). These observations may indicate that the Ainu is less adaptable to heat than the non-Ainu Japanese, presumably in part due to their genetic make up. This observation may correspond to the findings of Itoh et al. [35] that the Ainu is cold adapted, showing ethnic differences in metabolic responses of non-shivering thermogenesis from those of ordinary Japanese.

A definite sex difference was demonstrated in frequency distribution both in the Ainu and non-Ainu Japanese. Females differ remarkably from males in the absence of types

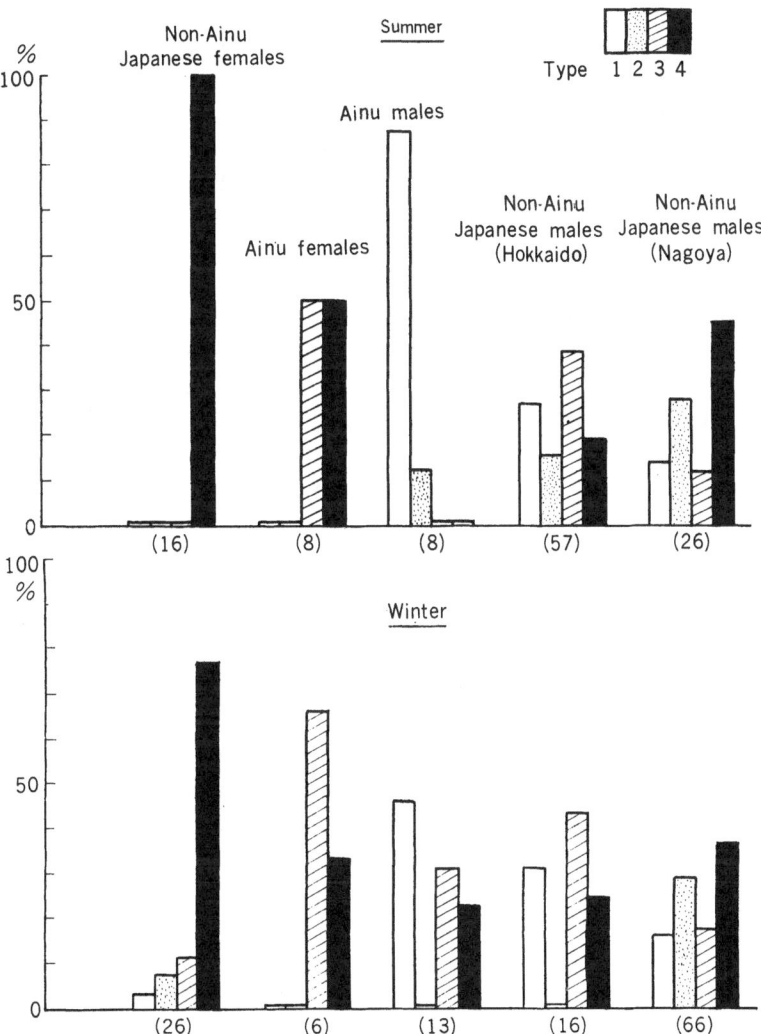

Fig. 68. Frequency distribution of sweating types in various groups in summer and winter. Numbers under each group indicate numbers of persons.

1 and 2 in any season. In non-Ainu Japanese almost all females tested were assigned to type 4, showing low sweat volume and low salt concentration. Regarding heat tolerance in females, reports previously made show conflicting results. Fox *et al.* [36], Hertig *et al.* [37], and Hirokawa *et al.* [38] reported that females are less tolerant of heat than males, while Weiman *et al.* [39] and Morimoto *et al.* [40] observed more efficient thermoregulation in women during heat stress. Wyndham *et al.* [41] and Bar-or *et al.* [42] found no difference between the sexes. When the observations regarding the relationship between sweating type and heat adaptability previously discussed are extended to include women, it may be concluded that women are more heat tolerant than men.

The representation of sweating function presented here was further studied by Osada *et al.* [13] in reference to heat tolerance. In this study sweating type was determined by using a modification of the original method described above, using the angle and length of the segment connecting the population mean and individual measures in a figure plotted as in Fig. 63.   Twenty parameters for thermoregulatory, circulatory and hormonal functions were studied together with sweating type.   It was reported by the authors that the respective rises in body temperature, heart rate and pulse pressure as well as sweating type are recommendable parameters to be used in studying heat tolerance, and that sweating type is of a higher reproducibility than other factors.   Inoue and Hori [43] proposed to classify sweating ability into five sweating types, in which individuals should be classified as type 5 whose values of sweat volume and salt concentration are within the range of a standard deviation from the respective population means.   They also proposed a new index for heat tolerance which is calculated as index $= \sqrt{A^2 + B^2 + C^2}$, where A is the loss of water in sweat measured by loss of body weight, B is an increase in body temperature and C is the salt lost in sweat.

SUMMARY

There are many reports which deal with sweating ability, both as to sweat volume and salt concentration in sweat, in its relation to heat adaptability or heat tolerance.   However, owing to great individual fluctuations in these parameters, even in a group of approximately equally acclimatized men, it is essentially impossible to predict with accuracy the degree of heat adaptability of individuals using the absolute value of the parameters investigated.   Ladell [44] proposed the use of a regression calculated from the improvement of sweating by successive exposure to heat in a group as a standard of comparison, or 'scale' against which the degree of heat acclimatization of other groups can be estimated.   In the present studies, loss of salt in sweat (salt concentration in sweat) and that of water (sweat volume) were evaluated not by their absolute values but relatively in comparison with the respective population means, namely, according to their ranking orders in the population.   In addition, the result of evaluation of the two parameters were cross related to determine "sweating type," which can represent sweating ability as a whole.   The characteristics of sweating type were investigated for individual as well as groups, resulting in findings which related closely to heat adaptability.   Studies on those lines are in progress, and it is expected that the relationship between sweating and heat adaptability will be elucidated more clearly from the new conceptional basis presented here.

REFERENCES

1. WEINER, J.S. and J.A. LOURIE (eds.) (1969): Human, Biology Backlwell Scient. Publ., Oxford.
2. KUNO, Y.: Human Perspiration, Charless C. Thomas, Springfield, Illinois.
3. KYUTOKU, T. (1940):   *J. Physiol. Soc. Japan* 5: 395–410 (in Japanese).
4. KAWAHATA, A., and S. ITOH (1943):   *J. Physiol. Soc. Japan* 8: 648–662 (in Japanese).
5. ROBINSON, S., R.K. KINCAID, and R.K. RHARY (1950):   *J. Appl. Physiol.* 3: 55–62.
6. KAWAHATA, A. (1951):   *Igaku-to-Seibutsugaku* 21: 65–68 (in Japanese).
7. TSUJI, T. (1962):   *Bull. Inst. Constit. Med. Kumamoto Univ.* 13: 29–48 (in Japanese).
8. WYNDHAM, C.H., N.B. STRYDOM, J.F. MORRISON, C.G. WILLIAMS, G.A.G. BREDELL, M.J.E. VON RAHDEN, L.D. HOLDSWORTH, C.H. VAN GRAAN, A.J. VAN RENSBURG, and A. MUNRO (1964):   *J. Appl. Physiol.* 19: 598–666.
9. SARGENT II, F., C.R. SMITH, and D.L. BATTERTON (1965):   *Int. J. Biometeor.* 9: 229–231.
10. DILL, D.B., F.G. HALL, and W. VAN BEAUMONT (1966):   *J. Appl. Physiol.* 21: 99–106.
11. OHARA, K. (1966):   *Jap. J. Physiol.* 16: 274–290.

12. KOSAKA, T., and S. TAKEUCHI (1967): *Niigata Med. J.* **81:** 114–120 (in Japanese).
13. OSADA, Y., S. TSUNASHIMA, K. YOSHIDA, S. OGAWA, A. HIROKAWA, K. NAKAMURA, and K. HARUTA (1969): *Bull. Inst. Public Health* **18:** 187–201 (in Japanese).
14. IKAI, K., K. SATO, K. SUGIYAMA, Y. OTSUKA, and H. NITTA (1969): *Nagoya Med. J.* **15:** 47–66.
15. LOBITZ, W.C., and A.E. OSTERBERG (1947): *Arch. Dermat. Syph.* **56:** 462–467.
16. VAN HEYNINGER, R., and J.S. WEINER (1952): *J. Physiol.* **116:** 395–403.
17. OHARA, K. (1968): *Nagoya Med. J.* **14:** 133–144.
18. COLLINS, K.J., and J.S. WEINER (1962): In: Biometeorology. p. 280 Pergamon Press, Oxford.
19. SIBINGA, M.S., and G.J. BARBERO (1961): *Pediatrics* **27:** 912–920.
20. ROBINSON, S., J.R. NICHOLAS, J.H. SMITH, J.W. DALY, and M. PEARCY (1955): *J. Appl. Physiol.* **8:** 159–165.
21. SIGAL, C.B., and R.L. DOBSON (1968): *J. Invest. Dermat.* **50:** 451–455.
22. SCHWARTZ, I.L., and J.H. THAYSEN (1956): *J. Clin. Invest.* **35:** 114–120.
23. PEARCY, M., S. ROBINSON, D.L. MILLER, J.T. THOMAS, and J. DEBROTA (1956): *J. Appl. Physiol.* **8:** 621–626.
24. CAGE, G.W., S.M. WOLFE, R.H. THOMPSON, and R.S. GORDON (1970): *J. Appl. Physiol.* **29:** 687–690.
25. ROBINSON, S., S.D. GERKING, E.S. TURRELL, and R.K. KINCAID (1950): *J. Appl. Physiol.* **2:** 654–662.
26. LADELL, W.S.S. (1951): *J. Physiol.* **115:** 69.
27. VAN HEYNINGER, R., and J.S. WEINER (1952): *J. Physiol.* **116:** 404–413.
28. CAGE, G.W., and R.L. DOBSON (1965): *J. Clin. Invest.* **44:** 1270–1275.
29. KUNO, Y. (1965): *Proc. 3rd Internat. Congr. Physiol. Sci.* Series No. **87:** 3–16.
30. KOSUGE, T., and A. KAWAHATA (1939): *J. Physiol. Soc. Japan* **4:** 212–220 (in Japanese). Also cited by Kuno [2].
31. HENSEL, H. (1964): In: Handbook of Physiology Section IV: Adaptation to the environment. p. 55 D.B. Dill, E.F. Adolph and C.G. Wilber (eds.). Am. Physiol. Soc., Washington.
32. GLASER, E.M., and G.C. WHITTOW (1957): *J. Physiol.* **136:** 98–111.
33. SARGENT, F., T. MORIMOTO, and K. OHARA (1966): *Biometrie Humaine* **3–4:** 97–137.
34. KAWAHATA, A., and H. SAKAMOTO (1951): *Jap. J. Physiol.* **2:** 166–169.
35. ITOH, S., K. DOI, and A. KUROSHIMA (1970): *Intern. J. Biomet.* **14:** 195–200.
36. FOX, R.H., B.L. LÖFSTEDT, P.M. WOODWARD, E. ERIKSSON, and B. WERKSTROM (1969): *J. Appl. Physiol.* **26:** 444–453.
37. HERTIG, B.A., H.S. BELDING, K.K. KRANING, D.L. BATTERTON, C.R. SMITH, and F. SARGENT II (1963): *J. Appl. Physiol.* **18:** 383–386.
38. HIROKAWA, A., S. TSUNASHIMA, and K. HARUTA (1969): *Bull. Inst. Public Health* **18:** 113–122 (in Japanese).
39. WEIMAN, K.P., Z. SLABOCHOVA, E.M. BERNAUR, T. MORIMOTO, and F. SARGENT II (1967): *J. Appl. Physiol.* **22:** 533–538.
40. MORIMOTO, T., Z. SLABOCHOVA, R.K. NAMAN, and F. SARGENT II (1967): *J. Appl. Physiol.* **22:** 526–532.
41. WYNDHAM, G.H., J.F. MORRISON, and C.G. WILLIAMS (1965): *J. Appl. Physiol.* **20:** 357–364.
42. BAR-OR, O., H.M. LUNDEGREN, and E.R. BUSKIRK (1969): *J. Appl. Physiol.* **26:** 403–409.
43. Personal communication.
44. LADELL, W.S.S. (1951): *J. Physiol.* **115:** 296–312.

CHAPTER 9

DESERT SWEAT RATES

D. B. DILL

*Laboratory of Environmental Patho-Physiology, Desert Research Institute, University of
Nevada System, Boulder City, Nevada, U.S.A.*

INTRODUCTION

What determines the rate of sweating in the desert? How is sweat rate related to work
capacity? How is sweat rate related to composition of sweat? We have provisional
answers to these questions; our exploration of this field has raised other questions that
remain to be answered. I propose to describe some of our studies of exercise in desert
heat in honoring Professor Yas Kuno who on March 30, 1970 reached the 88th milestone
of his rich and happy life. His contributions and those of his students have widened
the boundaries of physiology. His *The Physiology of Human Perspiration* has been a classic
since its publication in 1934 [6]. He brought this up to date in 1956 [7].

METHODS AND SUBJECTS

In general the rate of sweating in the desert depends on the need for dissipating heat.
In one type of our experiments two subjects walk over a 711-meter course for about an
hour. The course with a maximum grade of 2% up and down passes the rear door of
our laboratory; each subject is weighed to ± 20 g at the start and at the end of laps
1, 3, 5, etc. Skin temperatures, Ts, are observed as the subject walks past the door
after laps 2, 4, 6, etc. The subject picks up the thermocouple and thermos bottle containing the cold junction, walks past the door trailing a 30 m lead. He places the thermocouple on four sites in turn while the observer reads the potentiometer. The method
was described originally by Aldrich [2]. Fuller details of its use have been given by
Dill, Hall and van Beaumont [3]. The subjects start about 200 meters apart so aside
from about 30 seconds delay while they are weighed they maintain the same metabolic
rate and are exposed to the same environmental conditions. Rectal temperatures, T_{re}
are observed before and after; heart rates are monitored throughout by telemetry using
the Parks instrument (Parks Electronics Laboratory, Beaverton, Ore.). In each lap of
each walk observations of meteorological condition are made using instruments set up
near the course.* For air temperature a mercury thermometer is supported one meter
from the ground in an open-ended wire-mesh cylinder covered with aluminun foil.
It is 10 cm in diameter and 45 cm long. At the same height on the other side of this

---

*The stress of walking in the hot desert is more closely related to black body temperature than to air tem-
perature so this is used as our index to heat stress. Wind can modify the response but wind speeds
generally were less than 15 km per hr and rarely 30 km per hr.

support is hung a thin-gauge copper sphere 20 cm in diameter and painted flat black; a mercury thermometer is fitted into an aperture at the top with its bulb near the center of the sphere. The readings on this thermometer are called black-body temperature, T_{bb}. For wind speed a portable anemometer is used.

The rate of walking in the experiments to be described is 100 m per min. This increases O_2 consumption to about five times the basal rate. In preliminary walks O_2 consumption and CO_2 production were determined for each individual. From these measurements a correction of the weight loss can be made for the excess weight of CO_2 over O_2. However this correction proved to be of negligible importance in the present experiments so it was disregarded. Other weight losses include water from the sweat glands, water that diffuses through the skin and water from the lungs and air-way. Water from all these sources is available for temperature regulation. Hence for our purposes weight loss has been used as a measure of total water evaporated.

The subjects besides my colleague Yousef and myself were students or recent graduates of the Boulder City High School. Two, Faulkner and Connors, were chosen because of excess weight; the others are honor students in science who are assistants in the laboratory. While all are fit, only one, Richardson is a member of an athletic team—basketball.

RESULTS

In one set of experiments the same two students walked together on 10 different days. Table 8 shows for each walk the mean black body and skin temperatures, the increments

TABLE 8   Observations on Evans and Loftis in 10 one-hr walks at 100 m/min

Date	T_{bb} °C	T_s °C		ΔT_{re} °C		Final HR		Wt Loss, g/m²		Δwt, g
		E	L	E	L	E	L	E	L	
7-27	51	35.6	35.6	0.9	1.9	112	136	446	537	+91
7-28	50	35.1	35.3	1.0	0.6	116	137	401	430	+29
7-29	43	34.7	35.4	0.7	0.3	107	118	435	396	−39
7-30	48	34.3	34.5	0.9	1.6	116	122	367	383	+16
7-31	53	36.1	37.0	0.9	0.6	129	135	542	564	+22
8-3	44	34.3	33.8	0.9	0.8	112	134	373	356	−17
8-4	37	32.5	33.1	0.4	0.9	106	127	232	174	−58
8-5	52	35.1	35.6	1.2	0.6	126	130	407	389	−18
8-6	58	35.6	36.4	0.9	0.9	134	138	486	497	+11
8-7	53	35.3	35.2	0.8	0.9	117	133	446	416	−30
Mean		34.9	35.2	0.9	0.9	118	131	414	414	0

Note: Evans—Male, age 18, wt 63 kg, bsa 1.77 m².
       Loftis—Female, age 15, wt 48 kg, bsa 1.49 m².

in rectal temperature, the final heart rates and the weight losses expressed in g per m² of body surface. Fig. 69 illustrates the heart rates throughout each walk.

In another set of experiments Yousef, Dill, seven boys, and three girls paired off in 10 different combinations for the walk. Table 9 includes mean T_{bb}, body wt, body surface and weight loss related to body surface. The heart rates for each pair of subjects are shown in Fig. 70. It will be noted that the range of T_{bb} values is from 44–58 C and that on the days the girls walked it is 47 C for Dewey, 44 C for Singleton and 47 and 52 C for Loftis.

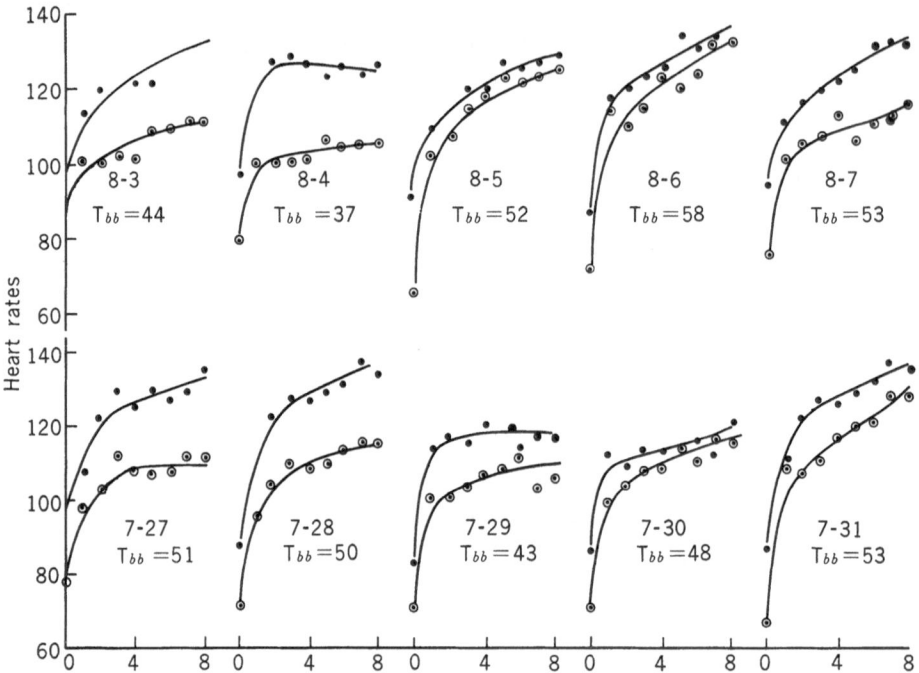

Fig. 69. Heart rates in Evans, circles, and Loftis, dots, walking for an hour at 100 m per min. Evans, male, was age 18 and Loftis, female, 15. The black body temperature, T_{bb} varied from 37 to 58 C. The heart rates remained below 140 but continued to rise, most rapidly on the hottest days.

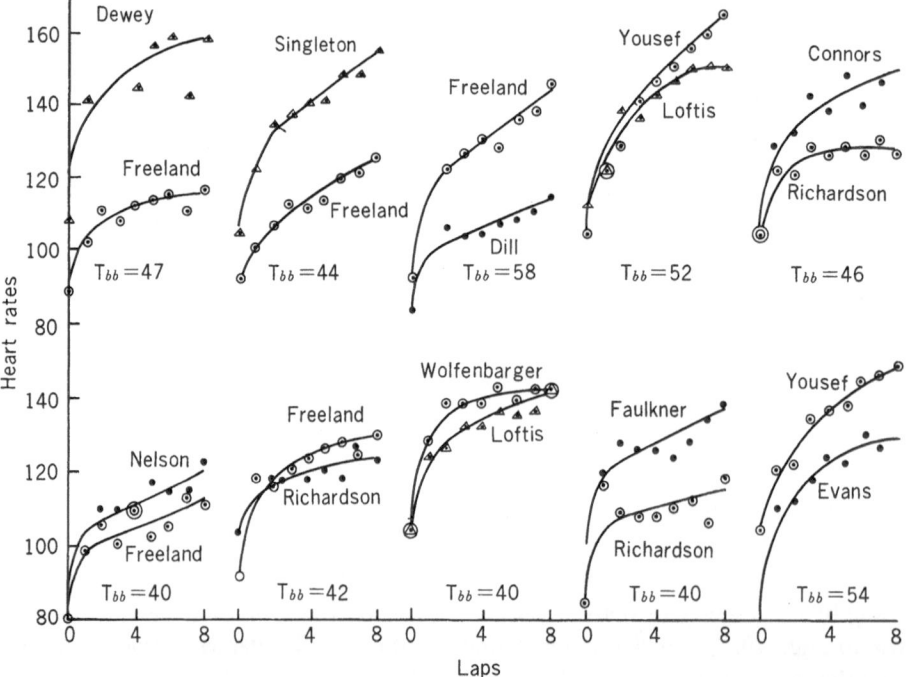

Fig. 70. Heart rates in 10 pairs including three girls, Dewey, Singleton and Loftis walking for an hour at 100 m per min. Note that in most subjects the heart rates continued to rise.

TABLE 9 Observations on 10 pairs of subjects, June and July, 1970. Ages 15–18
except Yousef, 34, and Dill, 79

Subjects and sex	T_{bb} °C	T_s °C	ΔT_{re} °C	Body wt. kg	Body surface m²	Wt. loss g/m²	ΔWt. g
Freeland, M	47	33.4	0.3	64	1.85	373	
Dewey, F		35.1	1.5	51	1.54	338	35
Freeland, M	40	32.3	0.3	64	1.85	341	
Nelson, M		32.7	0.9	59	1.71	327	14
Freeland, M	44	32.3	0.4	64	1.85	303	
Singleton, F		32.4		62	1.72	337	34
Freeland, M	52	35.3	1.4	64	1.85	395	
Richardson, M		32.9	0.8	70	1.90	468	73
Freeland, M	58	34.9	0.9	64	1.85	530	
Dill, M		33.4	1.4	71	1.88	626	96
Wolfenbarger, M	47	36.2	0.7	48	1.48	311	
Loftis, F		36.4	−0.1	48	1.49	302	9
Loftis, F	52	37.5	0.6	48	1.49	597	
Yousef, M		35.0	1.2	85	2.03	586	11
Evans, M	54	36.4	0.7	63	1.77	452	
Yousef, M		35.5	0.9	85	2.03	448	4
Richardson, M	40	32.7	0.5	70	1.90	478	
Faulkner, M		34.1	1.5	89	2.03	409	69
Richardson, M	46	33.3	0.8	70	1.90	566	
Connors, M		33.0	1.2	90	2.08	514	52

In the 10 experiments in which Evans and Loftis walked together T_{bb} varied from 37–58 C. Not all girls can walk for an hour at 100 m/min on our hotter summer days. Table 10 records the observations on three pairs with one girl of each pair dropping out with a heart rate of about 180.

TABLE 10 Observations on three pairs walking in early summer. One of each pair stopped short. Ages ranged from 15 to 18

Subjects and sex	T_{bb} °C	T_s °C	ΔT_{re} °C	Final HR	Duration min	Body wt kg	Body surface m²	Wt loss g/m²·min
Loftis, F	40	33.0	−0.3	142	58	48	1.49	6.4
Burk, F		33.2	0.7	177	37	69	1.80	4.1
Morris, M	51	36.0	1.2	152	59	84	2.10	8.9
Dewey, F			1.0	184	16	50	1.54	5.7
Morris, M	55		1.0	136	61	84	2.10	8.1
Burk, F			1.3	180	40	71	1.80	6.3

DISCUSSION

A major interest in these studies is rate of water loss measured by the rate of weight loss. The 10 comparisons of Evans and Loftis, Table 8, were made in mid-summer when both were well adapted to desert heat. Their weight loss as pointed out above is almost entirely water; no sweat runs off. On the hottest days some moisture may appear on the face but none accumulates so all water lost whether from the skin or from the lungs and airway is available for body cooling. In only two of these 10 paired walks did the weight losses in g/m² of body surface differ by more than 40 g. The mean weight loss was exactly the same, 414 g/m².

The 10 different pairs compared in Table 9 represent a wider range in fitness than the pair of subjects compared in Table 8. All but Faulkner and Connors had walked many times before; those two over-weight boys were persuaded to walk because we wished to compare fat and lean walkers. They showed some lack of acclimatization: Their weight losses were much less than Richardson's and their body temperature increases greater. But even including these two pairs the mean difference in weight losses, related to body surface, between members of each of the 10 pairs was 40 g, less than 10%.

The third set of observations were made on pairs with one of each pair failing to finish. These walks were in the early summer and probably reflect lack of full acclimatization. In the last column of Table 10 the losses are calculated to the basis of $g/m^2 \cdot min$. In Tables 8 and 9 everyone walked for an hour so the losses are expressed in $g/m^2 \cdot hr$. It is notable in Table 10 that those who failed to complete the hour show rates of water loss less by 22–36% than their partners' rates.

Observations on increases in rectal temperature are included in each table. No one, even of those who failed to complete the walk, shows an increase of more than 1.5 C. This is not exessive especially considering that a rise of 1.0 C is not unusual in an hour's walk at this rate even when T_b is low.

Since body temperature does not rise much in all those who walked for the full hour and since heat dissipation under the experimental conditions depends largely on water evaporation, it is not surprising that two subjects walking at the same rate in the dry heat of the desert evaporate about the same quantity of water. It would seem that in the person evaporating more than necessary T_{re} should drop and that in the person evaporating less than necessary T_{re} should rise. It must be admitted that the results of Table 10 seem to be at odds with the above conclusion: early in the summer three girls walking at 100 m per min show low rates of water loss and low increments in T_{re}. Yet high heart rates forced them to stop in from 16 to 40 min. The high heart rates in these three girls does not seem to relate to temperature regulation. While their rate of evaporation was low, it did not occasion an uncomfortable rise in T_{re}. Skin temperature was observed in only one; it was about the same as her partner's, another girl. The metabolic rate was not high—about one-half the maximal rate. These facts suggest that such a rise in heart rate is neurological in origin i.e. stimulation of the sympathetic nervous system.

The heart rate in desert walks generally gives an excellent measure of fitness and adaptation. The two subjects of Table 8 in 10 walks had final heart rates below 140, even when the T_{bb} reached 58 C. These walks were late in the summer after both had become well adapted. Loftis had taken part in earlier walks with higher rates: Fig. 70, 140 at T_{bb} 47 and 150 at T_{bb} 52 and in Table 10, 142 at T_{bb} 40. The rates shown in Fig. 69 illustrate how an individual varies from day to day even when well-adapted and in good health. Loftis always had a higher heart rate than Evans but the difference at the end of the walks ranged from two on 7–30 to 11 on 7–27 and 8–3.

A much greater difference in performance is indicated by the rates in Fig. 70. On one day when T_{bb} was 47 Freeland had a final heart rate of 118 while Dewey's was 159. Dill when T_{bb} was 58 walked the full hour with a final heart rate of 117 while Freeland's was 145. Dill's low heart rate compared with Freeland's does not imply greater fitness. Dill's maximum rate is about 140 and Freeland's about 200 so Dill was nearer his limit of performance than was Freeland. It would seem that Dill's low rate reflects virtual absence of sympathetic stimulation and that Freeland's higher rate depends in part on sympathetic stimulation.

In Fig. 71 we have compared terminal heart rates in the 10 pairs of Fig. 69 with T_{bb} values. As pointed out above the heart rate of an individual varies from day to day at the same work rate and with the same heat stress reflecting perhaps different levels of sympathetic stimulation. So we have used in Fig. 71 the mean heart rates of Evans and Loftis in each of their 10 walks; this minimizes the day-to-day individual variation. It seems that in well acclimatized individuals there is a roughly predictable heart rate for a given work rate, knowing the black body temperature. The heart rate is relatively unaffected by increases in T_{bb} from 36 to 44 C after which it increases rapidly but in these two fit and well-adapted subjects it remains below 140 up to T_{bb} 56.

Is performance in desert heat related to sex? Our evidence indicates that some girls are not capable of walking at 100 m per min on summer days when the black body temperature is above 50 C. Only one, Teresa Loftis, was able to do this easily. During the school year she walks five or more km per day between home and school. In one paired walk she had a lower heart rate than David Wolfenbarger and on another occasion, lower than Yousef's. Each of the other three girls had a higher heart rate than their partner's. While the evidence is inconclusive it appears that boys of high school age generally can out-walk girls in desert heat. At the same time it is certain there is some overlap in performance. Is the apparent superior performance of boys related to a greater capacity for sweating? Women have about 50% more sweat glands per unit area as shown by Kawahata [5]. Yet he also found that when exposed to a hot humid environment women are slower to begin sweating and produce less sweat than men. Morimoto *et al.* [8] studied this question in the climatic chamber under both dry and humid conditions. Sweat rates were significantly higher in men than in women especially at higher heat stresses. Their results suggest that the sweat rate of women approaches a limit of about 325 g/m²·hr in dry heat. Of the five girls who have been our subjects three reached about the same range at the end of the hour's walk: 302–338 g/m²·hr. On hotter days the three girls unable to finish because of high heart rates had rates of water loss ranging from 246 to 371 g/m²·hr. However, the girl who was a subject in the 10 walks of Table 8 lost water at rates up to 564 g/m²·hr. Even that high rate was

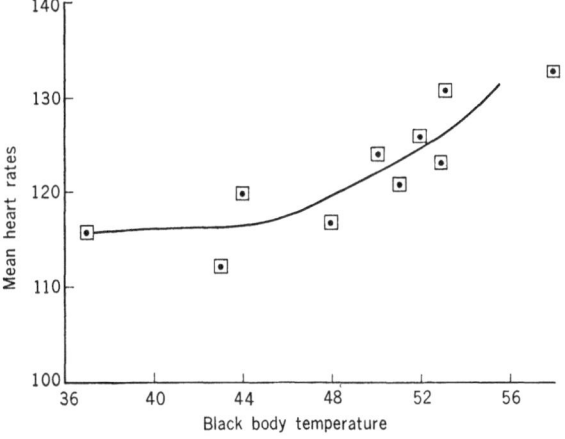

Fig. 71 Mean heart rates of Evans and Loftis in the 10 walks of Fig. 69. While the heart rate at a given metabolic rate is closely dependent on black body temperature other factors affect it.

well within her limit since her heart rate was 135 at the end of that walk. We have some other evidence still unpublished that a low capacity to produce sweat in exercise in desert heat is more common among women than among men. All of this evidence supports the findings of the above-mentioned investigators, Kawahata and Morimoto and his colleagues.

Is rate of sweating during exercise in desert heat related to skin temperature, T_s? The data of Table 9 can be used to give a provisional answer to this question. The five highest and the five lowest mean rates of water loss in Evans were 471 and 356 ml/kg·hr. In Loftis the corresponding values were 489 and 340. The corresponding mean T_s values were 35.5 C and 34.3 C in Evans and 35.9 C and 34.5 C in Loftis. In Evans a mean increase of 32% in rate of water loss was associated with an increase of 1.2 C in T_s. In Loftis a mean increase of 44% in rate of water loss was associated with an increase 1.4 C. These comparisons suggest a direct relation between T_s and rate of water loss. This is not always true when other pairs are compared as in Table 9. While T_s and rate of water loss go hand in hand in many of the 10 pairs there are some major divergences e.g. Freeland vs. Richardson. Still greater divergences are seen when metabolic rate varies. Dill, Hall and van Beaumont [3] compared sweat rates while sitting in the sun with sweat rates while walking at 100 m per min. They observed T_s but did not compare T_s and sweat rate. From their unpublished data this relation has been derived for two of their subjects. For van Beaumont the mean sweat rates expressed in ml/min were 13.8 walking and 8.7 sitting. The corresponding T_s values were 33.7 and 35.1. In Dill's case the corresponding values were 15.2 and 8.0 for sweat rate and 33.7 and 34.3 for T_s. It appears considering all the above evidence that when metabolic rate varies and in some cases when it is constant sweat rate does not depend directly on T_s. In fact sweat rate sometimes increases while T_s decreases.

The role of acclimatization has been mentioned above; even our subjects who live all year in the desert gained in acclimatization from early summer to late summer. Most people in Boulder City live in air-conditioned homes and are unaccustomed to walking far in midday. Our young subjects probably gained in acclimatization more from their walks in the sun than if they had been less active. The rate at which acclimatization can occur under controlled conditions was demonstrated by Robinson and associates [10]. Room temperature was about 40 C and relative humidity about 24%. Each of five men did a grade walk to exhaustion and repeated the walk for the same length of time every day for 10–23 days. Rectal temperature reached about 40 C on the first day and only reached 38–38.5 after 10 days, T_s declined from about 37–35 C. Heart rate at exhaustion on the first day was above 180 and between 140 and 160 at the end of the last walk. The initial stress, as judged by T_{re} was greater than in our walks but after the acclimatization period their subjects had about reached the capabilities of our group for exercising in the heat.

How do the foregoing observations agree with our earlier studies and with observation by others? Kuno has reviewed findings by many investigators that rate of sweating increases with acclimatization. Our present studies are not comparable since all of our subjects were partially acclimatized when the test began. We can say that by the latter half of the summer sweat rate per unit of body surface was approximately the same for all at a fixed rate of walking and with the same environmental stress. This holds true so long as the rate of sweating is below the capacity of the individual for sweating. Our studies are not comparable in another respect: In dry heat all sweat is utilized for cooling, the skin remaining dry while in humid conditions this need not be true; an increased rate of sweating serves to keep the body surface wetter and so contributes to cooling. As Kuno [6], has shown the distribution of sweat glands varies with the individual and is uneven. Hence sweat produced in excess on areas where sweat glands are abundant may spread and wet areas where sweat glands are few. At the same time some of the sweat runs off the body serving no useful purpose.

What is the state of our fitter subjects at the end of the hour? Their rate of energy expenditure has been well within their capacity and the depletion of energy reserves is relatively small. Increases in skin and rectal temperature are within tolerable limits. Only the heart rate provides a hint that a breakdown is approaching. With few exceptions the heart rate is rising at the end of the hour. The exceptions are on days when the T_{bb} is less than 40 or when clouds lowered the T_{bb} in the latter part of the walk. What does the increasing heart rate signify? Probably it depends chiefly on loss of body water, decrease in blood volume and decrease in venous return to the heart. As is well-known, under such circumstances the heart responds by an increased rate.

What evidence supports our suggestion that the rising heart rate seen throughout most of our walks relates to diminished blood volume? One might be inclined to question this since many investigations report an increase in blood volume in heat. But support comes from Gosselin's study [4] and Adolph's calculations [1]. Gosselin measured weight loss in the desert both in rest and work. Four men underwent dedydration while resting in the laboratory hot room at an air temperature of about 50 C. Over a six-hr period they sweat at a constant rate of about 1% of body weight per hour. In other words there was no diminution in sweat rate as body water was depleted. In such dehydration studies Adolph measured plasma volume. All lost, some more rapidly than others even at the same rate of water loss. He concluded that plasma generally contributes much more than its share of the water used for sweat secretion. He estimated that "*if all the tissues of the body lost water in the same proportion as the plasma loses water the loss from the whole body would be 2.5 times its actual value.*"

The report of some investigators that blood volume increases in heat has been resolved by Myhre and Robinson [9]. Their four subjects walked for two or more hours at 5.6 km per hr on a 2.5% grade. Room conditions were 50 C dry bulb and 26 C wet bulb. At the end of the walk they had lost 4.2% of their body weight and 17% of their plasma volume. They were kept dehydrated while resting at 25 C dry bulb. After five hours their water loss had increased to 4.5% but their plasma had regained 45% of the water it had lost during exercise. Hence while blood volume may increase in brief exposures to heat it decreases if significant dehydration occurs and decreases even more for the same degree of dehydration if the subjects exercise in the heat.

How soon is a constant rate of water loss attained? Our subjects were sweating before the walk started since our downstairs laboratory is open to the outdoors; its air temperature is about the same as the outdoor air temperature. As pointed out in *Methods* the subjects are weighed at the start, at the end of the first lap, about seven min, and every second lap thereafter to the final weighing. These measurements indicate that a uniform rate of water loss is reached during the first lap.

In what respects are our subjects in a steady state during the hour's walk? What is meant by steady state? In mammals a steady state includes rhythmic changes that involve drinking, eating, digesting, activity and sleeping. In a healthy man rhythmic changes begin when he awakes; the courses of these rhythms continue until he awakes the next morning. He then has regained the state of the previous morning barring stresses out of the ordinary: All rhythms have run their course. In our walks new levels of body and skin temperature are quickly reached and maintained. The metabolic rate is constant after the first minutes; this means a steady depletion of energy reserves during the walk but the percentage of stored energy used is small. Salt reserves also are depleted at a uniform rate but the depletion in an hour is of little importance. If no water is drunk reserves of body water undergo steady depletion with consequent disturbances. It appears that in an hour's walk at 100 m per min in the hot desert everyone undergoes cardiovascular embarrassment due to water loss. In some, particularly females, the heart rate becomes intolerably high in less than an hour without much increase in T_{re}. We guess that this may reflect an earlier sympathetic reaction to the heat stress than seen in those who finish the walk. This may manifest itself by an unusually rapid decrease in plasma volume and consequent circulatory handicap.

SUMMARY

The responses to walking for about one hr at 100 m per min in desert heat have been studied in pairs of subjects. All were between 15 and 18 yrs except Yousef, 34, and Dill, 79. Observations were made before and after of body weight and rectal temperature. The heart rate and skin temperature were monitored during the walk. When sweat rate increases skin temperature generally increases but sometimes the reverse is true, particularly when metabolic rate varies. Body weight was observed at occasional 30-sec breaks during the walk. Meteorological conditions were monitored; the black body temperature was considered the preferred best single index to heat stress. In aech pair finishing the hour's walk the rate of water loss was about the same when related to body surface. Three girls stopped short in early summer walks. Their rectal and skin temperatures were not high but their heart rates reached our arbitrary limit of about 180 within 16–40 min. Women generally have a lower capacity for sweating than men; as their limit is approached there appears to be a response of the sympathetic nervous system with increase in heart rate to the intolerable range. Nearly all subjects showed a continous increase in heart rate. This is interpreted as a response to decreased plasma volume, reduction in venous return and a dependent increase in heart rate. The heart rate in desert walks is an excellent index to fitness. Its rate of increase depends on the reserve capacity of the cardiovascular system and the rate of water loss.

ACKNOWLEDGEMENT

Thanks are due to my colleague M.K. Yousef and our laboratory assistants, named in the figures, who had essential roles in this study both as subjects and as collaborators.

This study was supported by Public Health Study Grant GM 15693-03, National Science Foundation Grant GB 17126 and the Nevada Heart Association.

REFERENCES

1. ADOLPH, E.F., and associates (1947): Physiology of Man in the Desert. Interscience Publishers, Inc. New York, 160–162.
2. ALDRICH, L.B. (1930): *Smithsonian Inst. Misc. Collections* **8**: 8–12.
3. DILL, D.B., F.G. Hall, and W. van BEAUMONT (1966): *J. Appl. Physiol.* **21**: 99–106.

4. GOSSELIN, R.E. (1947): Physiology of Man in the Desert. Interscience Publishers, Inc. New York, 58–63.
5. KAWAHATA, A. (1960): Essential Problems in Climatic Physiology. Yoshimura, H., K. Ogata and S. Itoh (eds.). Nankodo Publishing Co., Ltd. Kyoto, Japan, 171–184.
6. KUNO, Yas. (1934): The Physiology of Human Perspiration. J. and A. Churchill, London.
7. KUNO, Yas. (1956): Human Perspiration. Chas. C. Thomas, Springfield, Ill., 319.
8. MORIMOTO, T., Z. SLABOCHOVA, R.K. NAMAN, and F. SARGENT II (1967). *J. Appl. Physiol.* **22:** 526–532.
9. MYHRE, L.G., and S. ROBINSON (1969): *The Physiologist* **12:** 310.
10. ROBINSON, S., E.S. TURRELL, H.S. BELDING, and S.M. HORVATH (1943): *Am. J. Physiol.* **140:** 168–176.

CHAPTER 10

THE EFFECT IN MAN OF ACCLIMATISATION TO HEAT ON WATER INTAKE, SWEAT RATE AND WATER BALANCE

O. G. EDHOLM

Division of Human Physiology, National Institute for Medical Research, London, U.K.

The physiological changes which occur during acclimatisation to heat in man have been extensively studied (Eichna, Ashe, Bean and Shelley, 1945; Ladell, 1951; Bass and Henschel, 1956; Macpherson, 1960). One striking characteristic is an increase in sweat production. The majority of the many studies have been concerned with experiments in climatic chambers and have dealt with relatively acute effects, and there is some uncertainty whether the initial increase in sweat rate persists with continued exposure to hot conditions. Macpherson (1960) writes that 'perhaps the increased rate of sweating so often observed with acclimatisation is a transient phenomenon, the temporary nature of which escaped observation because laboratory experiments were of comparatively brief duration.' He expressed these doubts as a result of an experiment which was carried out over a period of 22 weeks with 12 subjects who were living in Singapore and were acclimatised to heat by daily exposure in a climatic chamber. After the initial acclimatisation routine, the men were variously exposed to a number of different combinations of climatic conditions, work, and clothing but at four-weekly intervals underwent a uniformity trial in which conditions were always similar (Adam, Ellis, John, Lee and Macpherson, 1953). The usual considerable increase in sweat loss occurred initially, but thereafter it declined gradually and at the end of 22 weeks was only slightly greater than it had been when the experiment began. However, these men were living in a hot and humid climate, and in an experiment in which British sailors living in Singapore were compared with a similar group living in England it was shown that the sweat loss of the Singapore subjects was significantly greater when the two groups were exposed to a similar hot and humid climate in a chamber (Hellon, Jones, Macpherson and Weiner, 1956).

An opportunity to re-examine this question arose in the course of an experiment in which the performance of two groups of men, one acclimatised and the other unacclimatised, were compared in the hot and humid climate of Aden (now the South Yemen Republic) (Edholm, Fox, Goldsmith, Hampton, Underwood, Ward, Wolff, Adam and Allen, 1964).

METHODS

1. Subjects

A total of 48 subjects were studied, divided into two groups of 24 men. Both groups were members of the Parachute Brigade who have to pass a severe test of physical fitness, which is maintained by arduous training.   One group consisted of men who were stationed in England and had either never experienced hot climatic conditions or had not been so exposed for a period of one year.   They were considered to be unacclimatised to heat.   The second group was drawn from men who had been stationed in Bahrein on the Persian Gulf for nine months and had therefore lived and trained in a hot and frequently humid climate.   The characteristics of the two groups are set out in Table 11.

TABLE 11   Characteristics of the subjects

	Unacclimatised	Acclimatised
Number of subjects	24	24
Age (yrs)	22.5 (range 19–28)	20.4 (range 19–23)
Height (cm)	175 (range 168.5–185.5)	174.5 (range 168.0–182.0)
Weight (kg)	70.5 (range 58.9–84.5)	69.5 (range 58.4–81.1)

2. Design

The experiment was carried out in three phases.   During the *first* phase the unacclimatised men were studied in England; this was followed closely by the *second* phase in Aden, where the unacclimatised and acclimatised men both carried out a similar programme.   After this both groups were flown to England and the *third* phase then began.   Each phase lasted for 12 days and a daily programme of activities was planned so that the first four days were occupied with hard or moderately hard physical activity, the second four days were spent resting and on light activities, and the last four days in hard work.   The planning of the detailed activities for each day included duration and timing, so they could be carried out in a virtually identical manner in each of the three phases and the first day in each phase had precisely the same programme, and so on for each succeeding day.   In this way it was expected that the energy expenditure for any particular day of the 12 days would be identical in each of the three phases.

The main objective of the experiment was to compare the performance of the two groups in the the hot climate of Aden, hence factors other than acclimatisation to heat had to be controlled as strictly as possible.   Both groups were, as shown in Table 11, of similar age, height and weight, were engaged in the same activities, had similar clothing, food and water.   It would, however, have been possible that the two groups differed in their physical fitness or in particular skills and such possible differences had to be assessed.   In Phase III, by comparison of the various details of performance and physiological responses of the two groups, any such differences could be detected; and by comparing the performance of the unacclimatised group in Phase I and Phase III, any effect of the intervening period in the hot climate of Aden could also be assessed.

3. Techniques and Measurements

Measurements were made throughout the whole experiment of every subject's daily food and water intake, urine output, faecal weight, body weight (a.m. and p.m.), skinfold thickness (a.m. and p.m.), body temperature and pulse rate (two-hourly intervals). Energy expenditure was assessed by detailed and continuous timed activity studies, and the climatic conditions in the immediate vicinity of the subjects were measured at one to two hour intervals.

Water intake: In the field during the period of hard work, water for drinking was carried by each subject in two water bottles each containing 1.14 litres. These were issued in the morning immediately after measuring body-weight, i.e., between 0530 and 0600. The subject was able to exchange his empty water bottles for full ones at each hour of the day. Before issue, the labelled bottles were weighed and the number of the subject to whom they were given was noted. The empty bottles were also weighed on collection. During the four 'rest' days, urns of cooled water and lemonade were available, and the quantity drunk by each subject was recorded. Each group of eight men had two observers attached, and continuous observation was maintained throughout the 24 hours. There were no sources of water other than those provided and recorded.

Food intake: Food intake was also recorded for each man throughout the experiment. During the days of hard work in the field, the men were issued with individual rations with items of known calorie value and water content. Unconsumed rations were collected each day before the next lot of rations were given. In this way the fluid intake and metabolic water derived from the food consumed was measured accurately.

Urine: Each subject was given a one litre stoppered polythene bottle labelled with his number. Bottles were issued in the morning at 0600 and collected at 1800 hours when a new bottle was provided. The subjects were instructed to urinate into the bottles, which were carried attached a belt worn round the waist. As the subjects were under constant observation at all times these instructions were followed.

Faeces: Portable fibreglass latrine seats were sited near the subjects at all times. Faeces were passed into a polythene bag attached to the underside of the seat. When used, the bag was detached by the subject, sealed and the subject's number written on a label attached to the bag. The full bags were collected and weighed. Subjects were instructed not to urinate into the bag, and this instruction was strictly adhered to.

Calculation of 'sweat loss': The equation used to calculate sweat loss was:
'Sweat' loss = [water intake (ml) + total food consumed (g)] — [urine (ml) + faeces (g)] ± body-weight change (g).

The term 'sweat' loss, as can be seen from the equation, includes water lost in the expired air and insensible perspiration.

Calculation of water balance:

Water balance = total water intake — total water loss

Total water intake = water drunk + water content of food + metabolic water

Total water loss = urine + sweat loss + faecal water.

The water content of faeces was taken to be 75% except in the case of liquid stools, when a figure of 95% was used.

Metabolic water was calculated using the figures:

1 g protein yields 0.41 g water

1 g fat   ″   1.07 g   ″

1 g starch   ″   0.60 g   ″   (Davidson and Passmore, 1966)

Apart from the 'errors' in calculating 'sweat' loss due to respiratory and insensible water loss, no allowance is made in these calculations for changes in body-weight due to calorie imbalance.

RESULTS

In this paper the only results to be considered in detail are those concerned with water intake, sweat rate and water balance.   Comparison of the various measurements made during Phase I and Phase III showed that there were no significant differences between the acclimatised and unacclimatised men after they had returned to England from Aden.   Furthermore, there were no evident differences between the results obtained in Phase I and Phase III as a result of the unacclimatised men's sojourn in Aden, apart from those which could be attributed to the small climatic difference between the first and last phase.   During the *first* phase in England, the weather was cool and wet, in the *second* phase in Aden it was hot and humid, and in the *third* phase in England the weather was mild.

1.   *Meteorological Measurements*

Dry-bulb, wet-bulb, air speed and globe thermometer measurements were recorded, using portable field equipment, at approximately hourly intervals in the immediate neighbourhood of the subjects (Underwood and Ward, 1964).

The mean dry-bulb temperature from 0600 to 1800 hr in each of the three phases ranged from 8.5–13.8 °C in Phase I, from 28.5–38 °C in Phase II and from 8.5–22 °C in Phase III.   Wet-bulb temperatures during the same hours were 7.2–9.5 °C in Phase I, 24.5–28 °C during Phase II in Aden, and in Phase III, 9–14 °C.   There was almost continuous sunlight in Aden, and the globe thermometer reading was fairly steady at about 45 °C, whereas in England sunshine was irregular and the globe thermometer readings varied from 10–22 °C in Phase I and from 14–35 °C in Phase II.   The wet-

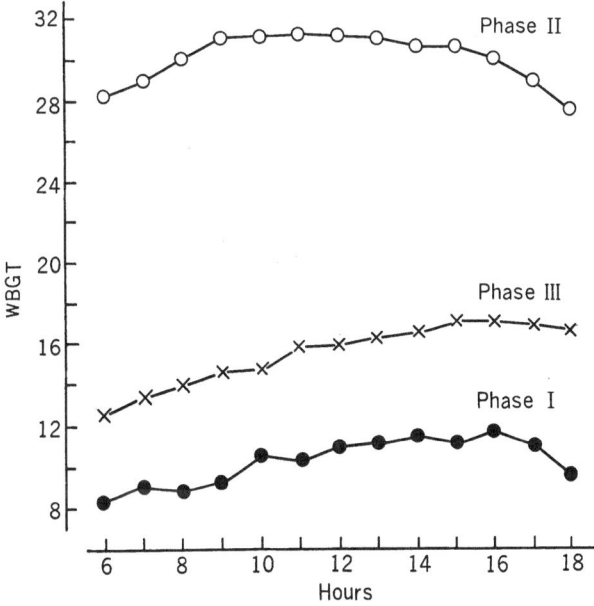

Fig. 72.   The wet-bulb globe thermometer index averaged for the 12 days of each phase for each hour from 0600 to 1800 hr, i.e. the period of daylight in Phase II in Aden.   All the active work was done during these hours.

bulb-globe thermometer index (WBGT) was calculated for each hour of each day, and
the averages are shown in Fig. 72.

2. Energy Expenditure

Energy expenditure was assessed from continuous timed activity. During the first
and last four days in each phase the subjects worked hard, or moderately hard. There
was a 10-mile march each morning, carrying kit which weighed approximately 25 kg.
The activities for the rest of the day varied in detail but included digging, carrying loads,
pushing vehicles, and playing games. The estimated mean energy expenditure for the
two groups in the different phases is set out in Table 12.

TABLE 12   Estimated mean energy expenditure (kcal) in the three Phases

	Phase I	Phase II		Phase III	
	A	A	B	A	B
1st 4 days	3640	3750	3610	3470	3450
2nd 4 days	2540	2560	2500	2340	2370
3rd 4 days	3790	3610	3440	3450	3330

Note: A = unacclimatised   B = acclimatised

The energy expenditure was similar in the three phases; the level during days of hard
work was well within the capacity of the men in England, and they could have carried
out a considerably more arduous programme. In the severe climate of Aden, the same
level of work was close to the maximum which could be tolerated, and it is unlikely that
the subjects could have endured a higher level of energy expenditure. Body temperatures were high (Wolff, Fox and Jack, 1964) and there were a considerable number who
were unable to complete their tasks (Edholm, 1969).

3. Water Intake

The average daily intake of water, including water content of food and water of metabolism is set out in Table 13. During Phase III, in England, the acclimatised and
unacclimatised men had average daily intakes which were virtually identical. Intake

TABLE 13   Average daily intake of water (ml) including water content of food and
            water of metabolism

PHASE I		PHASE II			PHASE III		
	Subj. 1–24		Subj. 1–24	Subj. 25–48		Subj. 1–24	Subj. 25–48
Day	Mean	Day	Mean	Mean	Day	Mean	Mean
1	4040	13	—	—	25	3980	3780
2	3760	14	6880	8180	26	4900	4930
3	3660	15	7460	8470	27	5130	5100
4	3470	16	8180	9310	28	3850	4090
5	3370	17	5240	5570	29	2930	3240
6	2490	18	4580	4850	30	2690	2320
7	2910	19	5350	5770	31	2720	2670
8	3380	20	4420	4940	32	2950	3060
9	3790	21	9360	10710	33	4640	4800
10	4310	22	9590	10730	34	4970	5270
11	3580	23	8510	9490	35	5190	5060
12	4130	24	7700	9300	36	3690	3820

Note: Subjects 1–24, unacclimatised; subjects 25–48, acclimatised.

during Phase I was less during the days of hard work than in the corresponding days of Phase III by approximately 500–750 ml/day. As indicated above, the weather was warmer in Phase III.

In Phase II, in the severe heat of Aden, water intake was much higher, and on the average was about twice as high as in the temperate condition of England. On each day the acclimatised men had a higher intake of water than the unacclimatised. During the 12 days in Aden total water intake averaged 77.25 litres in the unacclimatised and 87.00 litres in the acclimatised subjects, the overall range being 62 litres to 103 litres. (These figures should strictly refer to 11 rather than 12 days as the results for the first day in Aden are incomplete and have not been included).

The calculated average daily 'sweat' loss during the three phases is shown in Table 14. In Aden the acclimatised men had higher 'sweat' losses than the unacclimatised

TABLE 14   Average daily sweat loss (ml)

PHASE I		PHASE II			PHASE III		
	Subj. 1–24		Subj. 1–24	Subj. 25–48		Subj. 1–24	Subj. 25–48
Day	Mean	Day	Mean	Mean	Day	Mean	Mean
1	4150	13·	—	—	25	4090	3910
2	3310	14	6210	8030	26	5110	5290
3	3430	15	7520	8320	27	4700	4660
4	3040	16	8190	8760	28	3090	4000
5	600	17	4270	4670	29	1180	1690
6	1060	18	4640	4570	30	1490	1640
7	950	19	4840	5400	31	2010	1880
8	1180	20	4650	5070	32	1690	2030
9	4070	21	9990	11370	33	4860	5000
10	3950	22	10220	10670	34	5040	5230
11	3400	23	8640	8800	35	4670	4420
12	4220	24	7520	9200	36	2860	3660

Note: Subjects 1–24, unacclimatised; subjects 25–48, acclimatised.

on each day except for one day during the light activities period. But in England, during Phase III, the two groups had almost identical sweat losses on each day. The calculated 'sweat' loss also includes water lost in the expired air as well as insensible perspiration. No separate calculation has been made of these other channels of water loss as they are relatively small. During the days of active work, sweat losses were high in both groups and were greater during the last four days than in the first four days. Climatic conditions were similar in these two periods and energy expenditure, on the average, slightly lower during the last four days compared with the first four. These results suggest that acclimatisation had increased in both groups during the course of the 12 days.

The calculated daily water balance during Phase II in Aden is presented in Table 15, and the results show that there was a greater cumulative calculated deficit in the unacclimatised compared with the acclimatised subjects. Since changes in body weight are included in the calculation of water balance, calorie imbalance could, in part, be responsible for alterations attributed to differences in water balance. Calculated calorie balances show that both groups were in calorie deficit during the days of hard physical work. The cumulative calorie deficit for the unacclimatised men was calculated to be

TABLE 15 Average daily water balance (ml)

PHASE I			PHASE II			PHASE III	
	Subj. 1–24		Subj. 1–24	Subj. 25–48		Subj. 1–24	Subj. 25–48
Day	Mean	Day	Mean	Mean	Day	Mean	Mean
1	−635	13	—	—	25	−660	−440
2	−120	14	−65	−220	26	−875	−490
3	−220	15	−460	−225	27	−190	−15
4	10	16	−445	−150	28	350	−240
5	1585	17	250	−270	29	600	995
6	495	18	−725	−195	30	−55	−250
7	375	19	−200	−330	31	−635	−390
8	730	20	−945	−840	32	−230	−10
9	−1270	21	−1185	−1125	33	−995	−940
10	−130	22	−685	−485	34	−710	−565
11	−390	23	−210	425	35	−45	145
12	−580	24	−305	−85	36	235	−195

Note: Subjects 1–24, unacclimatised; subjects 25–48, acclimatised.

approximately 5000 kcal at the end of the 12 days. Assuming that 1 kg of body weight change is equivalent to 6000 kcal (Brozek, Grande, Taylor, Anderson, Buskirk and Keys, 1957) then an average loss of approximately 0.80 kg body tissue would be expected. In the case of the acclimatised men the calculated calorie deficit amounted to 1500 kcal or approximately 0.25 kg weight loss.

The relationship between calculated sweat loss and body weight has been examined. In the acclimatised men there is a significant relationship but not in the unacclimatised. Sweat loss has been calculated from many different measurements, so it is evident that there could be errors, random and/or systematic, which might obscure any relationship. A major component of the calculation is water intake, so this has been examined also in relation to body weight. Total water intake throughout the 11 days of measurement in Aden is highly correlated with body weight in the acclimatised men, but there is no evidence of any such relationship in the unacclimatised. The results obtained on each day spent in Aden have also been examined and on each occasion during days of hard work and high water intake in the acclimatised men there is a significant relationship between body weight and water intake. However, on no occasion was such a relationship evident amongst the unacclimatised men (Fig. 73–75). During the rest days the correlation coefficient was lower for the acclimatised men but still significant, although it remained insignificant for the unacclimatised subjects. The pattern of water drinking was examined by comparing the quantities drunk during daylight hours (0600–1800) with night hours (1800–0600). Although by far the greater proportion of the total water intake was consumed during the day in both groups, the amount drunk at night was greater amongst the acclimatised than the unacclimatised, being 17.2% of the total for the former and 12.8% for the latter.

Separate calculations were not made of sweat loss in these periods; urine volumes, however, were in general larger during the night hours than the days, a reversal of the more usual situation.

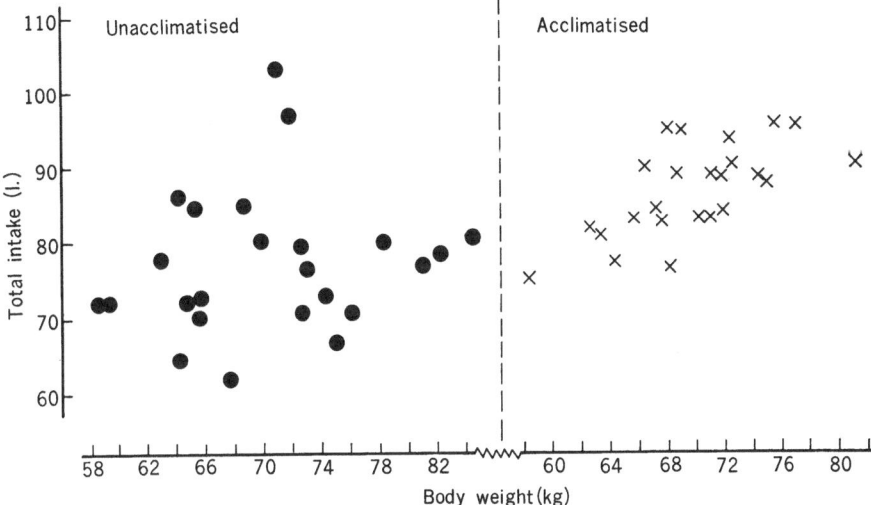

Fig. 73. Total water intake (litres) during the period of measurement in Phase II in Aden (the results for Day 1 are incomplete). Water intake has been plotted against initial body weight (kg). There is no significant relationship in the case of the unacclimatised subjects but there is a higlhy significant correlation in the acclimatised men ($r = 0.66$; $P<0.001$).

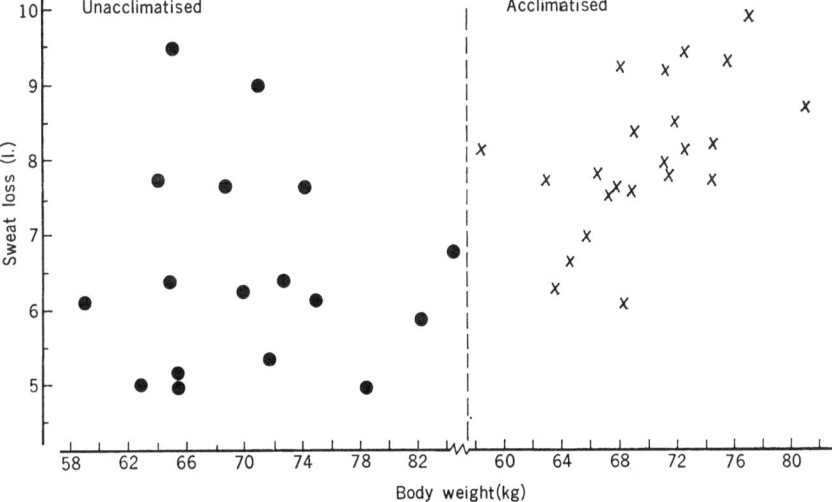

Fig. 74. Sweat loss for the unacclimatised and acclimatised men during the second day in Aden. This is highly correlated with body weight in the case of the acclimatised men with body weight in the case of the acclimatised men ($r = 0.556$, $P<0.01$); in the case of the unacclimatised men there is no correlation between sweat loss and body weight.

DISCUSSION

The two groups of men who were compared over a period of 12 days during both strenuous activity and days of low energy expenditure in a hot and humid climate were similar in age, height, weight and physical fitness (Edholm, 1969). They were engaged in identical activities and came from the same ethnic group. The only difference was that the members of one group had spent nine months immediately before the observa-

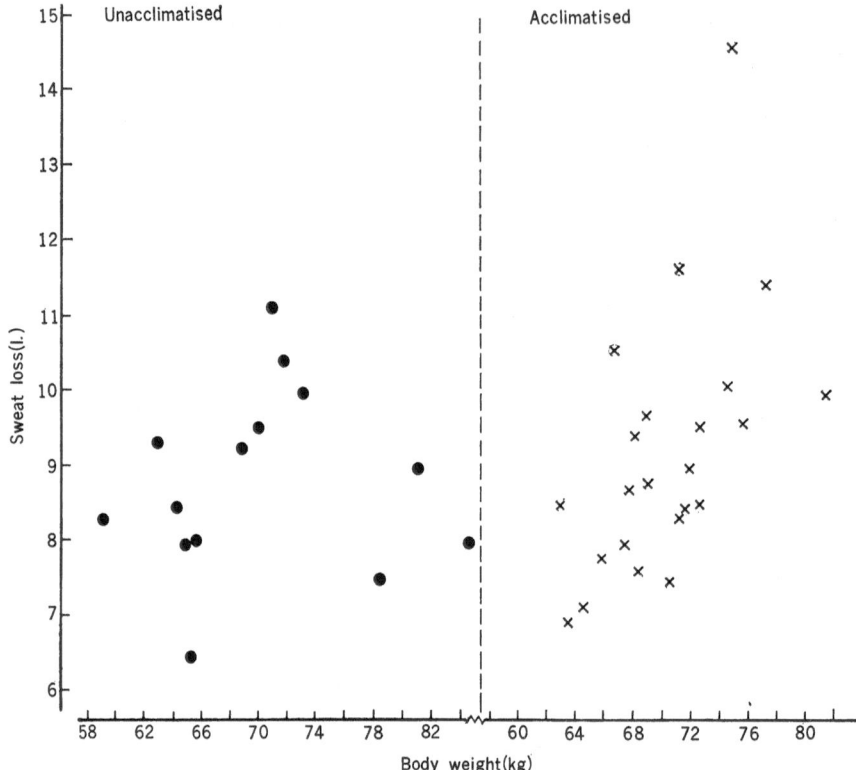

Fig. 75. Last day in Aden: Correlation of sweat loss and body weight. As on previous days, there is a significant correlation in the case of the acclimatised men (r = 0.544, P < 0.01); there is no correlation in the case of the unacclimatised men.

tions in Aden on the coast of the Persian Gulf, and the other group had not previously been exposed to hot conditions.

The sweat rate of people indigenous to a hot climate appears in some cases at least to be less than that of Europeans acclimatised to the local conditions (Macpherson, 1960). Ladell (1964) found that West Africans sweated less than residentially-acclimatised Europeans when exposed to a standard heat load in a climatic chamber, but the differences were small and might have been due to different patterns of activity in the two groups.

The natural state of acclimatisation of different ethnic groups has been compared by Strydom and Wyndham (1963), and they have found that the sweat rate of Bantu was lower than that of South Africans both in the unacclimatised and acclimatised state. The sweat loss of Indian subjects has also been shown to be less than that of British subjects exposed to the same standardised conditions (Edholm, Fox, Goldsmith, Hampton and Pillai, 1965; Edholm, 1966).

Yunusov (1970) has produced evidence that the water intake of men acclimatised to heat is lower than that of unacclimatised men. Furthermore, Yunusov and Makhmudov (personal communication) have claimed that restricting water intake of unacclimatised men speeds up the acclimatisation process. Altogether there is considerable evidence that long-term residence and work in a hot climate may not necessarily be accompanied by a persistence of the initial dramatic increase in sweat loss so commonly observed when unacclimatised men are first exposed to heat stress. Nevertheless, there are difficulties in accepting such a conclusion without more evidence. Comparisons between groups nearly always involve making a number of assumptions. If the subjects come from genetically distinct groups, then genetic factors may play a part. Furthermore, the results of comparisons can be difficult to interpret if there are anthropometric differences between the groups (Strydom and Wyndham, 1963, Discussion).

In the present experiment care was taken to ensure that the only difference between the two groups studied was in the experience of hot climatic conditions. The two groups were compared first in the severe heat of Aden and then in the temperate conditions of England. In the latter state there was virtually complete identity between the groups in the average results of many different measurements (water and food intake, energy expenditure, urine output, weight and skinfold changes, heart rate and body temperature) as well as performance in a wide variety of physically demanding tasks.

During the 12 days of the Aden part of the experiment there was free access to water at all times for all subjects. However, the acclimatised men on the average drank more than the unacclimatised on each day, and their calculated sweat rate was also higher. In this particular case, the conclusion is clear. Men acclimatised by living and working in a hot climate for a relatively long time (nine months) do not have lower water intakes or lower sweat rates than men otherwise similar but who were unacclimatised. It is, of course, not possible to conclude that longer residence in the heat might not have resulted in lower sweat rates, but this does not seem likely in view of observations on white Australians living in the hot and humid conditions of Queensland (Wyndham, Macpherson and Munro, 1964). Nor do the findings in the present experiment throw any further light on the significance of lower sweat losses in people indigenous to hot climates.

Amongst other features of the observations included in this paper are the relationships between body weight, sweat rate and water intake. Gosselin (1947) reported that in studies of men working in desert conditions of low humidity and high radient and air temperatures, sweat losses were significantly correlated with body weight. Although in the acclimatised men a similar relationship was found both with sweat rate and water intake compared with body weight, no such relationship was evident with the unacclimatised men. There is no clear reason for this difference between the two groups, but it is possible that this might be attributed to the more severe effects of the environment on the unacclimatised men. This was shown by the higher body temperatures and pulse rates of these men compared with the acclimatised and the much higher rate of heat illness amongst the unacclimatised (Edholm et al., 1964). It is possible that the differences between the two groups could also be attributed to a greater degree of 'voluntary dehydration' (Adolph, 1947) amongst the unacclimatised. However, the urine volume of the unacclimatised men was always larger than that of the acclimatised which is not consistent with a greater degree of dehydration. On the other hand, the calculated water balances show that there was a greater cumulative deficit in the unacclimatised men. These calculated water balances almost certainly exaggerate the water deficit in both groups, as the average weight changes were smaller. Even so, the overall weight loss of the unacclimatised men was greater than that of the acclimatised over the whole period of the 12 days, so it is reasonably certain that there was a degree of dehydration in the unacclimatised men. This, however, was small, being on the average about 1.5 litres, calculated from weight changes and allowing for calorie deficiency, or 3.5 litres calculated from the cumulative water balances, and also allowing for the calorie deficit. Clearly, the figure obtained from weight changes is more reliable, although it is possible that changes in body composition could put the figure nearer to 2.0 litres. Ladell (1964) has produced convincing evidence that there is approximately 2.5 litres of 'free' water, and there is no physiological evidence of dehydration until this is lost. As far as group mean results are concerned, the weight changes were very similar for the first eight days in the two groups. During this time there was on each day a higher water intake and calculated sweat loss amongst the acclimatised than the unacclimatised but no evidence of any difference as regards water deficit. It is unlikely that voluntary dehydration was different in the two groups and this cannot be evoked as responsible for the different relationship with body weight.

There is a considerable difference between the type of observation made by Gosselin (1947) and in the present work. Gosselin measured water intake and sweat loss during periods measured in hours, while activity was uniform. In the Aden experiment even when the water intake over a period of 11 days is compared with body weight a highly significant relationship emerges amongst the acclimatised men. The failure to find any such relationship in the unacclimatised men remains obscure, and only a tentative suggestion can be made attributing it to the greater strain experienced by these men.

It is not possible to draw any strict conclusions from these results regarding the relationship between water intake and sweat rate as the latter is calculated largely from the former.

The total water turnover during the 12 days spent in Aden was very large. Assuming that 70% of body weight is accounted for by water, the intake and loss of water ranged from 130 to 205% of total body water. Since most of the turnover would have taken place in the extracellular water, this would amount to a turnover of three to five times all the extracellular water in 11 days. There is no doubt that these subjects experienced unusually arduous conditions, and the rate of energy expenditure was exceptionally high for such a hot climate. The ability of the acclimatised men to endure can be considered a tribute to the process of adaptation of the human body.

ACKNOWLEDGEMENTS

The experiment was carried out by a large team, including: Colonel J.M. Adam, OBE, RAMC; Major J.R. Allen, RAMC: R.H. Fox, R. Goldsmith, I.F.G. Hampton, C.R. Underwood, E.J. Ward and H.S. Wolff, members of the Division of Human Physiology, National Institute for Medical Research, London. My thanks are due to many, but particularly to the members of the Parachute Brigade who acted as subjects. The main investigation was carried out under the auspices of the Army Personnel Research Committee.

REFERENCES

1. ADAM, J.M., F.P. ELLIS, R.T. JOHN, T.S. LEE, and R.M. MACPHERSON (1953): *Med. Res. Coun., Lond., R.N.P. Rep.* No. 53/750.
2. ADOLPH, E.F., and Associates. (1947): *Physiology of Man in the Desert.* Interscience Publishers, Inc., New York.
3. BASS, D.E., and A. HENSCHEL (1956): *Physiol. Rev.* **36**: 128.
4. BROZEK, J., F. GRANDE, H.L. TAYLOR, J.T. ANDERSON, E.R. BUSKIRK, and A. KEYS (1957): *J. Appl. Physiol.* **10**: 412.
5. DAVIDSON, S., and R. PASSMORE (1966): *Human Nutrition and Dietetics*, 3rd ed., Livingston; Edinburgh.
6. EDHOLM, O.G. (1966): In *Human Adaptability to Environments and Physical Fitness*, M.S. Malhotra (ed.), pp. 20–25. Defence Institute of Physiology and Allied Sciences: Madras.

7. EDHOLM, O.G. (1969): *Proc. Roy. Soc. Med.* **62:** Pt 2, 1175.
8. EDHOLM, O.G., R.H. FOX, R. GOLDSMITH, I.F.G. HAMPTON, C.R.U. UNDERWOOD, E.J.W. WARD, H.S. WOLFF, J.M. ADAM, and J.R. ALLAN (1964): *Med. Res. Coun., Lond., A.P.R.C. Rep.* No. 64/16.
9. EDHOLM, O.G., R.H. FOX, R. GOLDSMITH, I.F.G. HAMPTON, and K.V. PILLAI (1965): *J. Physiol.* **177:** 15P.
10. EICHNA, L.W., W.F. ASHE, W.B. BEAN, and W.B. SHELLEY (1945): *J. industr. Hyg.* **27:** 59.
11. GOSSELIN, R.E. (1947): In *Physiology of Man in the Desert*, Chap. IV, Adolph, E.F. and Associates, Interscience Publishers, Inc, New York.
12. HELLON, R.F., R.M. JONES, R.K. MACPHERSON, and J.S. WEINER (1956): *J. Physiol.* **132:** 559.
13. LADELL, W.S.S. (1951): *J. Physiol.* **115:** 296.
14. LADELL, W.S.S. (1964): In *Handbook of Physiology, Section 4: Adaptation to the Environment*, Chap. 39, American Physiological Society, Washington D.C.
15. MACPHERSON, R.K. (1960): *Physiological Responses to Hot Environments.* Med. Res. Coun., Lond., Special Report Series No. 298. H.M.S.O., London.
16. STRYDOM, N.B., and C.H. WYNDHAM (1963): *Fed. Proc.* **22:** 801.
17. UNDERWOOD, C.R.U., and E.J.W. WARD (1964): In Edholm *et al.* (1964): *Med. Res. Coun., Lond., A.P.R.C. Report* No. 64/16, Chap. 10.
18. WOLFF, H.S., R.H. FOX, and J.W. JACK (1964): In Edholm *et al. Med. Res. Coun., Lond., A.P.R.C. Report* No. 64/16, Chap 3.
19. WYNDHAM, C.H., R.K. MACPHERSON, and A. MUNRO (1964): *J. Appl. Physiol.* **19:** 1055.
20. YUNUSOV, A.Y. (1970): In *Proceedings of a Symposium on Adaptation of Man and of Animals to Extreme Natural Environments, 12–17 October, 1970, Novosibirsk*, p. 145. Siberian Branch of the Academy of Sciences of the USSR, Novosibirsk.

PART III

RESPONSES TO COLD AND COLD ADAPTABILITY

CHAPTER 11

PHYSIOLOGICAL ADAPTATIONS IN INFANT MAMMALS*

E. F. ADOLPH

Department of Physiology, The University of Rochester, Rochester, New York, U.S.A.

INTRODUCTION

How early in the life of a mammalian individual can physiological adaptations be induced? Are any capacities for adaptation present before or at birth? Can a schedule of ages be constructed to show the serial order in which various adaptations become available? Do the ontogenetic developments reveal general principles of physiological adaptations? These are questions that I will try to answer in this review.

Physiological *adaptation*, in the present study, is the process of change in an individual exposed to new circumstances. As it adapts it becomes different from a control individual that remains in the old circumstances. An *adaptate* is any quality or quantity by which the two individuals differ. Usually the difference is one of physiological regulations, the same processes being governed at different rates and setpoints. *Adaptability*, the capacity for physiological adaptation, is a chief factor relating animals to climate.

Physiological adaptations or acclimatizations have been widely investigated in adult animals; to a much smaller extent in infant animals. Indeed, numerous adaptations probably occur during embryonic differentiation, and others during fetal life. However, little progress has been made in prenatal studies, and new methods are needed for the investigation of adaptations in those stages.

Each natural environment induces specific modifications in young individuals, some of those modifications last a lifetime. Experimental manipulation also induces lasting modifications in the individual's physiological constitution. By comparison of the modified individual with its unmodified confrere, an observer measures the results of adaptations that have occurred.

Two classes of adaptations have been especially studied during development, those to cold air and those to high altitude. It is possible that the two classes, resulting from two types of treatment, may arouse common adaptates. What is the evidence for such overlap of adaptates in infant stages?

Other classes of adaptations will not be taken up here, such as, inductions of enzymes by hormones or substrates, inductions of immunities, blocking of communications or effectors, and others.

Most studies of physiological development have been made upon one species, the rat. In some respects the use of one species is unfortunate; however, this use makes it

*The National Science Foundation supported the preparation of this paper.

possible to recognize the times of onset of various adaptive capacities in one species. Where other species have been observed, developments of adaptations may be compared at ages measured from conception as well as at ages measured from birth.

I plan to mention known physiological adaptations, first those to cold air and later those to altitude; and then to interrelate the two. The sorts of tests by which the results of the two treatments have been measured will be indicated; details of the techniques can be found in the original reports.

COLD EXPOSURE

1. Heat Production

Mature mammals placed in cold air characteristically increase their heat productions, as measured by uptakes of oxygen. Immediately after birth such an increase is found in some species (Dawes, 1968, p. 194) but not in other species. In newborn rats the increase is absent while in air of 30°, until the individual has obtained milk from the mother (Baric, 1953). Therefore some factor connected with alimentation triggers a shift in the infant's response to immediate cooling. The shift confers on the individual a permanent modification of its response to cool air.

In guinea pigs the extra oxygen uptake in response to cool air is present at birth (Brück et al., 1969). The oxygen uptake represents an increase of metabolism without shivering. When the guinea pigs are reared at a neutral temperature most of the extra non-shivering thermogenesis is lost by 14 days of age. Instead the animals shiver, when placed in air of 8°. When the guinea pigs are reared in air of 3° they retain the non-shivering thermogenesis until somewhat older ages (Zeisberger et al., 1967). Therefore the type of response to cold exposure depends on the environment in which the animals live, and is an adaptate to cold air.

A large non-shivering thermogenesis in infants of various species is aroused not only by cold exposure but also by injections of norepinephrine (Moore and Underwood, 1963). Much of the extra thermogenesis occurs in brown fat (Dawkins and Hull, 1964) which is abundant in infant mammals.

In guinea pigs and rabbits (Blatteis, 1964) the heat production evoked by cold exposure and that evoked by norepinephrine are equal in amount. Both evocations are blocked by injection of pronethalol, a betablocker of catecholamine actions.

Newborn "miniature" pigs, in contrast, do not exhibit non-shivering oxygen uptake in response to cold exposure or to norepinephrine injection. However, individuals 28 days of age that are cold-adapted shiver more intensely, taking up more oxygen than non-adapted controls (Brück et al., 1969). Response by shivering is like that in the guinea pig whose adrenergic nervous system has been blocked by pronethalol, even on the day of birth (Mount, 1968).

In the following instances sharp onsets of physiological adaptations have been identified.

The temperature that prevails in rats' nests, and hence the temperature of the infants in them, may influence the subsequent response to sudden cold air (Gelineo, 1964, p. 272). If the nest temperature is 10°–16°, the increase of oxygen uptake in response to cold air is first found after seven days. This represents adaptation, since control infants kept in nests of 28°–32° do not increase their oxygen uptakes in response to cold air until 14 days of age.

In another type of pre-treatment, infant rats are placed in air of 3° for one hour daily (Hahn *et al.*, 1963). At the end of 10 days an increase of oxygen uptake, measured in air of 29°, is found in the pre-treated rats in contrast to control rats of the same age kept at 29°. The latter first respond to cold air at 14 days.

In both instances the infant rats, whether chilled daily or kept continuously in cold air, become sensitive and responsive to sudden cold air at younger ages than they otherwise would. Adaptation is induced by continued exposure to cold air.

Birth itself triggers an increase in oxygen uptake at rest. In various species the oxygen uptake when the newborn individuals are in neutral air temperatures increases during the first day or days after birth. Examples are given by Dawes (1968, p. 195). In this phenomenon, some change connected with birth acts as adaptagent; the just-born individual is a suitable control. Evidently the mechanical effects of air breathing alone are not responsible for the increase. The increase is complete in two to seven days in most species.

2. *Rate of Body Cooling*

Young rats that resided in air of 19° were pretreated by placement in air of 3° for one hour each day. When tested in air of 10° they cooled, at every age up to 14 days (Krecek *et al.*, 1957), at the same rate as those that resided in air of 34°. But at 18 days and older they cooled more slowly than the warm-reared controls. Evidently the control of body cooling is first modified by cold pretreatment at a later age than the oxygen uptake is modified. Consequently one may conclude that the greater resistance to body cooling is not merely due to faster heat production; it is also due to factors of insulation; indeed, hair has developed and shows piloerection. At still a later age (30 days) vascular controls become prominent; whether these controls also adapt during the days of cold pre-treatment is not yet certain. In any case, the adaptive responses become available stepwise, and not all at once.

Underfeeding, as might be expected, delays the development of thermoregulation in rats. At 16 days after birth, an under-fed rat in air of 30° takes up 17% less oxygen and gradually cools, as compared with a well-fed control rat that maintains its colonic temperature (Heim and Szelenyi, 1965). In air of 20° the under-fed rat increases its oxygen uptake by only a small amount and its colonic temperature falls to 30°, while a control rat doubles its oxygen uptake and levels its colonic temperature at 35°. In contrast, by 24 days of age, oxygen uptakes are alike in under-fed and control rats in spite of the fact that now the under-fed individuals weigh less than the control individuals weighed eight days previously. The authors conclude that the difference in nutritive state modifies the regulation of body temperature, and does not merely limit the use of substrate for energy conversion. Underfeeding is an adaptagent.

3. *Other Adaptates*

Lasting modifications also due to pre-treatments with low air temperatures are as follows.

a. Ascorbate content of adrenal glands is depleted in rats residing in cold air, beginning at 16 days of age (Jailer, 1950). Similar depletion is also found in rats handled daily from birth, at 12 days of age as contrasted with control individuals (not handled) at 16 days (Levine *et al.*, 1958). Handling appears to imitate cold air in its modifying effect. The adrenals of cold-exposed individuals are larger, beginning at 18 days of age (Vacek *et al.*, 1961).

b. Tails of cold-exposed rats are shorter, and devoid of dermal fat. Other areas of skin may be richer in fat beginning at 14 days of age (Vacek *et al.*, 1961).

c. Liver is heavier, relative to body weight, in cold-exposed rats as early as 18 days of age. As early as 10 days the livers are depleted of fat (Hahn *et al.*, 1963).

d. Follicles of the thyroid gland have higher columnar cells, and smaller follicles, at 10 days and earlier (Fig. 76). Even air of 23° is sufficiently cold to elicit these cellular changes in thyroid follicles (Vacek *et al.*, 1961).

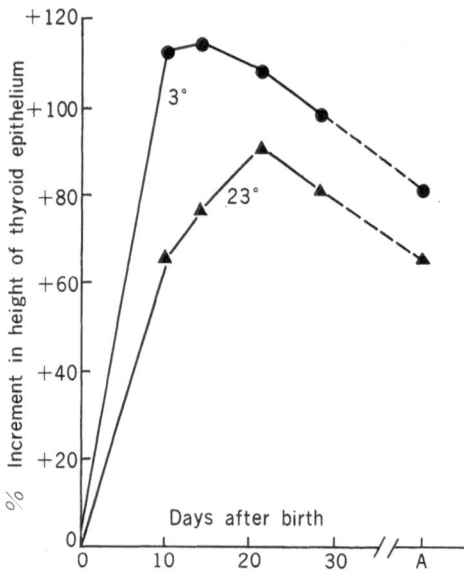

Fig. 76. Increment in height of thyroid epithelium in infant rats of various ages. Each point represents the mean $100(t_e/t_c)-100$, where t_e is the height of follicular epithelium in rats living from birth at 3° or 23 °C, and t_c that of control rats living at 33°. Data of Vacek *et al.* (1961).

e. The heart is heavier in cold-exposed rats beginning at 14 days of age (Vacek *et al.*, 1961).

Some other structural and chemical changes are known to be induced by cold exposure, but the above constitute a sample of the adaptates that become significant before weaning. Since all of the data reviewed concern rats, the onsets of various adaptates can be listed (Table 16) in the serial order of the ages at which they have first been detected.

Adaptates outlasting the treatment appear to be evoked earliest in a small range of ages, regardless of the exact method of cold exposure or of under-feeding. This range of ages is that in which control of body temperature develops. I conclude that adaptational processes become available along with regulational processes.

No adaptate has been detected before seven days after birth; exposed infants and control infants require that long to become different from one another. Further, some of the differences require 18 days to materialize. Biochemical differences and structural differences all are parts of the overall modifications of the whole individual.

TABLE 16   Adaptates (tests or modifications) in studies of adaptations
produced by pre-treatments in cold air, in infant rats

Adaptate	Age of onset, days after birth	Reference
Oxygen uptake at neutrality, incr.	7	Gelineo
"	10	Hahn et al.
Thyroid follicle size incr.	10	Vacek et al.
Heart weight incr./BW	14	Vacek et al.
Skin thickness incr.	14	Vacek et al.
Adrenal ascorbate decr.	16	Jailer
Rate of body cooling decr.	18	Krecek et al.
Liver weight incr./BW	18	Krecek et al.
Adrenal weight incr./BW	18	Vacek et al.
Kidney weight incr./BW	19	Vacek et al.

Deadaptations, or losses of evoked adaptates, have scarcely been observed in infant animals. In adult individuals adaptates are lost in a few days after exposures to cold air cease (Adolph, 1956). But, the same adaptates can be regained in subsequent exposures.

HYPOXIC EXPOSURE

The most widely studied adapting treatment (adaptagent) of animals and their infants has been diminished oxygen pressure. The effects are approximately the same whether total atmospheric pressure be reduced, or a mountain be scaled, or air be diluted with nitrogen or other inert gas.

Here I gather together some of the studies that have been done with infant mammals of various stages. Again, rats have been used more than any other species. What are the earliest effects (adaptates) that have been identified?

a. Tryptophan oxygenase in liver appears even at birth in hypoxic rats. Pregnant rats are kept in pO_2 of 76 mm mercury for four days before parturition, during delivery and several days thereafter. When born the infants have livers that are smaller but have oxygenase contents that are higher at all ages from zero to nine days (Francesconi and Mager, 1969). The data suggest that the program for build-up of this enzyme is shifted ahead by about three days. Glucocorticoids are known to enhance the development of this enzyme, and their early liberation may possibly mediate the premature onset activated by hypoxia.

b. Survival without oxygen. Infants of rats and other mammals survive total deprivation of oxygen for many minutes, even though their body temperatures be kept at 37°. When newborn rats are pre-treated by exposure to hypoxia for four hours or more, they maintain their breathing in absence of oxygen for 44% longer. This effect of the pretreatment can be demonstrated in rats only one to two days old, as well as in those up to 10 days old (Adolph, 1971). For example, at four days of age the rats keep gasping for 18 minutes without oxygen, instead of 12 minutes in control litter-mates. Usually the adapted individuals take more gasps, but not always.

Since this adaptate can be elicited by only a few hours of hypoxic exposure, it can be identified soon after birth. It is retained for two days after the exposure. It represents also a change in the manner in which anaerobic energy is expended, available only in infancy.

c. Fatty liver. Rats born in pO_2 of 96 mm mercury or less have high concentrations of fat in the liver by the third day of life (Chiodi and Bass, 1969). They are not present in fetuses. They develop also in rats or mice taken to altitude after birth at sea level. The condition usually kills the young unless they are placed at low altitude or are deprived of food for half of each day. After 10 days of age the fat is utilized faster and does not accumulate in the liver to a lethal extent. Fatty liver is clearly a modification that develops in response to hypoxia; whether it be favorable or unfavorable to survival need not be a criterion of physiological adaptation.

d. Non-righting. Rats placed in air of sufficiently low barometric pressure lose control of bodily equilibrium and become unable to right themselves. When infants are tested in pO_2 of 27 mm mercury on successive days, they decrease the time they can endure the test. If they have been also daily exposed to pO_2 90 mm mercury for several days after birth, they decrease the time to non-righting more slowly than do control infants (Barker, 1957). At seven days after birth they last twice as long as their controls, and retain the greater tolerance so long as the daily exposures to pO_2 90 mm continue, at least up to 84 days of age. This tolerance to hypoxia is believed to be partly due to increased oxygen delivery.

e. Hemoglobin affinity, which is the reciprocal of the pO_2 at which hemoglobin is half-saturated with oxygen, is a measure of the fraction of hemoglobin in the blood that is fetal hemoglobin. In infant rats the affinity for oxygen decreases during the first 10–12 days after birth, in parallel to the increase of the time the animals are able to right themselves after they are tilted. Individuals exposed daily to low pO_2 retain some of their high hemoglobin affinities, and at 17 days of age, if not earlier, differ significantly from control litter-mates (Barker, 1957). This adaptate, then, contributes to the tolerance revealed by the test of bodily righting.

f. Erythropoiesis is faster in adult animals exposed to hypoxia, and is ordinarily reflected in the high hematocrit ratios and the high hemoglobin concentrations of their blood. But in rats born at sea level and then exposed to hypoxia during the first two to three weeks of life, the concentrations of erythrocytes and hemoglobin do not differ from those in rats kept at sea level. The earliest inductions of erythremia of altitude are reported at 17–28 days after birth (Altland and Allen, 1952; Contopoulos *et al.*, 1954; Barker, 1957; Garcia, 1957 and 1961; Carmena *et al.*, 1966). Even injection of erythropoietin does not elicit erythremia at an earlier age. Altitude exposures of pregnant mothers do not induce erythremia of the offspring (Contopoulos *et al.*, 1955).

However, rats bred at altitude produce infants that show erythremia at eight days after birth (Timiras and Woolley, 1966) but not at birth (Fig. 77). This induction, earlier by 15 days, has not yet been attributed to a change in a specific control of erythropoiesis.

Dogs and sheep bred at high altitude, however, carry fetuses that have blood rich in hemoglobin. Dog fetuses delivered at term (63 days after conception) have such blood (Becker, 1955). In sheep, blood samples taken from fetuses of 115–137 days of gestation, show blood volumes and hemoglobin volumes per unit of body weight markedly greater than those in fetuses bred at sea level (Prystowsky *et al.*, 1960).

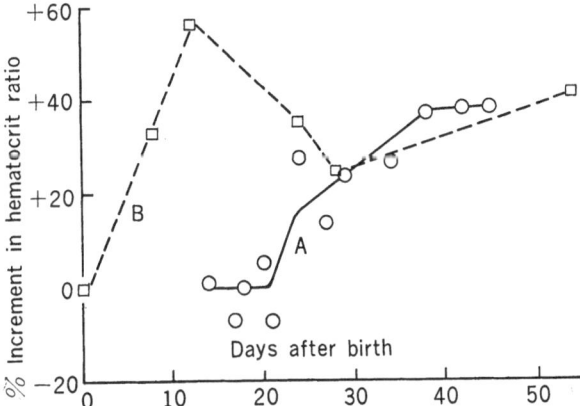

Fig. 77. Increment in hematocrit ratio in blood of infant rats of various ages. Each point represents the mean $100(h_e/h_c)$-100, where h_e is the hematocrit ratio of animals exposed to altitude, and h_c that of control animals kept at sea level. B, the F_2 generation born and maintained in pO_2 of 99 mm mercury (Timiras and Woolley, 1966); A, born at sealevel, exposed four hours daily in pO_2 of 59 mm mercury (Altland and Allen, 1952).

Humans born at high altitude have blood slightly richer in hemoglobin (Reynafarje, 1959). These three species have gestation durations much greater than those of rats, and possibly the long gestations furnish the fetuses with opportunity to adapt before their birth. But newborn bovines do not have blood richer in hemoglobin at altitude (Blatteis, 1963).

g. Heart weight. The organ most responsive to hypoxia is the heart. Especially the left ventricle hypertrophies in adults of various species at high altitudes. In infant rats born at altitude the heart is hypertrophied at eight and 12 days after birth, if not earlier (Timiras and Woolley, 1966).

In contrast, other organs including liver, kidneys and adrenals, maintain the same weights relative to total body weight in the very infant rats whose hearts hypertrophy. Whether the hypertrophy represents a response to more cardiac work in fetuses and infants at altitude is unknown. Part of the hypertrophy persists for three months after the rats are taken to sea level (Timiras, 1964).

h. Testes have been studied in rats born at sea level and taken to simulated altitude (59 mm mercury) intermittently. Their cells first become pycnotic at 14 days after birth (Altland and Allen, 1952). Various stages in the degeneration of testicular cells can be distinguished, the most critical stage being marked by the numbers of exfoliated cells present in the epididymis; these numbers were maximal after 29 days of age.

Although one may regard these testicular changes as representing an injury, the fact that they require the animal to develop to a certain stage before they take effect, fits them into the picture of onset and progression of adaptates with age.

i. Various adaptates. Adaptagents affecting the resistance of young rats to anoxia or hypoxia have been studied by Jilek and co-workers (1964). Such agents are: Ligation of both carotid arteries, repeated hemorrhages, and repeated centrifugations. The effects are tested variously, as, by survival times in nitrogen. For example, after three to six hemorrhages, there is no change in resistance to total anoxia (in nitrogen) at five days of age, but there is a loss of resistance at 10, 14, 18 and 21 days (Travnickova *et al.*, 1962).   Another example: Repeated centrifugations at 10 G induce adaptation as early as five days of age (Trojan and Jilek, 1964).   To what extent the tests of adaptation are standardized with respect to body temperature, absence of oxygen and other factors seems difficult to judge.   The general concept that pre-treatment with hypoxia forces developing rats to gain resistance to anoxia or hypoxia at early ages, is vigorously supported.

In summary, results of pre-treatments with hypoxia (Table 17) show that adaptates become available at diverse ages.   At least three of them (tryptophan oxygenase, fatty liver, anaerobic breathing) can be elicited within a day or two of birth.   Other adaptates might possibly be induced equally early if suitable pre-treatments were given before birth.   It is noteworthy that fetal erythremia and heart hypertrophy are not elicited by hypoxia of the rat mother, but develop soon after the fetuses have been born.   Hypoxia of the mother induced some change in the fetuses that came to light only after birth.

TABLE 17   Adaptates (tests or modifications) in studies of adaptations to hypoxia in infant rats

Adaptate	Age of onset, days	Reference
Tryptophan oxygenase in liver	0*	Francesconi
Fatty liver	1*	Chiodi and Bass
Duration of anaerobic breathing	2	Adolph (1971)
Duration of righting in pO₂ 27	7	Barker
Hemoglobin affinity	17	Barker
Hematocrit ratio	8*	Timiras and Woolley
	24	Altland and Allen
Heart weight incr./BW	8*	Timiras and Woolley
Testicular pycnosis	14	Altland and Allen

*Mother hypoxic during pregnancy

There is no doubt that some properties of the young rat, such as capacity for erythropoiesis, change with age, so that the newborn unaffected by hypoxia develops within eight days into an infant that is affected (erythremia, heart hypertrophy, fatty liver, non-righting time).   The transition means that the infant has gained capacities for adaptation.

COMMENT

1.   Ontogeny

Adaptations, by which animals are modified in response to extrinsic or environmental factors, depend on competences that resemble to a degree the results of inductions occurring during development of fetuses and embryos.   A physical or chemical factor impinges, and generates a modification that may last for hours, for days, or for a lifetime. In embryos the inductors operate chiefly through contacts among tissues; in fetuses and newborns some of the known inductors are also hormones, liberated in response to environmental influences.   In this view, physiological competences may postnatally embody the results of tissue interactions like those that prevail in embryos. Each adaptation utilizes and reveals a competence previously acquired. The adaptation goes into action when triggered by a specific extrinsic influence.

More specifically, it seems possible that RNAs produced under the influence of environments, may act on tissue targets during postnatal life in a manner similar to genetic endowments that act throughout development. Or, RNAs may mediate some competences and some adaptations. In an embryo the RNAs change their constitutions chiefly with the age program; in an infant the RNAs also change with specific environmental influences.

The existence of physiological adaptations shows clearly that at no age does the individual have to be exactly what its inherited constitution decrees. Its constitution is flexible within limits. These limits vary at different ages, but no age is without them.

Not only do constitutions vary, but each trait acquired corresponds to a specific environment. Some traits furnish a margin for survival in that very environment. These acquisitions reveal themselves only when environments of great variety are imposed.

Corticoadrenals. In adult rats both cold exposure and hypoxic exposure deplete the adrenal glands of ascorbic acid, an indication that cortical hormones have been liberated. This common effect has led to the supposition that either exposure can arouse the whole syndrome of physiological adaptates. But, the two exposures arouse other effects that differ (Adolph, 1956). Are the same effects produced by both these adaptagents in infants?

The earliest depletions of ascorbic acid elicited by cold exposures in rat infants are at 16 days (Jailer, 1950). It might have been supposed that adrenals do not react at all before this age. But Milkovic and Milkovic (1959a) found that ascorbate depletions could be elicited before birth by injections of epinephrine, which work through the pituitary gland to liberate ACTH which affects the corticoadrenals. Fetal hypophysectomy prevented the depletion of ascorbate. This finding led to the realization that the responding system is refractory for several days after birth, even premature birth (Eguchi and Wells, 1965). At five days after birth the ascorbate depletion once more responds to epinephrine injection (Milkovic and Milkovic, 1959b); in the interval between five and 16 days the response to cold exposure becomes installed.

A table showing the ages at which various stresses become effective in ascorbate depletion has been presented by Schapiro (1968). No adaptagent tested could elicit a response in postnatal rats until seven days of age. However, effects of hypoxia were not included in the table. Here (Table 17) I recognize three adaptates at zero to two days of age, thus demonstrating that they can appear at birth if not before. In addition, some effect upon the fetus in utero enables the individual after birth to adapt (hematocrit ratio, heart weight) earlier than an individual that was not hypoxic in utero. Whether ascorbate liberation from the adrenal glands is concerned in the production of these adaptates has not been tested.

In some other species (rabbit, dog, guinea pig) the adrenals of newborn individuals are depleted of ascorbate in response to epinephrine injection. The rat may be exceptional in suppressing the depletion after it has once gained it in the fetus.

In the rat Milkovic and Milkovic (1959a) found evidence that infants in small litters, which grew faster, responded to epinephrine two days earlier than those in larger litters. This suggests that the adaptive response matures in proportion as some factor of growth matures.

Possibly the lack of secretion of ACTH by the hypophysis limits the ascorbate depletion in early life, even after epinephrine injection becomes effective. Stimulation through electrodes implanted in the tuber cinereum of rats does not elicit the liberation of ACTH until 10–12 days after birth (Endröczi *et al.*, 1957).

The chain of responses through hypothalamus and hypophysis and adrenal may or may not be identified with that which results in physiological adaptation to cold exposure or to hypoxia or to both. If the links are identical, then parts of the chain are available before others; the adaptability arrives by steps. Several processes and tissues will fall into place, and until they do, the infant rat lives without the capacity to adapt to cold and to hypoxia through this chain.

Overlap. The series of adaptates that can be elicited by cold exposure (Table 16) may be compared with the series that can be elicited by hypoxic exposure (Table 17). The ages at which the two capacities for adaptation begin differ markedly; hypoxia becomes influential earlier in life. This fact suggests that the two means of elicitation actually differ.

The amounts of adaptates elicited also can be compared (Table 18). Only one of

TABLE 18   Increases in organ sizes or other adaptates in response to each of two adaptagents in infant rats. The % values are increments in experimental individuals relative to controlindividuals. N.S.=not significant.

	Air of 3°C		Hypoxia	
	Maximal	at age	Maximal	at age
Hematocrit ratio	N.S.		+44%	12 da
Adrenal ascorbate	−19%	16 da		
Adrenal wt/Body wt	+31%	20 da	N.S.	
Heart wt/Body wt	+86%	18 da	+138%	12 da
Liver wt/Body wt	+30%	20 da	N.S.	
Kidney wt/Body wt	+18%	18 da	N.S.	

Note: Data on 3° are from Vacek *et al.* (1961) and Jailer (1950). Data on hypoxia are from Timiras and Woolley (1966).

them is listed as aroused by both adaptagents, i.e., hypertrophy of the heart. The amounts of hypertrophy are about the same; the young heart doubles in weight. The maximal hypertrophy is reached about a week earlier under hypoxia than under cold exposure. The two ages could probably be made to match if an intermediate degree of hypoxia were applied.

Differences of adaptates are more prominent than similarities. Hypoxia arouses erythremia; hypothermia arouses hypertrophy of thyroid epithelial cells. Further explorations of other organs are needed, however, before it is certain that organ weights become any greater after one pre-treatment than after the other. Still further, both adaptagents may be imposed simultaneously or in succession. For the present, I conclude that the two lists of adaptates are specific, one for hypoxia and one for cold exposure, and differ significantly, exactly as was found for adult rats (Adolph, 1956).

2. Some Speculations

The information available about the ontogeny of physiological adaptations is obviously fragmentary. Even the study of the ontogeny of physiological regulations (Adolph, 1968) is still in a primitive stage. Techniques need to be standardized, animals standardized, ages chosen more critically, treatments less drastic, and control conditions more explicit.

Under natural conditions a fetal or newborn individual may be subjected to hypoxia at any age, but is usually subjected to low temperature only after birth. Hence one might anticipate that adaptation to hypoxia would appear at earlier ages than adaptation to cold air, and this is the actual case. Further, adaptive response to cold air may be disadvantageous to a poikilotherm such as a newborn rat, becoming practical only when the individual later acquires insulation, bulk, blood-flow controls and thermogenesis that make feasible the maintenance of a warm body. These factors suggest that the early acquisition of hypoxic adaptability and the later acquisition of thermal adaptability have each resulted under the cumulative experience of natural selection, and that each capacity for adaptation becomes available at an age when selection would influence it.

The relation between physiological regulation and adaptability is also evident. Until the body temperature is internally regulated, adaptation to cold air is either not possible, or undetectable. Maturation of regulatory arrangements depends on dif-ferentiations of function, which are now shown to be available at birth or before when hypoxia is the adaptagent, but only a week or two later when cold air is the adaptagent.

The chief *principles* illustrated in this paper are: (a) Specific properties of individuals are modified under the influence of particular environmental factors. (b) The capacity to be modified is not present at all ages but is acquired by the individual during development. (c) While the individual is acquiring its regulatory devices one by one, it also acquires one by one the capacities to shift those regulations in accord with the prevailing environment. (d) These capacities are the basis of specific interactions between physiological constitution and effective environment.

3. Concept of Superfunction

Finally, I would like to extend the concept of physiological adaptation. (a) Adaptation can be said to be elicited by a stress, from body or from environment, that works particular processes to their limit or near their limit. (b) Each adaptate grows, after a latent period, up to an asymptote. (c) It stays at asymptote as long as continuous or intermittent stress impinges. (d) It decays gradually after stress ceases.

These four statements also apply to a hypertrophy, a hyperplasia and a regenera-tion of an excised tissue. I suggest that all these processes are one and the same. Some are visible to the naked eye, some require microscopic examination, some require chemical analysis, some require physiological measurement. Often all super-activities are concurrent. They could be aspects of a common phenomenon.

Upon the view that these phenomena are similar in nature, one can look at what is known about hypertrophy and about regeneration for additional light upon physiological adaptations. A prominent feature is that all are responses to increase of work or to decrease of supply (Goss, 1964). The discrepancy between supply and demand con-stitutes a deficit of function. This deficit serves to arouse an increase in the tissue and the process; such a functional deficit triggers the hypertrophy and the regeneration and the adaptation. Varied examples are: The long-term responses to muscular exercise, to liver excision, or to dermal wound.

The chemical means of arousal of hypertrophy or of physiological adaptation in the tissue is little comprehended. It is specific, it is local, it is limited in amount. But the kinetics of the resultants are alike in hypertrophy, regeneration and adaptation; indeed the time constants are in the same range. All these facts suggest that physiological adaptation is understood exactly in proportion that hypertrophy and regeneration are understood. All suggest that each adaptation need not be a separate invention in the tissue, but that there may be a generalized capacity for response that becomes specific whenever a particular adaptagent impinges.

REFERENCES

1. ADOLPH, E.F. (1956): *Am. J. Physiol.* **184**: 18.
2. ADOLPH, E.F. (1964): *Am. Physiol. Soc.* **4**: 27.
3. ADOLPH, E.F. (1968): Origins of Physiological Regulations. Academic Press, New York.
4. ADOLPH, E.F. (1971): *Am. J. Physiol.* **221**: 123.
5. ALTLAND, P.D., and E. ALLEN (1952): *J. Morphol.* **91**: 541.
6. BARIC, I. (1953): *Arch. Biol. Nauk Beograd* **5**: 143.
7. BARKER, J.N. (1957): *Am. J. Physiol.* **189**: 281.
8. BECKER, E.L., M.G. COOPER and G.D. HATAWAY (1955): *J. Applied Physiol.* **8**: 166.
9. BLATTEIS, C.M. (1963): *Proc. 3rd Internat. Biometerol. Congr.* **176.**
10. BLATTEIS, C.M. (1964): *J. Physiol.* (London) **172**: 358.
11. BRÜCK, K., W. WÜNNENBERG, and E. ZEISBERGER (1969): *Fed. Proc.* **28**: 1035.
12. CARMENA, A., G. LUCARELLI, C. CARNEVALI, and F. STOHLMAN, JR. (1966): *Proc. Soc. Exp. Biol. Med.* **121**: 652.
13. CHIODI, H.P., and R. BASS (1969): *Fed. Proc.* **28**: 1080.
14. CONTOPOULOS, A.N., D.C. VAN DYKE, M.E. SIMPSON, J.H. LAWRENCE, and H.M. EVANS (1954): *Proc. Soc. Exp. Biol. Med.* **86**: 713.
15. CONTOPOULOS, A.N., D.C. VAN DYKE, S. ELLIS, M.E. SIMPSON, J.H. LAWRENCE, and H.M. EVANS (1955): *Blood* **10**: 115.
16. DAWES, G.S. (1968): Foetal and Neonatal Physiology. Yearbook, Chicago.
17. DAWKINS, M.J.R., and D. HULL (1964): *J. Physiol.* (*London*) **172**: 216.
18. EGUCHI, Y., and L.J. WELLS (1965): *Proc. Soc. Exp. Biol. Med.* **120**: 675.
19. ENDRÖCZI, E., J. SZALAY, und K. LISSAC (1957): *Endokrinol.* **34**: 331.
20. FRANCESCONI, R.P., and M. MAGER (1969): *Science* **166**: 1412.
21. GARCIA, J.F. (1957): *Am. J. Physiol.* **190**: 25.
22. GARCIA, J.F., and D.C. VAN DYKE (1961): *Proc. Soc. Exp. Biol. Med.* **106**: 585.
23. GELENIO, S. (1964): Handbook of Physiology, *Am. Physiol. Soc.* **4**: 272.
24. GOSS, R.J. (1964): Adaptive Growth. Academic Press, New York.
25. HAHN, P., O. KOLDOVSKY, J. KRECEK, J. MARTINEK and Z. VACEK (1963): *Fed. Proc.* **22**: 824.
26. HEIM, R., and Z. SZELENYI (1965): *Acta physiol. Hungaric.* **27**: 247.
27. JAILER, J.W. (1950): *Endocrinol.* **46**: 420.
28. JILEK, L. (1964): Progress in Brain Research, ed. W.A. Himwich, **9**: 115.
29. KRECEK, J., J. KRECKOVA and J. MARTINEK (1957): *Physiol. Bohemoslov.* **6**: 329.
30. LEVINE, S., M. ALPERT, and G.W. LEWIS (1958): *J. Compar. Physiol. Psychol.* **51**: 774.
31. MILKOVIC, K., and S. MILKOVIC (1959a): *Endokrinol.* **34**: 151.
32. MILKOVIC, K., and S. MILKOVIC (1959b): *Arch. Internat. Physiol. Biochem.* **67**: 24.
33. MOORE, R.E., and M.C. UNDERWOOD (1963): *J. Physiol.* (*London*) **168**: 290.
34. MOUNT, L.E. (1968): The Climatic Physiology of the Pig. Williams and Wilkins, Baltimore, 64.
35. PRYSTOWSKY, H., A. HELLEGERS, G. MESCHIA, J. METCALFE, W. HUCKABEE, and D.H. BARRON (1960): *Quart. J. Exp. Physiol.* **45**: 292.
36. REYNAFARJE, C. (1959): *J. Pediat.* **54**: 152.
37. SCHAPIRO, S. (1968): Early Experience and Behavior. ed. G. Newton and S. Levine. Thomas, Springfield, 198.
38. TIMIRAS, P.S. (1964): The Physiological Effects of High Altitude. ed. W.H. Weihe. Macmillan, New York, 21.

39. TIMIRAS, P.S., and D.E. WOOLLEY (1966): *Fed. Proc.* **25**: 1312.
40. TRAVNICKOVA, E., J. MOUREK, and S. TROJAN (1962): *Physiol. Bohemoslov.* **11**: 231.
41. TROJAN, S., and L. JILEK (1964): *Physiol. Bohemoslov.* **13**: 473.
42. VACEK, Z., P. HAHN, and O. KOLDOVSKY (1961): *J. Anat.* **95**: 210.
43. ZEISBERGER, E., K. BRÜCK, W. WUNNENBERG, und C. WIETASCH (1967): *Pflügers Arch. gesam. Physiol.* **296**: 276.

CHAPTER 12

MAN AND COLD STRESS*

STEVEN M. HORVATH

Institute of Environmental Stress, University of California, Santa Barbara, California, U.S.A.

It is only fitting that on the occasion of Professor Kuno's 88th birthday recognition be given to one of the first scientists to consider the necessity and importance of studying man in his natural environments. Professor Kuno and his students initiated many studies on man living and working in hot and cold climates. The successful response (adaptation) of man to a cold ambient environment is dependent upon behavioral and physiological mechanisms. Behavioral factors involve a complex interplay utilizing other elements of the environment to protect against the impacting one. The use of external and internal energy sources, properly designed clothing with improved insulation, reduction of effective areas for radiation, convective and conductive losses as well as limiting the duration of exposure illustrate the many behavioral responses utilized by man. However, physiological responses, i.e., modification of internal adaptative mechanisms are also involved. These physiological alterations which occur in man when chronically exposed to cold have been of interest for an understanding of man's capability to withstand cold environments. The experimental approaches which have been utilized to study this problem have been through three types of exposed subjects: those living in polar regions, those who have been exposed to cold (from minutes to days) in temperature regulated chambers, and those exposed to normal seasonal environmental cold. These three types of exposure have been assumed to result in either adaptation, acclimation, or acclimatization to cold, respectively. Adaptation to cold implies changes of a genetic nature which have occurred due to the natural selection processes in a cold environment. Acclimation refers to physiological changes occurring in response to temperature changes separated from contaminating factors such as activity, diet, etc. which may affect acclimatized subjects. Physiological acclimatization to cold refers, then, to any change in physiological mechanisms or regulatory systems which better enable an individual to survive effectively in a cold environment.

Horvath *et al.* [10] studied five men who lived continuously over a period of eight days in a cold room at an ambient temperature of $-29\,°C$. No evidence for acclimatization to a cold environment were obtained for either metabolic or body temperature parameters. Carlson *et al.* [3] observed seven subjects who were exposed for 14 days, 16–18 hours daily, to an ambient of -7 to $-5\,°C$. These subjects were supposedly adequately clothed so as to prevent uncomfortable cold sensations. These investigators concluded that acclimatization had occurred as evidenced by a diminution in heat

*Research sponsored by the Air Force Office of Scientific Research, Air Force Systems Command, under Grant No. AFOSR-69-1653. The United States Government is authorized to reproduce and distribute reprints for Governmental purposes notwithstanding any copyright notation hereon.

elimination. Davis [6] reported that men artificially acclimatized to cold in the summer had decreased heat production and lower mean skin and rectal temperatures as a consequence of eight-hour daily exposures to an ambient temperature of 13.5 °C. Dahms and Horvath [4] have summarized available evidence on acclimatization to cold from data obtained during studies involving seasonal alterations in physiological responses correlated with climatic temperature changes. The trends of seasonal changes in the common indices of temperature regulation in the cold: Mean skin temperature, rectal temperature, metabolic heat production, tissue conductance, shivering, and extremity temperature are summarized in Table 19. Because of the small number of subjects studied and the large interindividual variability, statistical evaluation was impossible and trends are only indicated. In all parameters measured, except basal metabolism and degree of shivering, changes in all three possible directions have been reported, i.e., increased, decreased, or no change. The BMR either decreased or did not change while shivering activity apparently decreased in all reported instances. The tissue conductance as recalculated by us appeared to be the best index of cold acclimatization as in every study it was lower in the winter. A reduction in skin blood flow, an increased level of vasoconstriction, occurred in the coldest portion of the year.

TABLE 19 Seasonal changes in acclimatization to cold

Reference	Location	Annual temperature range	Test procedure	T_{re}	$\bar{T}_s$	Extremity temp.	Extremity	Metabolism	Tissue* Conductance	BMR	Shivering
9	Pusan, Korea	10 to 27°C**	Water bath	↓	NI†	NI	NI	NI	↓	↑	↓
5	Fort Knox, Kentucky	−5 to 28°C	1 hr @ 14°C monthly	→	→	↓	Toe	↓	↓	→	↓
8	Toronto, Ontario	−4 to 21°C	1 hr @ 8.5°C monthly	→	→	→	Foot and hand	↓	↓	NI	↓
21	Kyoto, Japan	2.7 to 26.4°C	3 hr @ 10°C summer and winter	↑	↓	NI	NI	→	↓	NI	NI
1	Philadelphia Penn.	−5 to 30°C	Water bath summer and winter	NI	NI	NI	NI	NI	↓	NI	↓
18	Antarctica	−40 to 30°C	1.5 hr @ 5°C summer and winter	↓	↓	→	Toe and finger	↓	↓	→	NI
7	Canadian Arctic	−46 to 27°C	Overnight @ 0–3°C fall and spring	→	↓	↓	Arm and leg	→	↓	→	NI
11	Kyoto, Japan	3 to 27°C	Ambient conditions weekly for 1 yr	NI	↓	NI	NI	↑	↓	↑	NI

*Where specific conductances were not reported, calculations were made based upon available data.
**Water surface temperature range.
†NI indicates that there was no information presented.

Davis [5] exposed nude subjects to a constant cold stress (14 °C) for a period of one hour each month over a period of one year. The ambient environmental conditions represented an annual mean monthly temperature range of 31 °C with a maximum of 28 °C in August and a minimum of −3 °C in February. He reported a positive correlation between environmental temperature and shivering response to cold. Since shivering is a means of increasing metabolic heat production, there was a similar correlation to ambient temperature. However, while metabolism decreased 50%, shivering decreased 95%. Girling [8] performed a similar study in Toronto, Canada, where the annual mean daily temperature range was 25 °C with a maximum of 21 °C in July and a minimum of −4 °C in February. His subjects also exhibited no pattern of change in mean skin or rectal temperatures over the year when subjects were studied at 8.5 °C. These subjects exhibited a 90% reduction in metabolism after one hour at the test temperature and this decrease was correlated with the decrease in shivering activity. However, the maximal decrease in metabolic heat production had a two month lag when compared with the minimum environmental temperature. Yoshimura [21] has also reported seasonal changes in acclimatization to cold in Japanese soldiers living in Kyoto. The subjects were exposed nude to a 10 °C environment for three hours twice in winter (February) and twice in summer (August). The annual mean temperature range in Kyoto is 23.7 °C with a low of 2.7 °C in January and a high of 26.4 °C in August. All subjects showed a lower mean skin temperature and a higher mean rectal temperature in winter. The metabolic heat production increased to the same level in winter and summer after two hours of exposure but the rate of increase was slower in winter. Thus cold acclimatization was accomplished by lowering the $\bar{T}_s$ and consequently decreasing the heat loss which in turn minimized the metabolic cost of the thermal stress in winter.

Dahms and Horvath [4] have studied seven young men exposed in the nude to an ambient temperature of 4.5 °C for a period of two hours. Exposures were made at monthly intervals for a calendar year. The annual monthly range of ambient temperature at Santa Barbara was 8.8 °C with a minimum of 10.9 °C in December and a maximum of 19.7 °C in August. The reported indices of cold acclimatization, i.e., decreased tissue conductance, decreased shivering, decreased heat production, delayed rise of heat production, and elevated extremity temperatures, were not observed during an acute cold stress in Santa Barbara subjects. A seasonal change in tissue conductance, K_{tis}, was noted reaching its highest value, 7.4 kcal/m²-hour/C, during March and April with the lowest values of 5.0 being found in October to December. This and other evidence suggested that cold acclimatization did not occur in Santa Barbara residents. According to the data obtained from previous studies [5, 8, 21] it was hypothesized that due to every 10 °C change in mean monthly environmental temperature, a cold acclimatized subject should show a 15% reduction in total heat production after one hour of cold exposure. A reduction of 10–15 kcal/m²-hour per 10 °C change in environment should occur. No such change occurred after one hour cold exposure in Santa Barbara subjects, again suggesting that no cold acclimatization had occurred. However, some of the evidence collected appeared to imply that Santa Barbara subjects were still heat acclimatized in the winter months. An indication that an increased sensitivity to cold occurred during the winter months, contrary to observations on subjects residing in more northern latitudes, was obtained from the higher values obtained from the slope of the regression equation $\log_{10}$ kcal/m²-hour versus $\log_{10} \bar{T}_M$. It would appear that changes in physiological parameters depended not only upon the change in environmental temperature but also upon the absolute levels of the annual mean temperature.

These studies indicated that considerable confusion could ensue in determining the responses of man to seasonal variations in ambient temperatures due in part to selection of subjects, temperature at which subjects are tested, duration of test cold exposure, behavioral responses of subjects to the ambient temperatures of their locality, and the precise physiological response considered to be most representative of cold sensitivity. A most serious deficiency in all known studies relates to the precise amount of cold exposure experienced by test subjects. Davis's [5] subjects worked in air-conditioned facilities but their living quarters were not air-conditioned. Girling's [8] subjects lived and worked in heated facilities during the winter. Yoshimura's [21] soldiers were assigned to outdoor patrol duty but the insulative value of their clothing was not known nor was the degree of heating in their quarters indicated. However, this group had apparently the greatest cold exposure. In Santa Barbara there was little tendency to increase clothing insulation during cold months but living quarters were usually heated.

Evaluation of the response of the temperature regulatory system to an acute cold stress requires that the stress be of sufficient duration to permit the attainment of a relative steady state. The necessity for a test exposure of sufficient duration to obtain a steady state was first demonstrated by Yoshimura who used a three hour exposure. He reported no differences in steady state heat production in men studied during either summer or winter months. However, the rise to the steady state level was more gradual in the winter period. Buskirk *et al.* [2] stated that observations of subjects during a single hour of exposure failed to yield a full picture of cold adaptation. O'Hanlon and Horvath [14] concurred with this view point based on their studies of 34 men exposed for two hours to an ambient temperature of 7.7 °C. They also showed that older subjects generally tended to maintain higher body temperatures than younger subjects. Since many of the more recent cold exposure and acclimatization studies have been using an ambient temperature of 5 °C for their stress test, Raven and Horvath [15] made a careful metabolic and temperature response study of 11 men exposed to this environment (Fig. 78). The heat production increased during the cold exposure attaining an approximately stable level during the final 30 minutes of a 120 minute exposure. The group variability in response to the cold was greatest during the first 30 minutes and became less with continued exposure. All skin temperatures approached a stable value during the final 30 minutes. Rectal temperature was initially elevated and remained at the highest point throughout the exposure. Tissue conductance (with or without the inclusion of heat exchanges due to changes in body heat content and respiratory losses) was in agreement only during the final quarter of the exposure, indicating a state of physiological equilibrium. Thus steady states with minimal individual variability occurred only after some 90 minutes of exposure to 5 °C.

Wyndham *et al.* [19, 20] studies on racial, sexual, and adaptation differences utilized a two hour exposure but unfortunately base much of their evaluation of responses on a single measure of metabolic heat production obtained at the beginning of the second hour. Newman based his conclusions on the responses of subjects given a one hour cold stress. His [13] black subjects (American Negro) showed evidences of cold acclimatization following six weeks of daily four hour cold exposures. Interestingly the only changes reported in contrast to Davis's results were in a reduced amount of shivering with no change in metabolic heat production and warmer skin temperatures. He [12] also found a similar response in three continental Puerto Ricans. These

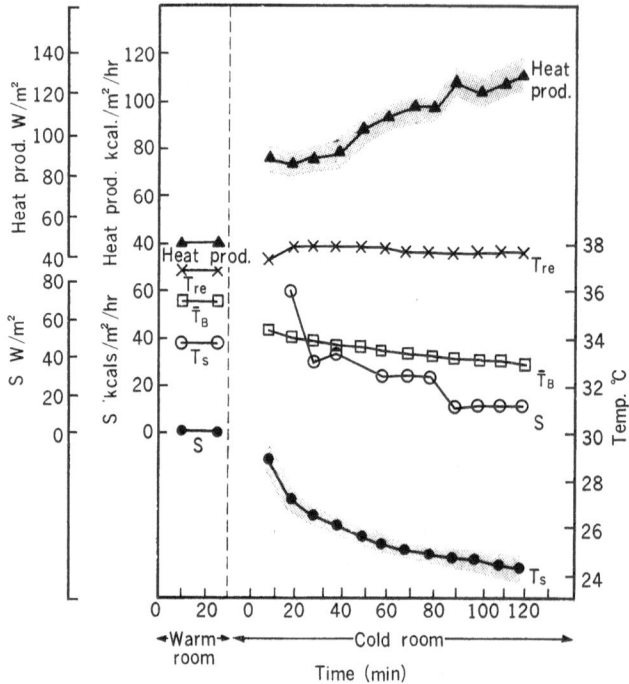

Fig. 78. Average rectal, mean body, mean skin temperatures, storage, and heat production as functions of time in the cold. One standard deviation for each mean function is shown by shading.

studies may have produced more interesting information if the cold. exposure had been longer as noted earlier by Yoshimura [21].

The scarcity of information on other physiological changes during cold exposure induced O'Hanlon and Horvath [14] to evaluate the heart rate response. They found as had Yoshimura *et al.* [22] earlier that the heart rate remained constant or was slightly increased during cold exposures. This constancy of heart rate and the marked increase in oxygen uptake during these cold stresses suggested to us that this high oxygen uptake could be accomplished by an elevation in cardiac output, greater oxygen extraction, or a combination of both. However, Wezler and Thauer [17] had reported that in a single subject exposed to a 5 °C ambient the oxygen uptake increased three fold without any alteration in cardiac output. Raven *et al.* [16] studied 11 males exposed to a 5 °C ambient for two hours. The data obtained is summarized in Table 20. Cardiac output was significantly elevated by as much as 95% above control levels obtained in a neutral environment. Within the first hour of exposure, the $(A-V)_{O_2}$ difference increased 30% with a concomitant elevation of cardiac output of 73%. During the next hour both parameters continued to increase. The $(A-V)_{O_2}$ difference had attained a stable level by 90 minutes while cardiac output continued to rise slightly until the termination of the exposure. The increased cardiac output was primarily due to an increased stroke volume. This response was quite different from that observed during exercise where at oxygen uptake levels of one to two liters, the increased cardiac output was primarily accomplished by elevating the heart rate and keeping stroke volume at its resting level. The direct relationship

TABLE 20 Group means and standard deviations of all cardiovascular and metabolic parameters for each thirty minute time period*

Parameter	28°C 30 min	5°C 30 min	5°C 60 min	5°C 90 min	5°C 120 min
Heat production (kcal/m² per hr	40 ± 5	78 ± 17	88 ± 12	103 ± 15	107 ± 17
Oxygen uptake, ml/min	260 ± 47	510 ± 150	580 ± 100	680 ± 110	710 ± 120
Cardiac index, liter/min per m²	2.6 ± 0.4	4.0 ± 1.0	4.5 ± 1.4	4.7 ± 1.0	5.1 ± 1.1
Stroke index, ml/beat per m²	41 ± 7	58 ± 11	65 ± 18	67 ± 13	73 ± 15
Heart rate, beat/min	64 ± 6	70 ± 7	69 ± 7	71 ± 6	70 ± 7
(A-V)O₂ difference, ml O₂/liter	54 ± 12	68 ± 22	70 ± 26	77 ± 23	75 ± 22
Total peripheral resistance (dynes. sec)/cm⁻⁵	1525 ± 354	1326 ± 760	1269 ± 715	1087 ± 395	1058 ± 409
Systolic blood pressure, mm Hg	119 ± 10	135 ± 11	138 ± 15	139 ± 16	141 ± 18
Diastolic blood pressure, mm Hg	76 ± 10	86 ± 5	88 ± 8	90 ± 9	90 ± 9
Mean blood pressure, mm Hg	88 ± 6	101 ± 5	103 ± 8	105 ± 9	105 ± 9

*Group Body Surface Area = 1.87 ± 0.04 SEM.

between cardiac output and oxygen uptake reported by many investigators to occur at certain levels of exercise was maintained during the cold stress. These studies on the cardiovascular responses to cold stress could well be expanded to consider the changes occurring in this system with acclimatization to cold. It would appear that such increases in cardiac output could not be maintained for excessively long periods of time, days, weeks, or months, without imposing an excessive load on this system.

It would appear from this brief review of some physiological responses of men to an acute cold stress—men who are either naive to or accustomed to cold environments—that there are many more aspects of physiological adjustment and adaptations that need to be studied. This area of physiology, so well initiated by Professor Kuno, has as he predicted no ending but just a beginning.

REFERENCES

1. BURTON, A.C., and H.C. BAZETT. (1936): *Amer. J. Physiol.* **117**: 36.
2. BUSKIRK, E.R., R.H. THOMPSON, and G.D. WHEDON (1963): *J. Appl. Physiol.* **18**: 603.
3. CARLSON, L.D., H.L. BURNS, T.H. HOLMES, and P.P. WEBB (1953): *J. Appl. Physiol.* **5**: 672.
4. DAHMS, T.E., and S.M. HORVATH: *Unpublished observations.*
5. DAVIS, T.R.A., and D.R. JOHNSTON (1961): *J. Appl. Physiol.* **16**: 231.
6. DAVIS, T.R.A. (1961): *J. Appl. Physiol.* **16**: 1011.
7. ELSNER, R.W., K.L. ANDERSON, and L. HERMANSEN (1960): *J. Appl. Physiol.* **15**: 659.
8. GIRLING, R. (1967): *Can. J. Physiol. Pharmacol.* **45**: 13.
9. HONG, S. (1963): *Fed. Proc.* **22**: 831.
10. HORVATH, S.M., A. FREEDMAN, and H. GOLDEN (1947): *Amer. J. Physiol.* **150**: 99.
11. KENZO, M. (1958): *J. Physiol. Soc. Japan* **20**: 204.
12. NEWMAN, R.W. (1968): *J. Appl. Physiol.* **25**: 277.
13. NEWMAN, R.W. (1969): *J. Appl. Physiol.* **27**: 316.
14. O'HANLON, J.F., and S.M. HORVATH (1970): *Can. J. Physiol. Pharmacol.* **48**: 1.
15. RAVEN, P.B., and S.M. HORVATH (1970): *Int. J. Biometeor.* **14**: 309.
16. RAVEN, P.B., I. NIKI, T.E. DAHMS, and S.M. HORVATH (1970): *J. Appl. Physiol.* **29**: 417.
17. WEZLER, K., and R. THAUER (1943): *Z. Ges. Exp. Med.* **112**: 345.
18. WYNDHAM, C.H., R. PLOTKIN, and A. MONRO (1964): *J. Appl. Physiol.* **19**: 593.
19. WYNDHAM, C.H., J.F. MORRISON, C.G. WILLIAMS, G.A.G. BREDELL, P.D. VAN RAHDEN, J.E. HOLDSWORTH, L.D. VAN GRAAN, A.J. VAN RENSBURGH, and A. MONRO (1964): *J. Appl. Physiol.* **19**: 877.
20. WYNDHAM, C.H., C.G. WILLIAMS, and H. LOOTS (1968): *J. Appl. Physiol.* **24**: 282.
21. YOSHIMURA, H. (1960): "Acclimatization To Heat and Cold." in *Essential Problems in Climatic Physiology* H. YOSHIMURA (ed.), Tokyo, Nankodo Co., Ltd.
22. YOSHIMURA, H., S. YSAMI, K. MAKIHATA, and S. SHIOMI (1962): *J. Physiol. Japan* **24**: 81.

CHAPTER 13

THYROID ACTIVITY AND COLD ADAPTABILITY

Mitsuo SUZUKI

Department of Physiology, Institute of Endocrinology, Gunma University, Maebashi, Japan

INTRODUCTION

It is a well attested fact that the body temperature of thyroidectomized animals exposed to cold decreases much more rapidly than that of controls with intact thyroids. Also the indispensability of the thyroid gland for the survival of homeothermic animals in a cold environment is beyond debate (Ershoff, 1948; LeBlond and Eartly, 1952; LeBlond and Gross, 1943; Ring, 1942; Sellers and You, 1950; Hsieh, 1966).

For survival in cold for a long period of time, non-shivering thermogenesis which accompanys increased oxygen consumption was found to be essential (Cottle and Carlson, 1956; Hsieh and Carlson, 1957; Depocas, 1960). The rapid response of the thermogenesis is obtained after an exposure of rather long duration, that is a cold-acclimated state. It is inferred that the thyoid hormone is indispensable for this acclimatization. The cold-acclimated rat in a cold environment can exert an acute non-shivering thermogenesis even after thyroidectomy (Hsieh and Carlson, 1957).

Acute thermogenesis is known to be increased by noradrenaline (Depocas, 1960; Hsieh and Carlson, 1957) which mimics the response to acute cold exposure. This indicates that the sympathetico-adrenomedullary system is also essential for survival in cold.

On the other hand, it has been widely recognized that the pituitary-adrenocortical axis counteracts rapidly such stress as exposure to cold since Selye (1950) who proposed a concept of "stress."

Therefore neural and endocrine responses of homeotherms to cold consist of an enormously complicated and integrated mechanism in which change in thyroid activity has to be evaluated.

RESPONSE OF HUMAN ENDOCRINE FUNCTION TO ACUTE COLD EXPOSURE

We carried out an experiment to observe the initial response of not only the thyroid but also the sympathetico-adrenal system and adrenal cortex of human subjects to acute cold exposure (Suzuki *et al.*, 1967).

Nine healthy young men were exposed nude to an environmental temperature of 10–15 °C for one hour in summer. Blood and urine specimens collected before, immediately after and six hours after the cold exposure were analyzed for hormone and electrolyte content.

Thyroid function has been evaluated by many methods such as protein-bound iodine (PBI) concentration, resin uptake of ^{131}I-triiodothyronine (T_3) and plasma thyrotropin (TSH) level. To assess these indices for the accurate evaluation of thyroid function, special care was taken to evaluate change in the metabolism of water and electrolytes due to the cold exposure. Also, estimation of hormone concentrations other than thyroid were made, e.q. cortisol in plasma and catecholamines and 17-ketosteroid in urine. The indices should throw light on understanding the feature of thyroid function which plays a role in the extensive response of the homeothermic animal in a cold environment.

The subsequent experimental schedule, cold exposure, diet, collection of urine and blood specimens, is shown in Table 21. During cold exposure, the volunteers were sitting on benchs and after exposure they were allowed to lie supine or in any other relaxed position. Blood pressure, both systolic and diastolic, heart rate, and rectal temperature were measured at appropriate intervals.

TABLE 21   Schedule of experiment

9 a.m.	Breakfast (milk, 3 ml/kg and cracker, 1 g/kg
10	Urination and water intake (2 ml/kg)
11	Urination and blood sampling
	Exposure to cold
12 noon	Urination and blood sampling
	Lunch (milk and crackers)
1 p.m.	
2	
3	Urination and water intake (3 ml/kg)
4	
5	Urination and water intake (2 ml/kg)
6	Urination and blood sampling

All nine volunteers suffered a chill during the cold exposure and four of them shivered markedly. One subject continued violent shivering even after the end of exposure, followed by a high fever of 39 °C, which made the subsequent assessments impossible.

1. Physical Response to Cold

Fig. 79 shows changes in blood pressure, heart rate, and rectal temperature during the course of the experiment. The blood pressure, both systolic and diastolic, rose significantly 15 minutes after the onset of cold exposure, remained high during it, and returned to normal six hours after the exposure. The salient change in the blood pressure shows an acute stimulation of the sympathetico-adrenal system. The increased blood pressure in turn probably stimulated the baroreceptors which caused bradycardia as shown in the figure (Marey's law). After exposure, the heart rate increased for a time and then decreased gradually. The temporary reflexed tachycardia may result from an acute disappearance of the stimulation of the baroreceptors. The rectal temperature rose significantly 15 minutes after the onset of exposure, then decreased slowly during it, returning to the normal level six hours after exposure. This quick response in the "core" temperature indicates an acute increase in thermogenesis. Girling (1963) reported that nude human subjects exposed to cold showed two different responses. The first group demonstrated shivering accompanying increased oxygen consumption 15 minutes after exposure, while the other group showed an immediate increase in oxygen consumption on exposure.

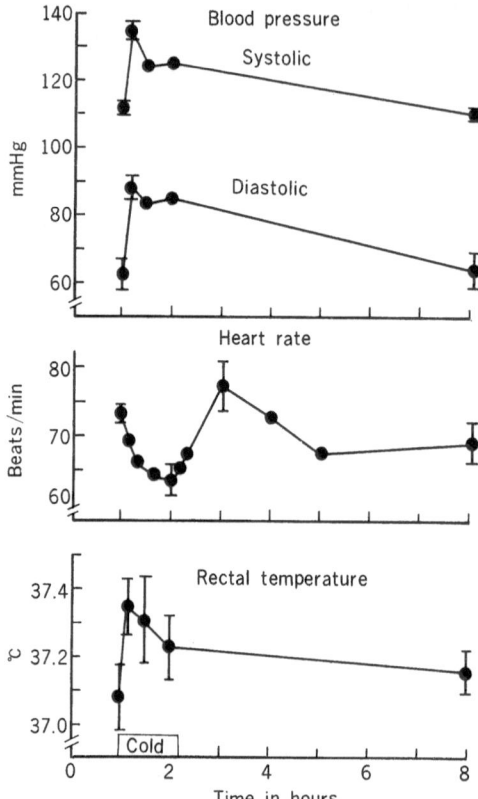

Fig. 79. Changes in blood pressure, heart rate, and rectal temperature before, during, and after cold exposure at 10–15°C for one hour. Mean ± S.E. is shown.

2. Cold Diuresis and Hemoconcentration

Fig. 80 shows changes in urine volume and urinary excretion of electrolytes during the experiment. Urine volume increased significantly during exposure (cold diuresis), decreased to a subnormal level, and then returned to normal at the end of observation (Adolph *et al.*, 1946; Bader *et al.*, 1952). Mean urine volume during exposure was 2.1 times that of the pre-exposure period. The diuresis was accompanied by an increase in electrolytes, particularly sodium and chloride, confirming both earlier and more recent observations (Bass, 1954; Bazett, 1924; Budd and Warharft, 1970). Phosphate excretion was also increased clearly during exposure, whereas the increase in potassium and calcium excretion was not so evident. The diuresis could be completely inhibited by a small dose of Pitressin (Bader *et al.*, 1952) and it would therefore appear that cold diuresis in man results from a diminished secretion of antidiuretic hormone (ADH). Itoh (1954) reported that secretion of ADH is reduced in rats on exposure to cold. Recently, Segar and Moore (1968) showed that the ADH level in human blood increases after exposure to heat and inversely decreases shortly after cold exposure. The rapid change in ADH secretion rate could be interpreted as due to mediation caused by the activity of the intrathoracic stretch receptors (the "volume receptors") in response to redistribution of blood. Namely, cold exposure caused hypertension resulting from vasoconstriction in the "shell," which

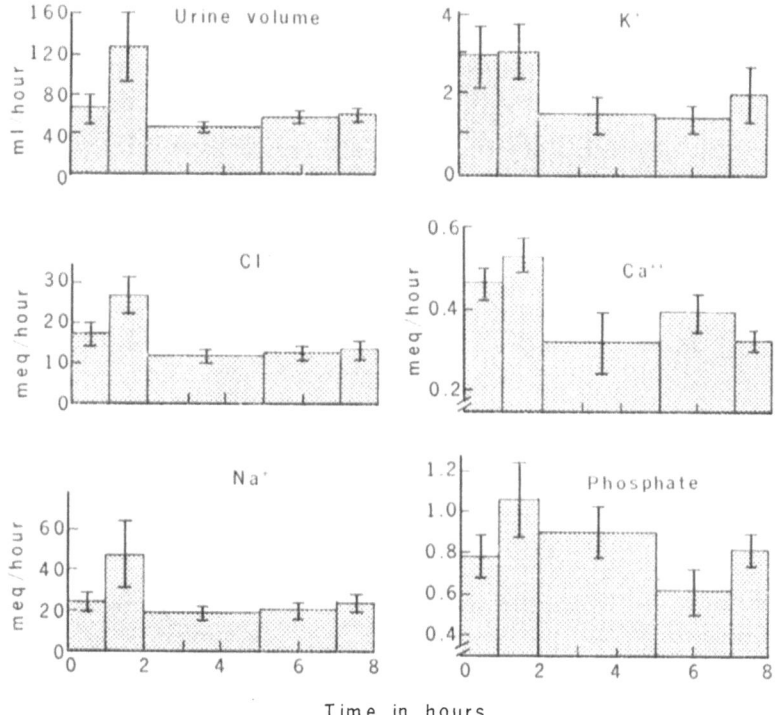

Fig. 80. Changes in urine volume and urinary content of some electrolytes. Subjects were exposed to cold for one hour after a one-hour pre-exposure period.

in turn increased the intrathracic blood volume. The natriuresis accompanying cold diuresis may be explained by a supposed substance, a third factor which has natriuretic potency (De Wardner *et al.*, 1961; Johnston *et al.*, 1967). Concentration of plasma protein and hematocrit values increased significantly (Fig. 81), indicating hemoconcentration during the cold exposure. The increase in plasma concentration was 10.7%, and the increase in hematocrit value was 10.8%. This distinct hemoconcentration should be taken into account in evaluating the change in concentrations of hormones in the plasma. In the following experiments, plasma concentration of cortisol and PBI was expressed in terms of micrograms per gram of plasma protein to make clear the actual changes in concentration of the substances in question.

The hemoconcentration and cold diuresis previously described, which are well-known accompaniments to acute cold exposure in human (Bass and Henschel, 1956; Baker, 1959) were clearly shown in this experiment. This conspicuous hemoconcentration was particularly noticeable in the present experiment which was undertaken in summer, because hemodilution takes place in at a high ambient temperature (Young *et al.*, 1920; Barcroft *et al.*, 1923; Bass *et al.*, 1955). It is inferred that hemodilution is available for facilitation of increased evaporation and perspiration in a hot environment (Kuno, 1946).

3. Response of the Adrenocortical Function

Plasma cortisol increased significantly during the cold exposure and approached the

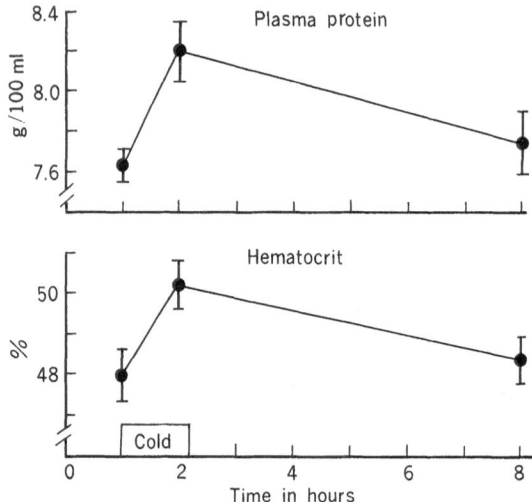

Fig. 81. Changes in plasma protein concentration and hematocrit values.

pre-exposure level six hours after exposure (Fig. 82). The increase in the ratio of plasma cortisol to plasma protein (μg cortisol per g protein) was also significant. On the other hand, urinary 17-ketosteroid (17-KS) decreased during the cold exposure, continued to decrease after exposure, and approached the normal level at the end of the experiment. However, the amount of 17-KS excreted in urine does not necessarily represent a real functional state of the adrenal cortex, as only five to 10% of total cortisol converts to 17-KS (Dorfman and Ungar, 1965). Actually, Yoshimura *et al.* (1958) and Tatai (1964) found a remarkable increase in urinary 17-hydroxy-corticosteroid in man after cold exposure, though Thorn *et al.* (1953) failed to observe any noticeable increase in corticosteroid excretion in the urine of two adult male humans after a four hour exposure to cold. Recently, Budd and Warhaft (1970) also reported the increase of 17-KS and 17-hydroxysteroid excretion in urine from four men who were exposed to cold both in normal and cold-acclimatized states.

4. *Response of the Sympathetico-adrenomedullary System*

Fig. 83 shows the free catecholamines excreted in the urine. Excretion of nor-adrenaline was much greater, by about four times, than that of adrenaline during the pre-exposure period. During cold exposure, catecholamine excretion increased sharply: noradrenaline increased from 16.3 to 44.6 μg. After exposure, the increased level again decreased rapidly to normal (noradrenaline) or to below normal (adrenaline) and remained at a low level until the end of the experiment. The increased excretion is not simply due to increased urine volume, since the urinary concentration of total catecholamines was increased from 3.7 to 4.5 μg/dl by exposure and also since the clearance rate of secreted catecholamines is rapid, indicating that the increased excretion of catecholamines may be due to increased secretion of the amines and not derived from the same pool as the extracellular fluid for cold diuresis. The marked increase in the excretion of noradrenaline was clearly in accordance with the increased diastolic blood pressure (vasoconstriction) which was probably caused by noradrenaline secreted from the sympathetic nerve endings rather than

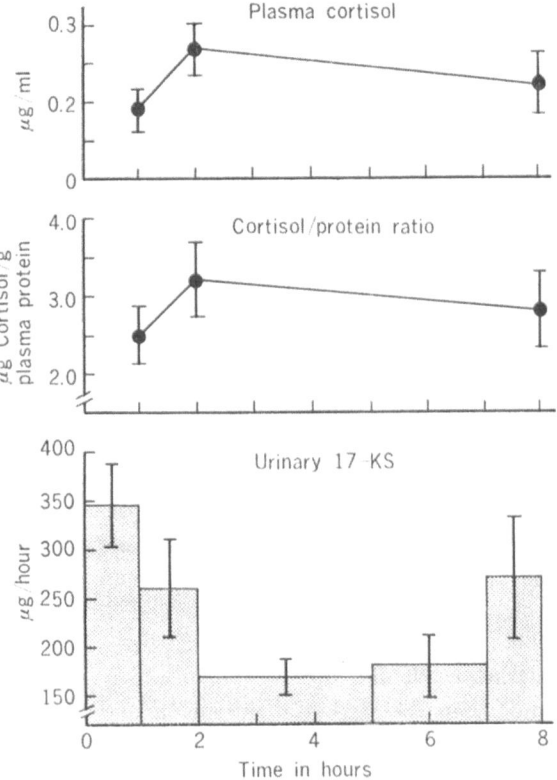

Fig. 82. Changes in plasma corticoid level, ratio of cortisol to plasma protein, and excretion of 17-ketosteroid (17-KS) in the urine.

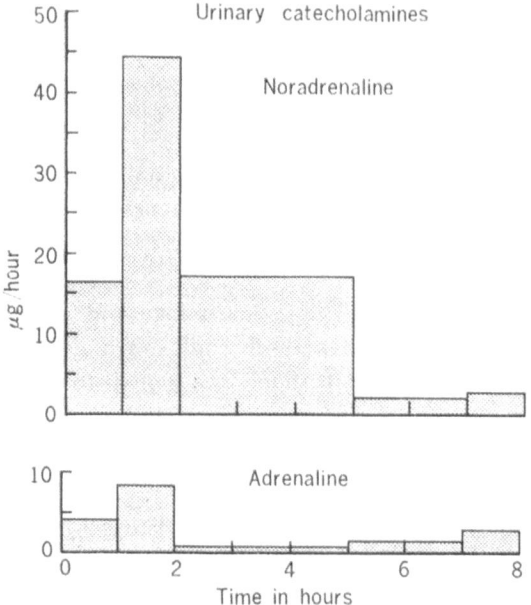

Fig. 83. Changes in excretion of free noradrenaline and adrenaline in the whole urine of eight subjects.

from the adrenal medulla (Hsieh *et al.*, 1957; Axelrod, 1962; Johnson, 1963; Pouliot, 1966). The acute response in raising noradrenaline secretion was more rapid and distinct than that in the case of adrenaline in the present experiment, similar to results reported previously in experiments with animals (Johnson, 1966; Le Blanc *et al.*, 1967; Leduc, 1961; Motelica, 1969) and human subjects. Tsunashima (1959) reported a similar increase in urinary catecholamines in young men after cold exposure at 10 °C for two hours. Arnett and Watts (1960) showed that catecholamine secretion in humans, especially adrenaline secretion, increased markedly on exposure to a low temperature, 6.5 °C for one hour. However, the present results, which showed a much more marked increase in noradrenaline excretion than in that of adrenaline during cold, were confirmed recently by Budd and Warhaft (1970).

Hsieh and Carlson (1957) demonstrated that noradrenaline plays a role in the acute calorigenic response (non-shivering thermogenesis) to cold. Later, it was shown by Depocas (1960) that by exposure to cold, cold-acclimated rats, both normal and eviscerated, showed a much more profound calorigenic response than normal rats. It is supposed that catecholamines facilitate not only non-shivering thermogenesis but also shivering due to direct action on the nervous system (Dell *et al.*, 1954) and by the effect on the muscle resulting from the increase in local blood circulation, glucose supply and cellular oxidation (Chatonnet and Minaire, 1966; Dallam and Reed, 1960; Sellers *et al.*, 1954).

There is much literature on the correlation between thyroid hormone and the adrenal medullary and sympathetic post-ganglionic agents, adrenaline and noradrenaline (Barker *et al.*, 1936; Bacq, 1949; Brewster *et al.*, 1956; Smith and Hoiger, 1962; Swansan, 1956, 1957; Hsieh and Carlson, 1957; Carlson, 1960; Tanche and Therminarias, 1969; Lutherer *et al.*, 1969). Thyroid hormone elevates the basal metabolic rate (BMR) and also potentiates oxygen consumption and thermogenesis which are initiated by catecholamine particulary in cold-acclimated animals.

In view of this, thyroid hormone, in addition to playing an important role in maintaining the BMR at a certain level, has a "permissive" role in acute thermogenesis caused by cold, probably via an increased rate of catecholamine secretion.

5. *Response of the Thyroid Function*

Plasma PBI was increased significantly upon exposure to cold and after six hours decreased to a lower level than that before exposure (Fig. 84). However, the increase was not statistically significant when hemoconcentration was taken into consideration (Fig. 84).

Percentage uptake of $^{131}I\text{-}T_3$ into the resin sponge was clearly decreased by cold exposure (Fig. 84). Normally, such a result indicates a decreased thyroid hormone content in the plasma. However, it should be noted that even if PBI does not change, or even increases, the resin uptake can decrease when hemoconcentration occurs. When the plasma protein concentration is increased, the binding sites of serum proteins for iodothyronines per unit volume of the plasma increase, thus resulting in a low uptake of $^{131}I\text{-}T_3$ by the resin, as seen in the case of pregnancy (Dowling *et al.*, 1956).

Urinary iodide (I^-) excretion increased significantly during cold exposure (Fig. 85). It has been noticed that the rate at which thyroxine is removed from the blood is increased in cold acclimated rats (Rand *et al.*, 1952; Bondy and Hagewood, 1952;

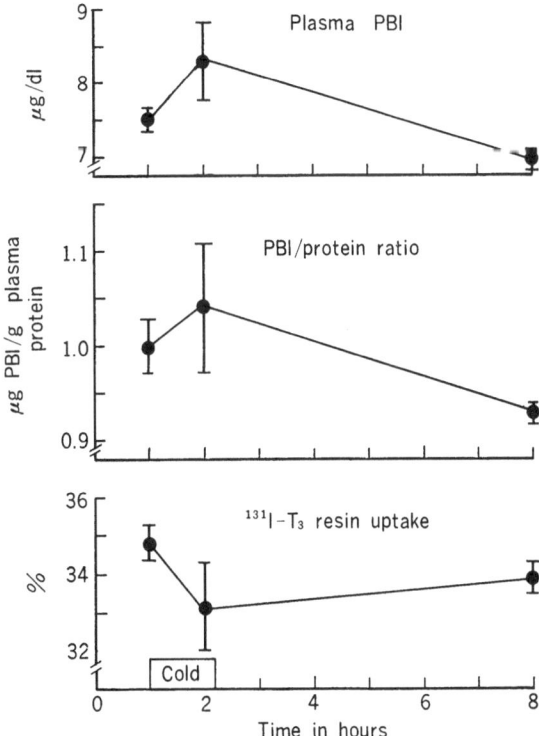

Fig. 84. Changes in plasma protein-bound iodine (PBI), ratio of PBI to plasma protein, and percentage uptake of radioactive triiodothyronine (T_3) into resin.

Cottle and Carlson, 1956; Yamamoto *et al.*, 1963). Hillier (1968 b) observed that the urinary radio-iodide ($^{131}I^-$) excretion following injection of ^{131}I-thyroid hormones is increased in cold-exposed and thyroidectomized rats for 30 hours. However, since the pattern of I^- excretion was so similar to that of Cl^- as a monovalet anion (Fig. 80), the question arose as to whether the increase simply results from the excretion of I^-, which is distributed in the same space as Cl^-, or derived from the increased degradation of thyroid hormones. An I^-/Cl^- ratio was calculated, and is shown in Fig. 85. The ratio was not changed by cold exposure, as far as comparison with the pre-exposure level showed, suggesting that deiodination of thyroid hormone did not markedly increase during the cold exposure. Halmi *et al.* (1958) reported that the administration of a higher amount of Cl^- to rat induces an increase in renal I^- clearance. However, this was not confirmed by Cottle (1966). In the present experiment, the volunteers did not take a large amount of NaCl. Thus, it is most probable that the increased excretion of urinary I^- was accompanied by the cold diuresis which induced increased excretion of NaCl.

On the other hand, during cold exposure, the fecal excretion of thyroxine was accelerated in the cold-acclimated rat (Intoccia and Van Middlesworth, 1959) and later this was confirmed to be due to a higher biliary thyroxine excretion accompanied by a large volume of feces resulting from an increased food intake in cold (Cottle, 1964; Hillier, 1968 a; Magwood and Heroux, 1968; Galton and Nisula, 1969; Cadot *et al.*, 1969). These observations were obtained from experiments using

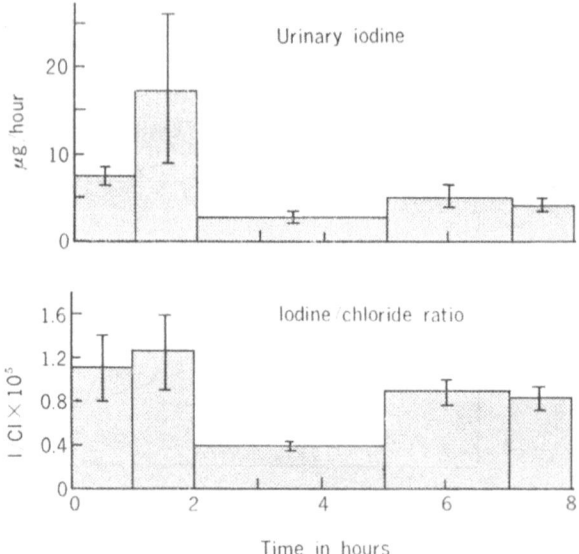

Fig. 85. Changes in excretion of iodide in the urine, and iodide-chloride ratio.

rats in which the entero-hepatic circulation of thyroid hormone was quite large (Myant, 1957). Presumably, this made it easy to increase the fecal loss of thyroid hormone, due to an increased fecal volume which might interfere with the reabsorption of the hormone. However, human subjects excrete a relatively small amount of thyroxine in bile and reabsorb it from the intestine to a lesser extent (Johnson and Beierwaltes, 1953), resulting in a low fecal excretion of thyroxine (Berson and Yalow, 1954).

Although the characteristic features of thyroid hormone metabolism in each human and rat must be taken into account in evaluating the present data, the results do not exclude the possibility that the hormone is secreted into the bile and eliminated in the feces at a higher rate in cold than at a warm ambient temperature.

Plasma TSH was increased upon cold exposure (Fig. 86). A 100% increase was observed at the end of one hour of the cold exposure and the TSH level did not return to the pre-exposure level after six hours. Knigge (1960) reported that TSH concentration in the normal hamster pituitary was less 30 minutes after cold exposure and a 60% decrease in TSH concentration was found after one hour. The increased level of plasma TSH shortly after cold exposure has been also observed in the case of rabbit (Bottari, 1957) and rat (Jobin and Fortier, 1965; Konno and Oseki, 1967; Washio, 1970).

Tonoue *et al.* (1963) reported that TSH stimulates T_4 uptake by the mouse abdominal muscle *in vitro*. This finding was confirmed later by Yamada *et al.* (1969) employing the guinea pig muscle in the presence of plasma. From the results of the present experiment, it might be inferred that the increase in plasma TSH during the exposure has an effect on a transfer rate of T_4 into peripheral tissues.

Circadian variations have been reported for many of the phenomena described above, as reviewed by Kleitman (1949), Kärki (1956) and Sollberger (1965). In general, however, the circadian variations were rather small during pre-exposure

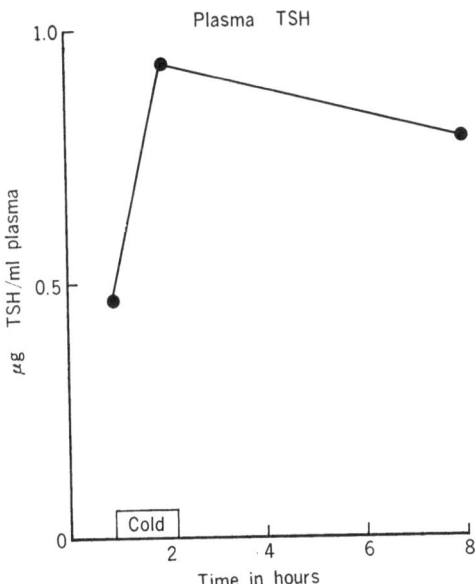

Fig. 86.   Changes in thyroid-stimulation hormone (TSH) in the plasma.

and exposure (10–12 a.m.) in the present experiment, and the effect of cold exposure, when observed, was beyond that of the circadian rhythm. For instance, urinary sodium, potassium, and chloride were reported to be at a broad peak between 9 a.m. and 1 p.m., decreasing gradually towards 3–6 a.m. (Doe *et al.*, 1960; Imrie *et al.*, 1963). Plasma cortisol was reported to be at a peak between 5 and 9 a.m. and to decrease gradually towards 8–12 p.m. (Doe *et al.*, 1960; Migeon *et al.*, 1956). These circadian variation would not have influenced the significance of the results obtained during the one hour cold exposure. However, the variations might have altered to a certain extent the significance of the post-exposure results. For precise evaluation of this influence, it will be necessary to carry out control measurements on a day on which no cold exposure is carried out.

MECHANISM OF INITIATING THYROID RESPONSE TO COLD

As has already been well-documented (D'Angelo and Traum, 1958; Knigge, 1960; Pitt-Rivers and Tata, 1959; Solomon and Dowling, 1960; Smith and Hoijer, 1962), exposure to cold leads to histological signs of thyroid activation within one hour, particularly in experiment with guinea pigs (Del Conte and Stux, 1954), and to an increased rate of rabbit thyroidal ^{131}I release (Brown-Grant *et al.*, 1954 a) and of guinea pig PB^{131}I secretion (Yamada *et al.*, 1965). More recently, the increase in rabbit, rat and human plasma TSH level shortly after exposure were repeatedly reported (Bottari, 1957; Jobin and Fortier, 1965; Konno and Oseki, 1967; Suzuki *et al.*, 1967; Washio, 1970).

The histological response of the thyroid to cold is prevented by hypophysectomy; also this pituitary-thyroid response to cold needs an intact connection between the pituitary and the hypothalamus. It has been demonstrated that section of the pituitary stalk in the rat (Uotila, 1940; Brolin, 1945) and transplantation of the pituitary into the anterior chamber of the eye in the rabbit (von Euler and Holmgren, 1956) abolish the activity of the response to cold. The experiments with lesions in the hypothalamus result in prevention of the response of the thyroid to cold (Knigge and Bierman, 1958; Van Beugen *et al.*, 1961; Yamada *et al.*, 1965). Localization of a proper area, the preoptic region in the hypothalamus, which is responsible for the cold-induced thyroid response through the anterior pituitary was suggested (D'Angelo 1960). A lesion in the preoptic region was reported not to affect the "baseline", level of plasma TSH. However, it was concluded that thyroid inhibition was caused by a lesion of the hypothalamus between the paraventicular nucleus and the anterior limit of the infundibulum (Reichlin, 1960). It is noteworthy that thermosensitive areas in the hypothalamus for the regulation of the body temperature are found to be closely related to the anterior part of the "thyrotropic area" (McClure and Reichlin, 1964).

Andersson *et al.* (1962, 1963) reported the curious finding that local cooling of the "heat loss center" in the hypothalamus of goats induces an acute increase in $PB^{131}I$. However, it is hardly conceivable that exposure to cold decreases the temperature in the hypothalamus because of a rapid rise in the "core" temperature due to cold in the present experiment with human subjects. However, these findings suggest a possible mechanism in which cold stimulates a neuroendocrine reflex, consisting of the skin thermoreceptor and the hypothalamic "thyrotropic area," responsible for the activation of the pituitary.

On the contrary, the other probable mechanism in activating the thyroid function of the cold-acclimated rat in a low ambient temperature was put forward by Rand *et al.* (1952) who attributed it to increased breakdown and excretion of the hormone. This is, in turn, felt to lead to a compensatory increase in TSH secretion, that is, a feedback control on the thyroid hormone homeostasis. The increased breakdown and excretion of thyroid hormone via fecal and urinary loss has been confirmed by Intoccia and Van Middlesworth (1959), Kassenaar *et al.* (1959), Cottle (1964), Hillier (1968 a,b), Magwood and Heroux (1967) and Cadot *et al.* (1969). Recently, Galton and Nisula (1969) obtained rather conclusive results in support of the theory.

The observations mentioned above indicate that two mechanisms work to increase the rate of thyroid hormone secretion in animals exposed to cold: The first is a mechanism of the neuroendocrine reflex excited by the thermoreceptors and the second is a feedback mechanism to maintain the level of plasma thyroid hormone which tends to decrease via increased breakdown and excretion. The latter mechanism is likely to operate in cold-acclimated animals which have accomplished a metabolic reconstruction ready for active thermogenesis to meet greater heat loss in a cold environment.

However, it may then be asked whether an acute exposure to cold could induce lowering level of plasma thyroid hormone through a peripheral mechanism which could be stimulated by the nervous reflex. Actually, Hillier (1968 b) reported that cold leads to an increase in the deiodinating activity of the rat exposed acutely to cold and the enhanced deiodination during cold exposure is mediated by the release of noradrenaline from the sympathetic nervous system. Thus, there is still a possibility that in an initial phase during cold exposure the level of plasma thyroid hormone might decrease, resulting in stimulation of the second mechanism, that is, the feedback control. Lang and Reichlin (1961) demonstrated a rapid response in thyroid hormone release, which had been suppressed by higher levels of T_4 previously injected, after diminishing below a certain critical concentration. In the case of thyroid activation in cold, however, surprisingly little evidence on this point has been reported.

INITIAL RESPONSE OF THE THYROID AND ADRENAL FUNCTIONING OF RATS

We next attempted to find early changes in rat thyroid and adrenal functioning on acute exposure to cold (Suzuki, 1971). In this experiment, special care was taken to avoid stimulation other than cold. Male Wistar rats weighing about 220 g were used. The animals were maintained in individual cages for eight days before the experiment to accustom them to the new environment, consisting of a constant temperature $25 \pm 1°C$, feedings of Oriental chow (MR) and water *ad libitum*, and 12 hours of light and 12 hours of darkness. Forty-eight hours before sacrifice, 10 μc of carrier free $^{131}I^-$ was given with intraperitoneal injection and the chow and the water bottle were removed three hours before decapitation. The rats in the same individual cages, were moved into a big, quiet cold room at $4°C$ under similar lighting conditions to the warm animal room. A part of each cage was cooled with flaked ice to keep the inside temperature below $4°C$. Cages containing controls were also moved to other places in the animal room. All the animal were killed at about 11.00–12.00 a.m. exactly 48 hours after the $^{131}I^-$ injection. Blood samples were collected in heparinized tubes after decapitation for estimation of $PB^{127}I$, $PB^{131}I$, $^{131}I^-$, corticosterone and also plasma protein concentration and hematocrit values. The longest exposure to cold was 220 minutes.

Table 22 shows changes in whole body and liver weight and liver glycogen content

TABLE 22   Whole body, liver weight and liver glycogen content in control and cold-exposed rats

Rats	Body weight (g)	Persent decrease of body weight	Liver weight (g/100 g)	Liver glycogen (mg/g)
Control (5)	228.4±6.1	0.89±0.30	4.49±0.40	62.99±3.65
Cold-exposed				
50 min. (5)	238.4±8.9	3.11±0.33††	4.12±0.11	50.10±5.05
100 min. (5)	230.8±9.3	3.08±0.73††	4.23±0.11	48.14±3.42
150 min. (5)	226.0±5.5	2.19±0.32††	4.05±0.07*	44.05±3.42†
220 min. (5)	237.0±7.9	3.15±0.34††	4.08±0.17	35.88±8.86**

*, **, †, ††: Defferences are statistically significant at the level of 5, 2, 1 and 0.1%, respectively.
Note: Number of animals is shown in parenthesis.

after the cold exposure. A small but significant decrease in body weight in the all groups exposed to cold was noticed, which was due to acute excretion of feces and urine. Liver weight of the exposed group tended to decrease and liver glycogen content was significantly diminished after exposure, confirming previous reports (Barnett *et al.*, 1960; Klain and Hannon, 1969).

Pituitary and thymus weight showed no change after exposure but adrenal weight increased slightly 50 minutes after exposure.

It was observed that the plasma protein concentration and the hematocrit value of the exposed group did not change within 220 minutes in cold, as reported by Baker (1960), in distinct contrast with the previous experiment on human subjects.

Changes in the thyroid function assessed by PB^{131}I and PB^{127}I after the cold exposure are shown in Fig. 87. PB^{131}I increased gradually and significantly after 90

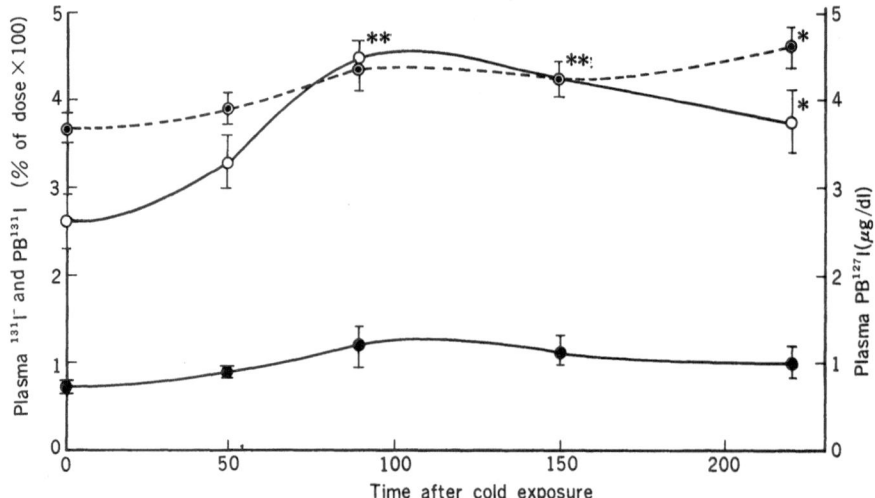

Fig. 87. Effects of cold on ^{131}I$^-$, PB^{131}I, and PBI^{127} in rat plasma. O–O: PB^{131}I, ●–●: Plasma^{131}I$^-$, ⊙–⊙: PB^{127}I, *, **: Differences are statistically significant at the level of 5 and 1% respectively.

minutes. On the other hand the PB^{127}I in question did not decrease but tended to increase and it was statistically significant 220 minutes after the exposure, which differed from the results obtained in experiments on longer duration of cold exposure than that in the present experiment (Bondy and Hagewood, 1952; Freinkel and Lewis, 1957; Ingbar and Bass, 1957; Stevens *et al.*, 1955; Kassenaar *et al.*, 1959). Table 23 shows changes in thyroid weight, ^{131}I in thyroid gland, ratio of ^{131}I-diiodotyrosine (DIT) to ^{131}I-monoiodotyrosine (MIT) which is a sensitive indicator of thyroid function. No change were observed in the weight and ^{131}I in the gland. However, DIT/MIT ratio increased, suggesting a thyroid activation by TSH.

Fig. 88 shows striking change in rapid decrease in ascorbic acid content in the adrenal and increase in plasma corticosterone level in particular, 50 minutes after exposure, as already demonstrated (Sellers, 1957; Heroux, 1960; Schönbaum, 1960;

TABLE 23   Thyroid function in control and cold-exposed rats

Rats	Thyroid weight (mg/100 g)	^{131}I in thyroid (% of dose)	DIT/MIT (^{131}I)
Control (5)	5.48±0.63	6.73±0.58	1.599±0.065
Cold-exposed			
50 min. (5)	4.69±0.53	6.96±0.50	1.497±0.121
100 min. (5)	5.12±0.30	6.67±0.69	1.847±0.102
150 min. (5)	4.97±0.76	6.32±0.42	1.812±0.070*
220 min. (5)	5.94±0.65	7.44±0.75	2.001±0.089**

*, **: Differences are statistically significant at the level of 5 and 2%, respectively.
Note: Number of animals in shown in parenthesis.

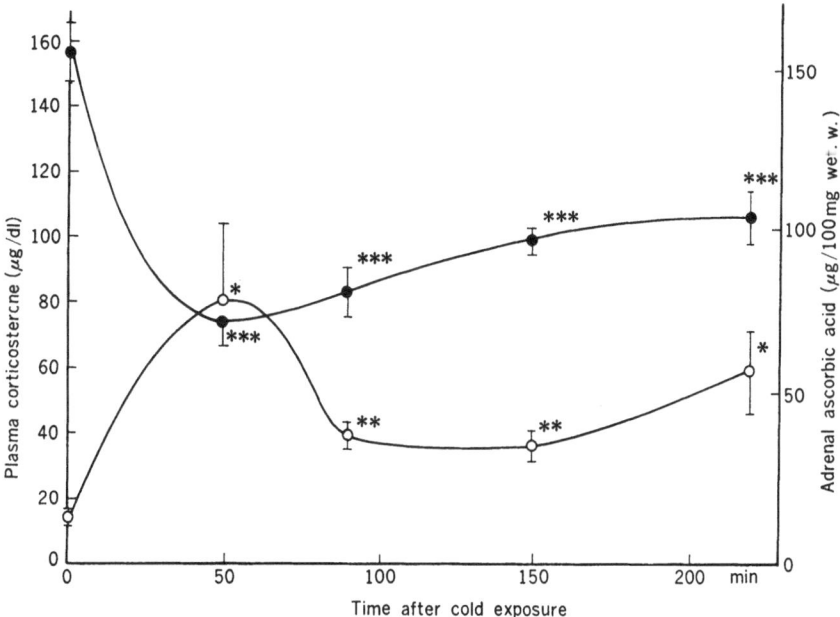

Fig. 88. Effects of cold on plasma corticosterone level and ascorbic acid concentration of rats. O–O: Plasma corticosterone, ●–●: Adrenal ascorbic acid, *, **, ***: Differences are statistically significant at the level of 5.2 and 1% respectively.

Smith and Hoijer, 1962). The ascorbic acid tended to recover gradually to a small extent and the corticosterone levels were much lower after 90 minutes than after 50 minutes. Administration of ACTH and cortisone or such a "stress" as severe cold in rabbits and rats caused a marked inhibition of release of ^{131}I from the thyroid gland. (Myant, 1953; Brown-Grant et al., 1954 b; Brown-Grant, 1956). The latter group found that this was also observable in adrenalectomized rabbit, probably through the hypothalamohypophyseal system (Brown-Grant et al., 1954 b). Thus, antagonism was suggested between the regulation of secretion of ACTH and that of TSH (Harris and Woods, 1956). However, this was not the case in the present experiment. The extraordinary increase in the activity of the pituitary-adrenocortical axis was found to be compatible with the stimulation of TSH secretion in exposure to cold, particularly in the experiment with rats.

Generally speaking the results coincided with those observed in the case of human subjects, that is, the initial response of the thyroid activation to cold was mediated mainly by the first mechanism described in this paper. The adrenocortical function of rat, however, seems to be much more sensitive to cold as compared with that of humans.

THE ROLE OF THYROID HORMONE IN COLD ACCLIMATION

In a cold environment, homeotherms maintain their body temperature through increased heat production and prevent heat loss with insulation. The response to cold which overcomes the increased heat loss has many mechanisms such as muscullar activity (that is, exercise and shivering) and non-shivering thermogenesis. Continued exposure to cold produces an acclimated state after some length of time. The cold-acclimated animal produces heat mainly through non-shivering thermogenesis, though interspecies differences in this thermogenesis have been reported (Jansky *et al.*, 1969). Even in human subjects, two types of increased heat production due to cold, namely shivering and non-shivering thermogenesis, were reported by Girling (1963).

Hypothyroid animals are unable to survive at low ambient temperature for a long time, indicating that thyroid hormone is essential in the acclimation to cold. A characteristic feature of the thermogenesis of acclimated rats is a rapid response which is "switched on" in cold and "switched off" in a neutral temperature (Sellers and You, 1950). Evidence accumulated recently indicates that the brown adipose tissue is responsible for acute thermogenesis both in the acclimated and normal rat though in the latter only to a lesser extent (Itoh and Hiroshige, 1971; Kuroshima and Itoh, 1971).

It was demonstrated by Weiss (1957) that the metabolic response to cold is observed in the same tissues, such as muscle, liver, heart and kidney, in which the oxygen consumptions are stimulated by T_4 administration. This indicates that thyroid hormone is involved in a stimulation of calorigenesis in the tissues of cold-exposed rats.

In general, one of the most conspicuous features of the thyroid hormone action *in vivo* is the latent period. Possible explanation for the latent period was extensively discussed by Tata (1965). However, latent period for function such as heart rate, BMR and weight of liver and body differ from each other. Among them, the latent period of BMR is about 30–36 hours when the hormone is administered to thyroidectomized rats (Tata, 1965).

The non-shivering thermogenesis in cold is initiated by catecholamines secreted in the sympathetico-adrenomedullary system (Cottle and Carlson, 1956 b; Hsieh and Carlson, 1957; Depocas, 1960; Steiner *et al.*, 1969; Jansky *et al.*, 1969). Tanche and Therminarias (1969) showed clearly that spinal- and thyroidectomized dogs can demonstrate calorigenic response to cold and catecholamines infusion though the basal level of calorigenesis of the thyroidectomized dog is lower than that of normal controls. The clear synergism between thyroid hormone and catecholamines has been repeatedly proved in their calorigenic action (Ring, 1942; Swanson, 1956). This was also proved in cold-acclimated rats by Swanson (1957) who attributed the effect of thyroid hormone to the facilitation of the calorigenic action by endogeneous adrenaline. Explanations for the synergism in cold were postulated by Lutherer *et al.* (1969) using rats and by Nagasaka and Carlson (1965) from their experiment with dogs. The former group suggested that thyroid hormone increases tissue sensitivity to catecholamines and the latter ascribed it to the increase of noradrenaline content in the blood. The exact nature of the synergism remains to be elucidated. However, it could be easily supposed that thyroid hormone facilitates a metabolic reconstruction which enables homeotherms to compensate a heat loss in cold through metabolic changes in carbohydrates, lipids and proteins as precisely reviewed by Smith and Hoijer (1962). The facilitation by thyroid hormone needs the presence of catecholamines and probably of TSH, ACTH, and corticoids. Thus, the induction time for cold acclimation must be related to the latent period of the thyroid hormone action.

Hsieh and Carlson (1957) demonstrated that cold acclimated rats can still respond to cold exposure by increasing non-shivering heat production even 12 days after thyroidectomy. This indicates that the metabolic pattern reformed in a cold environment remains responsible for a rapid increase in catecholamines level even in the absence of thyroid hormone. Considering this, an equivocal meaning of the thyroid hormone action in cold adaptability may be the most comprehensive; that is both the "permissive" action (Cottle, 1966; Tanche and Therminarias, 1969) and on the other hand, the indispensable action. Namely, the hormone action is "permissive" of the prompt increase in thermogenesis to cold, which is initiated by catecholamines, while the role of the hormone is "indispensable" for survival in cold for a long time.

Another question has been raised as to whether the *increased* thyroid activity in cold is essential for an elevation in metabolic rate or not (Sellers and You, 1950; Hsieh, 1960; Cottle, 1966; and Galton and Nisula, 1969). They demonstrated that thyroidectomized rats given a small constant daily dose of T_4 can not only survive in cold indefinitely but also show stimulated oxygen consumption. So far, no contrary evidence has been offered. It has been noticed that the growth promoting effect of thyroid hormone in the hypothyroid rat is observed with a much smaller daily dose of T_4 and T_3 than that for maintaining the normal metabolic rate in neutral temperatures (Evans *et al.*, 1960, 1964; Stasilli *et al.*, 1961). The growth promoting action seems to be mediated by an action of thyroid hormone on the synthesis of pituitary growth hormone (Suzuki and Shibasaki, 1970). Eartly and Leblond (1954) described that pituitary function is maintained by thyroid hormone for the secretion of gonado- and adreno-trophic hormones in addition to growth hormone. The amount of thyroid hormone available for effects on the pituitary is less than that available for calorigenesis (Tata, 1965; Contopoulos and Koneff, 1963; Escobar del Rey *et al.*, 1968). Hsieh (1966) reported that a larger dose of T_3 is required for maintaining a good growth rate in cold than for survival. In fact, the growth rate of rats exposed to cold for several weeks decreases to a considerable extent as shown by Galton and Nisula (1969). These findings suggest that the cold-exposed rats need higher amount of thyroid hormone for maintaining a physical states good enough to withstand the severe environment. Therefore, it should be noted that the amount of thyroid hormone required to have an effect on survival, acute increase in thermogenesis and normal growth rate in cold, and on the other hand, on growth promotion and calorigenesis in neutral temperatures, has its proper and minimal level.

CONCLUSION

1) The present systematic observation on the physical and endocrine response of human subjects and rats to cold exposure indicates the presence of a complex sequence as follows:

i) Through the afferent impulse from the skin thermoreceptors in acute exposure to cold, an excitation of the nervous reflex arcs stimulates shivering, discharge of noradrenaline probably from the sympathetic post-ganglionic nerve endings and secretion of catecholamines from the adrenal medulla.

ii) The increased secretion of catecholamines stimulates baroreceptors resulting in bradycardia. This increase of catecholamine secretion is known to facilitate shivering and non-shivering thermogenesis. A rise in blood pressure due to catecholamines also causes hemoconcentration and cold diuresis resulting from inhibited ADH secretion presumably through the intrathoracic stretch receptor.

iii) To a lesser extent, the function of the human adrenal cortex is also stimulated by cold exposure. The adrenocortical functioning of rats, however, was found to be much more sensitive to cold.

iv) Although change in water and electrolyte metabolism made it difficult to assess the human thyroid function, cold stimulation caused increased secretion of TSH shortly after exposure. However, within one hour after the exposure, the period was too latent to discover increases in thyroid functioning directly. The increased TSH level in plasma should subsequently stimulate thyroid hormone secretion which will induce a metabolic reconstruction for acclimation to a cold environment. The activation of TSH release due to cold was mediated mainly by the neuroendocrine mechanism rather than by the second mechanism, the feedback mechanism which was prevalent in the cold-acclimated state.

2) Some aspects of the role of thyroid hormone and thyroid activity in cold adaptability were surveyed and discussed.

REFERENCES

1. ADOLPH, E.F., and G.W. MOLNAR (1946): *Am. J. Physiol.* **146:** 507.
2. ANDERSSON, B., L. EKMAN, C.C. GALE, and J.W. SUNDSTEN (1962): *Life Science* **1:** 10.
3. ANDERSSON, B., L. EKMAN, C.C. GALE, and J.W. SUNDSTEN (1963): *Acta Physiol. Scand.* **59:** 12.
4. ARNET, E.L., and D.T. WATTS (1960): *J. Appl. Physiol.* **15:** 499.
5. AXELROD, J. (1962): The formation, metabolism, uptake and release of noradrenaline and adrenaline. Symposium on the clinical-chemistry of monoamines. Edited by Vailey, H. and Gowenlock, A.H., Elsevier Publ. Co. Amsterdam.
6. BACQ, Z.M. (1949): *Pharmacol. Rev.* **1:** 1.
7. BADER, R.A. J.W. ELIOT, and D.E. BASS (1952): *J. Appl. Physiol.* **4:** 649.
8. BAKER, D.G. (1959): *Fed. Proc.* **13:** 8.
9. BAKER, D.G. (1960): *Fed. Proc.* **19:** (Suppl. 5) 125.
10. BARCROFT, J., J.C. MEAKINS, H.W. DAVIES, J.M. DANCAN-SCOTT, and W.J. FETTER (1923): *Phil. Trans. Roy. Soc. London B.* **211:** 455.
11. BARKER, S.B., J.F. FEZIKAS, and H.E. HIMWICH (1936): *Am. J. Physiol.* **115:** 415.
12. BARNETT, S.A., E.M. COLEMAN, and B.M. MANLY (1960): *Quart. J. Exptl. Physiol.* **45:** 40.
13. BASS, D.E. (1954): *Fed. Proc.* **13:** 8.
14. BASS, D.E., C.R. KLEEMAN, M. QUINN, A. HENSCHEL, and A.H. HEGNAUER (1955): *Medicine* **34:** 323.
15. BASS, D.E., and A. HENSCHEL (1956): *Physiol. Rev.* **36:** 128.
16. BAZETT, H.C. (1924): *Am. J. Physiol.* **70:** 412.
17. BERSON, S.A., and R.S. YALOW (1954): *J. Clin. Invest.* **33:** 1533.
18. BONDY, P.K. and M.A. HAGEWOOD (1952): *Proc. Soc. Exptl. Biol. Med.* **81:** 328.
19. BOTTARI, P.M. (1957): *Ciba Found. Colloq. Endocrinol.* **11:** 52.
20. BREWSTER, W.R. JR., J.P. ISAACS, P.F. OSGOOD, and T.L. KING (1956): *Circulation* **13:** 1.
21. BROLIN, S.E. (1945): *Acta Anat.* **2:** suppl. 3.
22. BROWN-GRANT, K., C. VON EULER, G.W. HARRIS, and S. REICHLIN (1954a): *J. Physiol.* **126:** 1.
23. BROWN-GRANT, K., G.W. HARRIS, and S. REICHLIN (1954b): *J. Physiol.* **126:** 41.
24. BROWN-GRANT, K. (1956): *J. Physiol.* **131:** 58.
25. BUDD, G.M., and N. WARHAFT (1970): *J. Physiol.* **210:** 799.
26. CADOT, M. M.F. JULIEN, and L. CHEVILLARD (1969): *Fed. Proc.* **28:** 1228.
27. CARLSON, L.D. (1960): *Fed. Proc.* **19:** (suppl. 5), 25.
28. CHATONNET, J., and Y. MINAIRE (1969): *Fed. Proc.* **28:** 1348.
29. CONTROPOULOS, A.N., and A.A. KONEFF (1963): *Acta Endocrinol.* **42:** 275.
30. COTTLE, W.H., and L.D. CARLSON (1956 a): *Proc. Soc. Exptl. Biol. Med.* **92:** 845.
31. COTTLE, M., and L.D. CARLSON (1956 b): *Endocrinology* **59:** 1.
32. COTTLE, W.H. (1964): *Am. J. Physiol.* **207:** 1063.
33. COTTLE, W.H. (1966): *Gunma Symp. Endocrinol.* **3:** 249.
34. DALLAN, R.D., and J.M. REED (1960): *Biochim. Biophys. Acta* **37:** 188.
35. D'ANGELO, S.A., and R.E. TRAUM (1958): *Ann. N.Y. Acad. Sci.* **80:** 500.
36. D'ANGELO, S.A. (1960): *Am. J. Physiol.* **199:** 701.

37. DEL CONTE, E., and M. STUX. (1954): *Nature* **173**: 83.
38. DELL, P., M. BONVALLET, and A. HUGELIN (1954): *Electroencephalog. Clin. Neurophysiol.* **6**: 599.
39. DEPOCAS, F. (1960): *Fed. Proc.* **19**: (Suppl. 5) 106.
40. DEWARDNER, H.E., I.H. MILLS, W.F. CLAPMAN, and C.J. HAYTER (1961): *Clin. Science* **21**: 249.
41. DOE, R.P., J.A. VENNES, and E.B. FLINK (1960): *J. Clin. Endocrinol, Metabol.* **20**: 253.
42. DORFMAN, R.I., and F. UNGAR (1965): Metabolism of Steroid Hormones, New York and London, Academic Press.
43. DOWLING, J.T., N. FREINKEL, and S.H. INGBAR (1965): *J. Clin. Invest.* **35**: 1263.
44. EARTLY, H., and C.P. LEBLOND (1954): *Endocrinology* **54**: 249.
45. ERSHOFF, B.H. (1948): *Endocrinology* **43**: 36.
46. ESCOBAR DEL REY, F., G. MORREALE DE ESCOBAR, J. JOLIN, and C. LOPEZ-QUIJADA (1968): *Endocrinology* **83**: 41.
47. EVANS, E.S., L.L. ROSENBERG, and M.E. SIMPSON (1960): *Endocrinology* **66**: 433.
48. EVANS, E.S., L.L. ROSENBERG, A.B. EVANS, and A.A. KONEFF (1964): *Endocrinology* **74**: 770.
49. FREINKEL, N., and D. LEWIS (1957): *J. Physiol.* **135**: 328.
50. GALTON, V.A. and B.C. NISULA (1969): *Endocrinology* **85**: 79.
51. GIRLING, F. (1963): *Can. J. Physiol. Pharmacol.* **42**: 319.
52. HALMI, N.S., L.T. KING, R.R. WINDER, A.C. HAAS, and R.C. STUELKE (1958): *Am. J. Physiol.* **193**: 379.
53. HARRIS, G.W., and J.W. WOOD (1956): *Nature* **179**: 80.
54. HEROUX, O. (1960): *Fed. Proc.* **19**: (Suppl. 5) 82.
55. HILLIER, A.P. (1968 a): *J. Physiol.* **197**: 123.
56. HILLIER, A.P. (1968 b): *J. Physiol.* **197**: 135.
57. HSIEH, A.C.L., and L.D. CARLSON (1957): *Am. J. Physiol.* **188**: 40.
58. HSIEH, A.C.L., L.D. CARLSON, and G. GRAY (1957): *Am. J. Physiol.* **190**: 247.
59. HSIEH, A.C.L. (1966): *Gunma Symp. Endocrinol.* **3**: 239.
60. IMRIE, M., J.N. MILLS, and K.S. WILLIAMSON (1963): *Mem. Soc. Endocrinol.* **13**: 3.
61. INGBAR, S.H., and D.E. BASS (1957): *J. Endocrinol.* **15**: ii.
62. INTOCCIA, A., and L. VAN MIDDLESWORTH (1959): *Endocrinology* **64**: 462.
63. ITOH, S. (1954): *Japan. J. Physiol.* **4**: 185.
64. ITOH, S., and T. HIROSHIGE (1971): In this book.
65. JANSKY, L., J. BARTUNKOVA, J. KOCKOVA, J. MEJSNAR, and E. ZEISBERGER (1969): *Fed. Proc.* **28**: 1053.
66. JOBIN, M., and C. FORTIER (1965): *Fed. Proc.* **24**: 149.
67. JOHNSON, D.G. (1966): *Acta Physiol. Scand.* **68**: 129.
68. JOHNSON, G.E. (1963): *Acta Physiol. Scand.* **59**: 438.
69. JOHNSON, P.C., and W.H. BEIERWALTES (1953): *J. Lab. Clin. Med.* **41**: 676.
70. JOHNSTON, C.I., J.O. DAVIS, S.S. HOWARDS, and F.S. WRIGHT (1967): *Circulation Res.* **20**: 1.
71. KÄRKI, N.T. (1956): *Acta Physiol. Scand.* **39**: suppl. 132.
72. KASSENAAR, A., L.D.F. LAMEYER, and A. QUERIDO (1959): *Acta Endocrinol.* **32**: 575.
73. KLAIN, G., and J.P. HANNON (1969): *Fed. Proc.* **28**: 965.
74. KLEITMAN, N. (1949): *Physiol. Rev.* **29**: 1.
75. KNIGGE, K.M., and S.M. BIERMANN (1958): *Am. J. Physiol.* **192**: 625.
76. KNIGGE, K.M. (1960): *Fed. Proc.* **19**: (Suppl. 5) 45.
77. KONNO, N., and T. OSEKI (1967): *Folia Endocrinol. Japon.* **42**: 1227.
78. KUNO, Y. (1946): Perspiration (Ase) Yotokusha, Nara.
79. KUROSHIMA, A., and S. ITOH (1971): *Gunma Symp. Endocrinol.* **8**: (In press).
80. LANG, S., and S. REICHLIN (1961): *Proc. Soc. Exptl. Biol. Med.* **108**: 789.
81. LE BLANC, J. A., D. ROBINSON, D.F. SHARIMAH, and P. TOUSIGNAUT (1967): *Am. J. Physiol.* **213**: 1419.
82. LEBLOND, C.P., and J. GROSS (1943): *Endocrinology* **33**: 155.
83. LEBLOND, C.P., and H. EARTLY (1952): *Endocrinology* **51**: 26.
84. LEDUC, J. (1961): *Acta Physiol. Scand.* **53**: suppl 183.
85. LUTHERER, L.O., M.J. FREGLY, and A.H. ANTON (1969): *Fed. Proc.* **28**: 1238.
86. MAGWOOD, S.G.A., and O. HEROUX (1968): *Can. J. Physiol. Parmacol.* **46**: 601.
87. McCLURE, J.N., and S. REICHLIN (1964): *Fed. Proc.* **23**: 109.
88. MIGEON, C.J., F.H. TYLER, J.P. MATHONEY, A.A. FLORENTIN, H. CASTLE, E.L. BLISS, and L.T. SAMUELS (1956): *J. Clin. Endocrinol. Metabol.* **16**: 622.
89. MOTELICA, I. (1969): *Acta Physiol. Scand.* **76**: 393.
90. MYANT, N.B. (1953): *J. Physiol.* **120**: 288.
91. MYANT, N.B. (1957): *J. Physiol.* **136**: 198.
92. PITT-RIVERS, R., and J.A. TATA (1959): The Thyroid Hormones, London, Pergamon Press.

93. POULIOT, M. (1966): *Acta Physiol. Scand.* **68:** 164.
94. RAND, G.G., D.S. RIGGS, and N.B. TALBOT (1952): *Endocrinology* **51:** 562.
95. REICHLIN, S. (1960): *Endocrinology* **66:** 340.
96. RING, G.C. (1942): *Am. J. Physiol.* **137:** 582.
97. SCHÖNBAUM, E. (1960): *Fed. Proc.* **19:** (Suppl. 5) 85.
98. SEGAR, W.E., and W.W. MOORE (1968): *J. Clin. Invest.* **47:** 2143.
99. SELLERS, E.A., and S.S. YOU (1950): *Am. J. Physiol.* **163:** 81.
100. SELLERS, E.A., J.W. SCOTT, and N. THOMAS (1954): *Am. J. Physiol.* **177:** 372.
101. SELLERS, E.A. (1957): *Rev. Can. Biol.* **16:** 1751.
102. SELYE, H. (1950): *Stress, Acta Med. Inc.*, Montreal.
103. SMITH, R.E., and D.J. HOIJER (1962): *Physiol. Rev.* **42:** 60.
104. SOLLBERGER, A. (1965): Biological Rhythm Research. Elsevier Publ. Co., Amsterdam.
105. SOLOMON, D.H., and J.T. DOWLING (1960): *Ann. Rev. Physiol.* **22:** 615.
106. STASILLI, N.R., R.L. KROC, and P.L. NEMITH (1961): *Endocrinology* **68:** 1068.
107. STEINER, G., G.E. JOHNSON, E.A. SELLERS, and E. SCHÖNBAUM (1969): *Fed. Proc.* **28:** 1017.
108. STEVENS, C.E., S.A. D'ANGELO, K.E. PASCHKIS, A. CANTAROW, and F.W. SINDERMAN (1955): *Endocrinology* **56:** 143.
109. SUZUKI, M., T. TONOUE, S. MATSUZAKI, and K. YAMAMOTO (1967): *Can. J. Physiol. Pharmacol.* **45:** 423.
110. SUZUKI, M., and K. SHIBASAKI (1970): *Endocrinol Exper.* **4:** 187.
111. SUZUKI, M. (1971): *Gunma Symp. Endocrinol.* **8** (In press).
112. SWANSON, H.E. (1956): *Endocrinology* **59:** 217.
113. SWANSON, H.E. (1957): *Endocrinology* **60:** 205.
114. TANCHE, M., and A. THERMINARIAS (1969): *Fed. Proc.* **28:** 1257.
115. TATA, J.R. (1965): Action of Hormones on Molecular Processes, edited by Litwack, G. and Kritchevsky, D., John Wiley & Sons, Inc., N.Y., London, Sydney 58.
116. TATAI, K. (1964): *Bull. Inst. Public Health Tokyo* **13:** 205.
117. THORN, G.W., D. JENKINS, and J.C. LAIDLAW (1953): *Rec. Progr. Hormone Res.* **8:** 171.
118. TONOUE, T., M. SUZUKI, and K. YAMAMOTO (1963): *Endocrinology* **72:** 345.
119. TSUNASHIMA, S. (1959): *J. Physiol. Soc. Japan* **21:** 1256.
120. UOTILA, U.U. (1940): *Endocrinology* **26:** 129.
121. VAN BEUGEN, L., and J.J. VANDER WERFFTEEN BOSCH (1961): *Acta Endocrinol.* **38:** 585.
122. VON EULER, C., and B. HOLMGREN (1956): *J. Physiol.* **131:** 137.
123. WASHIO, S. (1970): *Folia Endocrinol. Japan.* **45:** 1652.
124. WEISS, A.K. (1957): *Am. J. Physiol.* **188:** 430.
125. YAMADA, T., A. KAJIHARA, T. ONAYA, I. KOBAYASHI, Y. TAKEMURA, and K. SHICHIJO (1965): *Endocrinology* **77:** 968.
126. YAMADA, T., H. FUKUDA, Y. TAKEMURA, and K. SHICHIJO (1969): *Metabolism* **18:** 339.
127. YAMAMOTO, K., M. SUZUKI, I. ISHIKAWA, M. NAGASHIMA, and N. KURIHARA (1963): *Japan. J. Physic. Fit.* **11:** 168.
128. YOSHIMURA, H., S. USAMI, K. MAKIHATA, S. SHIOMI, and M. MORISHIMA (1958): *J. Physiol. Soc. Japan* **20:** 603.
129. YOUNG, W.J., A. BREINL, J.J. HARRIS, and W.A. OSBORNE (1920): *Proc. Roy. Soc.*, London, Series B **91:** 111.

Chapter 14

MECHANISMS INVOLVED IN THERMOREGULATORY HEAT PRODUCTION IN BROWN ADIPOSE TISSUE

Tsutomu HIROSHIGE, Keiichi YOSHIMURA
and Shinji ITOH

Department of Physiology, Hokkaido University School of Medicine, Sapporo, Japan

Marked increment in heat production is well documented in cold-acclimated animals [67]. General attention has been drawn to the role of adipose tissue, special interest being focused on the significance of brown adipose tissue. There is now ample evidence that brown adipose tissue is involved in one way or another in non-shivering thermogenesis in a cold environment in the rat [69], newborn rabbit [32] and newborn human infant [1]. Mechanisms by which cold induces an increased heat production in this tissue, however, remain largely unknown. Several possibilities were previously proposed [4, 5, 43]. These topics have been dealt with excellently in several recent reviews [34, 35, 68]. In this report, therefore, we will confine our discussion mainly to the neurohumoral regulatory mechanisms involved in the enhanced thermogenesis in brown adipose tissue, primarily on the basis of observations made in our laboratory.

CATECHOLAMINES

It has been claimed [5, 68] that catecholamines released from the sympathetic nerve endings within brown adipose tissue are physiologically important in activating the high metabolic capabilities of this tissue. Therefore, the role of catecholamines was examined before and after cold acclimation [33].

Male Wistar rats, weighing from 150 to 220 g, were used. They were housed at a constant ambient temperature of $20 \pm 2\,^\circ\text{C}$. Rat biscuit and water were given freely. Interscapular brown adipose tissue was trimmed virtually free of adhering muscle and white adipose tissue. Adequately cubed pieces of brown adipose tissue or white fat pad were incubated at $37.5\,^\circ\text{C}$ in the Krebs-Ringer phosphate buffer (pH 7.4), glucose added to a final concentration of 100 mg per 100 ml and bovine albumin (Armour) added to a final concentration of 2 g% in Warburg vessels, using 100% oxygen as the gas phase.

1. Effect of Norepinephrine or Theophylline

First, the effects of norepinephrine or theophylline addition *in vitro* were examined on oxygen consumption and free fatty acid (FFA) and glycerol release, using epididymal adipose tissue. The results obtained are summarized in Table 24. FFA was determined by the colorimetric method of Duncombe [19] and glycerol by the method of Korn [39]. It is apparent from the table that addition of the catecholamine or theophylline caused

TABLE 24 Effects of *in vitro* addition of norepinephrine or theophylline on lipolytic and respiratory activities in epididymal white adipose tissue of non-adapted control and cold-adapted rats. All values are given as mean ± standard error of the mean.

Non-adapted control:

In vitro addition	Series No.	No. of rats	Tissue FFA level (μEq/g)		Medium FFA (μEq/g/hr)	Medium glycerol (μM/g/hr)	O_2 consumed (μl/100 mg/30 mim)
			initial	final			
None	I	7	5.7±0.46	2.8±0.21	3.5±0.57	3.2±0.49	10.8±1.19
Norepinephrine*	II	6	7.1±0.78	3.3±0.21	15.4±1.90	11.7±1.09	—
				vs. I	vs. I	vs. I	
				NS	P<0.001	P<0.001	
Theophylline**	III	6	7.1±0.64	4.2±0.73	15.2±1.99	11.3±1.01	16.4±2.13
				vs. I	vs. I	vs. I	vs. I
				NS	P<0.001	P<0.001	P<0.05
				vs. II	vs. II	vs. II	
				NS	NS	NS	

Cold-adapted:

In vitro addition	Series No.	No. of rats	Tissue FFA level (μEq/g)		Medium FFA (μEq/g/hr)	Medium glycerol (μM/g/hr)	O_2 consumed (μl/100 mg/30 mim)
			initial	final			
None	IV	11	9.3±0.42	4.2±0.19	4.8±0.99	6.0±1.13	21.4±1.81
			vs. I	vs. I	vs. I	vs. I	vs. I
			P<0.001	P<0.001	NS	P<0.10	P<0.001
Norepinephrine*	V	13	10.5±0.54	4.2±0.37	15.4±1.42	11.3±1.08	22.3±1.41
				vs. IV	vs. IV	vs. IV	vs. IV
				NS	P<0.001	P<0.01	NS
Norepinephrine* plus theophylline**	VI	6	9.8±0.48	6.5±0.18	39.7±1.76	20.4±0.96	19.8±2.93
				vs V	vs. V	vs. V	vs. V
				P<0.01	P<0.001	P<0.001	NS

*Norepinephrine 2 μg/ml
**Theophylline 5 X 10^{-4}M

a marked increase not only in FFA and glycerol release but also in oxygen consumption. The release of FFA appears to increase parallel to that of glycerol in both cases. In order to see the effect of cold exposure on the metabolic parameters of white adipose tissue, rats were exposed to cold of 5 °C for seven days. It was found (Table 24) that the initial level of tissue FFA was much higher in these groups than in the control, accompanied by a corresponding increase in oxygen consumption. It will be seen that FFA and glycerol release remained relatively low without the added hormone but showed a marked increase after the addition of norepinephrine. This increment was further amplified when the catecholamine was fortified with theophylline, although the oxygen consumption was not essentially affected.

Similar experiments were repeated with brown adipose tissue. It will be seen (Table 25) that tissue FFA levels were much higher in brown adipose tissue than in white. The most striking feature of brown adipose tissue was its enormously high rate of oxygen consumption, even in the control without the added hormone, while the rate of FFA and glycerol release remained quite low. Norepinephrine or theophylline caused, as in white fat, a marked increment both in FFA and glycerol release accompanied by a corresponding increase in oxygen consumption. When both were added simultaneously, further increase in FFA and glycerol release was observed, while oxygen consumption did not increase significantly. Next, the effect of cold exposure was examined. Contrary to our expectation, all the parameters except that of oxygen consumption were found unaffected by cold exposure, although initial level of tissue FFA was

TABLE 25 Effects of *in vitro* addition of norepinephrine or theophylline on lipolytic and respiratory activities in interscapular brown adipose tissue of non-adapted control and cold-adapted rats. All values are given as mean ± standard error of the mean.

Non-adapted control:

In vitro addition	Series No.	No. of rats	Tissue FFA level (µEq/g)		Medium FFA (µEq/g/hr)	Medium glycerol (µM/g/hr)	O₂ consumed (µl/100 mg/30 min.)
			initial	final			
None	I	11	10.4±0.21	8.7±0.38	1.6±0.29	1.9±0.19	73.1±5.61
Norepinephrine	II	9	8.9±0.65	7.8±0.43	3.9±0.56	3.6±0.57	120.2±11.27
				vs. I	vs. I	vs. I	vs. I
				NS	P<0.002	P<0.01	P<0.001
Theophylline	III	6	9.9±0.88	7.3±0.67	6.0±0.92	4.1±0.88	106.7±15.18
				vs. I	vs. I	vs. I	vs. I
				NS	P<0.001	P<0.01	P<0.05
				vs. II	vs. II	vs. II	vs. II
				NS	P<0.10	NS	NS
Norepinephrine plus theophylline	IV	6	7.5±0.31	4.9±0.55	10.2±0.34	7.3±0.46	129.4±2.06
				vs. II	vs. II	vs. II	vs. II
				P<0.002	P<0.001	P<0.001	NS

Cold-adapted:

In vitro addition	Series No.	No. of rats	Tissue FFA level (µEq/g)		Medium FFA (µEq/g/hr)	Medium glycerol (µM/g/hr)	O₂ consumed (µl/100 mg/30 min.)
			initial	final			
None	V	10	7.4±0.59	8.8±0.53	2.6±0.35	1.8±0.24	110.2±9.21
			vs. I	vs. I	vs. I	vs. I	vs. I
			P<0.001	NS	P<0.05	NS	P<0.01
Norepinephrine	VI	13	7.0±0.38	8.1±0.33	3.2±0.37	2.3±0.22	130.5±7.35
				vs. V	vs. V	vs. V	vs. V
				NS	NS	NS	NS
Norepinephrine plus theophylline	VII	8	6.6±0.47	6.7±0.34	3.7±0.37	2.0±0.23	132.0±5.81
				vs. VI	vs. VI	vs. VI	vs. VI
				P<0.10	NS	NS	NS

generally lower in cold-adapted animals than in the non-adapted group. Furthermore, the addition of norepinephrine or theophylline separately or in combination affected neither FFA and glycerol release nor oxygen consumption significantly.

2. Relationship between Oxygen Consumption and Fatty Acid Utilization

Calculations were made in order to assess the relation of FFA utilization to increased oxygen consumption in the adipose tissues of cold-adapted and non-adapted rats. The amount of FFA consumed was calculated from the difference between the expected production of fatty acids, i.e. three times the glycerol value, and that actually found. The latter was obtained from net change in tissue level added to the amount released into the medium. The rate of oxygen consumption was converted to µM/g/hr, using 25.4 L as the volume of one mole of oxygen at 37.5 °C. The results obtained were plotted in Fig. 89 for epididymal white adipose tissue, and Figs. 90 and 91 for interscapular brown adipose tissue. It is apparent from Fig. 89 that in both the control and cold-adapted groups the increase in oxygen consumption coincided well with the amount of FFA utilized. In both cases, the correlation was highly significant. The relationship between oxygen consumption (Y) and fatty acid utilization (X) was given as $Y = 0.44 X + 4.59$ for the non-adapted group, and $Y = 0.41 X + 10.59$ for the cold-adapted group. The slopes of both lines were essentially identical, while the ordinate intercepts were significantly different. When a similar analysis was

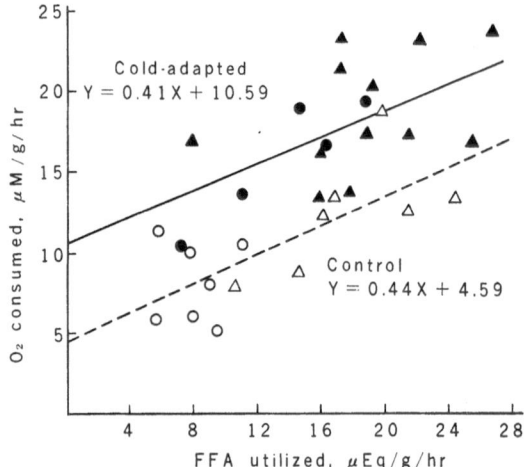

Fig. 89. Correlation between oxygen consumption and FFA utilized in epididymal white adipose tissue obtained from non-adapted control and cold-adapted rats. Open circles represent basal rates without added hormone, open triangles the addition of norepinephrine or theophylline, solid circles the basal rate in the cold-adapted rats, and solid triangles the addition of norepinephrine or theophylline into the medium.

performed on the data obtained with brown adipose tissue on the assumption that no glycerol was consumed in this tissue, there was again found a high correlation between oxygen consumption and fatty acid utilization, as given above, Y = 4.50 X + 40.85 for the non-adapted control group (Fig. 90).

Thermogenesis in adipose tissue is assumed to depend finally on one or both of the following metabolic mechanisms: a) utilization of ATP as heat, or b) uncoupling of oxidative phosphorylation. As to the possible utilization of ATP as heat, special

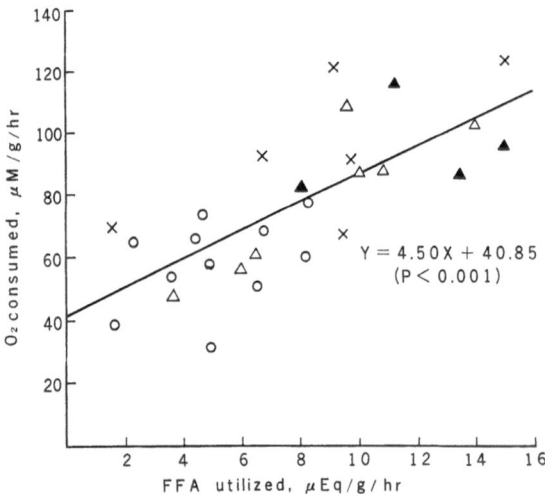

Fig. 90. Relationship between oxygen consumption and FFA utilized in brown adipose tissue of non-adapted control rats. Open circles stand for the basal rate without addition of hormone, crosses for theophylline addition, open triangles for epinephrine addition, and solid triangles for simultaneous addition of epinephrine and theophylline.

emphasis has been given to the following two aspects of the intermediary metabolism of lipids, i.e. one, described by Masoro [42], termed the fatty acid synthesis-oxidation cycle, the other, described by Ball and Jungus [4], called the lipolysis-reesterification cycle. Still another possibility is the oxidation of fatty acid after enhanced lipolysis.

If biosynthesized fatty acids are not stored but equivalent amounts are catabolized, the fatty acid synthesis-oxidation cycle could, by decreasing the net generation of ATP from glucose, provide for an increased utilization of substrate as heat [43]. For this cycle to be an effective means for increased heat production in cold-acclimated animals it must function at an increased rate in these animals and, if so, an augmented incorporation of labelled carbon from glucose or acetate into fatty acids would be expected. The available data on this point however are contradictory. Masoro et al. [44] found that adipose tissue of cold-adapted animals converted in vitro three times as much acetate-1-C^{14} to fatty acids as did adipose tissue from control rats [51]. Baumber and Denyes [6, 7] similarly observed an increased incorporation of acetate-1-C^{14} into C^{14}-lipids in vitro with both white and brown adipose tissues from cold-acclimated hamsters. It is noteworthy, however, that the increased lipogenic capacity was accompanied by decreased CO_2 production from acetate. Moreover, the lipogenic capacity of white adipose tissue was found to increase approximately sevenfold, while that of brown adipose tissue increased threefold at best. They concluded that increased lipogenic capacity is not a primary response of brown adipose tissue to cold exposure, but that some other pathway becomes active. In fact, Patkin and Masoro [52], by administering a large load of glucose-C^{14} to rats, found an unaltered fatty acid synthesis in the brown adipose as well as white adipose tissue of cold-acclimated rats. On the other hand, Steiner and Cahill [71] reported that the incorporation of glucose-C^{14} into neutral lipids, glyceride glycerol and fatty acids was increased in vivo and in vitro in the brown adipose tissue of cold-acclimated rats. These findings would be consistent with Masoro's proposal mentioned above [42]. Ball and Jungus [5] also remarked a necessary increase in oxygen consumption during active fatty acid synthesis in adipose tissue and gave an excellent discussion of the biochemical regulatory mechanisms involved [2]. It should be remembered, however, that fatty acid synthesis is known to proceed poorly in a phosphate buffer, presumably because of the lack of CO_2 needed for the conversion of acetyl CoA to malonyl CoA [5]. Since a Krebs-Ringer phosphate buffer was used in the present experiment, the possibility of utilization of ATP through fatty acid synthesis appears unlikely.

As to the lipolysis and reesterification cycle, i.e. another aspect of lipid metabolism specifically linked to nonshivering thermogenesis, Steiner and Cahill [71] and Himms-Hagen [26] showed that there was a greatly increased incorporation of glucose carbon into the glyceride glycerol of brown adipose tissue of cold-acclimated rats. These results suggest that the lipolysis-reesterification cycle is an important thermogenic mechanism in the brown adipose tissue of cold-acclimated rats. But, in white adipose tissue no evidence is available for the increased activity of this cycle during cold exposure. In the present study increments in oxygen consumption were shown to be highly correlated with amounts of FFA utilized. It should be noted here that FFA utilization includes FFA reesterification and oxidation. The slope of the line shows the value of micromoles of fatty acid utilized per each micromole of oxygen consumed, i.e. 2.27 for the control group and 2.44 for the cold-adapted group. If we assume a P:O ratio to be 3, this yields values, respectively, of 2.6—P and 2.5—P required for each molecule of fatty acid utilization.   Since it is known that 7 high-energy phosphate bonds are needed to esterify one mole of triglyceride, a theoretical value for P would be $7/3 = 2.3$ assuming the P:O ratio to be 3.   This can be considered excellent confirmation.   It is thus probable that FFA reesterification may account for a major portion of the total FFA utilization observed.   Earlier, Ball and Jungus [5] estimated the value, from a similar *in vitro* experiment, to be 3.8—P, higher than the present result.

Although oxygen consumption in the cold-adapted group was found significantly higher than that in the control group, this increase was evidently not related to the lipolysis-reesterification cycle, for it is apparent in the absence of esterification, as well, as shown by ordinate intercepts (Fig. 89).   In the cold-adapted animals, wet weight of white adipose tissue is well known to decrease mainly because of depletion of lipid content [47].   This in turn renders the tissue relatively rich in fat-free dry matter. Thus, an increment in oxygen consumption may well be ascribable to the relative increase in dry mass.   This factor would also explain an apparent parallel increase in the amount of esterification in the cold-adapted rats as compared to that of the control group.   Consequently, it appears reasonable to conclude that in white adipose tissue the basic mechanism responsible for nonshivering thermogenesis is essentially unaffected by cold adaptation.

Similar analysis of the brown adipose tissue of non-adapted control rats revealed a high correlation between oxygen consumption and fatty acid utilization as given in Fig. 90.   The ordinate intercept 40.85 which shows the oxygen consumption independent of fatty acid utilization is about 9 times greater than that of white adipose tissue under the similar conditions.   This value corresponds to the ratio of fat-free dry mass between brown and white adipose tissues [47, 67].   On the other hand, calculations from the slope show that high-energy bonds required for each molecule of fatty acid utilized in brown adipose tissue amount to 27.0—P, assuming a P:O ratio of 3. In other words, when calculated back from the theoretical value of 2.3, an expected ratio in brown adipose tissue would be 0.234.   This extremely low P:O ratio, though presumably due partly to underestimation of FFA utilization because of the neglect of glycerolkinase activity, may suggest the participation of a third mechanism operative in nonshivering thermogenesis, that is, the uncoupling of oxidative phosphoyrlation.   In fact, several workers [41, 70] reported low P:O ratio with isolated brown fat mitochondria and also an apparent absence of elementary particles which are hypothesized by Racker *et al.* [57] to contain the factor that couples phosphorylation to oxidation.   Joel *et al.* [36] however presented evidence against the above hypothesis. They observed in rat brown fat mitochondria that the mean P:O ratio in the absence of dinitrophenol (DNP) was 1.00 and the ratio in the presence of DNP was 0.54, the difference being highly significant.   Nevertheless, the values still remain low as compared with those obtained from other tissues.   This may be due to uncoupling action of FFA [10] that exists in a relatively high concentration in brown adipose tissue (Table 25).   Himms-Hagen in her recent review [27] discussed this problem more thoroughly and arrived at a similar conclusion.

It will be noticed (Fig. 91) that in the brown adipose tissue of cold-adapted rats rates of FFA utilization remain low in spite of the high rate of oxygen consumption.

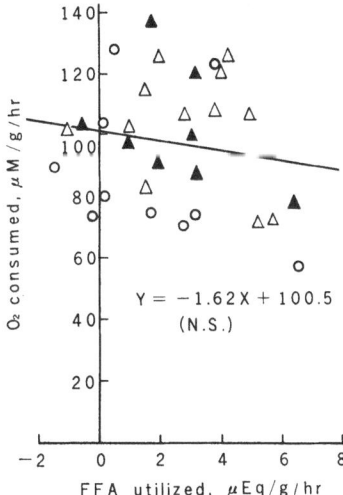

Fig. 91. Relationship of oxygen consumption to FFA utilization in brown adipose tissue of cold-adapted rats. For details of explanation, see Fig. 90. Note apparent low rates of FFA utilization in spite of high rates of oxygen consumption.

It should be remembered that in the calculation of FFA utilization in these experiments it is assumed that glycerol is not consumed. This may not be the case, since Treble and Ball [73] found a significant glycerolkinase activity in the brown adipose tissue of the rat, making this tissue well equipped to carry out the cycle of fat breakdown and resynthesis, although Dawkins and Hull [14] denied the presence of enzyme activity in the brown adipose tissue of newborn rabbits. Recently, Ball [3] and Kornacker and Ball [40] failed to obtain evidence for this cycle in brown adipose tissue, even though they admitted that the possibility cannot be excluded entirely. On the other hand, an accumulated body of evidence appears to indicate that brown fat mitochondria under basal conditions are able to carry out oxidative phosphorylation in an almost normal fashion [24, 28, 55, 56, 59], and yet are liable to uncoupling during cold exposure or catecholamine stimulation, probably due to a loosening in the coupling of phosphorylation to respiration [22, 53]. It is now generally believed that intracellular concentration of FFA is probably the controlling link between substrate supply and utilization in brown fat [30, 31, 54]. Recently, Williamson [79, 80] emphasized the extreme sensitivity of brown fat mitochondria to the release of respiratory control by FFA, drawing our attention also to the role of substrate level phosphorylation for the generation of high energy phosphate in this tissue.

All these findings may suggest that brown adipose tissue, in contrast to white adipose tissue, possesses mitochondria inherently liable to uncoupling of oxidative phosphorylation and, when exposed chronically to cold, that it shows an acceleration of fatty acid oxidation as well as of the fat breakdown and resynthesis cycle. It is assumed that by virtue of these features brown adipose tissue performs an important role in non-shivering thermogenesis during cold acclimation.

SEROTONIN

As to the metabolic activity of serotonin which is known to exist in brown adipose tissue in large amount [72], Vaughan [76, 77], using epididymal white fat, failed to demonstrate a lipolytic effect *in vitro*. On the other hand, Bieck *et al.* [8] claimed that a significant increase in lipolysis was demonstrable following the addition of serotonin *in vitro* in the presence of pargyline, a potent monoamine oxidase inhibitor. Since no report had been made on the effect of serotonin on brown adipose tissue, we performed the following experiments [83].

1. Lipolytic Action of Serotonin

Lipolytic effects of serotonin were compared among epididymal, mesenteric white adipose tissues and the brown fat of the rat. Observations were extended to the oxygen consumption of brown adipose tissue *in vitro*. Under basal conditions *in vitro*, the release of FFA from brown adipose tissue amounts to a 3-fold magnitude (6.9 μEq FFA/g/hr) as compared with white adipose tissue (2 μEq/g/hr). Difference between these values and previous ones (Tables 24 and 25) is probably due to the difference in the incubation conditions [33, 83]. The addition of serotonin (final concentration $5 \times 10^{-4}M$) caused a slight, though significant, increment in FFA release from the mesenteric adipose tissue, while in brown and epididymal adipose tissues serotonin had no effect. Failure to demonstrate a lipolytic effect of serotonin in these tissues might be due to a rapid inactivation of the amine by monoamine oxidase (MAO) as claimed by Bieck *et al.* [8]. The effect of serotonin was then examined under the effective (90%) inhibition of MAO activity by safrazine (final concentration 1 mM). MAO activity was assayed by the method of Sjoerdsma *et al.* [65]. It was found that safrazine did not affect the serotonin action at all. Thus, it is most unlikely that under the experimental conditions used the degradation of the amine by MAO is rate-limiting.

Since it is assumed [8, 77] that some metabolic effects of serotonin are mediated through a specific nucleotide, cyclic 3′, 5′-AMP, the effect of theophylline was examined. Theophylline itself, when given in a final concentration of 1 mM, caused a

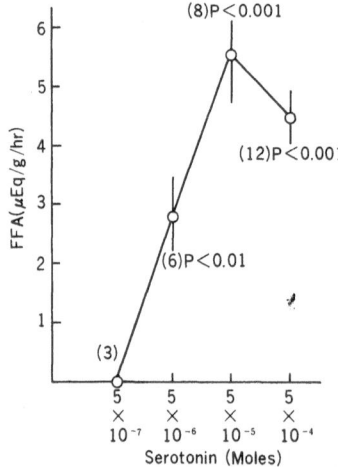

Fig. 92. Effect of serotonin on the FFA release from brown adipose tissue slices in the presence of theophylline. Theophylline was added in a final concentration of 1 mM. The amount of FFA release induced by serotonin was given as difference between control (theophylline alone) and experimental (theophylline plus serotonin) in paired determinations. Numbers in parenthesis indicate numbers of determination. Data are presented as mean and standard error.

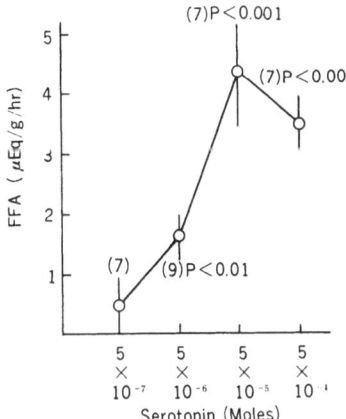

Fig. 93. Effect of serotonin on the release of FFA from mesenteric adipose tissue in the presence of theophylline. See the legend to Fig. 92 for further explanation.

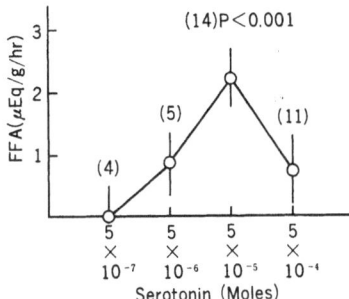

Fig. 94. Effect of serotonin on the release of FFA from epididymal adipose tissue in the presence of theophylline. See the legend to Fig. 92 for further explanation.

significant increase in FFA release from all the tissues examined. The effect of theophylline was several times greater in white than in brown adipose tissue. Next, the serotonin effect on FFA release was studied in the presence of theophylline in the incubation medium. As shown in Figs. 92, 93 and 94, a marked increase in FFA release was observed in all adipose tissues examined. It will be seen that in the presence of theophylline the lipolytic effect of serotonin was dose-dependent with a maximum response at a final concentration of the amine of 5×10^{-5}M. The magnitude of the maximal response to serotonin was the greatest in brown adipose tissue and the smallest in epididymal white adipose tissue, mesenteric adipose tissue being the intermediate. In all tissues dosages of serotonin above this maximal level tended to decrease the response. Since it was reported that serotonin content in brown adipose tissue was 1.07 µg/g of wet weight [72], a final concentration of the amine in the tissue, assuming a homogeneous distribution, is calculated to be of the order of 10^{-6}M which is well within the range where a linear dose-response relationship was proved.

Furthermore, it was found that although serotonin alone did not cause an increase in either oxygen consumption or FFA release, it increased both parameters

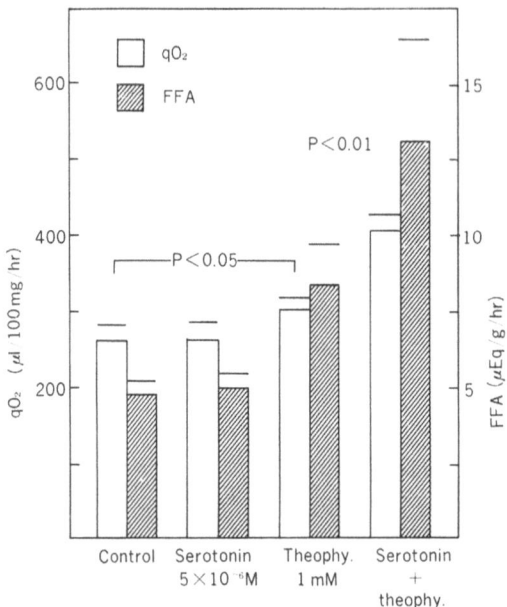

Fig. 95. Increase of oxygen consumption and FFA release in brown adipose tissue due to serotonin plus theophylline.   Data are given as mean of seven paired determinations with standard error.

significantly in the presence of theophylline (Fig. 95).   Serotonin was found to be potent also in eliciting an increase in glycerol release from mesenteric adipose tissue. Theophylline was also found again potent in causing a significant increase in glycerol release.   When both agents were combined in the test system, a much more pronounced effect was observed.   Thus, it may be inferred that serotonin may participate in the enhanced thermogenesis in brown adipose tissue through mechanisms similar to those of catecholamines.

2.   Serotonin and Thermogenesis in Brown Adipose Tissue

In order to understand the role of serotonin in an increased heat production in brown adipose tissue, comparison was made of the lipolytic effect of serotonin and

TABLE 26   Effect of serotonin and epinephrine on the oxygen consumption and glycerol release by brown adipose tissue.   Values are means $\pm$ S.E.

	No. of paired expt.	Hormone concentration	Without hormone	With hormone	% Stimulation
O_2 consumption (μl/100 mg/hr)	5	Serotonin 5×10^{-5}M	80.2 ± 6.2	232.6 ± 18.8	290.2
	6	Serotonin 5×10^{-4}M	83.0 ± 9.3	236.9 ± 23.5	285.6
	11	Epinephrine 1 μg/ml	120.2 ± 7.4	370.1 ± 25.0	308.0
Glycerol release (μM/g/hr)	5	Serotonin 5×10^{-5}M	0.87 ± 0.07	2.54 ± 0.40	292.0
	6	Serotonin 5×10^{-4}M	0.96 ± 0.13	2.52 ± 0.25	262.4
	10	Epinephrine 1 μg/ml	1.11 ± 0.07	3.95 ± 0.34	355.8

catecholamine [84]. These *in vitro* experiments were done in the absence of albumin in the incubation medium, since bovine albumin was sometimes found to interfere with the colorimetric determination of glycerol in the medium. It will be seen from Table 26 that increases in oxygen consumption under the influence of serotonin or epinephrine were of similar magnitude and varied in parallel with those of glycerol release. It should be mentioned here that serotonin in similar dosage exhibited no effect on the respiration of liver or brain slices *in vitro*.

To examine the relation between total oxygen consumption and FFA utilization, calculations were made as described above. The amount of FFA release was obtained from changes in tissue FFA content, because no FFA was released into the medium in the absence of albumin. The results obtained were plotted in Fig. 96 for serotonin and Fig. 97 for epinephrine. It is apparent that in both cases oxygen consumption

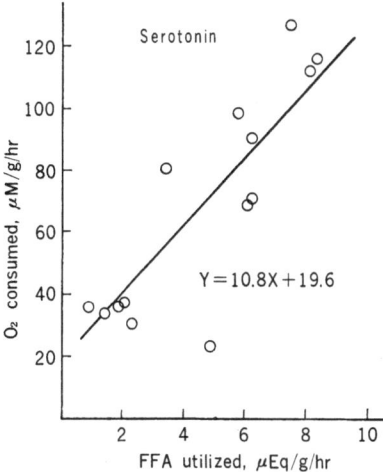

Fig. 96. Relation between oxygen consumption and FFA utilized in brown adipose tissue under the influence of serotonin. Incubation was performed in the absence of albumin in the medium.

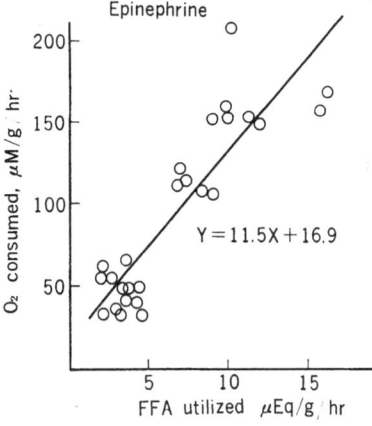

Fig. 97. Relationship between oxygen consumption and FFA utilization in brown adipose tissue under the influence of epinephrine. Incubation was carried out in the absence of albumin in the medium.

(Y) was highly correlated with the amount of FFA utilized (X). Correlation lines were given by $Y = 11.5 X + 16.9$ for epinephrine and $Y = 10.8 X + 19.6$ for serotonin. Slopes of both lines and their ordinate intercepts were essentially identical. This result may indicate the participation of serotonin in thermogenesis through a mechanism analogous to that of the catecholamines. Steeper slopes in these experiments than in the previous one (Fig. 90) may indicate higher rates of FFA utilization, probably linked with a higher degree of uncoupling of oxidative phosphorylation presumably due to a higher concentration of tissue FFA.

In order to know which of the amines, catecholamine or serotonin, is of primary importance as a means of activating metabolic machinery, the effects of both of the hormones were examined in the adipose tissue of reserpinized or denervated rats. Reserpine was injected subcutaneously at a dose of 2.5 mg per kg body weight. Denervation of interscapular brown adipose tissue was performed following the description of Weiner et al. [78]. The left lobe was exposed and the nerves were transected four days before the experiment, the right lobe serving as the control. Table 27 shows the data on the metabolic parameters of brown adipose tissue in vitro from

TABLE 27   Effect of serotonin and theophylline on the oxygen consumption and lipolysis in brown adipose tissue of reserpinized rats. Values are means ± S.E.

	No. of paired expt.	Control	Serotonin $(5 \times 10^{-4}M)$	Theophylline (1 mM)	Theophylline plus Serotonin
O$_2$ consumption (μl/100 mg/hr)	6	76.3±8.8	67.3±10.1	160.8±36.8	183.5±31.9
Glycerol release (μM/g/hr)	6	0.67±0.08	0.60±0.08	0.88±0.02	0.85±0.02
FFA release (μEq/g/hr)	6	0.88±0.41	1.43±0.31	3.99±0.31	3.84±0.42

reserpinized rats and the effects of serotonin and theophylline on them. Comparison of these data with those obtained from normal rats disclosed marked differences. First, reserpinization caused a marked reduction in FFA release in the control group (without added hormone). In spite of this, the lipolytic effect of added norepinephrine or theophylline was not affected at all, whereas serotonin effects on these parameters were completely abolished, even in the presence of theophylline. Similar results, though quantitatively different, were obtained with denervated brown adipose tissue. The basal rate of FFA release by the denervated lobe was significantly reduced (54.9% decrease). The lipolytic effect of serotonin in the presence of theophylline was similarly diminished (% decrease of 54.3), whereas the lipolytic action of theophylline was little affected.

It is of particular interest that serotonin effects on FFA release and oxygen consumption were completely abolished by reserpinization or significantly diminished by denervation, though effects of epinephrine or theophylline were not influenced by these treatments. Reserpine is known to cause a marked depletion of norepinephrine in various tissues. For instance, Bieck et al. [9] reported that either reserpinization or denervation of brown adipose tissue caused a marked decrease in norepinephrine content in it. Our results, therefore, clearly indicate the dependency of the serotonin effect on the presence of catecholamine in brown adipose tissue.

Next, interaction of norepinephrine and serotonin in their lipolytic effect was investigated, using the brown adipose tissue of reserpinized as well as normal rats. It was found that the combination of serotonin with catecholamine caused a marked increase in oxygen consumption, though either of the hormones alone had litte or no effect. In other words, norepinephrine effects were markedly potentiated by the addition of serotonin which by itself was ineffective in the amount used. From these results it may be concluded that catecholamines are of primary importance in the regulation of active thermogenesis in adipose tissues, whereas serotonin in brown adipose tissue plays a role in the presence of catecholamines. Nevertheless, serotonin present in abundance in brown adipose tissue appears to be an important though subsidiary means, regulating the delicate, high metabolic capabilities of this tissue in responding to demands for increased heat production.

ROLE OF POTASSIUM IONS

The importance of electrolytes for the manifestation of the hormonal effect on various tissues has been repeatedly emphasized [63, 75, 87]. As to the influence of potassium ions on the action of lipolytic hormone, Mosinger and Kujalova [48] first showed that the lipolytic action of catecholamine was significantly reduced in a potassium free medium, thus demonstrating the necessity of potassium for lipolytic hormone action. Since this effect of potassium was markedly reduced by the presence of ouabain, they suggested that the epinephrine effect on adipose tissue might be linked with the actively transported potassium or sodium pump. This view was supported by similar findings obtained by other investigators. [20, 29] Since these investigations were mainly concerned with the influence of potassium on hormonal effect in white adipose tissue, we examined this effect of potassium on brown adipose tissue [85].

To begin with, we confirmed that norepinephrine-induced lipolysis in epididymal white adipose tissue was markedly, though not completely, reduced by the presense of ouabain or the omission of potassium from the medium. Then, observations were extended to brown adipose tissue. Again, catecholamine-induced lipolysis was significantly reduced by the omission of potassium (Table 28). The basal rate of lipolysis in brown adipose tissue, as in white fat, was not influenced significantly by these conditions. It is of interest to note that the lipolytic effect of theophylline on brown as well as white aidpose tissues was increased by the omission of potassium from the medium.

TABLE 28   Effect of potassium free medium on glycerol release induced by norepinephrine or theophylline in interscapular brown adipose tissue. Control medium denotes Krebs-Ringer phosphate buffer. P shows the level of statistical significance of the difference between two values indicated by an arc.

	Basal	Norepinephrine (1.0 µg/ml)	Norepinephrine effect	P
Experiment I (9 paired determinations)				
K-free medium	1.32±0.09	1.68±0.11	0.37±0.13	} <0.005
Control medium	0.88±0.08	3.29±0.50	2.41±0.42	
	Basal	Theophylline (1 mM)	Theophylline effect	P
Experiment II (4 paired determinations)				
K-free medium	0.93±0.23	1.55±0.26	0.62±0.03	} <0.025
Control medium	0.87±0.26	1.05±0.24	0.18±0.05	

Further, it was found that potassium omission almost completely abolished the catecholamine-stimulated increase of respiration in brown adipose tissue as shown in Fig. 98. Similarly, ouabain effectively blocked the respiration (Fig. 99). In both cases, the basal rate of oxygen consumption remained almost unaffected. Omission of sodium ions from the medium likewise was found effective in blocking the hormone-induced lipolysis. These findings therefore may suggest the involvement of an active transport system for electrolytes in the lipolytic effect of norepinephrine on brown adipose tissue, since the active process is known in various tissue preparations to be

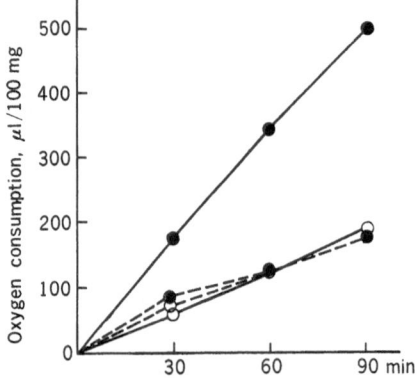

Fig. 98. Potassium dependency of hormone-stimulated increase of respiration of brown adipose tissue. Open circles stand for control without added hormone, and solid ones for added norepinephrine (1.0 μg/ml). Solid lines represent values in control medium (Krebs-Ringer phosphate buffer) and broken lines those of K$^+$-free medium. Note that the marked increment in respiration due to catecholamine stimulation was almost completely abolished in the absence of potassium ions. Average values of nine paired determinations are shown.

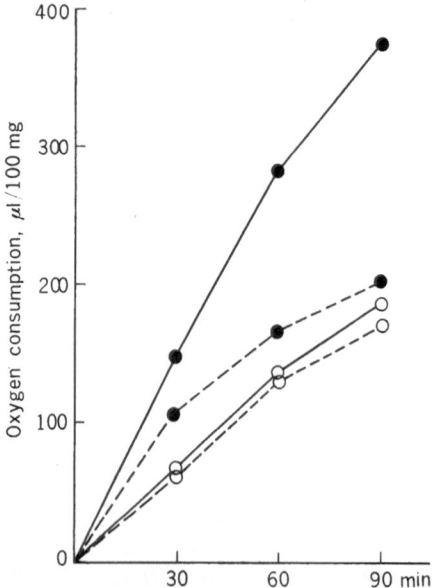

Fig. 99. Inhibition by ouabain of norepinephrine-stimulated respiration in brown adipose tissue. The same notations are used as in Fig. 98 except that a broken line stands for ouabain addition (5 X 10^{-4}M). Average values of six paired determinations are given.

inhibited by ouabain or omission of potassium or sodium from the medium [66]. A body of evidence indicates that specific Na-K dependent ATPase participates in the active transport of these cations. In fact, evidence has recently been presented for the existence of a Na-K dependent ATPase, though in extremely small amounts, in epididymal white adipose tissue [46].

It is interesting to note that the lipolytic action of theophylline was not suppressed at all by ouabain but rather increased in the absence of potassium ions. Similar potentiation of theophylline effects by potassium omission was reported by Fain [20, 21] in experiments using isolated white fat cells. Since theophylline is believed to activate lipolysis by inhibiting phosphodiesterase, the potentiation may be due to an enhancement of lipase activation by cyclic AMP. In fact, Mosinger and Vaughan [50] reported that lipolytic action of cyclic AMP was enhanced by the omission of potassium ions from the phosphate buffer medium. They stressed variable responses of adipose tissue to this nucleotide depending on animal conditions and also on the ionic compositions of the incubation medium. In spite of this complexity, it may be surmised that the enhanced lipolysis by theophylline is mediated through stimulation of cyclic AMP formation. Comparison of the lipolytic action of both catecholamine and theophylline revealed some interesting contrast. As was repeatedly shown [33, 60], both agents are lipolytic and also synergistic. And yet, difference in their mode of action is apparent. Norepinephrine effect is clearly ouabain sensitive and potassium dependent, whereas the reverse is true for the theophylline effect. Thus, it is assumed, as was first suggested by Mosinger and Vaughan [49], that there may be two mechanisms involved in the enhanced lipolysis in adipose tissues: one linked somehow to a Na-K dependent ATPase, the other related to production of cyclic AMP. Since potassium ions exhibited influence on both of them, i.e., potassium omission was inhibitory in the former while rather stimulatory in the latter, it may be surmised that potassium ions play some essential role in the operation of these two mechanisms. Although transport ATPase and adenyl cyclase are believed to be localized in cell membranes, their anatomical relationship as well as functional similarity and dissimilarity is yet to be elucidated.

LIPOLYSIS BY EXCESS POTASSIUM

There is evidence that various cellular secretory activities are stimulated by excess potassium in the solutions which bathe tissues. For example, the addition of excess potassium to perfusion fluid stimulated insulin release from the isolated pancreas [23] and norepinephrine release from the adrenal medulla [16]. Similarly, excess potassium in the incubation medium induced the release of luteinizing hormone from the adenohypophysis [62] and vasopressin from the neurohypophysis [15]. Although the lipolytic action of catecholamine has been shown to require potassium ions, no studies have yet been made on the effect of excess potassium alone on adipose tissues. On the other hand, stimulation of various secretory activities is known to be dependent on the presence of calcium ions [23, 45, 58]. Therefore, we examined the influence of excess potassium on the lipolytic and respiratory activities of brown adipose tissue in comparison with the norepinephrine effect, special attention being focused on their calcium dependency [81, 86].

The effect of excess potassium on lipolysis and oxygen consumption in brown

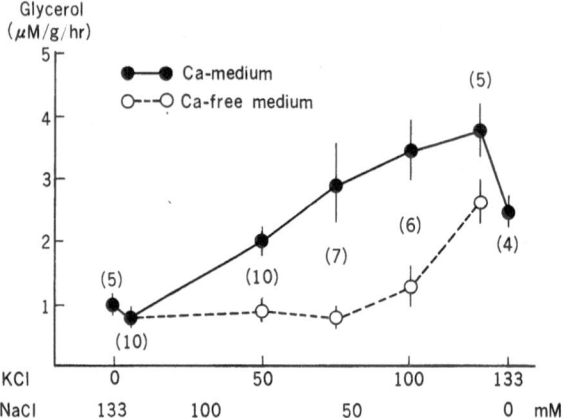

Fig. 100. Effects of various concentrations of potassium and sodium ions on the glycerol release from rat brown adipose tissue in the presence or absence of calcium ions. Sodium chloride was replaced to various extents by equimolar amounts of potassium chloride to produce a final concentration of 133 mM, other components of Krebs-Ringer phosphate buffer being kept constant. Numbers in parentheses show the number of paired determinations.

adipose tissue is shown in Figs. 100 and 101. The concentration of potassium chloride in the incubation medium was increased from 0 to 133 mM and glycerol release into the medium was measured (Fig. 100). It is apparent that by increasing the potassium concentration a marked stimulation of glycerol release was obtained. This effect of excess potassium was "dose"-dependent and maximum response was attained at a concentration of 123 mM of potassium chloride. Similarly, excess potassium was found to stimulate respiration (Fig. 101). The increase of oxygen consumption was maximally stimulated at 75 mM of potassium ions and maintained at this level up to 123 mM of the ions. In the absence of sodium, however, both parameters showed a marked reduction. It is evident that the stimulation of lipolytic activity in brown adipose tissue by excess potassium was due not to the fall in sodium ions, but to the

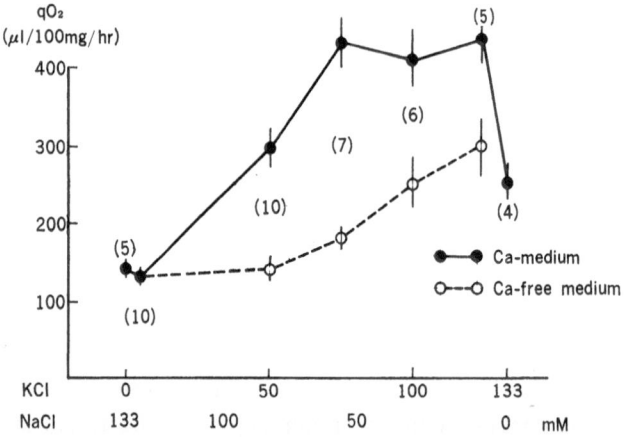

Fig. 101. Effects of various concentrations of potassium and sodium ions on the respiration of rat brown adipose tissue. Other conditions of incubation were the same as in Fig. 100.

rise of potassium ions, because the response was equally obtained in experiments where sodium was held constant at 10 mM, the medium being kept iso-osmotic by adding appropriate amount of sucrose.

In the absence of calcium, the stimulating effect of excess potassium was either completely inhibited or markedly diminished as shown in Figs. 100 and 101 (dotted lines). The effect of low doses of excess potassium (50 mM and 75 mM, respectively) was almost completely inhibited by calcium omission. By increasing the potassium concentration, however, excess potassium effects were partially recovered even in the absence of calcium. The effect of calcium omission was found reversible, namely, potassium always restored its stimulant effect on the oxygen consumption of brown adipose tissue after calcium had been added to the medium. Recently, Turtle et al. [74] and Rasmussen and Tenenhouse [58] independently claimed that the stimulating effects of excess potassium on various cellular secretory activities are mediated by formation of cyclic AMP. The latter authors [58] suggested that in the regulation of these secretory activities cyclic AMP and calcium ions are key elements and their effects are intimately related to membrane structure and function. An interesting feature is that these secretory activities are stimulated by excess potassium in the bathing solution and that this effect is also calcium dependent [23, 58, 62]. In this series of experiment, we could show that the lipolytic effect of excess potassium was potentiated by theophylline [86]. Therefore, we are inclined to suggest that the excess potassium effect in brown adipose tissue is mediated through an increased formation of cyclic AMP. In addition, the excess potassium effect was shown to be calcium dependent. This calcium dependency was further fortified by other findings with magnesium ions. That is, the response of brown adipose tissue to excess potassium was markedly inhibited by excess magnesium (13.3 mM) which is known to act as a calcium antagonist in many systems. [15, 17, 58]. These results therefore may, in line with the postulate of Rasmussen et al. [58], suggest the participation of cyclic AMP and calcium ions in potassium-induced lipolysis in the brown adipose tissue.

As to the role played by calcium ions, Mosinger et al. [49] showed that the lipolytic effect of theophylline and dibutyryl cyclic AMP was not affected by the presence or absence of calcium ions. They claimed that calcium ions are essential for cyclic AMP formation which is stimulated by lipolytic hormones. On the other hand, Rasmussen and Tenenhouse [58] arrived at a different conclusion, working with the rat parotid gland. They observed that omission of calcium or addition of excess magnesium into the medium had no influence on cyclic AMP formation in the gland, although the amylase secretion was markedly inhibited. From these results they concluded that calcium ions are essential for the effective action of cyclic AMP. Thus, although it was evident from the present experiment that both cyclic AMP and calcium ions are necessary for the manifestation of an excess potassium effect on brown adipose tissue, the exact role played by calcium ions therein still remained to be explored.

Further attempts were therefore made to clarify the mode of action of excess potassium and the role of calcium ions, by comparing it with the action of norepinephrine. First, we examined the calcium dependency of the norepinephrine effect. In contrast with the excess potassium effect, the stimulating effect of norepinephrine on lipolysis and oxygen consumption in brown adipose tissue was only partially, though signifi-

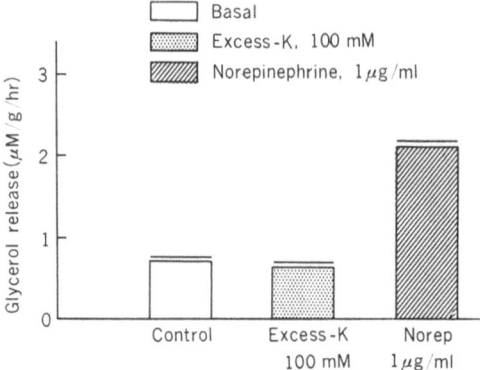

Fig. 102. Comparison of the lipolytic effect of excess potassium and norepinephrine in reserpinized rat brown adipose tissue. Average values of five paired determinations are shown with standard errors at the top of each column.

cantly, reduced in a calcium free medium. Thus, there appears to exist a dissociation between the mode of action of excess potassium and norepinephrine in brown adipose tissue. To further examine this point, the lipolytic action of excess potassium was compared with that of norepinephrine in brown fat slices obtained from reserpinized or denervated rats [82]. Fig. 102 shows the data obtained from reserpinized rats. Reserpinization had no significant influence on basal lipolysis as well as on the norepinephrine effect, even though the lipolytic effect of norepinephrine seems somewhat decreased. In contrast, the lipolytic effect of excess potassium was completely abolished by reserpinization. Similar results were also obtained with denervated rat brown adipose tissue (Fig. 103). It will be apparent that the lipolytic effect of excess potassium was markedly inhibited by denervation, whereas that of norepinephrine was little affected. Both reserpinization and denervation are known to cause a marked decrease in norepinephrine content in many tissues. These results therefore may suggest that the lipolytic effect of excess potassium on brown adipose tissue is dependent on the presence of norepinephrine in this tissue.

It should be mentioned here that in epididymal white adipose tissue excess potassium

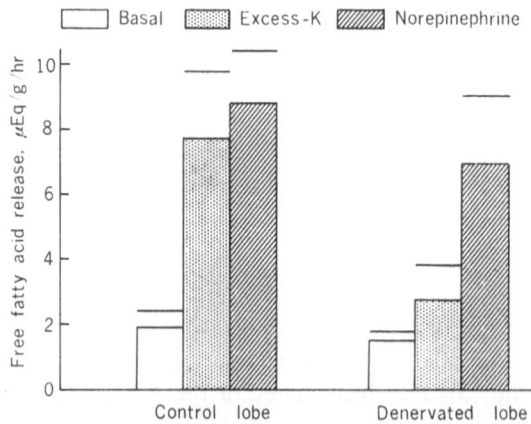

Fig. 103. Comparison of the lipolytic effect of excess potassium and norepinephrine in denervated rat brown adipose tissue. Average values of seven paired determinations are given with standard errors.

failed to show any significant effect not only on the basal rate of lipolysis but also on the enhanced rate after norepinephrine or theophylline addition. According to Stock and Westermann [72], norepinephrine content in epididymal adipose tissue and interscapular brown adipose tissue was 0.04 μg/g wet weight and 1.40 μg/g, respectively. Under our experimental conditions, the minimum effective dose of norepinephrine in epididymal adipose tissue and brown adipose tissue in vitro was 0.03 and 0.08 μg/ml, respectively. Rudman et al. [61] also reported similar results on the minimum effective dose for rat epididymal fat. Therefore, even if all the catecholamine contained in the adipose tissue is assumed to be released by excess potassium, norepinephrine concentration in the medium will at most be 0.002 μg/ml. This is far below the minimum effective dose. Similar calculation based on the hormone content in brown adipose tissue shows that a possible final concentration in the medium may reach about the level of minimum effective dose of catecholamine. Thus, failure to demonstrate the lipolytic effect of potassium in epididymal fat is due most probably to the extremely low content of norepinephrine in this tissue.

Kirpeker and Misu [37] reported that the removal of calcium from the incubation medium markedly reduced the amount of norepinephrine released by splenic nerve stimulation. They suggested that calcium is required as a link between excitation-secretion coupling at sympathetic nerve endings. Kirpeker and Wakade [38] also showed that norepinephrine was caused to be released from the spleen by injecting excess potassium into the splenic artery, and that the removal of calcium from the perfusion medium as well as addition of excess magnesium markedly reduced the norepinephrine release by excess potassium. From these results they concluded that the effect of excess potassium was probably due to depolarization of nerve membrane and the subsequent release of norepinephrine stored in the sympathetic nerve endings. Similar dependency on calcium ions of the release of catecholamine from adrenergic nerve endings was reported by Boullin [12], using the cat colon. Brown adipose tissue is known to be innervated by adrenergic fibers [35, 68] and contains as much norepinephrine as does the heart [64, 72]. Correll [13] reported that in vitro stimulation of nerve fibers supplying the interscapular brown fat of adult rabbits caused a marked rise in FFA content in the medium. Taking this evidence into consideration, our results may be interpreted to mean that the lipolytic effect of excess potassium on brown adipose tissue is due to norepinephrine release from the sympathetic nerve terminals as a consequence of depolarization of nerve membrane. In fact, we examined the rate of disappearance of norepinephrine in brown adipose tissue and found that the catecholamines disappeared more rapidly from adipose tissue in a high potassium medium [82]. The above interpretation is further supported by the result obtained with barium ions. These ions are known to be able to activate secretory mechanisms in many systems [12, 18, 25]. It was shown [82] that barium ions showed some intrinsic lipolytic effect on brown adipose tissue and this effect was more pronounced in high potassium medium. The latter finding is explained by the fact that barium ions act as an effective substitute for calcium ions in the norepinephrine release induced by nerve stimulation. Furthermore, lipolytic effect of excess potassium as well as norepinephrine on brown adipose tissue was almost completely abolished by propranolol, whereas the effect of ACTH and theophylline was not affected at all [82]. Blecher et al. [11] reported that the concentration of propranolol required to inhibit lipolysis due to ACTH and glucagon was several times greater than that for norepinephrine-induced lipolysis. Thus, these results may indicate a similarity of excess potassium effect to norepinephrine from the view point of propranolol inhibition.

Taking all of these findings into consideration, it may reasonably be concluded that the lipolytic effect of excess potassium on brown adipose tissue is mediated through norepinephrine release as a consequence of depolarization of adrenergic nerve endings within the tissue.

SUMMARY

Attempts were made to understand the neurohumoral regulatory mechanisms involved in enhanced heat production in the brown adipose tissue of the rat. Special emphasis was laid on the mode of action of catecholamine, which has been claimed to be a physiologically important means in activating thermoregulatory heat production in brown adipose tissue. The *in vitro* addition of norepinephrine or theophylline separately or in combination was used as a stimulant.

It was found that in epididymal white adipose tissue increment in oxygen consumption was highly correlated with amounts of FFA utilization. From analysis of the slopes of this correlation, high-energy phosphate bonds required for each molecule of fatty acid utilized were estimated to be 2.6—P, a value quite comparable to a theoretical value of 2.3—P on the assumption that major portion of FFA utilization is accounted for as FFA reesterification. Since the slope remained unchanged after chronic cold exposure, it is concluded that basic mechanisms responsible for non-shivering thermogenesis in white adipose tissue is not affected after cold adaptation. In contrast, in the brown adipose tissue of non-adapted rats the slope of the regression line yielded a very low P:O ratio, a finding strongly suggestive of the involvement of an uncoupling of oxidative phosphorylation which is most probably due to a high concentration of FFA in the tissue. After cold adaptation, in spite of high rate of oxygen consumption the correlation between oxygen consumption and FFA utilization was entirely lost. This may be mainly due to further acceleration of fatty acid oxidation as well as fat breakdown and resynthesis cycle.

Serotonin is another amine present abundantly in brown adipose tissue. The role of serotonin was examined in the control of thermogenesis. Serotonin was found to cause a marked, dose-dependent lipolysis in the presence of theophylline. Here again, increases in oxygen consumption correlated well with FFA utilization, a fact suggesting a participation of mechanisms analogous to that of norepinephrine. These serotonin effects, however, were completely abolished by prior reserpinization of rats or significantly diminished by denervation, whereas epinephrine or theophylline effects were not influenced. On the other hand, serotonin at the dose below its minimum effective dose was found to potentiate markedly the norepinephrine-induced lipolysis. It is therefore inferred that catecholamines are of primary importance in the regulation of active thermogenesis in brown adipose tissue, whereas serotonin appears to play a subsidiary role which is exhibited only in the presence of catecholamines.

During the course of these studies, it was found that excess potassium was a potent stimulant for enhanced lipolysis and oxygen consumption in the brown adipose tissue, but not in epididymal white adipose tissue. To understand the action of this, comparison was made of excess potassium effects with those of catecholamines in relation to calcium requirement and also to the influence of reserpinization or denervation. The results obtained may indicate that the lipolytic effect of excess potassium on brown adipose tissue is mediated through norepinephrine release from the sympathetic nerve terminals as a result of depolarization of adrenergic nerve membrane.

Finally, the role of potassium ions in physiological concentration was studied through the manifestation of a lipolytic hormone effect *in vitro*. It was shown that potassium omission from the medium resulted in a marked reduction of catecholamine-induced increases of lipolysis and respiration. Similar inhibition was obtained by sodium omission or the addition of ouabain. On the other hand, lipolytic action of theophylline was not affected at all by ouabain and was significantly increased in the absence of potassium ions. Thus, it is assumed that there may be two mechanisms involved in the enhanced lipolysis in adipose tissues: one linked to a Na-K dependent ATPase, the other related to production of cyclic AMP. Although it is surmised that potassium ions play some essential role in the operation of these two mechanisms, their exact action remains to be clarified in specific relation to transport ATPase and adenyl cyclase systems in cell membranes.

REFERENCES

1. Aherne, W., and D. Hull (1966): *J. Path. Bact.* **91**: 223.
2. Ball, E.G. (1966): In: Advances in Enzyme Regulation, Vol. 4, p. 3, G. Weber, ed., Pergamon Press, Oxord.
3. Ball, E.G. (1970): *Lipids* **5**: 220.
4. Ball, E.G., and R.L. Jungus (1961): *Proc. Natl. Acad. Sci.* **47**: 932.
5. Ball, E.G., and R.L. Jungus (1964): *Rec. Progr. Hormone Res.* **20**: 183.
6. Baumber, J., and A. Denyes (1963): *Am. J. Physiol.* **205**: 905.
7. Baumber, J., and A. Denyes (1964): *Can. J. Biochem.* **42**: 1397.
8. Bieck, P., K. Stock, and E.O. Westermann (1966): *Life Sci.* **5**: 2157.
9. Bieck, P., K. Stock, and E. Westermann (1967): *Naunyn-Schmiedebergs Arch. Pharmak. Exp. Path.* **256**: 218.
10. Björntorp, P., H.A. Ellis, and R.H. Bradford (1966): *J. Biol. Chem.* **239**: 339.
11. Blecher, M., N.S. Merlino, J.T. Ro'Ane, and P.D. Flynn (1969): *J. Biol. Chem.* **244**: 3423.
12. Boullin, D.J. (1967): *J. Physiol.* **189**: 85.
13. Correll, J.W. (1963): *Science* **140**: 387.
14. Dawkins, M.J., and D. Hull (1964): *J. Physiol.* **172**: 216.
15. Douglas, W.W., and A.M. Poisner (1964): *J. Physiol.* **172**: 1.
16. Douglas, W.W., and R.P. Rubin (1961): *J. Physiol.* **159**: 40.
17. Douglas, W.W., and R.P. Rubin (1963): *J. Physiol.* **167**: 288.
18. Douglas, W.W., and R.P. Rubin (1964): *Nature* **203**: 305.
19. Duncombe, W.G. (1963): *Biochem. J.* **88**: 7.
20. Fain, J.N. (1968): *Mol. Pharmacol.* **4**: 349.
21. Fain, J.N. (1968): *Endocrinology* **83**: 548.
22. Grav, H.J., J.I. Pedersen, and E.N. Christiansen (1970): *Europ. J. Biochem.* **12**: 11.
23. Grodsky, G.M., and L.L. Bennett (1966): *Diabetes* **15**: 910.
24. Guillory, R.J., and E. Racker (1968): *Biochim. Biophys. Acta* **153**: 490.
25. Hales, C.N., and R.D.C. Milner (1968): *J. Physiol.* **199**: 177.
26. Himms-Hagen, J. (1965): *Can. J. Physiol. Pharmacol.* **43**: 379.
27. Himms-Hagen, J. (1970): In: Advances in Enzyme Regulation, Vol. 8, p. 131, G. Weber, ed., Pergamon Press, Oxford.
28. Hittelman, K.J., O. Lindberg, and B. Cannon (1969): *Europ. J. Biochem.* **11**: 183.
29. Ho, R.J., B. Jeanrenaud, Th. Posternak, and A.E. Renold (1967): *Biochim. Biophys. Acta* **144**: 74.
30. Horwitz, B.A., P.A. Herd, and R.E. Smith (1968): *Can. J. Physiol. Pharmacol.* **46**: 897.

31. HORWITZ, B.A., P.A. HERD, and R.E. SMITH (1970): *Lipids* **5**: 30.
32. HULL, D., and M.M. SEGALL (1965): *J. Physiol.* **181**: 449.
33. IKEMOTO, H., T. HIROSHIGE, and S. ITOH (1969): *Japan. J. Physiol.* **19**: 293.
34. JOEL, C.D. (1965): In: Handbook of Physiology, 5: Adipose Tissue, p. 59, A.E. Renold and G.F. Cahill, Jr., eds., Am. Physiol. Soc., Washington, D.C.
35. JOEL, C.D. (1966): *J. Biol. Chem.* **241**: 814.
36. JOEL, C.D., W.B. NEAVES, and J.M. RABB (1967): *Biochem. Biophys. Res. Commun.* **29**: 490.
37. KIRPEKER, S.M., and Y. MISU (1967): *J. Physiol.* **188**: 219.
38. KIRPEKER, S.M., and A.R. WAKADE (1968): *J. Physiol.* **94**: 595.
39. KORN, E.D. (1955): *J. Biol. Chem.* **215**: 1.
40. KORNACKER, M.S., and E.G. BALL (1968): *J. Biol. Chem.* **243**: 1638.
41. LINDBERG, O., J. DE PIERRE, E. RYLANDER, and B.A. AFZELIUS (1967): *J. Cell Biol.* **34**: 293.
42. MASORO, E.J. (1963): *Feder. Proc.* **22**: 868.
43. MASORO, E.J. (1966): *Physiol. Rev.* **46**: 67.
44. MASORO, E.J., J.M. FELTS, and S.S. PANAGOS (1957): *Am. J. Physiol.* **189**: 479.
45. MILNER, R.D.C., and C.N. HALES (1967): *Diabetologica* **3**: 47.
46. MODOLELL, J.B., and R.O. MOORE (1967): *Biochim. Biophys. Acta* **135**: 319.
47. MORIYA, K., and S. ITOH (1969): *Japan. J. Physiol.* **19**: 775.
48. MOSINGER, B., and V. KUJALOVA (1966): *Biochim. Biophys. Acta* **116**: 174.
49. MOSINGER, B., and M. VAUGHAN (1967): *Biochim. Biophys. Acta* **144**: 556.
50. MOSINGER, B., and M. VAUGHAN (1967): *Biochim. Biophys. Acta* **144**: 569.
51. PATKIN, J.K., and E.J. MASORO (1961): *Am. J. Physiol.* **200**: 847.
52. PATKIN, J.K., and E.J. MASORO (1964): *Can. J. Physiol. Pharmacol.* **42**: 101.
53. PEDERSEN, J.I., E.N. CHRISTIANSEN, and H.J. GRAV (1968): *Biochem. Biophys. Res. Commun.* **32**: 492.
54. PRUSINER, S.B., B. CANNON, and O. LINDBERG (1968): *Europ. J. Biochem.* **6**: 15.
55. PRUSINER, S.B., R.H. EISENHARDT, E. RYLANDER, and O. LINDBERG (1968): *Biochem. Biophys. Res. Commun.* **30**: 508.
56. PRUSINER, S.B., J.R. WILLIAMSON, B. CHANCE, and B.M. PADDLE (1968): *Arch. Biochem. Biophys.* **123**: 368.
57. RACKER, E., B. CHANCE, and D.F. PARSONS (1964): *Feder. Proc.* **23**: 431.
58. RASMUSSEN, H., and A. TENENHOUSE (1968): *Proc. Natl. Acad. Sci.* **59**: 1364.
59. REED, N., and J.N. FAIN (1968): *J. Biol. Chem.* **243**: 2843.
60. ROBISON, G.A., R.W. BUTCHER, and E.W. SUTHERLAND (1968): *Ann. Rev. Biochem.* **37**: 149.
61. RUDMAN, D., S.J. BROWN, and M.F. MALKIN (1963): *Endocrinology* **72**: 527.
62. SAMLI, M.H., and I.I. GESCHWIND (1968): *Endocrinology* **82**: 225.
63. SCHRAMM, M. (1968): *Biochim. Biophys. Acta* **165**: 546.
64. SIDMAN, R.L., M. PERKINS, and N. WEINER (1964): *Nature* **193**: 36.
65. SJOERDSMA, A., T.E. SMITH, T.D. STEVENSON, and S. UDENFRIEND (1955): *Proc. Soc. Exp. Biol. Med.* **89**: 36.
66. SKOU, J.C. (1965): *Physiol. Rev.* **45**: 596.
67. SMITH, R.E., and D.J. HOIJER (1962): *Pyhsiol. Rev.* **42**: 60.
68. SMITH, R.E., and B.A. HORWITZ (1969): *Physiol. Rev.* **49**: 330.
69. SMITH, R.E., and J.C. ROBERTS (1964): *Am. J. Physiol.* **206**: 143.
70. SMITH, R.E., J.C. ROBERTS, and K.J. HITTELMAN (1966): *Science* **154**: 653.
71. STEINER, G., and G.F. CAHILL, JR. (1964): *Am. J. Physiol.* **207**: 844.
72. STOCK, K., and E.O. WESTERMANN (1963): *J. Lipid Res.* **4**: 297.
73. TREBLE, D.H., and E.G. BALL (1963): *Feder. Proc.* **22**: 357.
74. TURTLE, J.R., G.K. LITTLETON, and D.M. KIPNIS (1967): *Nature* **213**: 727.
75. VALE, W., and R. GUILLEMIN (1968): *Experientia* **23**: 855.
76. VAUGHAN, M. (1960): *J. Biol. Chem.* **235**: 3049.
77. VAUGHAN, M. (1961): *J. Lipid Res.* **2**: 293.
78. WEINER, N., M. PERKINS, and R.L. SIDMAN (1962): *Nature* **193**: 137.
79. WILLIAMSON, J.R. (1969): *J. Biol. Chem.* **245**: 2043.
80. WILLIAMSON, J.R., S. PRUSINER, M.S. OLSON, and M. FUKAMI (1970): *Lipids* **5**: 1.
81. YOSHIMURA, K., and T. HIROSHIGE (1970): *Japan. J. Physiol.* **20**: 483.
82. YOSHIMURA, K., and T. HIROSHIGE (1971): *Japan. J. Physiol.* **21**: 189.
83. YOSHIMURA, K., T. HIROSHIGE, and S. ITOH (1969): *Japan. J. Physiol.* **19**: 176.
84. YOSHIMURA, K., T. HIROSHIGE, and S. ITOH (1969): *Japan. J. Physiol.* **19**: 791.
85. YOSHIMURA, K., T. HIROSHIGE, and S. ITOH (1969): *Japan. J. Physiol.* **19**: 876.
86. YOSHIMURA, K., T. HIROSHIGE, and S. ITOH (1969): *J. Biochem.* **66**: 565.
87. ZOR, U., I.P. LOWE, G. BLOOM, and J.B. FIELD (1968): *Biochem. Biophys. Res. Commun.* **33**: 649.

CHAPTER 15

PARTICIPATION OF THE LIMBIC-HYPOTHALAMIC STRUCTURES IN COLD ADAPTATION

Masazumi KAWAKAMI, Katsuo SETO, Hideo NEGORO,
Sadao YAMAOKA and Motohiko MOHRI

2nd Department of Physiology, Yokohama City University School of Medicine, Yokohama, Japan

Since a heat production center was assumed to be present in the brain by Otto and Richet in 1884, a number of studies have been carried out to locate the center or to elucidate its mechanisms. The earliest experiment was performed by Aronsohn and Sachs using a "heat puncture" method to stimulate or cause lesions to develop in the brain. Following this experiment, many researchers attempted either a more extensive destruction or removal of a part of the brain and observed its effect on the body temperature. Isenschmidt (1912), Bard and Rioch (1937), Pinkston *et al.* (1934) found that the removal of the forebrain and midbrain, decortication or removal of neopallium and hippocampus resulted in a loss of ability to regulate body temperature in response to environmental temperature. Magoun, Harrison, Brobeck and Ranson (1938) assumed from their lesioning experiment that the heat loss center was located in the anterior hypothalamus and the heat production center in the posterior hypothalamus. The presence of a temperature receptor in the anterior hypothalamus was first claimed by Barbour in 1912. Kuno (1956) hypothesized that the center of thermal sweating is localized in the diencephalon upon which another center in the cortex has a tonic inhibitory influence. Progress in this field of study has been made by means of heating or cooling parts of the brain. Ogata (1961, 1966, 1971), Nakayama (1961), Murakami (1967), Eisenman (1967), and Hardy (1964) revealed the presence of receptor cells for temperature in the anterior hypothalamus through recording of unit discharge in the hypothalamic neurons.

Previous studies indicate that partial cooling or heating of the brain alters its hormonal environment. Andersson (1962) showed that direct cooling of the preoptic area caused an increase in the secretion of TSH and heating a decrease in it. Chowers *et al.* (1962) reported that cooling of the preoptic area evoked a rise in plasma cortisol concentration. These findings suggest that temperature stimuli act on the brain directly and control the secretion of hormones involved in body temperature regulation.

Hemingway and his associates (1963) have shown by their elaborate studies that shivering, which plays an important role in physical heat production, is controlled by the brain stem, especially the hypothalamus. Simon and Thauer (1964) and Trichi and Kosaka (1967) reported that shivering was evoked by cooling the spinal cord at the lower thoracal and lumbosacral level in an animal spinalized at Th_2-Th_8. This observation suggest that a temperature receptor is present also in the spinal cord.

It has been postulated by Huntington, Kuno and Shoji that a temperature exposure experience early in life influenced an individual's resistance to heat or cold in adult life. Presumably then, the body is able to memorize the experience of exposure to unusual temperatures and to condition its brain mechanism as well as that of peripheral organs to adapt readily to subsequent temperature changes. Although very few studies have been made concerning the brain mechanism, evidence points to the involvement of the brain in adaptation to temperature changes. Harri and Tirri (1969) have also reported that the serotonin level in the brain increased in a hot environment and decreased in cold.

The authors' study was an attempt to elucidate the thermoregulatory functions of the hypothalamus and the limbic system and their role in the adaptation mechanism to unusual temperatures. The following aspects were investigated; effect of cold exposure or heat exposure on the EEG activity; effects of brain stimulation on body temperature; effect of lesioning in the brain on the body temperature in the cold environment and effects of various hormones and brown adipose tissue on brain activity and on body temperature.

Experimental animals employed were adult New Zealand white rabbits and adult Wistar rats maintained in an air conditioned (20 ± 2 °C) light controlled (14 hrs. light, 10 hrs. darkness) room. For EEG recording or electrical stimulation of the brain, concentric bipolar electrodes (for rabbits) or side by side bipolar electrodes (for rats) were implanted stereotaxically into various parts of the hypothalamus and limbic systems and fixed to the skull with dental cement. Stereotaxic coordinates were obtained from the atlas of Sawyer, Everett and Green and the atlas of de Groot. Lesioning of the brain was made with tungsten monopolar electrode in order to avoid the electrochemical effect of ion released from steel electrode. Experiments were performed more than 2 weeks after the operation in order to allow the animal to recover. During the experiments, animals were free to move about and to eat and drink thus eliminating all acute stress factors except for cold.

Cold exposure was achieved by placing animals in a cold box (temperature controlled cabinet) at a temperature of −20 °C (for rabbits) and −15 °C (for rats) for 12 hours, while heat exposure was conducted in a hot box (temperature controlled cabinet) at a temperature of 40 °C for four hours. The body temperature of the rabbit was measured by a mercury thermometer placed in the rectum 75 mm inward from the anus. The body temperature of the rat was recorded by a thermister chronically implanted in the retroperitoneal cavity.

ELECTRICAL BRAIN ACTIVITY AT UNUSUAL ENVIRONMENTAL TEMPERATURE AND ITS THERMOREGULATION MECHANISM

Changes in the electrical activity of various parts of the brain during exposure to extreme cold or extreme heat may be caused by (1) variation in the activity of cold-sensitive neurons with elevated or lowerde blood temperature, (2) increased or decreased input from the peripheral sensory organs to the central nervous system, (3) emotional change or (4) feedback action on the brain of humoral factors, such as hormones. Probably all of these factors are more or less involved. The authors investigated responses of the electrical activity of certain parts in the hypothalamus and limbic system to the cold or heat stimulus.

Response of the body temperature to cold exposure both in rats and in rabbits showed a seasonal variation. In summer, body temperature was lowered by $0.7 \pm 0.3\,°C$ in the rabbit and by 0.5–$2.6\,°C$ in the rat during the cold exposure at $-20\,°C$ for 12 hours, whereas during the winter it was elevated by $0.4 \pm 0.3\,°C$ in the rabbit and by $0.7 \pm 0.4\,°C$ in the rat in the same experimental environment.

However, when this cold treatment was repeated every day in summer, the tendency of body temperature to decrease during the exposure gradually diminished and disappeared completely on the 3rd day. On the 4th day, the body temperature showed a slight rise $(0.2$–$0.5\,°C)$ during cold exposure. On the other hand, when the animals were exposed to heat $(40\,°C)$, body temperature immediately rose to 40.5–$41.5\,°C$ and was maintained at this level during the 4 hours of exposure. Neither seasonal variation nor change in response to the repetitive heat exposure was observed.

1. Hypothalamic Activity and Thermoregulation

Many studies have been done on the thermoregulatory function of the hypothalamus; its localization and functional role are fairly evident.

a) *Medial preoptic area and anterior hypothalamus*: The anterior hypothalamus first attracted attention as a probable site of thermoregulation in the brain (Arohnsohn and Sachs, 1885; Barbour, 1912). Frazier, Alpers and Lewy (1936) and Clark, Magoun and Ranson (1939) lesioned a large part of the preoptic area extending from the optic chiasma to the anterior commissure in the cat and monkey and observed that the animals lost their thermoregulatory response in a hot environment but not in a cold environment. Thus, they proposed this area as a heat loss center. The stimulation of the medial preoptic area inhibits the shivering elicited by an anesthetic drug, with the lowest threshold of any part of the brain (Hemingway and Birzis, 1954). It was also shown that stimulation of this area evoked panting in the goat (Andersson, 1956). In our study, the effect of stimulation of the medial preoptic area on the body temperature was examined both at normal temperature $(20\,°C \pm 2\,°C)$ and under extreme cold. Stimulation was applied for one hour, 60 sec on and 60 sec off at 2–2.5 V intensity, 0.5 msec duration and 100 Hz frequency. At normal temperature, the rabbit and rat showed a double-peaked rise in body temperature; an immediate rise during stimulation and a delayed rise after stimulation (Fig. 104-a). Under extreme cold the rabbit showed a single-peaked rise only during stimulation. As described above, body temperature in the intact rabbit rose immediately after cold exposure in winter or after repeated exposure in summer. The rabbit with a lesion in the medial preoptic area, on the contrary, showed an immediate fall in body temperature when exposed to extreme cold. This response was invariable although the exposure was repeated for more than seven days. These findings indicate that the medial preoptic area is also involved in thermogenetic function.

As for the electrical activity of the preoptic area, Curt von Euler reported in 1938 that the slow potential change in this area was dependent on body temperature, that the voltage increased by 1.0 mV per $1\,°C$ rise of the body temperature and that there was close correlation between this slow potential change and panting. In 1961, Nakayama and Eisenman found that the discharge rate of some neurons in the preoptic region in the cat increased in response to local warming. Hardy *et al.* (1964) showed that there are also cold-sensitive neurons in this area and stated that 20% of

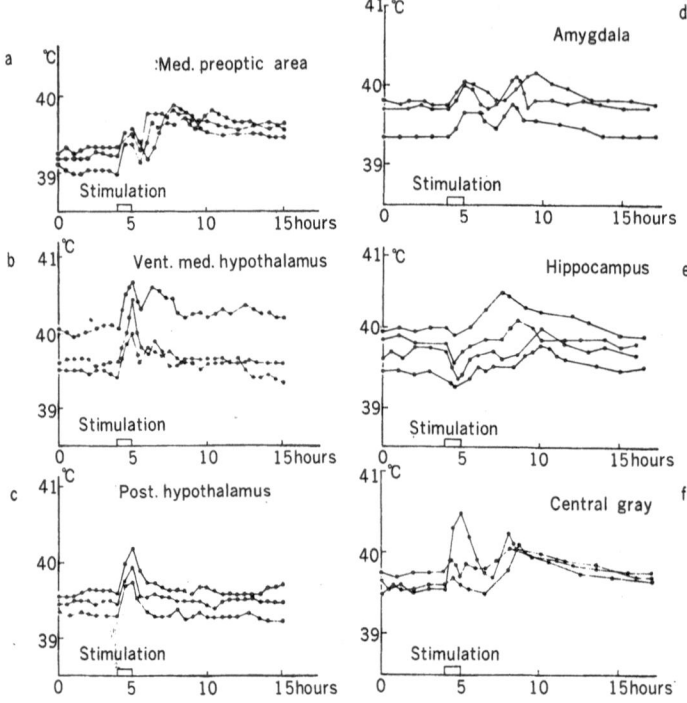

Fig. 104. Effects of electrical stimulation of the medial preoptic area (a), ventromedial hypothalamus (b), posterior hypothalamus (c), amygdala (d), hippocampus (e), and central gray (f) on rectal temperature.

Note that rectal temperature rises during stimulation of these areas except the hippocampus and rises again after cessation of stimulation except in the case of posterior hypothalamic stimulation.

thermosensitive neurons in the preoptic region were cold-sensitive and 80% of them were heat-sensitive.

In our experiment, EEG activity was recorded from this area and its frequency components observed with a frequency band analyzer. The effect of cold exposure on the electrical activity of the preoptic area was studied, and differences in response to the cold stimulus were observed between its medial and lateral part. Activity in the border area between the medial and lateral preoptic area did not show any significant change in the first two or three hours of cold exposure but then it increased gradually and the fast wave component started to augment markedly. On the other hand, in the EEG activity recorded from the inner part of the medial preoptic area, marked synchronization and increase in amplitude of theta wave were brought about at the beginning of cold exposure. Thereafter the theta wave component showed a tendency to decrease and returned to the control level after 12 hours of exposure to extreme cold. Seasonal variation was hardly observed at all in the response of the activity in this area to the cold stimulus. The EEG activity here was increased also by heat stimulus and no accomodative change in its activity was observed in repeated heat exposure (Fig. 105). Similar results were obtained also in the rat.

Local cooling of the preoptic region was reported to activate the thyroid function (Andersson, 1961); to increase plasma cortisol level (Chowers et al., 1962) and urinary cathecholamine secretion (Andersson, 1964); and to cause a rise in blood pressure (Hayward and Baker, 1968). Conversely, local heating of this area was shown to block the effect of cold stimulus or the activation of the thyroid function (Chowers *et al.*, 1962). It was also reported that electrical stimulation of the ventral anterior hypothalamus augmented the plasma TSH level (Averill and Salaman, 1967).

These observations suggest that the preoptic region is not only a heat loss center as Ranson and his associates claimed but may also be involved in heat production mechanism through its neural influence or endocrine function. Furthermore it is evident that the preoptic region is closely related to the function of the brown adipose tissue, which is an important heat producing organ in some species. This point is dealt with elsewhere in this article.

b) Ventromedial hypothalamus and arcuate nucleus: Ogata (1966, 1971) has suggested

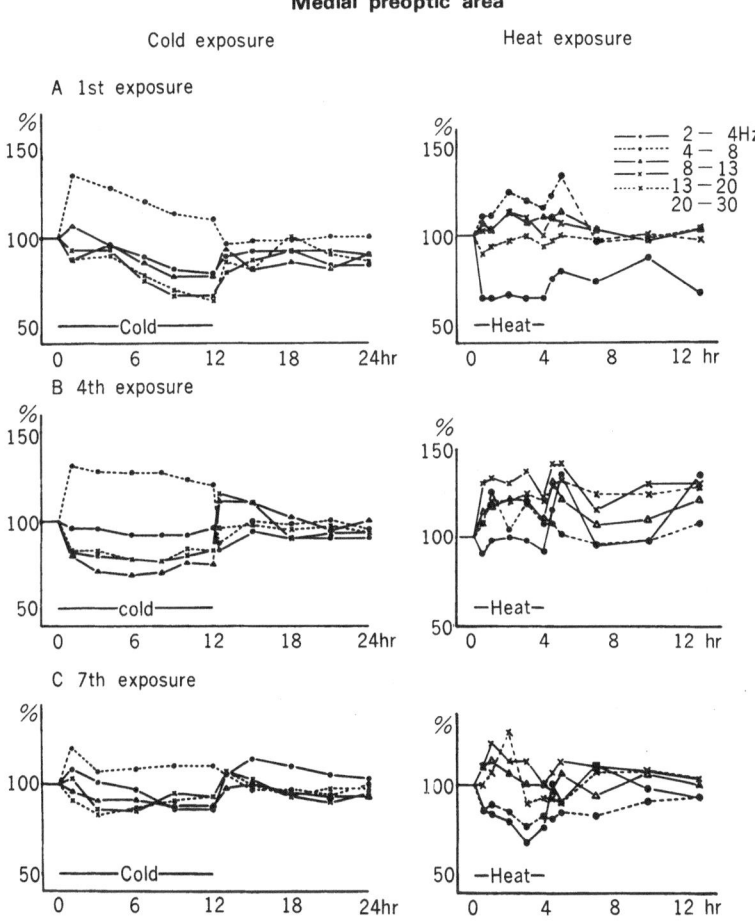

Fig. 105. Left: The changes in the EEG frequency components (band analysis) recorded from the region in rabbits repeatedly exposed to cold (−20°C), 12 hours per day.

Right: The changes in the EEG frequency components (band analysis) recorded from the region in rabbits repeatedly exposed to heat four hours per day.

The ordinate indicates the changes as compared with the control (100%) in integration of band passed frequency components every 10 seconds in percentage. The abscissa is time in hours.

that the ventromedial hypothalamus directly affected on neural thermoregulation from various experiments. While Taylor and Blackburn (1967) reported that elevation of body temperature increased the EEG activity in the ventromedial hypothalamus and suppressed the activity in the lateral hypothalamus. These authors assumed that the heat regulating center might have an influence on the feeding and satiety centers, since the environmental temperature influenced food intake, which then affected heat production, and furthermore, that suppression of activity in the ventromedial hypothalamus (satiety center) or activation of activity in the lateral hypothalamus (feeding center) affected food intake. Furthermore, ventromedial hypothalamus facilitated the adrenocorticoid synthesis, which then affected body temperature (Kawakami et al., 1971). Therefore, the activity in the ventromedial hypothalamus might have some indirect relation, as well as direct one, to body temperature regulation.

In our experiment, stimulation of the ventromedial nucleus was followed by a double-peak elevation of the body temperature similar to the effect of medial preoptic region stimulation. But the rise during stimulation of the former was greater than that resulting from the stimulation of the latter (Fig. 104-b). Environmental temperature had no effect on the change of body temperature evoked by the ventromedial hypothalamic stimulation.

The rabbit with a lesion in the ventromedial hypothalamus showed a slight drop in body temperature at the beginning of cold exposure which was seen even after repetition of the exposure for seven days, while the intact rabbit usually showed "initial rise of body temperature."

The obese rat with a lesion in the ventromedial hypothalamus showed a gradual fall in the body temperature throughout the period of exposure to cold. The body temperature reached $36\,°C$ ($3\,°C$ lower than that of control group) after seven hours of exposure to cold at a temperature of $-5\,°C$ and $34.5\,°C$ ($3.5\,°C$ lower than control group) after seven hours of exposure to cold at $-15\,°C$.

The EEG activity in the ventromedial hypothalamus in the rabbit was increased during cold exposure and almost no seasonal variation was observed. The change in activity was gradually reduced after repetition of the exposure and almost no activation was observed in the EEG of this area during the fourth or fifth exposure.

The EEG recorded from this area in the rat showed marked activity only at the beginning of the cold exposure and returned to the normal activity level after six to seven hours of exposure. The activity of the ventromedial hypothalamus was reduced by heat exposure. However, when the heat exposure was repeated, the activity increased. The physiological implication of the reversal is not clear.

The ventromedial hypothalamus has been shown to control various humoral factors; for example lesioning of the area decreased 17-OHCS level in the adrenal venous blood (Ganong et al., 1961), reduced corticosterone level in the blood during cold exposure (D'Angelo, 1960) and delayed increase in response of 17-OHCS to cold stimulus (Brodish, 1969), while electrical stimulation of this area increased the plasma corticosterone and biosynthesis of adrenocorticoids under both normal and stressful conditions (Kawakami et al., 1970).

It seems reasonable to assume that the ventromedial hypothalamus is involved in the temperature regulation mechanism and in the mechanism of adaptation to usual environmental temperature, both through its control of humoral factors and through nervous control of autonomic functions.

c) Lateral hypothalamus: It was reported by Frazier *et al.* (1936) and Clark *et al.* (1939) that bilateral lesion in the lateral hypothalamus interferred with the regulation response to heat and cold. Stimulation of the lateral hypothalamus is known to evoke, in general, parasympathetic responses. Ban (1964), however, reported that a part of the posterior lateral hypothalamus showed sympathetic response when stimulated. In our experiment, when the lateral hypothalamus between the premammillary area and the optic tract was stimulated at normal environmental temperature (20 $\pm$ 3 °C), the body temperature of the rabbit gradually rose and reached a peak (0.4–0.8 °C higher than control level) 0.5–2 hours after the stimulation. It then slowly fell to the control level. Stimulation of the lateral hypothalamus above the supraoptic nucleus caused a slight fall in body temperature (0.3–0.5 °C) during the stimulation which disappeared immediately after stimulation. No special behavioral change was observed during the stimulation. When this area was stimulated under extreme cold, the fall of the body temperature became more remarkable (around 1 °C fall) and recovery time was longer.

The EEG responses to cold exposure were also different in the anterior and the posterior lateral hypothalamus. The EEG recorded from the rostral part of the lateral hypothalamus was activated by cold exposure, while that recorded from the caudal part was suppressed. The increase in activity in the rostral part of the lateral hypothalamus was either not changed or tended to intensify after repetition of the cold exposure. On the other hand, the EEG change in the caudal part during cold exposure gradually decreased and almost disappeared after seven or eight exposures.

d) Posterior hypothalamus and premammillary area: The posterior hypothalamus has been thought to be a heat production center. A number of studies have been done on its function in temperature regulation. It was reported that bilateral lesion of the posterior lateral hypothalamus inhibited shivering (Clark *et al.*, 1939; Blair and Keller, 1946; Birzis and Hemingway, 1956; Keller and Bostel, 1952) and the larger destruction of the posterior hypothalamus not only interferred with body temperature regulation at low environmental temperatures but also elevated the threshold of reaction to high environmental temperatures. Ranson and Thompson showed that administration of pyrogen could induce hyperthermia even in the animal with a lesion in the posterior hypothalamus, in which hypothermia was easily induced under a low ambient temperature, but that the degree of increase in the body temperature varied according to the environmental temperature or size of the lesion. Pyrogen raised the body temperature in the intact animal independent of the environmental temperature. Stimulation of the posterior hypothalamus is known to evoke an intense sympathetic response (Kurotsu, 1949). Ogata (1971) reported that a moderate cooling and heating in the posterior hypothalamus caused no thermoregulatory response, while an intensive cooling even inhibited shivering which had been observed previously, and that on the contrary the animal shivered vigorously with an intensive warming if it had already started to shiver. From these results it could be inferred that there is no thermoreceptor in the posterior hypothalamus which drive the heat production system. But it is already reported that unit activity of some neurons in this area varied synchronizing with shivering (Birzis and Hemingway, 1956). Besides, electrical stimulation of this area was found to have a facilitatory effect on release of ACTH and epinephrine which are related to heat production.

In our experiment, stimulation of the posterior hypothalamus evoked an immediate rise in body temperature (0.5–0.7 °C), either at normal environmental temperature or under extreme cold (Fig. 104-c). It took 30 minutes to one hour in the rabbit and two to four hours in the rat for the body temperature to return to the normal level.

When the rabbit with a lesion in the posterior hypothalamus was exposed to cold repeatedly for seven days, coincident with the exposure it showed an initial fall in body temperature (by 0.3–0.5 °C), which returned to the control level during the next three to five hours of continued exposure. This response was similar to that observed in the medial preoptic area. The EEG recorded from this area in the rabbit was activated by cold exposure in summer, showing a synchronized high amplitude theta wave. The change was most remarkable during the initial exposure and the elevated activity returned to normal during a six or nine hour-exposure. In winter the change was less remarkable. When the rabbit was exposed to cold repeatedly, the activation of the EEG in the posterior hypothalamus was gradually reduced; however, the initial activity level remained even at the 7th exposure.

By exposure to heat, the EEG activity of the posterior hypothalamus was suppressed. However, when the exposure was repeated, the change was gradually reduced and finally reversed to induce activity (Fig. 106).

Thus the posterior hypothalamus increases its activity in a cold environment and maintains body temperature, mobilizing neural mechanisms such as shivering or vasoconstriction and humoral mechanisms such as the release of epinephrine or ACTH, while in a hot environment it reduces its activity as well as contributes to the maintenance of body temperature through the suppression of heat production or enhancement of heat loss.

The response of the activity in the premammillary area and the effect of its stimulation were quite similar to those of the posterior hypothalamus.

2. *Limbic System*

The limbic system has generally been considered to have some role in thermo-regulation from various experiments.

a) Hippocampus: When the hippocampus was stimulated in the rabbit and rat at normal environmental temperature, body temperature showed no change or a slight fall during the stimulation, but rose 30 minutes to four hours after applying the stimulation (Fig. 104-e). On the other hand, when this area was stimulated under extreme cold, body temperature rose during the stimulation. Pinkston (1935) reported that the body temperature of the animal with a lesion in the hippocampus, neopallium and fornix became dependent on environmental temperature. In this point, Ogata (1966) suggested that the hippocampus took part in the regulation of body temperature against cold from various experiments. Authors recorded and analyzed the EEG activity of the hippocampus during cold and heat exposure. The theta wave in the hippocampal EEG was markedly synchronized with and increased in amplitude by exposure to cold in summer. This increased activity returned to normal immediately after returning the environmental temperature to 20 °C. In winter, the activation of the hippocampal EEG was not induced by the cold stimulus. In addition, when the animals were exposed to cold repeatedly in summer, the EEG response was reduced and was not observed in the third or fourth exposure. Apparently, an accomodative change occurred in the hippocampus earlier than in the hypothalamic

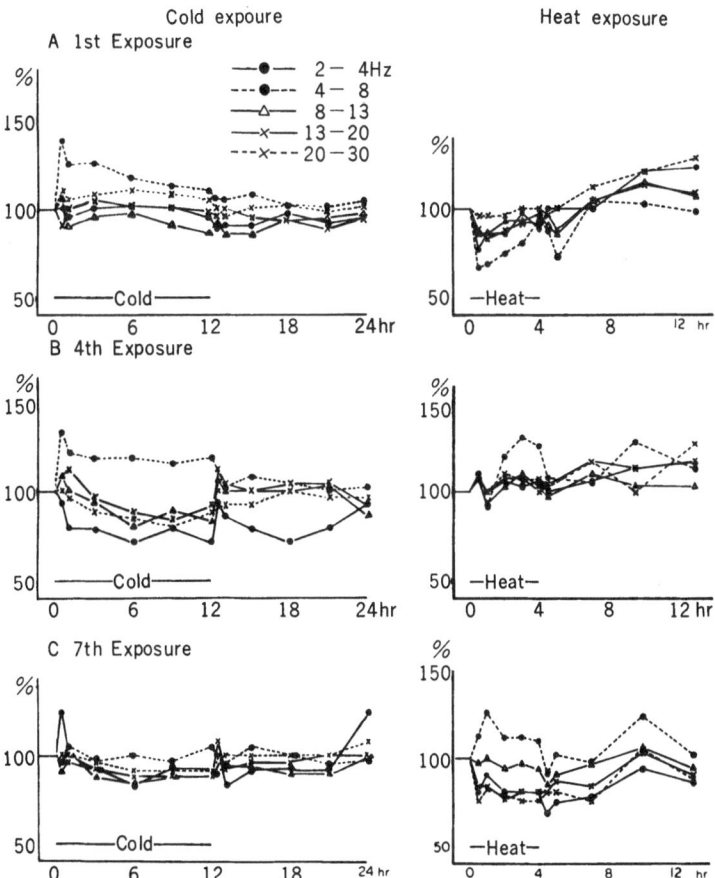

Fig. 106. Left: The changes in the EEG frequency components (band analysis) recorded from the posterior hypothalamus in rabbits repeatedly exposed to cold ($-20\,°C$) 12 hours per day.

Right: The changes in the EEG frequency components (band analysis) recorded from the region in rabbits repeatedly exposed to heat ($40\,°C$) four hours per day.

areas. The hippocampal EEG response to cold in the immature rabbit was opposite to that of the mature rabbit. The immature rabbit, less than 15 days old, showed a marked reduction of the hippocampal activity accompanied by a fall in body temperature by 6–$8\,°C$ in the four hours of cold exposure; at a body temperature of around $32\,°C$, the hippocampal EEG showed an activated pattern transiently and as body temperature fell further, the hippocampal EEG as well as the EEG patterns recorded from all part of the brain were characterized by flattening. The response in body temperature to exposure to cold became gradually milder as the animal got older, until it could endure extreme cold of $-20\,°C$ for 12 hours at around 30 days of age. Thereafter, the EEG activity in the hippocampus or other areas responded to the cold exposure in the same fashion as the adult rabbit.

The change in the hippocampal EEG activity in the young rat caused by exposure to cold was similar to that observed in the adult, but the increased activity was more marked during the exposure.

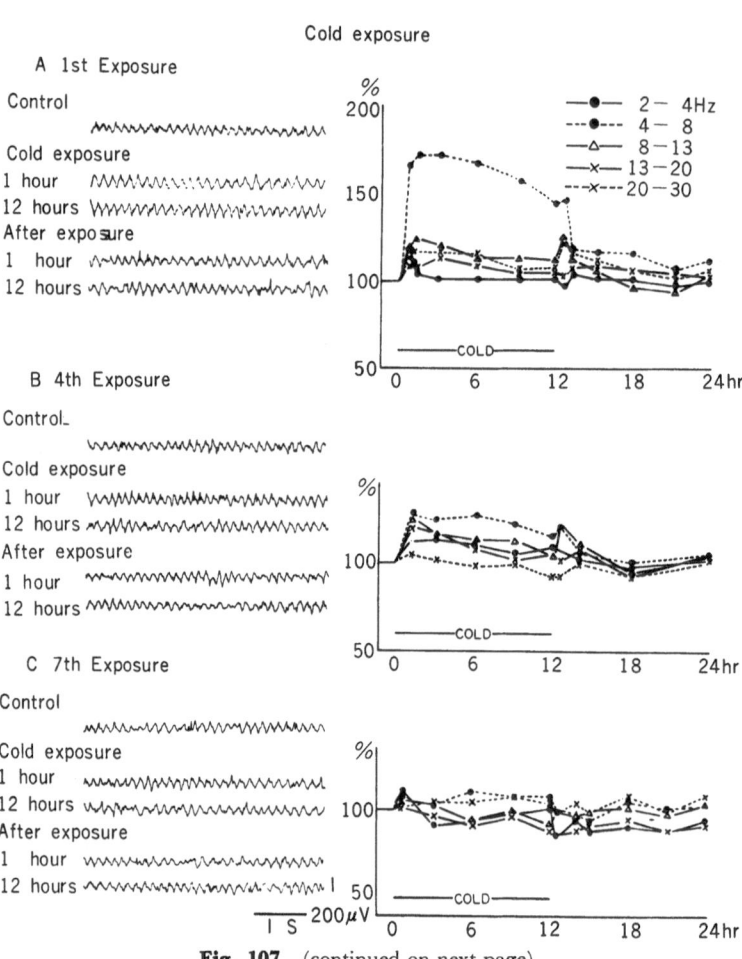

Fig. 107   (continued on next page)

On the other hand, when the animals were exposed to heat, the EEG activity in the hippocampus was reduced and the change was not influenced by repeated exposure (Fig. 107).

It has been reported that stimulation of the hippocampus facilitated the release and biosynthesis of 17-OHCS and corticosterone (Endröczi and Lissák, 1960; Kawakami et al., 1968), enhanced TSH secretion (Shizume et al., 1962; Kawakami et al., 1967) and increased blood sugar level (Kaada, 1951).

Presumably, the activation of the hippocampus by cold stimulus promotes heat production through some humoral mechanisms such as the hypothalamo-pituitary-adrenal axis, hypothalamo-pituitary-thyroid axis or brown adipose tissue as well as through neural mechanisms of the autonomic nervous system.

In addition, the activity in the hippocampus was characterized by seasonal variation, positive inclination to adaptation to cold exposure and negative inclination to adaptation to heat exposure.

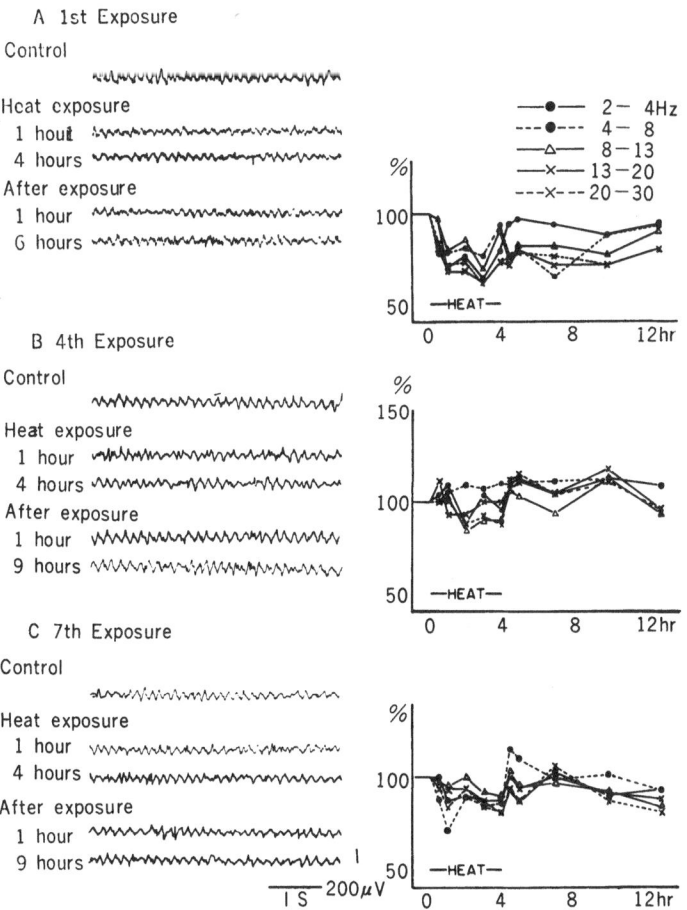

Fig. 107. The frequency analysis of the hippocampal EEG in rabbits repeatedly exposed to cold 12 hours per day (left) and to heat four hours per day (right).

b) *Amygdala:* It was suggested by Ogata (1966) that the amygdaloid complex also had some role in thermoregulation. On this point, the medial part of the amygdala has been shown to have a sympathetic function, but a rise in body temperature was found to be induced most intensely by stimulating the lateral part of the amygdala (Koikegami *et al.*, 1952), whereas lesioning the amygdala and its neighboring area was reported to induce a fall in body temperature (Anand and Brobeck, 1952). We also examined the effect of amygdalar stimulation on body temperature. Body temperature in the rabbit rose during an hour of on-off stimulation in the medial part of the amygdala, and after returning to the control level immediately after stimulation, it started to rise again and reached a peak three to five hours afterwards (Fig. 104-d). When the medial amygdala was stimulated under extreme cold the elevation of body temperature during stimulation was less remarkable, but after stimulation showed almost the same changes as were seen under normal environmental temperature. The rat showed a single-peak change in body temperature with stimulation of the medial amygdala; body temperature rose during stimulation and was maintained at a high level until it returned to the normal level seven hours after stimulation.

The EEG response of the medial part of the amygdala to exposure to cold was different in summer and in winter; in summer, the fast wave component markedly increased during the exposure; it decreased in winter. On the other hand, the EEG activity in the lateral part of the amygdala decreased in amplitude in the cold exposure in summer and showed almost no change in winter. When repeated exposure to cold was attempted in summer, the responses both in the medial and lateral amygdala were gradually reduced and were not observed in the seventh exposure.

The amygdalar EEG of the immature rabbit mainly increased in amplitude during exposure to cold, unlike that of the hippocampus. This change indicated that activity in the area was still maintained when the body temperature fell to 34°C. The EEG activity gradually decreased with increased exposure and the curve flattened at a body temperature of 32°C. The rabbit older than 30 days of age showed a change in amygdalar activity in response to exposure to cold, as the adult did. The amygdalar activity in the rat responded to exposure to cold in the same manner as did the rabbit.

When the rabbit was exposed to heat, the EEG activity in the amygdala also increased. This response was gradually reduced by repetition of the exposure, and no change or only a slight reduction of activity was observed in the seventh heat exposure (Fig. 108).

In summary, the medial amygdala was activated both by cold and heat stimuli, which was different from response of the hippocampus, and the change was characterized by ready adaptation to these stimuli. It might be assumed that the medial amygdala takes part in the initiation of thermoregulation at unusual environmental temperature and that it plays an important role in the maintenance of the body temperature and in the development of thermoregulatory mechanism well ahead of other areas in the brain.

c) *Septum:* The septum has been studied in terms of thermoregulation for a long time compared with other areas in the limbic system. It was reported by Bond et al., (1957) that an animal with bilateral lesions in the posterior septum, including part of the anterior thalamus, showed hypothermia in a relatively cold environment (19–28°C). They assumed that the hypothermia resulted from disturbance of heat producing functions such as shivering. But Stuart et al. (1962) showed that shivering could be induced by cold exposure in an animal with a lesion in the septum. These two results seem to conflict, but the former experiment was done soon after lesioning and the latter was done more than 26 days after lesioning. The stimulation of the septum was shown to evoke constriction of the peripheral blood vessel, shivering and piloelection resulting in an elevation of body temperature by 0.5°C. The effects became undetectable as the body temperature rose. It was also reported by Andersson (1957) and Stuart et al. (1961) that shivering occurring in a cold environment was intensified by the stimulation of the septum. But the stimulation of some part of the septum was shown to inhibit shivering (Stuart et al., 1961).

The authors also observed the effect of stimulation in the septum on the body temperature of the rabbit. Body temperature rose by 0.2–0.3°C during an hour of on-

AMYGDALA

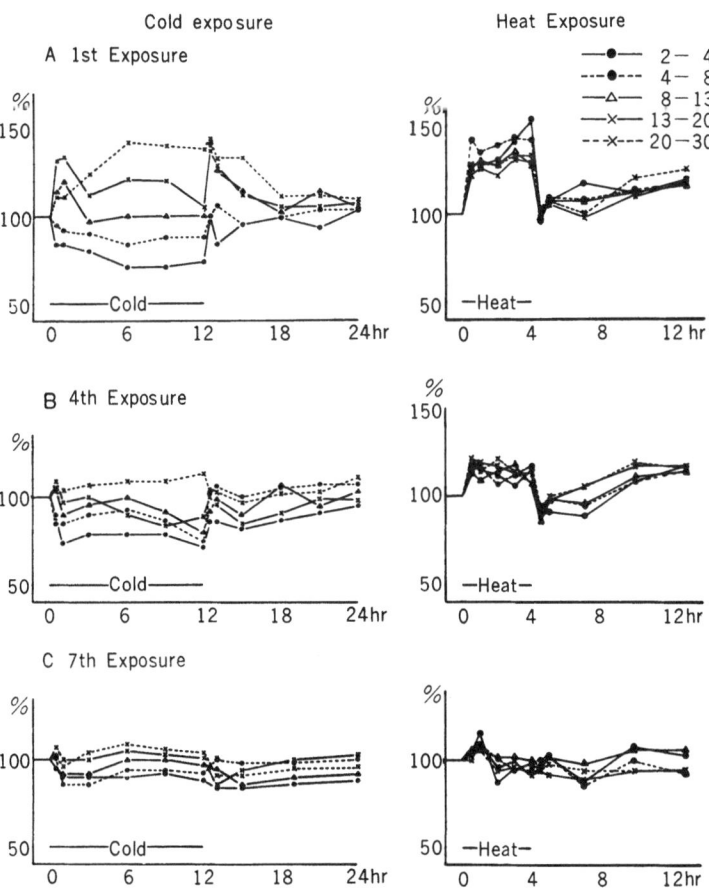

Fig. 108. Left: The changes in the EEG frequency components (band analysis) recorded from the amygdala in rabbits repeatedly exposed to cold 12 hours per day.

Right: The changes in the EEG frequency components (band analysis) recorded from the region in rabbits repeatedly exposed to heat four hours per day.

off stimulation. After the stimulation, it returned to the control level and rose again with a latency of 30 minutes to one hour reaching a peak 1.5–2 hours afterwards. The stimulation of the medial septum had almost no influence on body temperature. The EEG recorded from the lateral septum was activated in extreme cold. The change was most marked in the initial exposure to cold and was gradually reduced thereafter. Immediately after releasing the rabbit from the exposure the activity increase again transiently. Such a transient increase in activity after release from cold exposure was also observed in the septum, lateral hypothalamus, posterior hypothalamus in the rat and the amygdala and hippocampus in the immature rat and rabbit. But its physiological significance is not clear. The response in the lateral septum to cold exposure was rapidly reduced in the repetition of the exposure and it was hardly observed at all in the fourth or fifth exposure.

The EEG activity in the medial septum was decreased during exposure to cold and returned to the control level immediately after release from the exposure.

The EEG activity in the lateral septum was reduced under heat exposure and the response was not influenced by the repetition of the exposure. Many studies also suggest involvement of the septum in hormonal control; the stimulation of this area inhibited the secretion of TSH and ACTH and lesioning facilitated it (Endröczi and Lissák, 1960; Slusher and Hyde, 1961; Kawakami *et at.*, 1969). These findings seen to contradict the activation of the lateral septum under extreme cold. The lateral septum evidently takes part in thermoregulation under a cold environment chiefly through the neural mechanism of shivering or sympathetic responses. A characteristic feature of our observations is that the activity of this area, as well as that of the hippocampus and amygdala, adapted to the cold stimulus before the hypothalamus. Therefore, this limbic area might have an important role in thermoregulation involving the hypothalamus in the initial adaptation to cold; in hot environment, on the other hand, the lateral septum reduces its activity and serves to reduce heat production and/or to increase heat loss.

d) *Midbrain reticular formation and central gray:* In 1938, Magoun and Ranson showed that the midbrain and central gray played an important role in the thermoregulatory function.

Since 1957 Ogata has done elaborate studies on the thermoregulatory function of the midbrain reticular formation. He concluded that the reticular ascending activating system was one of the major factors controlling the afferent impulses which were the generators of somatic reactions to cold.

Massopust *et al.* (1965) have demonstrated that the anterior reticular formation resists the depressant effect of cold and helps maintain minimal metabolic and possibly circulatory conditions to protect the vital processes of nonhibernating species. In our experiments, contradictory results were obtained concerning the changes in midbrain reticular formation activity during exposure to cold; i.e. a decline and elevation of activity level during cold. In the former case, theta components decreased by 14–52% at the first exposure; then by 12–18% at the third and finally by only 10% at the seventh exposure. The latter case did not show the adaptation like effect in spite of repeated exposure, persisting in showing an increase in the theta component during cold.

In the present experiment involving the central gray, there appears to be a species difference in the thermoregulatory function between the rabbit and the rat. The stimulation of the central gray in the rabbit induced a double-peak elevation of the body temperature; a peak (0.45–1.1 °C higher than control level) during one hour of on-off stimulation and another peak (0.4–0.6 °C higher than control level) three to four hours after the stimulation (Fig. 104-f). On the other hand, when the central gray in the rat was stimulated, the body temperature fell by 0.2–0.6 °C during the stimulation and it showed another bottom 2.5–3 hours after the stimulation. The EEG activities of the central gray in the rabbit and rat also showed opposite responeses to cold exposure. The EEG in the rabbit was activated by exposure to cold, showing marked synchronization and augmentation in the amplitude of the theta wave. The most remarkable change occurred in the initial exposure and then was gradually reduced in subsequent exposure. After repetition of the cold exposure, the response was decreased and was undetectable or reverted to suppression in the 8th or 9th exposure. The EEG of the central gray in the rat showed a decrease in amplitude and desynchronization in exposure to cold which was indicative of reduced activity.

When the rabbit was exposed to heat, EEG activity in the central gray was reduced. And it became less responsive with repetition of the exposure, until the response was undetectable at the seventh cold exposure.

Thus, the effect of stimulation and response to the cold stimulus in the central gray was species specific. The anatomical feature of this area is that various ascending and descending pathways such as the bundle of Schütz, Stratum periventriculare hypothalami and medial forebrain bundle pass through it. Furthermore, this area connects not only with the midbrain reticular formation but also with the hypothalamus and the limbic system. Accordingly, the effect of stimulation or response in the activity in the central gray might be vastly dependent upon activities and functions of other areas in the brain.

3. Changes in EEG Arousal Threshold and Induced-spindle Response in Both Cold and Heat Environment

The arousal threshold which was characterized by desynchronization in the neocortical EEG during electrical stimulation of midbrain reticular formation (square wave of 0.5 ms pulse duration at a frequently of 100 Hz) decreased markedly, when animals were exposed to both cold and heat environments. On the contrary, the arousal threshold in the neocortical EEG upon high frequency electrical stimulation of the CM increased, when animals were exposed to cold environment. Thus a diffuse ascending excitatory system was enhanced by either cold or heat environment. The changes did not show adaptation in spite of repeated exposure to cold or heat at least seven times during one week (Fig. 109-A).

The threshold of induced-spindle response was tested by induction of the spindle burst in the EEG of frontal cortex by a single shock of the caudate nucleus. The threshold during cold exposure lowered to about 65% of the control value, while the threshold during heat exposure rose to about 25% of the control (Fig. 109-B). Thus exposure to cold environment in the rabbit seems to facilitate the activity of the inhibitory system described by Gellhorn (1957).

4. Limbic Activity as Indicated by Evoked Potentials

These results revealed that the activity of some limbic structures rises in response to extreme cold. The next experiment was designed in order to see the details of the functional changes in the synaptic connection between limbic structures during cold exposure as indicated by evoked potentials. The stimulus used was a square wave of duration 0.1 ms and intensity 5.2–12 V.

The hippocampally evoked potentials were recorded in the cental gray of the midbrain consisting of the first positive and second negative components. The first component showed an increase in amplitude by 13–23% compared with that before the application of cold exposure but no change in latency. The second component decreased in latency. The evoked potentials recorded in the hippocampus induced by the stimulation of the central gray consisted of the first negative, the second positive and the third negative components. During cold exposure all of the components showed an increase in amplitude, the first by 31–50%, the second by 12–18% and the third by 20–25%. The latencies was observed not to be affected. The evoked potentials recorded in the central gray by stimulating the medial amygdala consisted

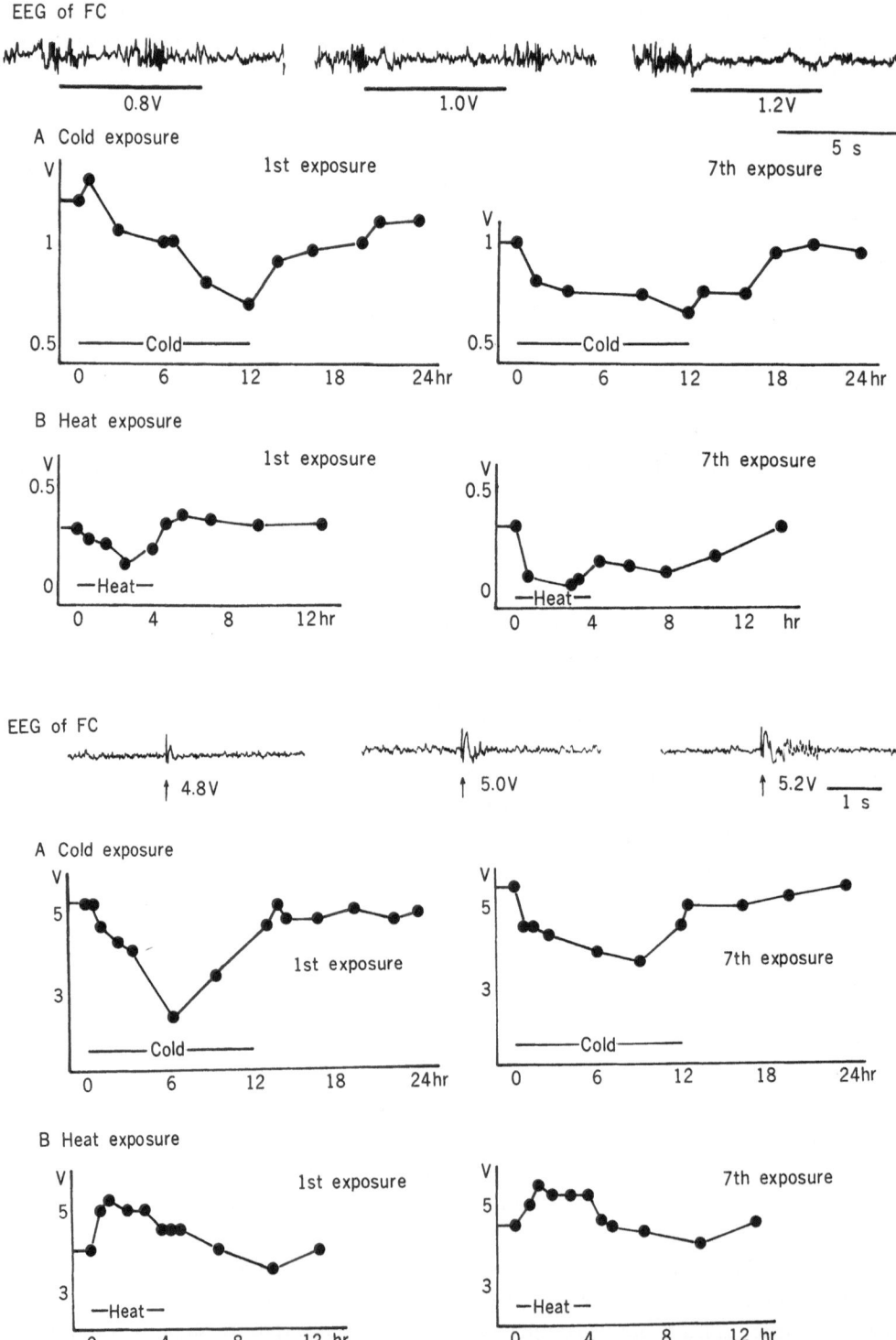

Fig. 109. Effects of repeated cold and heat on the cortical EEG arousal threshold by stimulation of the midbrain reticular formation (A) and on the spindle burst induced by the caudate stimulation (B) in rabbits.

of the first negative and the second positive components. During cold exposure only the second component was influenced, showing an increase in amplitude of 50–72%. The latency did not show change.

The evoked potential recorded in the dorsal hippocampus by the stimulation of ventral hippocampus showed an increase in amplitude of the first component during cold. Thus the synaptic connection as well as the local activity of the limbic structures were facilitated during extreme cold.

The change in synaptic connection between limbic structure and the hypothalamus during extreme cold was examined.

The hippocampally evoked potential recorded in the medial preoptic area consisted of first positive and the second negative components. During cold exposure the first component did not show significant change, while the second component decreased in amplitude by 20% without a change in latency. Repetition of exposure did not result in adaptation phenomenon.

The amygdalarly evoked potential recorded in the ARC of the hypothalamus showed an increase in the amplitude of the first component without a change in latency during cold exposure. On the other hand, the hippocampally evoked potential recorded in the ARC showed either no change or only a slight decrease of 8–16% in amplitude in the first component without a change in latency during cold exposure.

Thus, it is concluded that during extreme cold the synaptic connection from the amygdala to the basal hypothalamus is facilitated while the connection from the hippocampus to the basal hypothalamus is inhibited.

BROWN ADIPOSE TISSUE AND CENTRAL THERMOREGULATION

The participation of various humoral factors in the regulation of the body temperature has been studied by numerous researchers. These studies were recently introduced in detail in the papers of Smith and Hoijer (1962), Collins and Weiner (1968) and Benzinger (1969). Among the humors related to thermoregulation one unique factor is brown fat. Recently an excellent review was written on the relation between fat and thermogenesis by Smith and Horwitz (1969).

Brown adipose tissue was first described by Conrad Gesner in 1551 in the interscapular area of the marmot. Hatai (1902) identified fat pads on the back and neck in the human foetus to be brown adipose tissue. The tissue is distributed in the interscapular, axillar and perinephric region and around larger vessels in various kinds of hibernators, rat, mouse, monkey and in the immature rabbit. Brown fat cells differ characteristically from white fat cells in that they are smaller in size; polygonal rather than round in shape; multilocular rather than unilocular in the manner of distribution of lipid, and in that they possess a high concentration of mitochondria. Brown fat is well vescularized and is richly innervated by autonomic nerves. Ochi et al., (1969) have shown through electron microscopic and fluorescence microscopic studies that the nerves supplied to brown adipose tissue are sympathetic nerves. The morphology and chemical composition of brown fat varies according to age, environmental temperature, season, or diet. In the younger animal, more multilocular cells are found in the tissue and the trigriceride and phosphotide constituents are high (Smalley et al., 1969; Spencer and Dempster, 1962). The short-term exposure of the animal to cold decreases the weight and decolorizes brown fat, whereas chronic exposure

(0.5 °C for 60–90 days) leads to hypertrophy of brown fat (Page and Babineau, 1950). On the contrary, exposure of the animal to high temperature induces essentially the reverse of the response of brown fat to cold. Brown fat has been shown to be sensitive to changes in the hormonal environment. Adrenalectomy leads to a progressive loss of glycogen and lipid from the brown fat with an increase in water content (Lachance, 1953), while administration of cortisone to the adrenalectomized rat result in an increase in the fat content and weight of the brown fat. The changes in fat content after hypophysectomy are similar to those observed in the adrenalectomized animals and this change can be prevented by daily injection of ACTH or cortisone (Fawcett and Jones, 1949). Moreover, administration of cortisone or ACTH significantly increases the blood flow in the brown fat of the rats (Kuroshima et al., 1968). The thyroid hormone also exerts a facilitatory influence on the activity of the brown fat. The thyroid hormone administered by feeding induces hypertrophy of the brown fat with an increased lipid level (Lachane, 1953), while the hypothyroid rat treated with thyouracil shows a lipid depletion of brown fat (Fawcett and Jones, 1949). The catecholamines have been shown to play a particularly important role in the thermogenesis of the brown fat. Norepinephrine content and its turnover are significantly high in the brown fat. Intravenous injection of norepinephrine, epinephrine, or isoprenaline leads to an increase in the venous outflow from the brown adipose tissue and in the temperature of the tissue in the newborn rabbit (Heim and Hull, 1965, 1966). Stimulation of the sympathetic nerves which are supplied to the brown fat is followed by a rise in temperature of the tissue (Hull and Seagull, 1965). On the other hand, denervation of the brown fat blocks the effect of exposure to cold on the brown fat (Hull and Seagull, 1965), accordingly, lipids stored in the brown fat cannot be utilized without the sympathetic nerve supply.

Thus, numerous studies have been carried out on brown fat from anatomical, hormonal and metabolic points of view, and it is now clear that brown fat is under the control of various humoral factors and the sympathetic nervous system. No study, however, has been attempted on the central nervous control of the brown fat. We therefore investigated the participation of the brain, especially the hypothalamus and limbic system, in the thermogenesis of the brown adipose tissue.

1. Effect of Electrical Stimulation of the Hypothalamus and Limbic System on Brown Fat

The effect of electrical stimulation of various parts of the brain, using the same parameters as were mentioned above, on changes in the weight of brown fat and the incorporation of ^{14}C-1-acetate into lipid in the brown fat was studied by Yamaoka and Seto in our laboratory. In addition, the effects of the stimulation on the incorporation of ^{14}C-1-acetate into adrenocortical hormones were observed at the same time.

The hippocampal stimulation was followed by an increase in the brown fat in the incorporation of ^{14}C-1-acetate into lipids, especially into phospholipid and sterol of the ester type, and a decrease in the incorporation of ^{14}C-1-acetate into 17-OHCS and corticosterone in the adrenal. The stimulation of the medial amygdala, medial preoptic area or posterior hypothalamus led to a marked decrease in the incorporation of ^{14}C-1-acetate into phospholipid in the brown fat with an increase in the incorporation of ^{14}C-1-acetate in 17-OHCS in the adrenal (Table 29). This indicates that the former (the hippocampus) and the latter areas (the medial amygdala, medial preoptic area and posterior hypothalamus) have a reciprocal relationship regarding lipid formation in brown fat and in steroid synthesis in the adrenal which varies according to ACTH secretion; excitation of the former suppresses the lipid formation in the brown fat and facilitates ACTH release and that of the latter acts in the opposite way. The phospholipid attracts attention especially in terms of the relation between lipid metabolism and brain activity, for it was characteristically influenced by the stimulation of the brain among lipid fractions in the brown fat.

2. Electrical Activity of the Brain and Brown Adipose Tissue

The following experiments dealt with the effects of removal of the intrascapular brown fat and administration of lipids extracted from brown fat on the EEG activity of the rat exposed to cold, and the relation between brain activity and brown adipose tissue.

As is mentioned previously, the EEG activities in the hippocampus, medial amygdala, lateral septum, medial preoptic area, anterior hypothalamus, ventromedial hypothalamus and posterior hypothalamus were increased by exposure to cold, while those

TABLE 29-a   Effect of brain stimulation on the weight of brown adipose tissue

Site of stimulation	No. of rat	Weight of brown adipose tissue		
		Body weight g	mg	mg/100g B.W.
Control	9	247.2±19.6	254.7±41.7	110.7±21.7
HPC	8	235.7± 5.8	122.8±14.0	56.2± 4.4
AME	6	213.3± 3.4	267.0±39.6	126.0± 4.4
AL	6	202.4±22.5	176.0±14.0	88.0± 3.6
CG	5	276.7±18.4	218.0±21.4	80.0±10.3
MPO	7	210.0±14.2	138.6±16.7	66.0± 6.4
VMH	6	212.6±10.9	248.0±24.7	116.5±10.4
LHA	5	223.4±12.5	303.4±16.2	136.0± 3.6
PHY	7	260.6±12.3	202.0±13.5	77.8± 4.3
PMA	7	200.0± 4.3	144.2±24.5	72.1±11.7

Mean ± S.D.

Note: HPC: hippocampus, AME: medial principal nucleus of amygdala, AL: lateral nucleus of amygdala, CG: central grey, MPO: medial preoptic area, VMH: ventromedial hypothalamus, LHA: lateral hypothalamus, PHY: posterior hypothalamus, PMA: premammillary area.

TABLE 29-b   Effects of brain stimulation on biosynthesis of adrenal steroid and lipid of brown adipose tissue.

Site of stimulation	No of rats	Acetate-1-C-- incorporation into steroid		Acetate-1-C¹⁴ incorporation into lipid of brown adipose tissue			
		A	B	Total lipid	C	D	E	F
Control	10	737±34 (100%)	85±2 (100%)	1460±21 (100%)	35±3 (100%)	389±15 (100%)	66±2 (100%)	815±14 (100%)
HPC	6	610±14 (82.7)	63±3 (74.1)	1518±99 (104.0)	49±5 (142.5)	486±27 (125.0)	70±2 (106.2)	901±15 (110.5)
m-AMYG	6	782±14 (106.0)	95±3 (111.8)	1266±23 (86.6)	32±2 (93.0)	244±9 (62.7)	58±2 (87.8)	718±6 (88.1)
MPO	6	800±21 (108.4)	100±3 (117.7)	1385±43 (94.8)	23±2 (66.8)	289±9 (74.2)	60±2 (90.9)	713±10 (87.4)
PHY	6	828±21 (112.2)	102±3 (120.0)	1239±40 (84.9)	31±3 (90.1)	222±9 (57.1)	55±4 (83.4)	712±9 (87.4)

The mean value of dpm/1 hr per mg of protain of brown fat N±SD

Note: Fraction A and B were composed principally of corticosterone and of 17-hydroxycorticosterone. Fraction C,D,E and F were composed principally of esterified sterol, of phospholipid + compound lipid, of free sterol and of trigriseride.

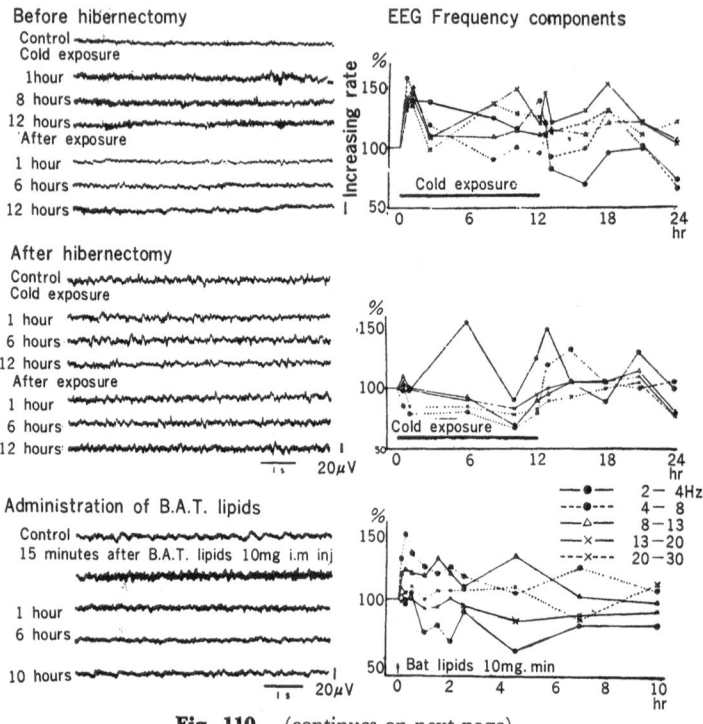

Fig. 110. (continues on next page)

in the central gray, lateral preoptic area and lateral hypothalamus were reduced (Fig. 110). Among the areas which exhibited increased activity in cold exposure, the hippocampus and medial amygdala showed no response to the stimulus, the lateral septum, medial preoptic area and ventromedial hypothalamus reduced activity and the anterior hypothalamus and posterior hypothalamus the same response as that of the intact animal during cold exposure after removal of brown fat. On the contrary, the central gray, lateral preoptic area and lateral hypothalamus showed diminished activities during cold exposure, and responded less to the same stimulus after extirpation of the interscapular brown fat than before.

Administration of lipids extracted from the brown fat stimulated the activities of the hippocampus, medial amygdala, lateral septum, medial preoptic area and posterior hypothalamus and suppressed the activity of the midbrain central gray. The activities of the anterior hypothalamic area, ventromedial hypothalamus, arcuate nucleus and lateral hypothalamus did not show any response to the lipid extract.

Evidently, some parts of the brain are sensitive to certain components of brown fat which are released during cold exposure; lipids are among such components that act on the brain. The action of the components in brown fat is specific to each part of the brain; conducive to the activity of some areas and inhibitory or ineffective in others. Although the EEG of the posterior hypothalamus was activated by administration of lipids extracted from brown fat, it showed almost the same enhanced activity during cold exposure both in the intact and hibernectomized rat. This fact might suggest an

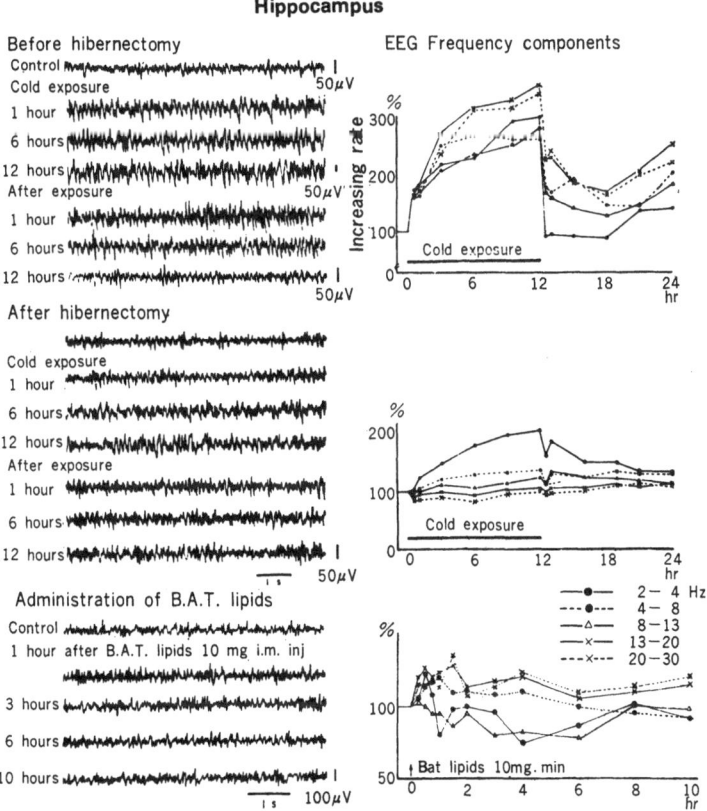

Fig. 110. Changes of EEG patterns and frequency analysis in the pippocampus (right) and the medial preoptic area (left) of the rat during and after cold exposure (−5°C), and after the administration of the lipid (10 mg i.m.) from brown adipose tissue.

essential role for this area in thermoregulation. The activities of other areas which evidenced involvement in thermoregulation in the previous experiment were more or less influenced by the components of the brown fat, which indicates that brown fat contributes to thermoregulation not only directly through its thermogenesis at the tissue in situ but also indirectly through its action on the central nervous system.

ACTION OF SEROTONIN ON BODY TEMPERATURE

It is known that various humoral factors such as ACTH, TSH, thyroid hormone, adrenocortical hormone and some components in brown fat participate in thermoregulation. Moreover, some transmitter substances have also attracted the interest of researchers in temperature regulation. Feldberg and Myers (1964) observed in the cat that intraventricular injection of 5-hydroxytryptamine (5-HT) was followed by hyperthermia, while that of noradrenaline was followed by hypothermia. Similar results were obtained in the dog (Feldberg, Hellen and Myers, 1966) and in chickens (Allen and Marley, 1966). In the rabbit, sheep, goat and cow, however, the intraventricular administration of 5-HT was reported to cause lowering of rectal temperature (Cooper *et al.*, 1965; Bligh, 1966; Andersson *et al.*, 1966; Findlay and Robertshaw, 1967). This discrepancy was supposedly attributable to species difference. Conversely, Cranston and Rosendorff (1967) offered the view that neither 5-HT nor norepinephrine has an influence on "resting temperature" on the basis of their experiment in which a monoamine oxydase inhibitor was used.

It is also known that various amines including 5-HT are found in the brain, especially in the hypothalamus. The quantity was shown to be influenced by a lesion in the medial forebrain bundle or septum (Heller *et al.*, 1962; Heller and Harvey, 1963; Heller and Moore, 1965). Moreover, it is reported that the 5-HT level in the brain shows an initial brief increase followed by gradual decrease to normal levels within a day in the cold environment; the reverse is true at high ambient temperatures.

The foregoing data suggest the possible involvement of serotonin (5-HT) in the thermoregulation mechanism. We then investigated the effect of exogenous serotonin on body temperature with special reference to previous exposure to unusual ambient temperature.

Serotonin (5-HT) injected intravenously at a dose of 20 γ per Kg exerted no influence on the body temperature of the rabbit reared at the room temperature (20 ± 2 °C). Even a dose of 200 γ per Kg under the same condition had no influence. However, i.v. injection of 5-HT at a dose of 20 γ per Kg elevated the body

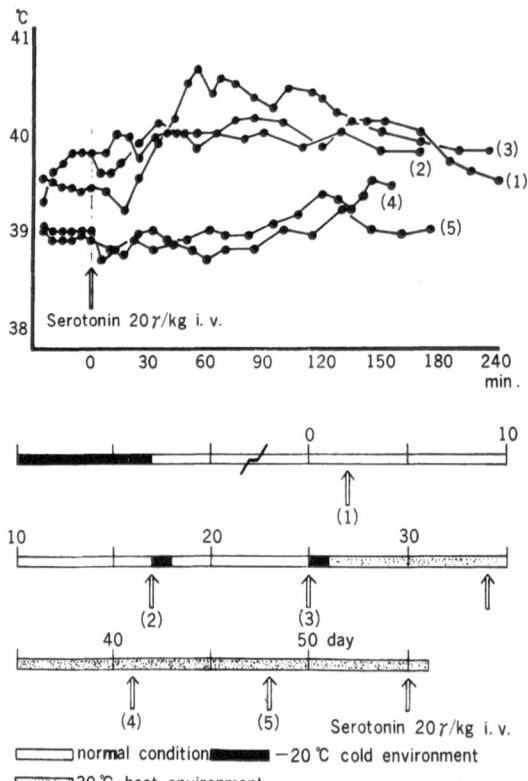

Fig. 111. The changes in body temperature after administration of 5-HT in the normal (20 ± 2 °C), cold (−20 °C) and heat (30 °C) environment after repeated exposure to cold 12 hours per day.

temperature of seven rabbits out of eight which were born the previous spring and had been exposed to extreme cold ($-20\,°C$) 12 hours a day for a period of seven days during autumn and winter. When 5-HT was administrated to the rabbit, the body temperature rose rapidly, reached a peak ($0.7–1.6\,°C$ higher than the control level) and then gradually fell. The remaining one rabbit showed no remarkable change. On the first, third and seventh day of cold exposure, 5-HT was administrated to the rabbit four hours after the beginning of cold exposure when the body temperature had reached a constant level. 5-HT induced no change except in a few cases in which on the seventh day injection tended to raise body temperature slightly (Fig. 111).

These facts may suggest that the effect of 5-HT upon body temperature is a multiplication effect together with ACTH, adrenocorticosteroids and other substances which increase in their secretion under extreme cold. The multiplication effect of 5-HT with ACTH and TSH upon the body temperature was examined in following experiments.

Single injection of ACTH at a higher dose (1.5–2.0 u i.v.) induced a biphasic change in the body temperature; the body temperature fell within five minutes after injection and reached its trough ($0.4–0.6\,°C$ lower than the control level) after about 60–90 minutes, then rose again and reached a peak ($0.5–0.7\,°C$ higher than control level) after about 2.5 hours. On the other hand, single injection of ACTH in a smaller dose (0.07–0.1 u i.v.) had no influence upon the body temperature of seven rabbits out of ten. But one rabbit showed the same biphasic change of the body temperature as that caused by 2.0 u injection of ACTH. The other two rabbits showed only a monophasic change; the body temperature rose 30–40 minutes after the injection and reached its peak ($0.6–0.7\,°C$ higher than control level) about 75 minutes after the injection and then gradually fell to its control level.

Injection of ACTH (0.07–0.1 u), followed by 5-HT injection at a dose of 20 γ per Kg after 50–60 minutes induced a monophasic change in body temperature in the seven rabbits previously mentioned, which had showed no change after a single ACTH injection. The body temperature rose gradually to reach a peak ($0.6–1.4\,°C$ higher than control level) 60–90 minutes after the 5-HT injection and returned to the control level about six hours after the injection. Of course, in all the cases no remarkable change was observed in the period between the injection of ACTH and 5-HT (Fig. 112). This experiment suggests that 5-HT, cooperating with ACTH, may result in vasodilation or an increase in energy metabolism. This assumption may be supported by following facts; 5-HT stimulates ACTH secretion when administered parenterally to animals, and hypophysectomy, hypothalamic lesions, midbrain section and predonisolone pretreatment prevent this action of 5-HT (Moussatche and Alvares-Pereira, 1957; Smelik et al., 1958; Fischer et al., 1959; Sapeika, 1959; Miyawaki et al., 1961; Dixit and Buckley, 1969).

A single injection of TSH (0.25 u/kg i.v.) induced no change in the body temperature of the rabbit reared at room temperature. When a TSH injection of the same dose was followed by 5-HT (20 γ/Kg) 50–60 minutes later a very slight rise in body temperature was observed for six hours after the injection.

When a 5-HT injection (20 γ/Kg) preceded ACTH (0.1 u) by 50–60 minutes, the body temperature showed little change in contrast to the notable change when ACTH preceded 5-HT.

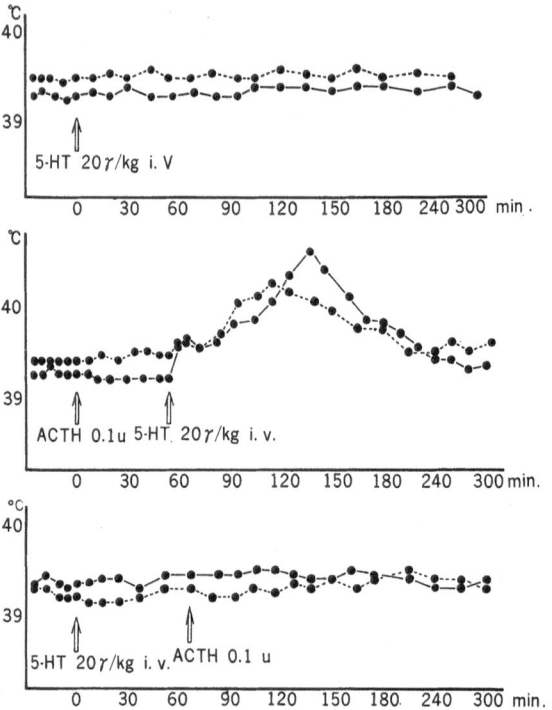

Fig. 112. Effects of 5-HT on the body temperature.
ACTH administration (0.1 u i.v.) was effective in elevating the temperature when it was injected previously to 5-HT (20/Kg, i.v.), while it was not when it followed 5-HT treatment.

Simultaneous intravenous injections of noradrenaline (20 γ/Kg) and 5-HT (20 γ/Kg) raised the body temperature (0.5–1.2 °C higher than control lever), with a latency of 45–70 minutes, while the injections of adrenaline (20 γ/Kg) and 5-HT (20 γ/Kg) lowered the body temperature (0.3–0.4 °C lower than control lever) a with latency of about 30 minutes. These results showed that 5-HT markedly inhibited the action of adrenaline and facilitated the action of noradrenaline. Therefore some interaction may be suggested between 5-HT and these catecholamines in thermoregulation.

The effect of 5-HT upon the EEG pattern was examined before and after the repeated exposure to extreme cold (−20 °C) 12 hours a day for a period of seven days. Injection of 5-HT after the exposure caused a rise in EEG activity in the LHA (A=2, Atlas of Sawyer) which remained for about five hours. Also slight vasodilation of the auris was observed for a few hours following the injection. It seems that small amount of 5-HT, which fails to cause any recognizable change in the EEG under normal conditions, can influence certain areas of the brain during exposure to extreme cold.

It is interesting to note that a substance can elicit different responses in an animal under the same experimental conditions, except in those responses involving previous experience. The mechanism of this phenomenon, however, remains to be elucidated.

It was shown by Hsieh and Carlson (1957) that noradrenaline had a similar effect on blood sugar level; 1-noradrenaline induced hyperglycemia in the cold adapted spinal rat but not in the nonadapted rat. Cranston and Rosendorff (1967) reported that injection of serotonin into the anterior hypothalamus was followed by slight fall or no change in the body temperature in the conscious rabbit; it was followed, however, further rise in body temperature in the rabbit in which the body temperature initially increased prior to pretreatment with noradrenaline or pyrogen. They postulated that the effect of serotonin on body temperature was dependent on the base level of the body temperature at the time of the administration.

It is clear that amines participate in thermoregulation and, if we may speculate, amines produced in the brain might possibly change the activity level in the autonomic or thermoregulatory center, which in turn may alter muscle tonus, initiate shivering, constrict or dilate the blood vessels. Amines released from sympathetic nerve ends may act not only on the peripheral organs but also on the physiological regulation system of heat production in the brain, and may possibly control its function.

SUMMARY AND CONCLUSION

A marked similarity was observed in the response of the medial preoptic area and medial amygdala to high and low ambient temperatures and the response of body temperature to stimulation of these areas. This finding suggests that the two areas might play similar roles in thermoregulation. The response to repeated exposure to heat and cold, however, differed in each case in that exposure to heat or cold resulted in accomodative change in the activity of the medial amygdala and hardly any at all in the medial preoptic area. Thus, the role of the medial preoptic area appears to be more essential to the thermoregulatory mechanism than the medial amygdala. Stimulation of this area caused a double peaked rise in body temperature, that is, an immediate response and a delayed response. This could mean that excitation of this area promotes heat production either through a neural mechanism or a humoral mechanism. However, at low ambient temperatures, when the heat productive mechanism was functioning or in which the set point of body temperature was at a higher level, excitation of the medial preoptic area resulted in decreased delayed response of this area and that of the medial amygdala decreased immediate response. Accordingly, the medial preoptic area might have a phasic action on heat production. The response of the activities in the ventromedial hypothalamus, posterior hypothalamus, hippocampus and lateral septum to unusual ambient temperatures may be considered as a group. These various areas seem to participate mainly in heat production. Of these areas the posterior hypothalamus showed the least accommodation to respeated cold exposure, suggesting that its role in heat production may be irreplacable. Moreover, stimulation of this area elicited an immediate rise in body temperature both at normal and low ambient temperatures. These observations indicate that the posterior hypothalamus has a phasic heat productive action and that it is one of the most essential areas to the thermogenetic mechanism together with the medial preoptic area. Results of the studies on the role of the lateral hypothalamus in thermoregulation appear to be inconsistent, especially regarding the effect of stimulation or lesion in this area on body temperature and the response of activity in this area to cold stimulus. Probably, the lateral hypothalamus participates both in heat production and heat loss not only through a neural mechanism but also through humoral regulation. The response of activity in the central gray and the effect of its stimulation on body temperature was characterized by species difference between the rabbit and the rat; following exposure to cold the activity in the rabbit was increased and decreased in the rat.   In the rabbit, however, the response was reversed from activation to suppression by repeated exposure to cold.   Stimulation of this area elicited no response in body temperature during the cold exposure.   Presumably then, the central gray in the rabbit participate in thermoregulation only during the initial period of exposure to cold and its role becomes less significant in prolonged exposures.

Apparently, the area involved in body temperature regulation is not limited to the hypothalamus but is also found in the limbic system and in other areas in the brain, and there is a functional differentiation in the brain as regards thermoregulation.   In addition, there are indications that these areas exert their thermoregulatory function by acting on the endocrine organs or brown adipose tissue as well as on the peripheral organs associated with production or heat loss, and that the hormones and components of brown fat also affect their activity.

In terms of seasonal variation of thermoregulatory activities in these areas, the limbic areas such as the hippocampus, amygdala and midbrain central gray responded much less to extreme cold in winter than in summer, while the posterior hypothalamus and medial preoptic area showed EEG activation during cold exposure even in winter, although the activity became shorter in duration.   In the other hypothalamic regions examined in our study such as the ventromedial hypothalamus, lateral hypothalamus, arcuate nucleus and periventricular nucleus no seasonal difference in response to the cold stimulus was seen.   Thus it seems that the limbic system is affected by seasonal changes much more than the hypothalamic area.   The hypothalamus appears to function in homeostasis regardless of seasonal influences, while the limbic system probably plays a role in the adaptation of the thermoregulatory mechanism to seasonal variations in the development of resistance to cold.   Moreover, the seasonal nature of the activity in the limbic system may be affected by several humoral factors, especially catecholamines secretion, which is known to fluctuate in summer and in winter.

ACKNOWLEDGEMENTS

The authors wish to thank Dr. Nelia P. Salazar for her kind help in correction of the English. This work was supported by a grant from the Ministry of Education, Japan.

REFERENCES

1. ALLEN, D.J., and E. MARLEY (1966):   *J. Physiol.* **183:** 61.
2. ANAND, B.K., and J.R. BROBECK (1952):   *J. Neurophysiol.* **15:** 421.
3. ANDERSSON, B., R. GRANT, and S. LARSSON (1956):   *Acta Physiol. Scand.* **37:** 261.
4. ANDERSSON, B. (1957):   *Acta Physiol. Scand.* **43:** 90.
5. ANDERSSON, B., L. EKMAN, C.C. GALLE, and J.W. SUNDSTEN (1962):   *Acta Physiol. Scand.* **54:** 191.
6. ANDERSSON, B., C.C. GALLE, B. HOKFELT, and A. OGHA (1964):   *Acta Physiol. Scand.* **61:** 182.
7. ANDERSSON, B., M. JOBIN, and K. OLSSON (1966):   *Acta Physiol. Scand.* **67:** 50.
8. AROHNSOHN, E., and J. SACHS (1885):   *Pflugers Arch. ges. Physiol.* **37:** 232.
9. BAN, T. (1964):   *Med. J. Osaka Univ.* **15:** 1.
10. BARBOUR, H.G. (1912):   *Arch. Exp. Pathol. Pharmak.* **70:** 1.
11. BARD. P., and D.Mck. RIOCH (1937):   *Johns Hopk. Hosp. Bull.* **60:** 73.
12. BENZINGER, T.H. (1969):   *Physiol. Rev.* **49:** 671.
13. BIRZIS, L., and A. HEMINGWAY (1956):   *J. Neurophysiol.* **19:** 37.
14. BLAIR, J.R., and A.D. KELLER (1946):   *J. Neuropathol. Exp. Neurol.* **5:** 240
15. BLIGH, J. (1966):   *J. Physiol.* **185:** 46.

16. BOND, D., C.T. RANDT, T.G. BIDDER, and V. ROWLAND (1957): *Arch. Neurol. Psychiat.* **78:** 143.
17. BRODISH, A. (1969): *Neuroendocrinol.* **5:** 33.
18. CHOWER, I., H.T. HAMMEL, S.B. STROMME, and S.M. MacCANN (1962) *Amer. J. Physiol.* **207:** 577.
19. CLARK, G., H.W. MAGOUN, and S.W. RANSON (1939): *J. Neurophysiol.* **2:** 61.
20. CLARK, G., H.W. MAGOUN, and S.W. RANSON (1939): *J. Neurophysiol.* **2:** 202.
21. COLLINS, K.J., and T.S. WEINER (1968): *Physiol. Rev.* **48:** 785.
22. COOPER, K.E., W.I. CRANSTON, and A.J. HONOUR (1965): *J. Physiol.* **183:** 61.
23. CRANSTON, W.I., and C. ROSENDORFF (1967): *J. Physiol.* **193:** 359.
24. D'ANGELO, S.A. (1960): *Amer. J. Physiol.* **199:** 701.
25. DIXIT, B.N., and J.P. BUCKLEY (1969): *Neuroendocrinol.* **4:** 32.
26. EISENMAN, J.S. (1967): *Physiologist* **10:** 160.
27. ENDOROCZI, E., and K. LISSAK (1960): *Acta Physiol. Acad. Sci. Hung.* **17:** 39.
28. FAWCETT, D.W., and I.C. JONES (1949): *Endocrinol.* **45:** 609.
29. FELDBERG, W., and R.D. MYERS (1964): *J. Physiol.* **173:** 226.
30. FELDBERG, W., R.F. HELLON, and R.D. MYERS (1966): *J. Physiol.* **186:** 416.
31. FINDLAY, J.D., and D. ROBERTSHAW (1967): *J. Physiol.* **89:** 329.
32. FISCHER, P., J. RENSON, and P. CICCARONE (1959): *Arch. int. Physiol. et Biochem.* **67:** 147.
33. FRAZIER, C.H., B.J. ALPERS, and F.H. LEWY (1936): *Brain* **59:** 122.
34. GANONG, W.A., A.M., NOLAN, A. DOWDY, and J.A. LUETOHER (1961): *Endocrinol.* **68:** 169.
35. GELLHORN, E. (1957): Autonomic Imbalance and the Hypothalamus, Minneapolis Univ. of Minnesota Press.
36. HARDY, J.D., R.F. HELLEN, and K. SUTHERLAND (1964): *J. Physiol.* **175:** 242.
37. HARRI, M., and R. TIRRI (1969): *Acta Physiol. Scand.* **75:** 631.
38. HATAI, S. (1902): *Anat. Anz.* **21:** 369.
39. HEIM, T., and D. HULL (1965): *J. Physiol.* **181:** 60.
40. HEIM, T., and D. HULL (1966): *J. Physiol.* **186:** 42.
41. HELLER, A., J.A. HARVEY, and R.Y. MOORE (1962): *Biochem. Pharmac.* **11:** 859.
42. HELLER, A., and J.A. HARVEY (1963): *Pharmacologist* **5:** 264.
43. HELLER, A., and R.Y. MOORE (1965): *J. Pharmac. Exp. Ther.* **150:** 1.
44. HEMINGWAY, A. (1963): *Physiol. Rev.* **43:** 398.
45. HEMINGWAY, A., P. FORGRAVE, and L. BIRZIS (1954): *J. Neurophysiol.* **17:** 375.
46. HSIEH, A.C.L., and L.D. CARLSON (1957): *Amer. J. Physiol.* **190:** 243.
47. HULL, D., and M.M. SEGALL (1965): *J. Physiol.* **173:** 226.
48. ISENSCHMIDT, R., and L. KREHL (1912): *Arch. Exp. Pahtol. Pharmac.* **70:** 109.
49. ITOH, S. (1970): Japanese Handbook of Physiology, Vol. IX, 307 (Ed. YOSHIMURA, H., TAKAGI, K. and IKAI, M.)Igaku Shoin, Tokyo.
50. KAADA, B.R. (1951): *Acta Physiol. Scand.* **24:** 285 (Suppl. 83).
51. KAWAKAMI, M., and H. NEGORO (1967): *Proc. XXXX Anual Meeting of Japan Endocrinological Society* **152.**
52. KAWAKAMI, M., K. SETO, E. TERASAWA, K. YOSHIDA, T. MIYAMOTO, M. SEKIGUCHI, and Y. HATTORI (1968): *Neuroendocrinol.* **3:** 337.
53. KAWAKAMI, M., H. NEGORO, M. YANASE, and M. MOHRI (1969): *Jap. J. Physiol.* **19:** 609.
54. KAWAKAMI, M., K. SETO, and F. KIMURA: Progress in Brain Research (In press)
55. KELLER, A.D., and H. BOSTEL (1952): *Army Med. Res. Lab. Rept.* **84:** 6-6-028.
56. KOIKEGAMI, H., H. KUSHIRO, and A. KIMOTO (1952): *Ibid.* **6:** 76.
57. KOSAKA, M., E. SIMON, and R. THAUER (1967): *Experientia* **23:** 385.
58. KUNO, Y. (1956): Human Perspiration Springfield, Thomas, 177.
59. KUROSHIMA, A., N. KONNO, K. DOI, and S. ITOH (1968): *Jap. J. Physiol.* **18:** 446.
60. KUROTSU, T. (1949): *No-Kenkyu (Brain Research)* **3:** 39.
61. LACHANCE, J.P., and E. PAGE. (1953): *Endocrinol.* **52:** 57.
62. MAGOUN, H.W., F. HARRISON, J.R. BROBECK, and S.W. RANSON (1938): *J. Neurophysiol.* **1:** 101.
63. MASSOPUST, L.C., L.R. WOLIN, and J. MEDER (1965): *Exp. Neurol.* **12:** 25.
64. MIYAWAKI, H., U. MICHIO, and B. KOBAYASHI (1961): *Endocrinol. Jap.* **8:** 148.
65. MOUSSATCHE, H., and N. ALVARES-PEREIRA (1957): *Acta Physiol. Lat. Amer.* **7:** 71.
66. MURAKAMI, N., J.A.J. STOLWIJK, and J.D. HARDY (1967): *Amer. J. Physiol.* **213:** 1015.
67. NAKAYAMA, T., J.S. EISENMAN, and J.D. HARDY (1961): *Science* **134:** 560.
68. OCHI, J., M. KONISHI, and H. YOSHIKAWA. (1969): *Z. Anat. Entwickl.-Gesch.* **129:** 259.
69. OGATA, K. (1961): *Bull. Res. Inst. Diath tic Med.*, Kumamoto Univ. Vol. XI, Suppl.
70. OGATA, K., T. SASAKI, and N. MURAKAMI (1966): *Bull. Inst. Const. Med. Kumamoto Univ.* Vol. XVI, Suppl.
71. OGATA, K. (1971): *Bull. Inst. Med. Kumamoto Univ.* Vol. XXI, Suppl.
72. PAGE, E., and L.M. BABINEAU (1950): *Rev. Can. Biol.* **9:** 202.

73. Pinkston, J.D., P. Bard, and D. McK. Rioch (1934): *Amer. J. Physiol.* **109:** 515.
74. Sapeika, N. (1959): *Arch. int. Pharmacodyn.* **122:** 196.
75. Shizume, K., F. Matsuki, S. Iino, K. Matsuda, S. Nagataki, and S. Okinaka (1962): *Endocrinol.* **71:** 456.
76. Simon, E., W. Rantenberg, R. Thauer, and M. Iriki (1964): *Pflügers Arch. ges. Physiol.* **281:** 22.
77. Slusher, M.A., and J.E. Hyde (1961): *Endocrinol.* **69:** 1080.
78. Smelik, D.G., and D. Wied (1958): *Experientia* **14:** 17.
79. Smith, R.E., and B.A. Horwitz (1969): *Physiol. Rev.* **49:** 330.
80. Smith, R.E., and D.J. Hoijer (1962): *Physiol. Rev.* **42:** 60.
81. Spencer, W.A., and G. Dempster (1962): *Can. J. Biochem. Physiol.* **40:** 1705.
82. Stuart, D.G., Y. Kawamura, and A. Hemingway (1961): *Exp. Neurol.* **4:** 485.
83. Stuart, D.G., Y. Kawamura, A. Hemingway, and W.M. Price (1962): *Exp. Neurol.* **5:** 335.
84. Taylor, R.A., and J.G. Blackburn (1967): *Exp. Neurol.* **23:** 91.

CHAPTER 16

THERMAL REGULATION DURING WATER IMMERSION

TARO INOUE

Central Hospital, Aichi Prefectural Colony-Welfare Center for the Mentally and Physically Handicapped, Kasugai, Japan

On exposure to a cold environment, man responds with a broad spectrum of physiological reactions to maintain a relatively constant body temperature. Although the individual mechanisms are numerous, they can be divided into two categories: i.e., heat conservation and heat production mechanisms.

Heat conservation mechanisms involve behavioral and other neurophysiological alternations, hemodynamic changes, and changes in thermal insulation. Of these, subcutaneous adipose tissue is an important factor in insulation since its heat conductivity is about one-third that of water.

Among heat production mechanisms, we note that cold exposure elicits a rise in the plasma concentration of free fatty acid as well as a lowered respiratory quotient (R. Q.) in the expired air. These facts suggest an increased rate of fat catabolism, since fat serves as fuel during cold exposure.

In an attempt to clarify the basic factors affecting human adaptability to cold to establish a method to investigate it, the critical temperature was determined in human adults using a water bath method, and the lipid metabolism was investigated in relation to the adaptability to the cold.

The original paper of this study has not yet been published elsewhere, and the experimental methods and discussions will be described in the respective parts of this paper.

COLD TOLERANCE AND CRITICAL TEMPERATURE

To analyse human adaptability to cold, many efforts have been made to establish a standard experimental procedure (Yoshimura and Weiner, 1966). Wyndham *et al.* (1964) proposed the two-hr. multi-temperature test. They noticed the difference in physiological reaction to cold between Caucasians and Bantus, natives of South Africa, with respect to the metabolic rate, skin and rectal temperature and the vascular response of the finger to cold.

Another parameter for comparison of cold tolerance is the critical temperature, i.e. the lowest temperature necessary to maintain the resting metabolism without any increment in heat production. Scholander *et al.* (1950), measuring the oxygen consumption of various kinds of animals at various air temperatures, reported that the critical temperature of tropical animals was mostly around 22 to 27°C and that of arctic animals from 15°C in small animals to −30°C in relatively large ones.

These observations indicate that the critical temperature is a reasonable parameter for estimation of human adaptability to cold. In this connection, comparative studies have been carried out among different ethnic groups, and it was shown that there are some differences between them in both critical temperature and cold tolerance. Yoshimura *et al.* (1969) reported that the critical temperature of the Japanese is approximately 24 °C, lower by 2–3 °C than that of the Norweigians and Nomadic Lapps, living in the northern part of Norway (Scholander *et al.*, 1957). The racial difference between the Japanese and the Caucasians may come from differences in living habits and in habitat, and also from differences in bodily constitution or nutritional habits.

1. Water Bath Method for Estimating Critical Temperature

There are at least two disadvantages in testing temperature tolerance through exposure to air. One is the difficulty in precisely controlling the ambient conditions. The second is the difficulty in measuring the skin temperatures, since the values obtained vary somewhat from time to time and from area to area of the skin. The validity of average skin temperature estimated by the best available means is questionable, and an average skin temperature seems necessary to estimate the degree of cold tolerance.

As already pointed out by Burton and Bazett (1936), the advantages of a water bath are:

(a) that skin temperature may be fixed and known.
(b) that the external environment is precisely known.
(c) that in the steady state the amount of heat loss can be estimated from metabolic heat production and body temperature.
(d) that it is relatively cheap to produce a portable, controlled temperature bath.

It should be remembered, however, that the production of a uniform temperature creates a somewhat abnormal physiological condition, which may be associated with abnormality of reflex responses.

In order to determine the critical temperature in a water bath, the level of body fat must be taken into consideration as well as the duration of the exposure in the cold bath (Carlson *et al.*, 1958; Keatinge, 1960).

Subcutaneous fat was determined by measuring skinfold thickness at ten sites (Skerlj *et al.*, 1953) with a caliper (Eiken type); 40 mm was subtracted from the total to allow for skin thickness and the remainder divided by 20 to determine mean fat thickness.

All subjects were at least 3 hrs. postprandial and control values of oxygen consumption and heart rate were measured before water immersion, at a room temperature of 25–27 °C.

The subjects in swimming suits were immersed until the level of the water was just below the chin anteriorly and the occipital ridge posteriorly, sitting on a perforated board. During the immersion the subjects were not permitted to cross their legs or hold their arms against the bodies.

The water bath was 0.8 m wide, 1 m long, and 1.5 m deep. The circulating pump and air bubbling pump assured adequate mixing and circulation of the water, and the temperature was controlled within ±0.05 °C.

All temperature measurements were made with Cu-Co thermocouples and registered on a electric automatic recorder. A flexible rectal probe was inserted between 15 and 20 cm into the rectum.

Calculations of heat exchanges were made on the assumption that there was a peripheral mass equal to 0.4 body weight.   During immersion the peripheral temperature was assumed to be water temperature.   The core temperature as measured by the rectal temperature was assumed to be the temperature of the remaining 0.6 of the body's mass (Rennie *et al.*, 1962).

In calculating thermoconductivity or its reciprocal, insulation index, it was assumed that 8% of the heat loss occurred through the respiratory tract.   When the core temperature continued to decline, the net loss of body heat (0.83 X $\varDelta$ rectal temperature X 0.6 X body weight) was added to the metabolic rate in estimating skin heat loss.

Tissue insulation (I) was computed from the formula

$$I = (\text{rectal temperature} - \text{bath temperature}) / \text{rate of skin heat loss}$$

where, skin heat loss = metabolic rate (m) — respiratory heat loss (0.08 X m) + (0.83 X $\varDelta$ rectal temperature X 0.6 X body weight).

2. Critical Water Temperature and Insulation Index

Fig. 113. shows a typical demonstration of experimental items and results.   After measuring control values in the standard temperature room (25–27°C), the subject

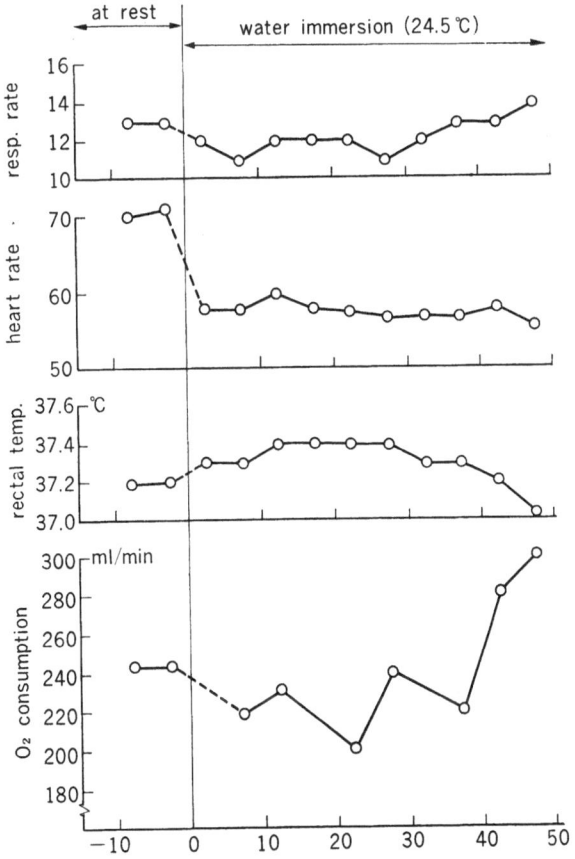

Fig. 113.   Measurement of critical water temperature (Subject: T.I.)

(a relatively fat man) was immersed in the water bath (in this case, at 24.5 °C).

After immersion, the respiratory rate ran parallel with the O_2 consumption. The heart rate decreased dramatically throughout the hour of immersion. This brady-cardia was accompanied by peripheral vasoconstriction (Rennie, 1965). As already pointed out by Craig *et al.* (1966), the cardiovascular functioning at the midrange of water temperature (24–35 °C) suggests that the blood flow to the skin is minimal and that the demands for cardiovascular output are also minimal under these resting conditions.

The rectal temperature showed an initial rise for about 20 minutes and then gradually decreased until below control value.

In the water bath, the oxygen consumption slightly decreased for 40 minutes and a greater amount of oxygen was retained than in the control at the end of the period of immersion. Therefore, for this subject the water temperature of 24.5 °C was not the critical temperature. Next time (two days later), the critical water tem-perature was established to be 24.7 °C, because the oxygen consumption did not exceed the control value throughout the hour of immersion.

The experimental results of seven subjects are summarized in Table 30. From this table, it is clear that the critical water temperature remains within the range 25 °C to 32 °C, depending largely upon the thickness of their subcutaneous fat.

TABLE 30 Relationship between critical temperature and subcutaneous fat thickness

| subject | age | body weight | critical temperature | | subcutaneous fat thickness |
			summer	winter	
Ma	34	56.0 Kg	31.9 °C	33.0 °C	1.2 mm
Y	20	50.0	31.5	32.0	2.3
O	20	58.0	30.6	31.8	1.3
A	25	58.0	30.5	32.0	1.0
N	20	53.5	30.5	31.5	2.5
M	20	60.5	27.1	28.5	5.1
I	42	67.5	24.7	26.8	6.8

In spite of the uniformity of the experimental conditions, the critical water tem-perature in winter was higher by 0.5–2.1 °C than that of summer.

Since body heat content differs from season to season, subjects were prewarmed in the bath to raise body heat in the winter experiment, but the critical water tem-perature still remained higher by 0.2–0.6 °C than that of summer.

The results suggest that seasonal variations exist in the physical regulation of tem-perature, and that chemical thermoregulation is enhanced in winter under the same degree of cold exposure.

According to Rennie *et al.* (1962), American female subjects whose mean sub-cutaneous fat thickness was less than 4 mm had a critical water temperature of 33–34 °C, similar to Burton's value (1936). For more obese Americans, it was 30 °C or lower. In contrast, Koreans had lower critical water temperature than Americans of comparable fat thickness. For the Koreans they were as follows: men, 33–31 °C; nondiving women, 31–30 °C; diving women, 30 °C or lower.

As already described above, the insulation index (I) includes the main factors which influence cold tolerance. Therefore, it is reasonable to compare the insulation index in analysing human adaptability to cold in different ethnic groups.

Burton and Bazett (1936) have previously noted that as water bath temperature was lowered, body insulation increased to a maximal value concomitant with cutaneous vasoconstriction and then decreased again as shivering supervened. They observed that at a critical water temperature of 33 °C the body insulation averaged 0.135 °C/ Kcal/m²/h, identical to maximal tissue insulation attainable during cool air exposure.

The individual I values of our seven male subjects, computed from body temperature and metabolism after one hour of immersion, are summarized in Table 31. The average I values for Americans and Koreans are also listed in Table 31.

TABLE 31   Comparison of insulation index

subject	subcutaneous fat thickness mm	critical temp. °C summer	critical temp. °C winter	insulation index °C/Kcal/m²/hr. summer	insulation index °C/Kcal/m²/hr. winter
Ma	1.2	31.9	33.0	0.140	0.088
Y	2.3	31.5	32.0	0.118	0.104
O	1.3	30.6	31.8	0.155	0.132
H	1.7	—	32.0	—	0.099
A	1.0	30.5	32.0	0.150	0.102
N	2.5	30.5	31.5	0.109	0.095
M	5.1	27.1	28.5	0.184	0.163
I	6.8	24.7	26.8	0.348	0.257
Americans (Craig)	5.4±1.4	30—32		0.098—0.111	
Americans (Rennie)	2.8±0.6	30—33		0.11±0.01	
Korean diving women	2.0±0.3	(30—31)		0.13±0.01	

As already pointed out by many authors the thickness of the subcutaneous fat play a prominent role in body insulation (Daniels and Baker, 1961; LeBlanc, 1954).

Pugh (1965) computed an I value of 0.25 °C/Kcal/m²/h on an obese male channel swimmer with a mean subcutaneous fat thickness of 7 mm.

A second factor affecting body insulation is a larger shell of non-fatty tissue, achieved by more severe vasoconstriction. This appears to be a cold-adaptive mechanism seen in Korean diving women as well as in naked Australian aborgines. According to Hammel et al. (1959), Australian aborgines, having fat thickness equal to their control subjects, were able to increase tissue insulation to values almost double those of the control.

With regard to the insulation of the non-fatty shell, Fig. 114 shows the correlation between insulation index (I) and subcutaneous fat thickness (F) of different ethnic groups. The slope of regression lines, which shows the fat dependency in the insulation, is larger in Japanese and Americans than that in Koreans. However, the intercept constant, which may give the insulation of the non-fatty shell, is larger in Japanese and Koreans than that in Americans. For Americans this intercept constant was 0.05 °C/Kcal/m²/hr. Assuming that this is composed of nonperfused muscle having an insulation of 0.03 °C/Kcal/m²/hr/cm (Hatfield et al., 1951), its thickness would be 1.7 cm. This is remarkably close to commonly accepted values for the

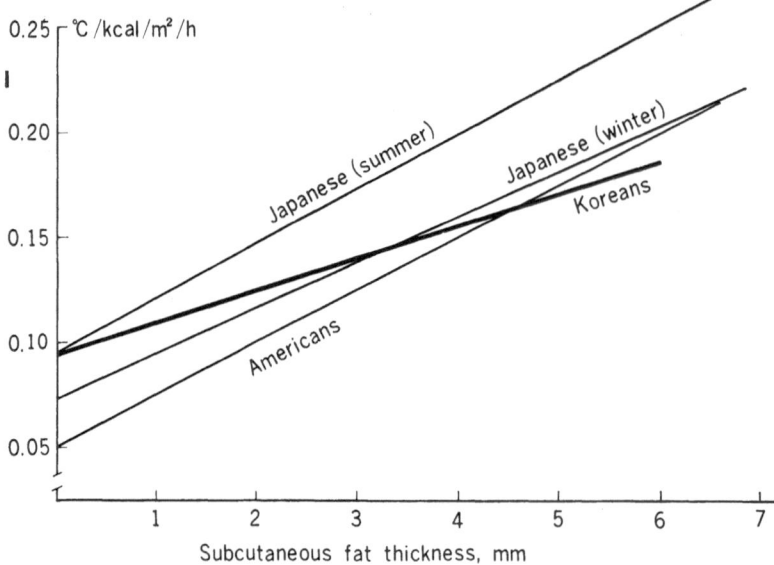

Fig. 114. Correlation between insulation index (I) and subcutaneous fat thickness (F).

Remarks:

Japanese (male)	summer	I = 0.026F + 0.097
	winter	I = 0.021F + 0.072
American (male and female)		I = 0.024F + 0.050
Korean (female) non-divers		I = 0.014F + 0.094

mean thickness of the insulation shell around the body (Burton *et al.*, 1955). Similarly, the intercept for Koreans and Japanese was 0.072–0.097°C/Kcal/m²/hr. This corresponds to an insulation of 2.4–3.2 cm of nonperfused muscle.

Thus the greater over-all insulation of the Koreans and Japanese, when compared to Americans of equal fat thickness, could be accounted for by a non-fatty shell.

By contrast, Alaskan Eskimos attain comparatively low maximal tissue insulation (Rennie *et al.*, 1962), and tolerate cold by metabolic increment.

These results suggest that racial differences exist in the physical regulation of body temperature.

LIPID METABOLISM IN WATER IMMERSION

As already well known, the Ama, diving women have significantly thicker subcutaneous fat than non-diving women (control) during the non-harvesting season (winter). The subcutaneous fat thickness decreases more markedly than in the control in close association with body weight loss (5–8 kg) during summer harvesting season (Iwasaki, 1970; Kohara, 1970). The women's actual diving days are roughly counted to be 60–80 days during the season, from spring to autumn. Thus they lose body weight of about 100 g every diving day.

On the other hand, on the diving day, according to the time study, the Ama consumes 2500–2800 Kcal/day, but her caloric intake is calculated to be only around 1800 Kcal/day. Assuming that the body weight decrease is mainly attributed to a loss of body fat, the caloric supply from the adipose tissue of 100 g, corresponds to

700–900 Kcal. Thus the difference between energy consumption and intake almost equals that of the fat catabolism.

In normal human subjects the plasma free fatty acid concentration (FFA) increases with fasting (Fredrickson *et al.*, 1958), after exercise (Carlson *et al.*, 1961), and during infusion of norepinephrine, epinephrine (Dole, 1958), and growth hormone (Raben *et al.*, 1959).

In our pilot experiments, water immersion elicited a similar rise in plasma FFA as well as a lowered R. Q. in the expired air, which suggests increased fat catabolism.

With this background, the lipid metabolism, especially the mobilization of fatty acids was studied during water immersion. Breath-hold diving contains at least three kinds of stress, i.e., muscle exercise, high pressure of the environment, and water immersion. In this paper, attention was focused on the effect of water immersion (cold stress) on the lipid metabolism, applying the water bath method to the subjects under resting conditions. Oxygen consumption, respiratory quotient (R. Q.), rectal temperature, plasma FFA and blood glucose were measured during as well as before and after immersion.

Plasma FFA was determined by the colorimetric method of Itaya and Ui, a modification of Duncombe's method (Itaya and Ui, 1965; Duncombe, 1963). Blood glucose was measured colorimetrically by o-toluidine method (Dubowski, 1962; Genba and Kobayashi, 1967).

Fig. 115 shows the data of a pilot experiment, using the water bath method in summer. Young (20–23 years old) female college students in swimming suits were immersed for 30–40 min. at 22–23 °C. As seen here, O_2 consumption increased in three subjects, while in others it did not change or even decreased during immersion. These results may be understood in terms of individual differences in sensitivity to cold. R. Q. of expired air showed a tendency to decrease during immersion.

Plasma FFA of the control showed remarkable individual difference and during

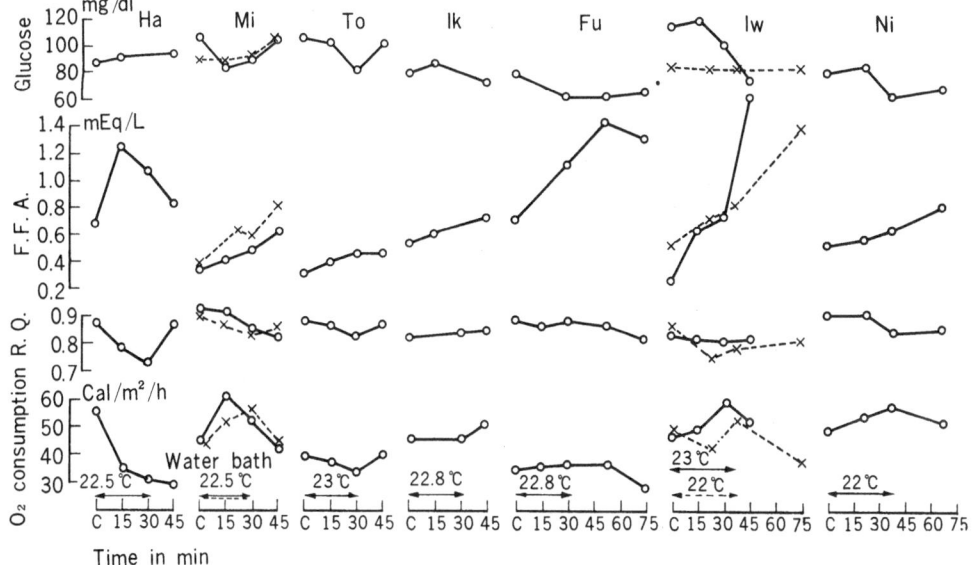

Fig. 115. Metabolic responses to water immersion

immersion it increased significantly.   It also remained at high level for more than 30
minutes after immersion.

On the other hand, blood glucose decreased during and after immersion, con-
trasting with the fact that it increased during exposure to cold air (5–10°C).

In the next experiment in winter, the immersion was carried out at 20°C and
the immersion time was shorter than that of the previous pilot experiments.

Fig. 116 shows the differences in FFA and glucose levels between Ama (23–34 years
old) and non-Ama (female college students, 20–23 years old) groups.

The elevations of the plasma FFA and the lowering R. Q. during immersion were
not demonstrated clearly in this experiment.   This may be attributed to the relatively
short duration of the immersion, and/or a seasonal effect of the immersion time on
lipid metabolism, assuming that the turnover rate of FFA had already accelerated for
winter (Ikemoto et al., 1969).

It is interesting that Fig. 116 demonstrates the relationship between low FFA—high
glucose in the Ama group and high FFA—low glucose in the non-Ama group.   Further
studies will be made to analyse the mechanism of human adaptability to cold from the
standpoint of lipid metabolism.

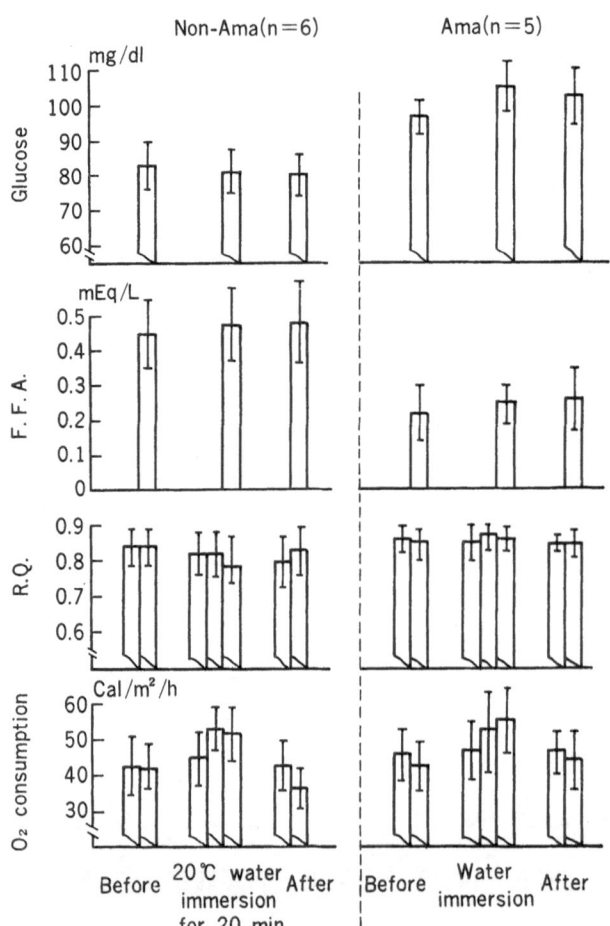

Fig. 116. Comparison between Ama and non-Ama in their responses to cold water.

These results suggested that FFA in plasma may be utilized as fuel material in cold, and the metabolic fate of FFA in plasma may be involved in the mechanism of cold acclimatization (Itoh *et al.*, 1970).

From these considerations, the following experiments were designed.

1. Changes in the Pattern of Fatty Acids of Plasma during Water Immersion

Changes in the pattern of fatty acids in blood plasma were studied to clarify the mechanism of FFA elevation during water immersion.

The fatty acids in blood plasma were analysed for their methyl esters by gas-liquid chromatography with a hydrogen-ionized detector (Okura electrochemical Co.). Diethylene glycol succinate 15% on dichrom AS 60/80 was chosen as the liquid phase to be used. The column temperature was maintained at 215 °C, and that of the injection block at 360 °C. Nitrogen gas was used as the carrier. Arachidic acid (C-20-0), found at trace levels in human blood plasma, was used as the internal standard for the calculation of fatty acid concentrations in the samples.

Fig. 117 shows the effect of water immersion (at 24 °C, for 30 min.) on the pattern of fatty acids in plasma. As seen in here, unsaturated fatty acids of long C-chains such as arachdonic acid (C-20-4) and linoleic acid (C-18-2) were attacked at first. By around the 30th minute of immersion, the total amount of fatty acids in plasma fell by about 10%, and the decrease continued even after the subject came out of the water. At the 30th minute after the emergence from water the total amount of fatty acids in plasma was about 80% of the original control value. It appears that, whereas in the short-term immersion, lasting for 30 minutes, only the plasma fatty acids are utilized, longer lasting submersion would cause mobilization of tissue fatty acids too.

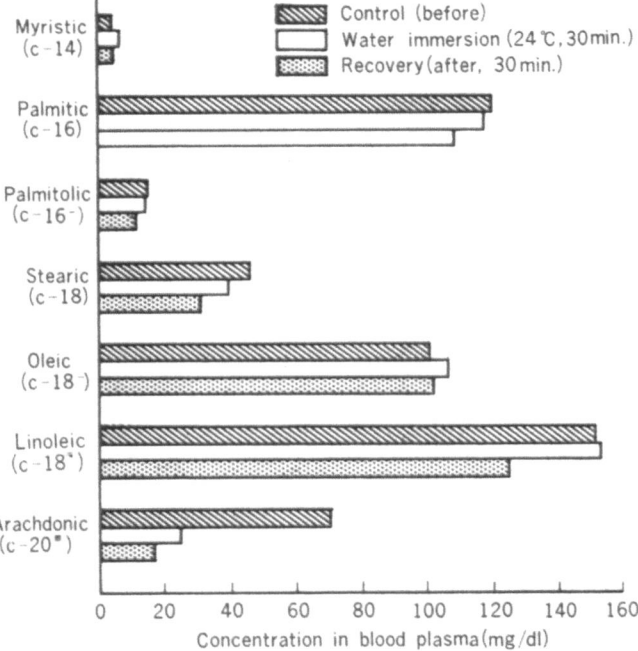

Fig. 117.   Effect of cold water immersion of whole body on fatty acid pattern in blood plasma.

Fig. 118 shows the effect of an actual diving performance (at 24°C, for 40 min.) on the fatty acid pattern. In the Ama, it is very remarkable that the total amount of fatty acids in plasma as well as the level of FFA was about half that of the non-Ama (refer to Fig. 116).

In these cases, arachdonic acid did not appear in the plasma.

At the end of the diving, the amount of total fatty acids fell to 82% (Nakayama) or 63% (Okuda), and the decrease remained for 90 minutes of the recovery period. With the diving performance, linoleic acid (C-18-2) and oleic acid (C-18-1) were perfectly or partly consumed.

As already pointed out, the stress caused by the diving performance are assumed to be more complicated and stronger than that of the water immersion. It takes more than 90 minutes for the perfect recovery of the fatty acid pattern.

From these results, it is assumed that mobilization of tissue fatty acids would be needed for a fairly long time.

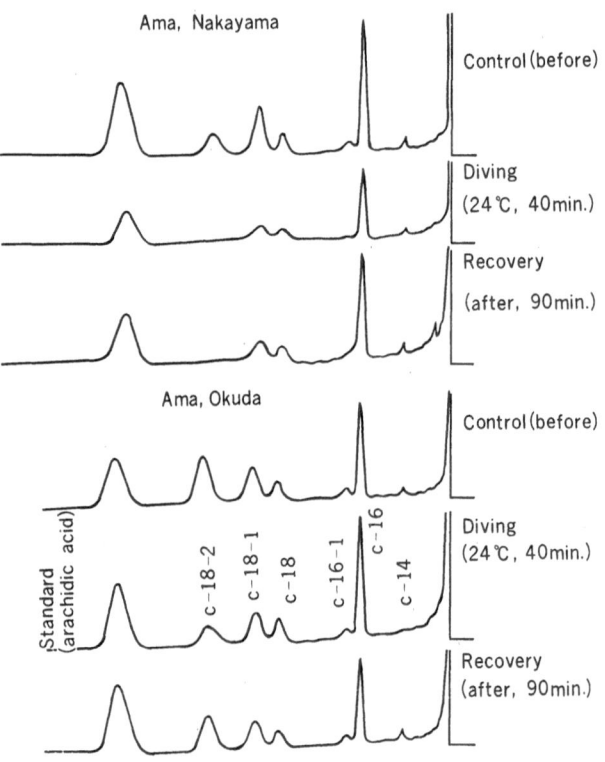

Fig. 118. Effect of diving on fatty acid pattern in blood plasma.

2. *Effect of Catecholamine on the Pattern of Fatty Acids in Plasma and Its Possible Role in Cold Tolerance*

In recent years it has become clear that one of the most striking metabolic effects of the catecholamines is their ability to stimulate mobilization of depot fat in the form of free fatty acids (Fredrickson *et al.*, 1958). Recently, Steinberg *et al.*, (1964) reported that the influence of norepinephrine increased the rate of oxygen consumption in man and that this was accompanied by an increase in the rate of conversion of labeled plasma FFA to respiratory $^{14}CO_2$.

In connection with these reports, Fig. 119 demonstrates the effect of norepinephrine (0.2 mg, subcutaneously injected) on the pattern of fatty acids in the plasma.

By around the 10th minute after the injection of norepinephrine, the total amount of fatty acids in the plasma decreased by about 15%. Fatty acids which decreased in the control were almost the same as those in the case of water immersion, i.e. unsaturated fatty acids of long C-chains such as arachdonic, linoleic, and oleic acid (C-18-1).

By the 30th minute after the norepinephrine, both the total amount of fatty acids and the pattern of fatty acids returned to the control level, due to the short-term action of norepinephrine.

On the other hand, the injection of epinephrine did not effect the total amount of fatty acids nor the pattern of fatty acids.

These facts suggest that the effect of water immersion on the acceleration of catabolism of fatty acids is triggered by norepinephrine.

It is well known since Cannon (1932) proposed the emergency theory that epinephrine may initiate a rise in blood glucose during cold exposure. Cannon emphasized that sympathico-adrenal system plays a very important role in survival in the cold.

Besides the metabolic roles of catecholamine in tolerating cold stress, Cannon pointed out that erection of hair and vasoconstriction of skin vessels play a role in cold tolerance.

On the other hand, the catecholamine also inhibits the motility of the digestive tract accompanying the vasoconstriction. Carlson (1919) pointed out that the hunger peristalsis is accompanied by appetite. Thus the loss of appetite in the Ama

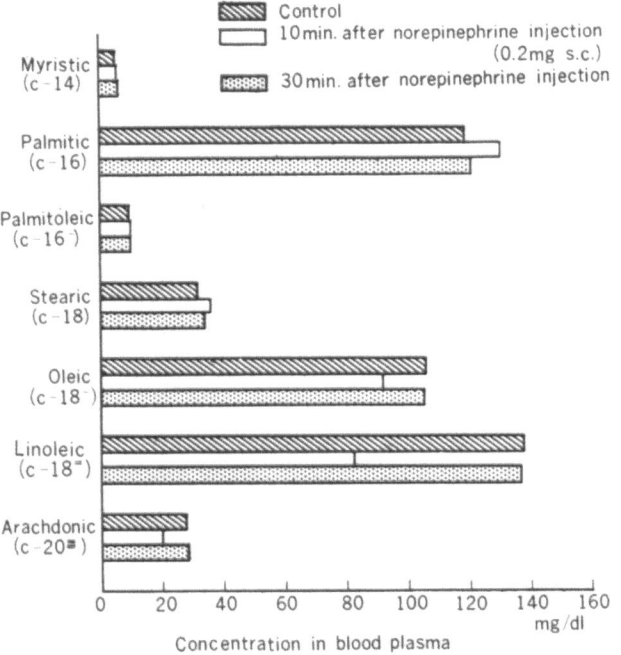

Fig. 119. Effect of norepinephrine injection on fatty acid pattern in plasma.

during the harvesting season might be partly attributed to an influence of the catecholamine which inhibits hunger peristalsis.

SUMMARY

By using a water bath method, both the critical temperature and the lipid metabolism were studied in relation to adaptability to cold.

Results are summarized as follows:

1) It was clarified that the critical water temperature is a reasonable parameter for estimating human adaptability to cold, and that body fatness might be considered in determining the critical temperature in the bath water.

2) By computing the tissue insulation (I value), it was suggested that racial differences exisit in man's physical regulation of body temperature.

The value of I contains at least two components; one is body insulation depending on the subcutanous fat thickness and the other is that of the non-fatty tissue.

The greater over-all insulation of the Koreans and Japanese, when compared to Americans of equal fat thickness, could be accounted for by the non-fatty shell.

3) When bath water temperature was lower than the critical temperature, the lipid metabolism was accelerated for chemical thermogenesis. Unsaturated fatty acids of long C-chains such as arachdonic acid and linoleic acid were attacked at first in the pattern of fatty acids in plasma.

The catabolism of fatty acids in plasma was assumed to be triggered by the catecholamine especially by norepinephrine, which was released due to the stress of the water immersion or the diving performance.

4) Possible roles of catecholamine in cold tolerance were discussed. It was suggested that the loss of appetite in the Ama (diving woman) during harvesting time might be partly due to the influence of catecholamine, which inhibits hunger peristalsis.

ACKNOWLEDGEMENTS

The author is indebted to Dr. S. Hori and Miss M. Ashida, Department of Physiology, Kyoto Prefectural University of Medicine, for their cooperation, and to Professor H. Yoshimura for his kind criticism in this study.

This study was carried out as a part of J-IBP/HA.

REFERENCES

1. Burton, A.C., and H.C. Bazett (1936): *Am. J. Physiol.* **117**: 36.
2. Burton, A.C., and O.G. Edholm (1955): Man in a cold environment, Williams and Wilkins, Baltimore.
3. Cannon, W.B. (1932): The wisdom of the body, Kegan Paul, Trench and Trubner, London.
4. Carlson, A.J. (1919): The control of hunger in health and disease, Univ. of Chicago Press.
5. Carlson, L.D., A.C.L. Hsieh, F. Fullington, and F.W. Elsner (1958): *J. Aviation Med.* **29**: 145.
6. Carlson, L.A., and B. Peronow (1961): *J. Lab. Clin. Med.* **58**: 673.
7. Craig, A.B. Jr., and M. Dvarak (1966): *J. Appl. Physiol.* **21**: 1577.
8. Daniels, F., Jr., and P.T. Baker (1961): *J. Appl. Physiol.* **16**: 421.
9. Dole, V.P. (1958): *Arch. Internal. Med.* **101**: 1005.
10. Dubowski, K.M. (1962): *Clin. Chem.* **8**: 215.
11. Duncombe, W.G. (1963): *Biochem. J.* **88**: 7.
12. Fredrickson, D.S., and R.S. Gordon, Jr. (1958): *J. Clin. Invest.* **37**: 1504.
13. Fredrickson, D.S., and R.S. Gordon, Jr. (1958): *Physiol. Rev.* **38**: 585.

14. GEMBA, T., and H. KOBAYASHI (1967): *Jap. J. Clin. Path.* **15:** 515 (in Japanese).
15. HAMMEL, H.T., R.W. ELSNER, D.H. LE MESSURIER, H.T. ANDERSON, and F.A. MILAN (1959): *J. Appl. Physiol.* **14:** 605.
16. HATFIELD, H.S., and L.G.C.E. PUGH (1951): *Nature* **168:** 918.
17. IKEMOTO, H., T. HIROSHIGE, and S. ITOH. (1969): *Jap. J. Physiol.* **19:** 293.
18. ITAYA, K., and M. UI (1965): *J. Lipid Research* **6:** 16.
19. ITOH, S., K. DOI, and A. KUROSHIMA (1970): *Hokkaido J. Med. Sci.* **45:** 206.
20. IWASAKI, S. (1970): Ecological situations of Japanese Ama (in Japanese) In: Human Adaptability in Japanese, Ed. by HA-section of JIBP, Kodansha, Tokyo.
21. KOHARA, S. (1970): Morphological adaptability in Ama (in Japanese) In: Human Adaptability in Japanese, Ed. by HA-section of JIBP, Kodansha, Tokyo.
22. KEATINGE, W.R. (1960): *J. Physiol.* **153:** 166.
23. LE BLANC, J. (1954): *Can. J. Biochem. Physiol.* **32:** 354.
24. PUGH, L.G.C.E. (1965): Temperature regulation in swimmers. In: Physiology of Breath-Hold Diving and the Ama of Japan. Ed. by RAHN, H. and T. YOKOYAMA, Natl. Acad. Sci., Natl. Res. Council, Washington, D.C.
25. RABEN, M.S., and C.H. HOLLENBERG. (1959): *J. Clin. Invest.* **38:** 484.
26. RENNIE, D.W. (1965): Thermal insulation of Korean diving women and non-divers in water. In: Physiology of Breath-Hold Diving and the Ama of Japan. Ed by RAHN, H. and T. YOKOYAMA, Natl. Acad. Sci., Natl. Res. Council, Washington, D.C.
27. RENNIE, D.W., B.G. COVINO, M.R. BLAIR, and K. RODAHI (1962): *J. Appl. Physiol.* **17:** 326.
28. RENNIE, D.W., B.G. COVINO, B.J. HOWELL, S.H. SONG B.S. KANG, and S.K. HONG (1962): *J. Appl. Physiol.* **17:** 961.
29. SCHOLANDER, P.F., R. HOCK, V. WALTERS, F. JOHNSON, and L. IRVING (1950): *Biol. Bull.* **99:** 237.
30. SCHOLANDER, P.F., K.L. ANDERSON, J. KROG, F.V. LORENTZEN, and J. STEEN (1957): *J. Appl. Physiol.* **10:** 2311.
31. SKERLJ, B., J. BROZEK, and E.E. HUNT JR. (1953): *Am. J. Phys. Anthropol* **11:** 577.
32. STEINBERG, D., P.J. NESTEL, E.R. BUSKIRK, and R.H. THOMPSON (1964): *J. Clin. Invest.* **43:** 167.
33. WYNDHAM, C.H., J.S. WARD, N.B. STRYDOM, J.F. MORRISON, C.G. WILLIAMS, G.A.G. BREDELL, J. PETER, M.J.E. VON RAHEN, L.D. HOLDSWORTH, C.H. VANGRAAN, A.J. VAN RENSBURG, and A. MUNRO (1964): *J. Appl. Physiol.* **19:** 583.
34. YOSHIMURA, H., and J.S. WEINER, (eds.) (1966): Human adaptability and its methodology, Japan Society for the Promotion of Sciences. Maruzen, Tokyo.
35. YOSHIMURA, M., and H. YOSHIMURA (1969): *Int. J. Biometeor* **13:** 163.

Chapter 17

LIPID METABOLISM OF COLD-ADAPTED MAN

Shinji ITOH and Akihiro KUROSHIMA

Department of Physiology, Hokkaido University School of Medicine, Sapporo, Japan

In regard to the effect of cold acclimatization on lipid metabolism, a large number of studies have been done on various mammals, but few on human subjects. According to Hicks [34], serum cholesterol showed some increase in April during one-year stay at an Antarctic station. Mager and Iampietro [56] found in human subjects that plasma cholesterol, phospholipids and total lipids increased during the early phases of cold and starvation, but returned to control levels by the end of the two-week period. Plasma free fatty acids (FFA) rose to over 200% of the control level within two days and remained constant thereafter. Since more knowledge is required to clarify the physiological significance of fat metabolism in human adaptation to cold, we have carried out a series of investigations on this problem. In this study particular attention was focussed on the biochemical characteristics of the Ainu, natives of Hokkaido, the northern island of Japan, since metabolic features of the Ainu are presumed to be related to the cold adaptability of this ethnic group.

SEASONAL VARIATIONS IN PLASMA LIPIDS

Extensive studies have been made by Yoshimura and his colleagues [82] on the seasonal variations of homeostatic mechanisms in relation to environmental temperature. However, no report appeared on plasma lipids in this regard. Therefore, seasonal variations of plasma lipid concentrations were observed under basal conditions in the morning on healthy male subjects [40].

Plasma concentrations of total lipids, esterified fatty acids, total cholesterol and phospholipids, and plasma lipase activity did not show appreciable seasonal changes, but plasma levels of FFA were high in the winter and low in the summer. Mean value in the winter was 21% higher than the summer level (P<0.05). The plasma concentration of free cholesterol was also high in the winter as compared with the spring level (P<0.05).

The observed seasonal change in the plasma level of FFA is interesting, since plasma FFA has been suggested to be of central importance in determining over-all rates of body metabolism. However, it is known that during fasting the release of FFA is increased as glucose entry into adipose tissue is decreased. Therefore, the plasma FFA might be affected by the time of blood sampling after food intake. In fact, the plasma FFA level began to increase 10 hours after a meal and thereafter rose progressively with the passing of time [39]. Accordingly, differences in the plasma FFA levels observed between winter and summer might be ascribed, at least in part, to the difference in elapsed time after dinner which might be longer in the winter due to the longer night. Hemoconcentration in the winter may also affect the plasma concentration.

PLASMA LIPID PROFILES IN THE WINTER

In the above experiment on the seasonal changes of plasma lipids, we noticed particularly high levels of plasma FFA, amounting to 626 and 741 μEq/l, respectively, in the winter in two subjects native to the main island of Japan. Accordingly, we compared the plasma FFA concentration as well as other lipid components in different groups of subjects in the winter in cold districts.

Eight groups, totaling 128 male subjects, including two groups of Ainus, were used for this study. They were group I: students who were born on the main island of Japan and living in Sapporo for two to three years; group II: students and professionals born on Hokkaido and living in Sapporo; group III: policemen in Asahikawa; group IV: farmers in Huren; group V: farmers in Niikappu; group VI: fishermen and fish factory workers in Monbetsu; group VII: Ainu in Asahikawa; and group VIII: Ainu in Niikappu. These Ainu were mostly of mixed descent. Among the places listed here, Huren is the coldest, followed by Asahikawa and Monbetsu. Niikappu and Sapporo are not very cold in the winter (Table 32). The study was made during the

TABLE 32   Mean temperature in °C (1957–1967)

Place	Jan	Feb	Mar	Apr	May	Jun	Jul	Aug	Sep	Oct	Nov	Dec
Nayoro*	−10.5	−10.0	−5.2	3.8	6.4	17.3	17.9	20.3	15.4	8.6	1.1	−6.1
Asahikawa	− 8.2	− 7.3	−2.4	5.1	11.7	15.9	20.0	20.7	15.4	8.7	2.0	−4.3
Monbetsu	− 6.5	− 6.7	−2.6	4.6	9.5	12.2	16.4	18.3	15.5	9.7	3.0	−2.4
Sapporo	− 4.8	− 3.8	0.0	6.5	12.5	15.8	19.9	21.6	18.5	10.6	4.2	−1.9
Urakawa**	− 2.9	− 2.7	−0.1	5.1	9.8	13.0	17.1	19.9	16.9	11.6	5.6	0.2

*Town adjacent to Huren.
**Near Niikappu.

period from January to the beginning of March. Blood samples were obtained in the morning before breakfast under resting condition [41, 43].

1. Total Lipids

Mean value of plasma total lipids in the Ainu (441 ± 21.2 mg/100 ml (Mean ± SEM)) was somewhat low, as compared with that of the non-Ainu Japanese (491 ± 18.4 mg/ 100 ml for group I; 457 ± 9.3 for group II–VI), but the difference was not significant. Values reported by Boyd [8] and Mager and Iampietro [56] are similar to ours. However, other investigators found considerably higher values. For instance, Lund et al. [55] reported 567 ± 11 mg/100 ml for males and 569 ± 15 for females, and Svanborg and Svennerholm [75] 610 ± 15.3 and 648 ± 21.1, respectively. The great differences between our results and these figures might be due mostly to differences in total cholesterol and phospholipids, as will be shown below.

2. Triglycerides

Plasma levels of triglycerides of the Ainu (79 ± 5.8 mg/100 ml) were not different from the levels of the non-Ainu Japanese (84 ± 10.6 mg/100 ml for group I; 75 ± 4.0

for group II–VI).   Values obtained in this study were similar to those of the Japanese on the main island [62] and of caucasians as reported by several investigators [10, 13, 21, 23, 26, 75], though higher average values amounting 138 and 152 mg/100 ml were also reported by Schwartz et al. [70] and Dunn and Moses [20], respectively.   Such differences may be due to different dietary habits.

3. Cholesterol

Appreciable differences in the plasma cholesterol concentrations were not observed among Japanese subjects born on the main island (171 ± 8.7 mg/100 ml), those born on Hokkaido (168 ± 3.6 mg/100 ml) and the Ainu (164 ± 4.7 mg/100 ml).   Values obtained in these groups were the same as reported by Okinaka [60] who summarized 6977 determinations of total cholesterol in the plasma of the Japanese in the main island and southern islands of Japan.   However, it should be noted that plasma cholesterol level was considerably higher in policemen in Asahikawa, averaging 193 ± 9.2 mg/100 ml.   The subjects are engaged in patrol of 24-hour duty every other day. Such occupational stress may cause an elevation of the plasma cholesterol level, as suggested by Friedman et al. [22].

Plasma cholesterol concentrations in the Japanese are markedly low in comparison with those of Americans and Europeans.   Although Svanborg and Svennerholm [75] and Stamp et al. [72] found average values of 192 and 195 mg/100 ml, respectively, others reported values of over 200 mg/100 ml [1, 20, 21, 52, 55].   Lewis et al. [53] who measured total serum cholesterol on 10,690 men and 3,404 women also reported average values higher than 200 mg/100 ml.   The principal cause of this difference in plasma cholesterol levels between the Japanese and Americans or Europeans may be difference in diet.

Plasma levels of free cholesterol in the three groups of the present study were on the same level (46 ± 3.1 mg/100 ml for group I; 47 ± 1.6 for group II–VI; 51 ± 3.1 for group VII and VIII); and the values were not very different from those found by others [8, 49, 56].

4. Phospholipids

Plasma phospholipid levels of subjects born on the main island (139 ± 5.0 mg/100 ml) were somewhat low, though differences were not significant when compared with the values of Japanese (149 ± 3.5 mg/100 ml) and Ainu (149 ± 7.1 mg/100 ml) who were born on Hokkaido.   However, in general the average values were found to be considerably lower than those reported in the literature.   This might be due, in part, to the method employed in this study.   Oyama et al. [62] found an average of 182 mg/100 ml in the Japanese in the main island, Gjone and Orning [24] showed 170 mg/100 ml for males and 182 for females, Svanborg and Svennerholm [75] 208 mg/100 ml for males and 232 for females, and Dunn and Moses [20] as high as 297 mg/100 ml. Adlersberg et al. [1] also described high average value of 249 mg/100 ml for males between the age of 23 and 27, and observed that the values increased gradually with age.

5. Esterified Fatty Acids

The average value of esterified fatty acids was somewhat lower in the Ainu (303 ± 10.9 mg/100 ml) than in the non-Ainu Japanese (340 ± 16.5 for group I; 350 ± 8.5 for group II–VI).   The difference between the Ainu and the Japanese born on

Hokkaido was significant (P<0.05). This is mostly ascribed to high levels of esterified cholesterol in Asahikawa policemen (148 mg/100 ml) and fishermen and fish factory workers in Monbetsu (138 mg/100 ml), in comparison with low average value of 113 mg/100 ml in the Ainu. As a whole, the values obtained in the present study were on the same level as those reported by Boyd [8] and Verheyden and Nys [79].

6. Free Fatty Acids (FFA)

The most striking finding of this study was the marked differences seen in the plasma FFA levels, which were highest in the Japanese subjects born on the main island, followed by those born on Hokkaido, and lowest in the Ainu (Table 33). The

TABLE 33   Plasma levels of FFA in the winter

Group	No. Subj.	Age (average)	FFA, μEq/l (Mean ± SEM)
I Students (Sapporo) born on the main island	15	21–26 (22)	598 ± 23.0
II Students and professionals (Sapporo) born on Hokkaido	24	20–34 (23)	481 ± 29.5
III Policemen (Asahikawa)	15	21–40 (27)	376 ± 32.5
IV Farmers (Huren)	15	28–39 (35)	393 ± 29.5
V Farmers (Niikappu)	11	20–50 (33)	357 ± 25.5
VI Fishermen and fish factory workers (Monbetsu)	21	20–50 (38)	382 ± 37.3
II–VI Total	86	20–50 (31)	407 ± 14.8
vs I			P<0.001
VII Ainu (Asahikawa)	17	17–45 (28)	314 ± 26.5
VIII Ainu (Niikappu)	10	22–58 (42)	294 ± 41.0
VII + VIII Total	27	17–58 (33)	306 ± 22.2
vs I			P<0.001
vs II–VI			P<0.001

differences between these groups were highly significant. It is of particular interest that the plasma levels of FFA showed stepwise changes paralleled with the subjects experience in cold exposure. The lowest levels were found in subjects who were considered to be well adapted to cold, the highest in subjects who were not so adapted. A similar difference was seen in females between the Ainu (234 ± 34.2 μEq/l) and non-Ainu Japanese (394 ± 18.4 μEq/l) in the same district (Asahikawa). Moreover, considerably higher levels of plasma FFA, amounting 634 ± 33.0 μEq/l, were observed in four students born on Okinawa, located between Japan and Formosa. As shown in Table 34, fasting levels of plasma FFA in normal subjects have been reported to range between 470 and 750 μEq/l. The values of Sapporo students obtained in this study were in this range, but the Japanese in rural districts showed considerably lower levels and the Ainu had a very low average value of 306 μEq/l. This might be offset by a higher turnover of the plasma FFA in cold-adapted subjects.

It is necessary to mention that Niikappu Ainu are living under the same conditions, including diet, as the non-Ainu Japanese in the same village, but that the plasma FFA levels of the Ainu group were lower (294 ± 15.7 μEq/l) than those of the

TABLE 34   Plasma levels of FFA (μEq/l)

Source	Sex	No. subj.	FFA
Trout et al. [77]		12	584 $\pm$ 11.2 (S.E.)
Svanborg and Svennerholm [75]	M	62	750 $\pm$ 34 (S.E.)
	F	29	781 $\pm$ 45
Anstall and Trujillo [3]	M	24	540
	F	6	514
	Total	30	534
Björntorp et al. [7]		8	631 $\pm$ 150 (S.D.)
Stamp et al. [72]	M	50	575 $\pm$ 160 (S.D.)
De Caro et al. [15]		12	460 $\pm$ 26 (S.E.)
Reitsma [64]		17	570
Glennon et al. [25]	M	21	474 $\pm$ 39 (S.E.)
	F	21	484 $\pm$ 43
	Total	42	482 $\pm$ 29
Harlan et al. [29]		38	471 $\pm$ 38 (S.E.)
Marks et al. [57]		6	731

Japanese group (357 $\pm$ 25.5 μEq/l), and that the values of the Ainu were on the same level as observed in Asahikawa Ainu (314 $\pm$ 26.5 μEq/l). Therefore, the low levels of plasma FFA in the Ainu are not attributable to diet. Furthermore, we failed to detect significant difference in the plasma FFA levels between younger and older subjects in the present study. This excludes the possibility that age difference in the group causes appreciable variation in the plasma FFA concentrations.

BASAL METABOLIC RATE IN RELATION TO PLASMA FFA CONCENTRATION

Recently there has been much argument regarding seasonal variations of the BMR. Japanese investigators [61, 69, 82, 83] saw a significant elevation of the BMR in the winter, while American investigators noted little or no seasonal change [67]. Underlying mechanisms may be concerned with various factors, including living conditions, food intake, physical activities, and so on. The elevated thyroid activity in the winter was proposed as the principal cause of the increase in basal energy metabolism [82]. According to Rich et al. [65], an elevation in the BMR was accompanied by an increase in plasma FFA level in human subjects with hyperthyroidism. These authors stated that increased plasma FFA concentration reflects the accelerated mobilization of fat necessary to support the greater metabolic requirement of hyperthyroid subjects. The significant increase in basal plasma FFA concentration in hyperthyroid subjects was confirmed by Marks et al. [57], Harlan et al. [29] and Vinik et al. [80]. It was thought that there might be some positive relationship between BMR and plasma FFA level in normal men. To test this possible relation, a series of experiments were carried out on 27 students in Sapporo, 16 farmers in Huren, 21 fishermen and fish factory workers in Monbetsu and 23 Ainu in Asahikawa [38, 41, 42].

In the Sapporo students the average value of BMR in the winter was 41.2 $\pm$ 0.50 kcal/m². hr, while that shown in the summer was 36.3 $\pm$ 0.22 kcal (P<0.001). A similar significant seasonal difference was observed in the BMR of Huren farmers (43.9 $\pm$ 1.57 kcal/m². hr in winter; 35.7 $\pm$ 0.96 kcal in summer; P<0.001), though differences in the plasma FFA levels between winter and summer were not significant in these groups, due to large individual differences in the concentration. When the values of the BMR were plotted against the levels of plasma FFA, significant correlations were obtained. Fig. 120 shows the result in the Sapporo students. In this group the relationship was given as an equation, $Y = 0.0097 X + 33.8$ ($r = 0.546$, $P < 0.01$). Similar correlations were obtained in the Huren and Monbetsu subjects. For these groups the relations were given as $Y = 0.0217 X + 31.7$ ($r = 0.508$, $P < 0.05$) and $Y = 0.0147 X + 36.0$ ($r = 0.720$, $P < 0.01$), respectively. These findings apparently indicate that the BMR is related to the availability of FFA as metabolic fuel.

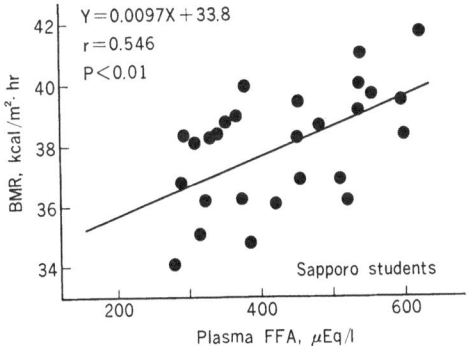

Fig. 120. Relation between BMR and plasma FFA concentration in Sapporo students.

However, it was surprising that the relationship was negative in the Ainu, as illustrated in Fig. 121. Here the correlation was given as $Y = -0.0158 X + 44.2$ ($r = -0.506$, $P < 0.05$). Namely, subjects who had lower levels of plasma FFA were found to show higher energy metabolism, and vice versa [18]. This may suggest that in the Ainu circulating FFA is very rapidly removed after it is mobilized from fat stores, bringing about a lowering of the plasma level, especially in subjects showing relatively high energy metabolism. Since the relationship of plasma FFA concentra-

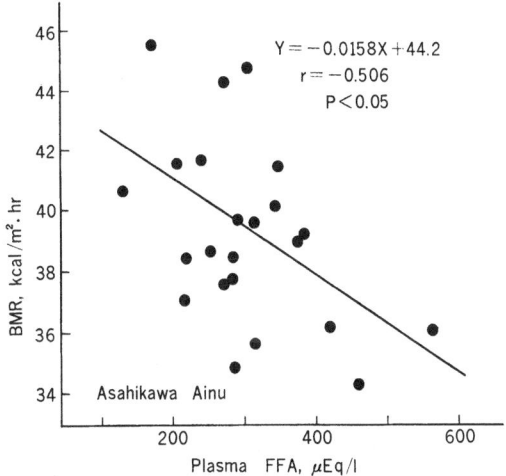

Fig. 121. Relation between BMR and plasma FFA concentration in Asahikawa Ainu.

tion to RQ was not significant in these subjects, it is unlikely that less FFA is utilized in subjects with low plasma FFA levels. The mean RQ values of 20 Ainu was 0.826 ± 0.0045, lower than the control values of the non-Ainu Japanese groups (0.843 ± 0.0043 in 14 Sapporo students; 0.840 ± 0.0055 in 21 Monbetsu fishermen and fish factory workers). It is suggested that the utilization of fat is not disturbed in the Ainu in spite of low plasma FFA concentration.

1. Effects of Nicotinic Acid

It is evident that the plasma level of FFA depends on the rate of FFA mobilization from adipose tissue and the rate of FFA removal from the blood or the oxidation of FFA. Nicotinic acid is known to lower the concentration of FFA in the plasma, but has no effect on the rate of its removal or oxidation [11, 12]. When the mobilization of FFA is inhibited by nicotinic acid, the plasma FFA concentration may reflect the rate of removal. Therefore, after administration of nicotinic acid the pattern of the BMR in relation to plasma FFA concentration in the Ainu might be different from that in the Japanese, if any difference exists in the rate of FFA utilization between these two groups. To elucidate this point the following experiment was performed on male volunteers; the subjects were eight students in Sapporo and 11 Ainu in Asahikawa [19].

The administration of nicotinic acid in an oral dose of 200 mg in fasting subjects produced a pronounced fall in the plasma FFA level. Changes in the BMR, RQ and in plasma FFA 60 minutes after administration were summarized in Table 35, where

TABLE 35   Effects of nicotinic acid on BMR, RQ, and plasma FFA concentration

Group	No. of subjects		BMR (kcal/m².hr)	RQ	FFA (μEq/1)
Japanese	8	Before	37.1 ± 0.67	0.82 ± 0.009	421 ± 48.6
		After	33.9 ± 0.52	0.86 ± 0.012	238 ± 16.1
Ainu	11	Before	39.2 ± 0.73	0.83 ± 0.006	310 ± 53.0
		After	33.9 ± 1.09	0.87 ± 0.010	180 ± 22.7

Mean $\pm$ SEM

the marked decrease in plasma FFA concentration is shown to be associated with a decrease in BMR and an increase in RQ. Although Havel *et al.* [30] reported that the basal energy metabolism was not altered by the lowered levels of plasma FFA after injection of nicotinic acid, a significant decrease in the BMR was observed in our subjects.

The correlation of BMR to plasma FFA concentration is shown in Fig. 122. In the Japanese subjects the values after nicotinic acid fit on the same regression line as that obtained with the values at rest. On the other hand, in the Ainu the values after nicotinic acid showed a very different distribution from those of the resting state. As illustrated in Fig. 123, a significant negative correlation was obtained; that is, in subjects who showed a relatively high metabolic rate after nicotinic acid the plasma FFA level was low, while subjects with a low metabolic rate showed a relatively high plasma FFA level.

From the results it was inferred that the rate of FFA oxidation depends upon its plasma concentration in the case of the non-Ainu Japanese, but that in the Ainu plasma FFA is likely to be oxidized effectively even when plasma concentration is

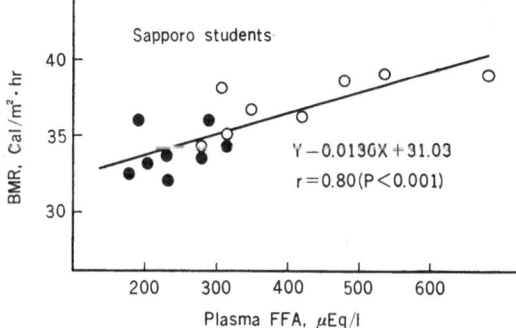

Fig. 122.   Effect of nicotinic acid on the relation between BMR and plasma FFA concentration in Sapporo students.

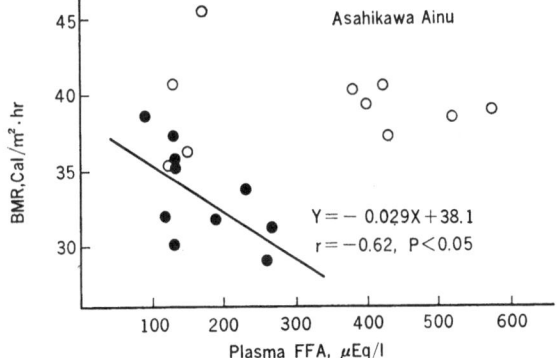

Fig. 123.   Effect of nicotinic acid on the relation between BMR and plasma FFA concentration in Asahikawa Ainu.

low.   It was interesting that in the Ainu the decrease of plasma FFA concentration was related to low RQ values (Fig. 124).   This suggests that lower concentration of plasma FFA reflects a higher rate of FFA utilization, maintaining a relatively high energy metabolism in subjects with a higher rate of FFA removal.   Moreover, since a greater decrease in BMR was associated with a higher elevation of RQ (Fig. 125), it would be inferred that a marked decrease in fat utilization is involved in the further reduction in the BMR.

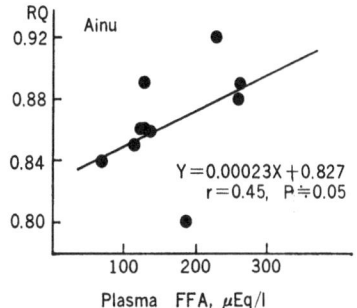

Fig. 124.   Effect of nicotinic acid on the relation between RQ and plasma FFA concentration in Asahikawa Ainu.

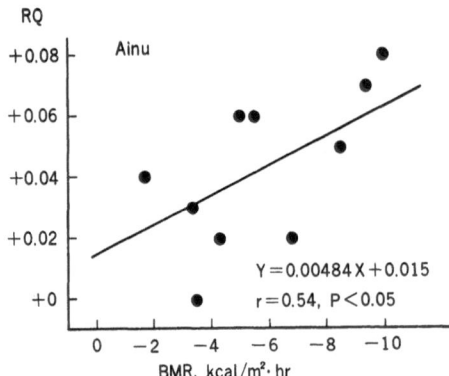

Fig. 125. Effect of nicotinic acid on the relation between increase in RQ and decrease in BMR.

EFFECTS OF NORADRENALINE

A striking sensitivity in cold-adapted rats to noradrenaline was demonstrated by Hsieh and Carlson [35] and confirmed by Depocas [17]. Further, white and wild rats kept outdoors were found to become more sensitive to noradrenaline during the winter [32, 33]. In man, Davis [14] suggested that cold acclimatization is accompanied by the development of nonshivering thermogenesis. Joy [46] found that noradrenaline produced a significant increase in oxygen consumption in cold-exposed men, and proposed that in man noradrenaline may be the direct mediator of nonshivering thermogenesis occurring with cold acclimatization. Budd and Warhaft [9] also observed the apparent development of a calorigenic response to noradrenaline in men after acclimatization to cold in Antarctica. According to Kang *et al.* [47], a slight calorigenic action caused by noradrenaline was demonstrated in the winter in Korean women divers who are daily exposed to severe cold water stress, while no significant changes were seen in controls. Consequently, it could be presumed that sensitivity to exogenous noradrenaline may be different among populations living under different climatic conditions. A higher sensitivity is expected to be observed in ethnic groups in cold areas. We attempted therefore to study sensitivity to noradrenaline in the Ainu, observing changes in metabolic rate, plasma FFA and total ketone body levels following injection of noradrenaline [37].

Three groups of subjects were used for this study. They were five students in Sapporo, 10 farmers in Huren, and six Ainu in Asahikawa. In the morning under basal conditions noradrenaline was injected subcutaneously in a dose of 0.025 mg/10 kg body weight in the Ainu and 0.025 and 0.05 mg/10 kg in the Japanese subjects.

As shown in Fig. 126, in the Ainu the injection of noradrenaline in a dose of 0.025 mg/10 kg produced a marked elevation in the energy metabolism from 40.6 $\pm$ 1.86 kcal/m². hr to 46.8 $\pm$ 1.77 (+15.3%) after 15 minutes and to 47.6 $\pm$ 1.47 (+17.2%) after 30 minutes, while in Sapporo students no change was effected by this dose of noradrenaline. When 0.05 mg/10 kg was injected into the Japanese subjects, the metabolic rate increased moderately. Percentages of the increment were 13.9% in Huren farmers and 4.1% in Sapporo students after 15 minutes and 8.7% and 9.7%, respectively, after 30 minutes.

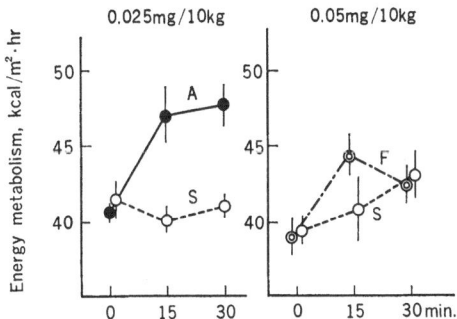

Fig. 126. Effect of noradrenaline on energy metabolism in Asahikawa Ainu (A), Sapporo students (S) and Huren farmers (F).

Plasma levels of FFA also markedly increased following the injection of noradrenaline in the Ainu (Fig. 127). The average concentration after 0.025 mg/10 kg (602 $\pm$ 53.7 μEq/l) was just double the initial level (301 $\pm$ 23.5 μEq/l). Although Sapporo students showed no increase in the plasma FFA due to this dose of noradrenaline, a higher dose of 0.05 mg/10 kg caused a significant elevation. Huren farmers responded to this dose as Sapporo students did (Fig. 127).

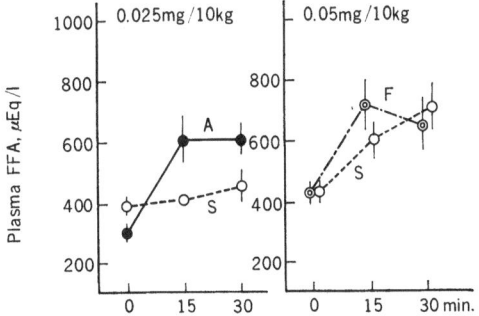

Fig. 127. Effect of noradrenaline on plasma FFA concentration in Asahikawa Ainu (A), Sapporo students (S) and Huren farmers (F).

Plasma levels of total ketone bodies in the fasting state were very high in the Ainu (1107 $\pm$ 86.0 μM/l) compared with the levels in the Japanese groups (586 $\pm$ 32.7 μM/l in Huren farmers; 778 $\pm$ 38.8 μM/l in Sapporo students). Injection of noradrenaline in a dose of 0.025 mg/10 kg caused a marked increase in the plasma ketone bodies to 1526 $\pm$ 64.8 μM/l after 15 minutes and to 1370 $\pm$ 52.1 after 30 minutes in the Ainu. On the other hand, in the non-Ainu Japanese groups the plasma concentration showed only a slight increase even after 0.05 mg/10 kg of noradrenaline (Fig. 128).

The effect of different doses of noradrenaline was also examined in the Ainu. However, injection of 0.01 mg/10 kg had no significant effect and 0.05 mg/10 kg produced marked subjective ill effects, for instance feelings of tightness in the chest and apprehension, weakness, numbness and/or heaviness in the extremities, pallor of the face, and so on. Increased rate and depth of the respiration and extra-systoles were

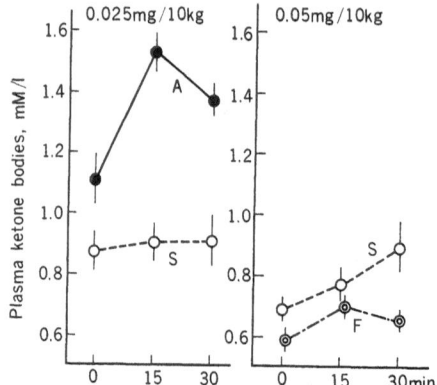

Fig. 128. Effect of noradrenaline on plasma total ketone bodies in Asahikawa Ainu (A), Sapporo students (S) and Huren farmers (F).

also noticed. Therefore, the study could not be carried through. In the Japanese subjects such ill effects were slight and scarce even after higher doses of noradrenaline.

A small dose of noradrenaline which was ineffective in the non-Ainu Japanese groups, was shown to produce marked elevations in the metabolic rate and plasma levels of FFA and total ketone bodies in the Ainu. These intense responses to exogenous noradrenaline might be concerned with inherent cold adaptability. It was suggested that this ethnic group is equipped with an adaptative mechanism characterized by noradrenaline-sensitive thermogenesis.

It has been shown that the calorigenic effect of noradrenaline is related to its FFA mobilizing action [74]. However, it is questionable whether the FFA mobilization is essential for the calorigenic effect, or whether the calorigenic action is only partially dependent on the simultaneous FFA mobilization [73]. Hsieh *et al.* [36] suggested that noradrenaline may stimulate the oxidation of fatty acids as well as lipolysis. According to the present theory, it is likely that noradrenaline elicits an increase in the oxygen consumption via two mechanisms, that is, by providing the substrate to support the effect and more directly by stimulating the oxidation of fatty acids, although no evidence is available for the latter concept. The striking elevation of plasma ketone bodies as well as the significant increase in plasma FFA following noradrenaline injection in the Ainu may suggest that the catecholamine not only stimulates the mobilization of FFA but accelerates the oxidation of FFA.

Although presently the anatomical sites and the biochemical mechanisms responsible for the nonshivering thermogenesis mediated by noradrenaline remain unknown, Hannon *et al.* [27] suggested that the liver might be a primary site of heat production during noradrenaline calorigenesis, while Depocas [16, 17] showed that the muscle may play a principal part in nonshivering thermogenesis. Further, the increased sensitivity to noradrenaline seen in cold-acclimated rats might be attributable to the enhanced thermogenic activity of hypertrophied brown adipose tissue. Not only in cold-acclimated rodents, but in a wide range of newborn mammals, including kittens [58], piglets [51], lambs [2, 76] and babies [48], a direct calorigenic action of noradrenaline was seen by a number of investigators. The increased response to the catecholamine in the newborn animals could be, at least in part, attributable to the noradrenaline stimulation on brown adipose tissue. In human adults the occurrence of brown adipose tissue is questionable. However, the striking responses to noradrenaline in the Ainu suggest that this ethnic group is possibly equipped with an adaptative mechanism characterized by noradrenaline-sensitive thermogenesis. The problem of ethnic differences in the distribution and development of brown adipose tissue in man should be examined in further experiments.

When the relation of energy metabolism to plasma FFA concentration was examined before and after noradrenaline injection in the above experiment, a significant positive correlation was proved not only in the control Japanese groups but also in the Ainu. Fig. 129 shows the results obtained from Sapporo students as an example. The figure indicates that the noradrenaline-induced increase of energy metabolism is supported by the increase in plasma FFA as metabolic substrate. However, in the Ainu

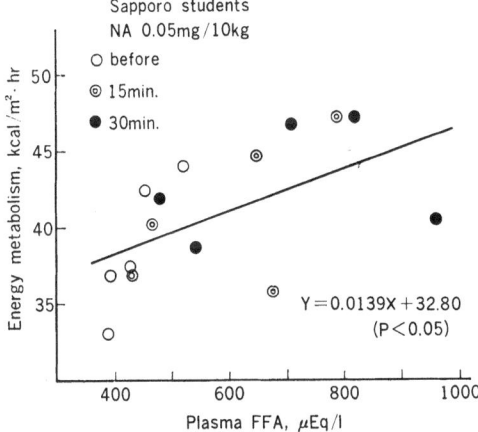

Fig. 129. Relation between energy metabolism and plasma FFA concentration before and after noradrenaline injection in Sapporo students.

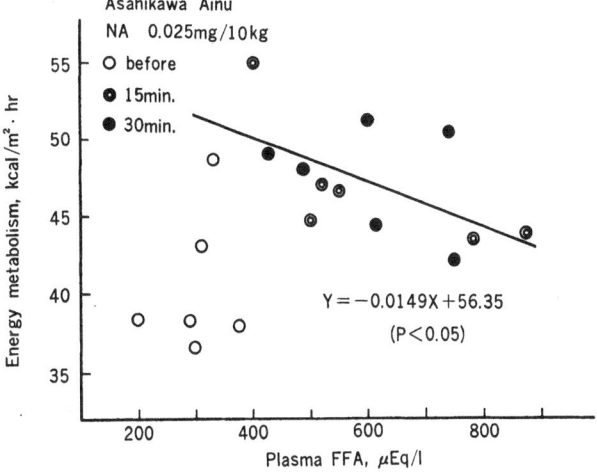

Fig. 130. Relation between energy metabolism and plasma FFA concentration after noradrenaline injection in Asahikawa Ainu.

when values of energy metabolism after noradrenaline were plotted against plasma FFA concentration, a negative correlation was obtained, as shown in Fig. 130. This may suggest that faster oxidation of FFA is related to raising of the metabolism.

In this connection, it is interesting to cite a report of Hsieh *et al.* [36]. They found a positive correlation between the elevation of plasma FFA concentration and an increase in oxygen consumption after noradrenaline infusion in warm-adapted rats, while in cold-adapted rats the relation was negative. The observation that an increase in oxygen consumption was associated with a decrease in plasma FFA in cold-adapted rats might be compatible with the present finding in the Ainu.

EFFECT OF WHOLE BODY COLD EXPOSURE

Biochemical changes in response to acute cold exposure were observed in nude subjects who were immersed in a cold water bath for 30 minutes. The subjects were 6 Asahikawa Ainu and 6 Huren farmers. The water temperature was 23 °C for the Ainu and 25 °C for the control Japanese. This study was done in the autumn.

Energy metabolism increased markedly in both groups. In Huren farmers the resting level was 39.6 ± 1.04 kcal/m². hr; it increased to 52.0 ± 5.10 kcal after 15 minutes and to 69.5 ± 7.68 kcal after 30 minutes at 25 °C. In the Ainu the metabolic rate increased from 39.4 ± 1.55 kcal to 62.4 ± 2.91 kcal after 30 minutes at 23 °C. Although the water temperature was lower in the Ainu's experiment than in the farmers' experiment, the increase in metabolism was almost the same or greater among the Japanese.

In Huren farmers plasma FFA increased markedly from 402 ± 44.5 μEq/l to 635 ± 83.5, while blood sugar decreased from 79 ± 4.5 mg/100 ml to 68 ± 2.8. On the other hand, in the Ainu plasma FFA increased only slightly from 252 ± 20.2 μEq/l to 336 ± 35.4 and no change was observed in the blood sugar level. Plasma ketone

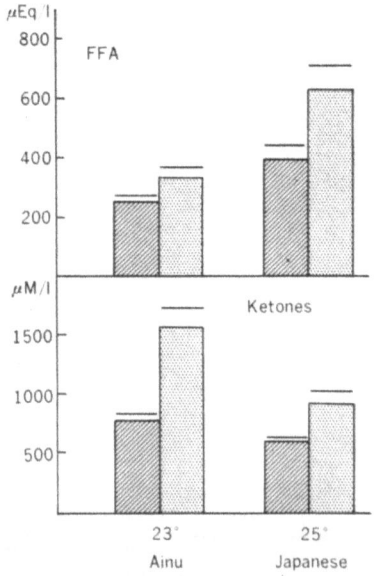

Fig. 131. Effects of whole body immersion in a cold water bath on plasma FFA and total ketone body levels in Asahikawa Ainu and Huren farmers. Oblique-lined columns show the levels before and dotted ones after the cold exposure.

bodies increased 102 percent in the Ainu, but only 50 percent in the control Japanese. Values were from 786 ± 44.0 μM/l to 1587 ± 147.6 in the Ainu and from 617 ± 36.4 to 925 ± 119.3 in the Japanese. Namely, in the Ainu a greater increase in plasma ketone bodies was associated with a smaller increase in plasma FFA (Fig. 131).

PLASMA KETONE BODIES

Several factors are known to affect ketosis [63]. Exposure to cold has been shown to increase the production of ketones [66, 68]. Johnson et al. [45] showed significant seasonal differences in the urinary excretion of ketone bodies in man, but the concentration in the serum was not different between winter and summer. Lloyd [54] measured total ketone body excretion rate on young men spending a year in the Antarctic, and found that there was no evidence of adaptation to sledging ketosis even after 7 months continuous sledging in the field. He noted, however, that energy expenditure, negative caloric balance and degree of cold exposure were all positively and independently associated with total ketone body excretion rate. Muir [59] also measured the excretion rate of total ketone bodies in men during winter sledging activities in Antarctica. According to this author, some acclimatization might have occurred, since a low excretion rate of ketone bodies was observed on the last and coldest journey. The possibility that cold acclimatization may prevent ketosis by an increased capacity to utilize ketone bodies, was suggested by Hanson and Johnson [28]. They exposed semi-nude men to 0 °C for 90 minutes once a week for three weeks. In the first week there was an increase in plasma ketones during the cold exposure, but plasma ketones did not increase during the second and third weeks. Further investigations may determine whether biochemical adaptation occurs in the metabolism of ketone bodies in man.

In the Ainu it was demonstrated that high level of ketone bodies in the plasma appeared to be associated with low plasma FFA (Table 36). The low plasma FFA

TABLE 36 Fasting levels of plasma FFA and ketone bodies

Group	No. of subjects	FFA (μEq/1)	Ketones (μM/1)
Farmers (Huren)	10	419 ± 35.9	612 ± 27
Students (Sapporo)	17	421 ± 15.6	695 ± 43
Policemen (Asahikawa)	14	376 ± 32.5	680 ± 63
Fishermen and fish factory workers (Monbetsu)	21	382 ± 37.3	528 ± 42
Ainu (Asahikawa)	11	285 ± 16.7	1063 ± 107

Mean ± SEM

might be, at least in part, a result of the high level of ketone bodies which may inhibit the mobilization of FFA from fat stores [4, 5, 6, 31, 44, 71]. However, this inference may not be the case with the Ainu, since a marked noradrenaline stimulation increasing plasma FFA concentration was observed together with a pronounced elevation in plasma ketone bodies (Figs. 127 and 128). Fig. 132 also shows a striking increase of ketone bodies and concomitant increase in the plasma FFA after administration of noradrenaline in the Ainu.

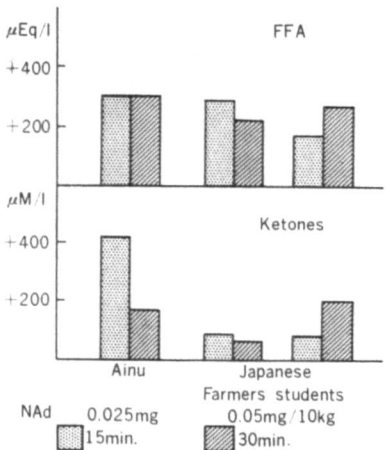

Fig. 132. Changes in plasma FFA and total ketone bodies after noradrenaline injection in Asahikawa Ainu, Huren farmers and Sapporo students. Dose of noradrenaline was 0.025 mg/10 kg body weight in the Ainu and 0.05 mg/10 kg in the non-Ainu Japanese.

Ketone bodies have been shown to be a substrate of respiration and their presence in the circulating blood serves to supply tissues with fuel for respiration. Their function in this respect is analogous to that of glucose and FFA [50, 81]. On the basis of this concept, a good correlation between energy metabolism and plasma ketone body level would be expected. In fact, the correlation between these parameters was significantly positive among Sapporo students and fishermen and fish factory workers in Monbetsu. The relation was also exmained with the values obtained after noradrenaline injection. A straight line correlation was obtained in Sapporo students, but not in Huren farmers. The relation was found highly significant in the Ainu, as indicated in Fig. 133. A similar positive correlation was also obtained in the Ainu in the case of the cold water bath, but no relation was seen in the control Japanese subjects. This may suggest that the ketone bodies are possibly utilized more effectively

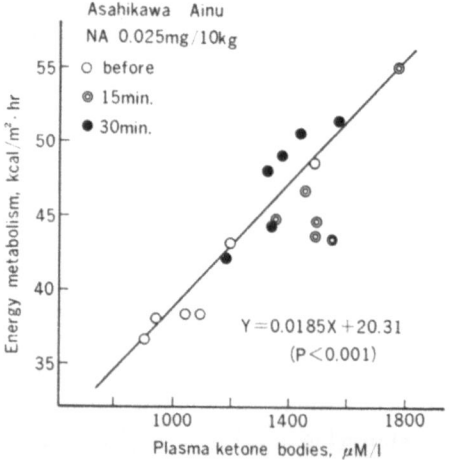

Fig. 133. Relation between energy metabolism and plasma total ketone bodies before and after noradrenaline injection in Asahikawa Ainu.

as metabolic fuel in the Ainu. Therefore, it would be assumed that fat is utilized more in the form of ketone bodies than in the form of FFA in this ethnic group.

SUMMARY

In the winter plasma lipid concentrations were determined under basal conditions on several groups of healthy male subjects, including two groups of Ainus. No appreciable differences were found in the concentrations of total lipids, triglycerides, phospholipids, total and free cholesterol and esterified fatty acids among the groups studied. The most striking finding was marked differences seen in the plasma FFA which were highest in non-Ainu Japanese subjects born on main island of Japan, followed by those born on Hokkaido, and lowest in the Ainu. A similar difference was also found between Ainu and non-Ainu Japanese females. It is likely that the plasma levels of FFA are low in subjects who are well adapted to cold and high in subjects who are not exposed to cold.

Under basal conditions a significant positive correlation was found between energy metabolism and plasma FFA concentration in Japanese groups, while the relation was negative in the Ainu. Administration of nicotinic acid which inhibits the mobilization of FFA from fat stores caused a decrease in the plasma FFA with concomitant decrease in BMR and increase in RQ. In the Japanese, the values of BMR after nicotinic acid in relation to plasma FFA fit on the same regression line as obtained with values at rest. On the other hand, in the Ainu values after nicotinic acid showed quite different patterns from those observed in the resting state. Here again a significant negative correlation was found when values of BMR after nicotinic acid were plotted against plasma FFA determined simultaneously.

A small dose of noradrenaline which was insufficient to produce any effects in the Japanese caused marked increases in the oxygen consumption and plasma levels of FFA and ketone bodies in the Ainu. The striking sensitivity to noradrenaline of the Ainu suggests that this ethnic group is possibly equipped with an adaptative mechanism characterized by noradrenaline-sensitive thermogenesis.

Immersion of the whole body in a cold water bath at 23°C for 30 minutes produced an increase in energy metabolism in the Ainu similar to or slightly less than the increase shown by the Japanese subjects immersed at 25°C. In the water bath the Ainu showed a small elevation of plasma FFA and a marked increase in plasma ketone bodies, while the control Japanese showed a pronounced increment in plasma FFA and a small rise of plasma ketones.

Under basal conditions plasma ketone body levels were significantly higher in the Ainu than in the non-Ainu Japanese, in contrast with the low levels of plasma FFA in the former group. Moreover, in the Ainu, plasma ketone bodies showed a pronounced elevation after noradrenaline and acute cold exposure, and a highly significant correlation was found between energy metabolism and plasma ketone bodies after noradrenaline administration and cold exposure. It was inferred that the ketone bodies may be effectively utilized as metabolic fuel in this ethnic group.

The above mentioned findings in the Ainu may indicate general features of cold-adapted men, but it is also possible that the observed biochemical characteristics might be specific to the Ainu. Further investigation is necessary to decide this point.

REFERENCES

1. ADLERSBERG, D., L.E. SCHAEFER, A.G. STEINBERG, and C.I. WANG (1956): *J.A.M.A.* **162**: 619.
2. ALEXANDER, G., and D. WILLIAMS (1968): *J. Physiol.* **198**: 251.
3. ANSTALL, H.B., and J.M. TRUJILLO (1965): *Clin. Chem.* **11**: 741.
4. BALASSE, E., and H.A. OOMS (1968): *Diabetologia* **4**: 133.
5. BJÖRNTORP, P. (1966): *Am. J. Physiol.* **210**: 733; *J. Lipid Res.* **7**: 621; *Metabolism* **15**: 191.
6. BJÖRNTORP, P. and T. SCHERSTEN (1967): *Am. J. Physiol.* **212**: 683.
7. BJÖRNTORP, P., A. JONSSON, and B. HOOD (1965): *Acta Med. Scand.* **178**: 175.
8. BOYD, E.M. (1942): *J. Biol. Chem.* **143**: 131.
9. BUDD, G.M., and N. WARHAFT (1966): *J. Physiol.* **186**: 233.
10. CARLSON, L.A. (1960): *Acta Med. Scand.* **167**: 377.
11. CARLSON, L.A., R.J. HAVEL, L.G. EKELUND, and A. HOLMGREN (1963): *Metabolism* **12**: 837.
12. CARLSON, L.A., and L. ORÖ (1962): *Acta Med. Scand.* **172**: 641.
13. CRAMER, K. (1962): *Acta Med. Scand.* **171**: 413.
14. DAVIS, T.R.A. (1961): *J. appl. Physiol.* **16**: 1011.
15. DE CARO, L.G., A. FATTORINI, and M. GORINI (1966): *Metabolism* **15**: 65.
16. DEPOCAS, F. (1958): *Can. J. Biochem. Physiol.* **36**: 691.
17. DEPOCAS, F. (1960): *Can. J. Biochem. Physiol.* **38**: 107.
18. DOI, K., A. KUROSHIMA, and S. ITOH (1969): *J. Physiol. Soc. Japan* **31**: 672.
19. DOI, K., A. KUROSHIMA, and S. ITOH (1969): *J. Physiol. Soc. Japan* **31**: 705.
20. DUNN, J.P., and C. MOSES. (1965): *Metabolism* **14**: 787.
21. FELDMAN, E.B., P. BENKEL, and R.V. NAYAK (1963): *J. Lab. Clin. Med.* **62**: 437.
22. FRIEDMAN, M., R.H. ROSEMAN, and V. CARROL (1958): *Circulation* **17**: 852.
23. FURMAN, R.H., R.P. HOWARD, K. LAKSHMI and L.N. NORCIA (1961): *Am. J. Clin. Nutr.* **9**: 73.
24. GJONE, E., and O.M. ORNING (1966): *J. Clin. Lab. Invest.* **18**: 209.
25. GLENNON, J.A., W.J. BRECH, and E.S. GORDON (1967): *Metabolism* **16**: 503.
26. HALLGREN, B., S. STENHAGEN, A. SVANBORG., and L. SVENNERHOLM (1960): *J. Clin. Invest.* **39**: 1424.
27. HANNON, J.P., E. EVONUK, and A.M. LARSON (1963): *Feder. Proc.* **22**: 783.
28. HANSON, P.G., and R.E. JOHNSON (1965): *J. appl. Physiol.* **20**: 56.
29. HARLAN, W.R., J. LASZLO, M.D. BODDONOFF, and E.H. ESTES (1960): *Metabolism* **9**: 1133.
30. HAVEL, R.J., I.A. CARLSON, L.G. EKELUND, and A. HOLMGREN (1964): *Metabolism* **13**: 1402.
31. HELLMAN, D.E., B. SENIOR, and H.M. GOODMAN (1969): *Metabolism* **18**: 906.
32. HÉROUX, O. (1961): *Can. J. Biochem. Physiol.* **39**: 1929.
33. HÉROUX, O. (1962): *Can. J. Biochem. Physiol.* **40**: 537.
34. HICKS, K.E. (1967): *Clin. Sci.* **33**: 527.
35. HSIEH, A.C.L., and L.D. CARLSON (1957): *Am. J. Physiol.* **190**: 243.
36. HSIEH, A.C.L., C.W. PUN, K.M. LI, and K.W. TI (1966): *Feder. Proc.* **25**: 1205.
37. ITOH, S., K. DOI, and A. KUROSHIMA (1970): *Int. J. Biometeorol.* **14**: 195.
38. ITOH, S., K. DOI, A. KUROSHIMA, and R. OTA (1967): *J. Physiol. Soc. Japan* **29**: 700.
39. ITOH, S., K. DOI, A. KUROSHIMA, I. WAKABAYASHI, and C. OGURA (1968): *J. Physiol. Soc. Japan* **30**: 181.
40. ITOH, S., N. KONNO, K. YOSHIMURA, A. KUROSHIMA, and H. IKEMOTO (1967): *J. Physiol. Soc. Japan* **29**: 266.
41. ITOH, S., A. KUROSHIMA, K. DOI, K. MORIYA, H. SHIRATO, and K. YOSHIMURA (1969): *Feder. Proc.* **28**: 960.
42. ITOH, S., A. KUROSHIMA, K. DOI, and K. YOSHIMURA (1968): *J. Physiol. Soc. Japan* **30**: 483.
43. ITOH, S., A. KUROSHIMA, K. DOI, K. YOSHIMURA, and K. MORIYA (1969): *Japan. J. Physiol.* **19**: 233.
44. JENKINS, D.J.A. (1967): *Lancet* **II**: 338.
45. JOHNSON, R.E., F. SARGENT II, and R. PASSMORE (1958): *Quart. J. Exp. Physiol.* **43**: 339.
46. JOY, R.J.T. (1963): *J. appl. Physiol.* **18**: 1209.
47. KANG, B.S., D.S. HAN, K.S. PAIK, Y.S. PARK, J.K. KIM, C.S. KIM, D.W. RENNIE, and S.K. HONG (1970): *J. appl. Physiol.* **29**: 6.
48. KARLSBERG, P., R.E. MOORE, and T.K. OLIVER (1962): *Acta Pediat.* **51**: 284.
49. KOMATSU, S. (1960): *Nisshin Igaku* **47**: 449 (in Japanese).
50. KREBS, H.A. (1961): *Biochem. J.* **80**: 225.
51. LEBLANC, J., and L.E. MOUNT (1968): *Nature* **217**: 77.
52. LEFFLER, H.H., and C.H. McDOUGALD (1963): *Am. J. Clin. Path.* **39**: 311.
53. LEWIS, L.A., F. OLMSTED, I.H. PAGE, E.Y. LAWRY, G.V. MANN, F.J. STARE, M. HANIG, M.A. LAUFFER, T. GORDON, and F.E. MOORE (1957): *Circulation* **16**: 227.

54. LLOYD, R.M. (1969): *Br. Antarc. Sur. Bull.* **20**: 59.
55. LUND, J.C., E. SILVERTSSEN, and H.C. GODAL (1961): *Acta Med. Scand.* **169**: 623.
56. MAGER, M., and P.F. IAMPIETRO (1966): *Metabolism* **15**: 9.
57. MARKS, B.H., I. LIEM, and A.G. HILLS (1960): *Metabolism* **9**: 1133.
58. MOORE, R.E., and M.C. UNDERWOOD (1963): *J. Physiol.* **168**: 290.
59. MUIR, A.L. (1969): *Br. Antarc. Sur. Bull.* **20**: 53.
60. OKINAKA, S. (1965): *Jap. Circul. J.* **29**: 505.
61. OGATA, K., T. SASAKI, and N. MURAKAMI (1966): *Bull Inst. Const. Med. Kumamoto Univ.* **16**: suppl.
62. OYAMA, K., H. UZAWA, M. MATSUDA, and K. IMAICHI (1965): *Jap. Circul. J.* **29**: 937.
63. PASSMORE, R. (1961): *Lancet* **II**: 839.
64. REITSMA, W.D. (1967): *Acta Med. Scand.* **182**: 353.
65. RICH, C., E.L. BIERMAN, and I.L. SCHWARTZ (1959): *J. Clin. Invest.* **38**: 275.
66. SARGENT, F. II, and C.F. CONSOLAZIO (1951): *Science* **113**: 631.
67. SARGENT, F. II, and S. ITOH (1965): *Science* **147**: 761.
68. SARGENT, F. II, R.E. JOHNSON, E. ROBBINS, and L. SAWYER (1958): *Quart. J. Exp. Physiol.* **43**: 345.
69. SASAKI, T. (1966): *Feder. Proc.* **25**: 1163.
70. SCHWARTZ, D., E. PATOIS, and J.L. BEAUMONT (1967): *J. Atheroscl. Res.* **7**: 537.
71. SENIOR, B., and L. LORIDAN (1968): *Nature* **219**: 83.
72. STAMP, T.C.B., J. LANDON, and V. WYNN (1965): *Metabolism* **14**: 1041.
73. STEINBERG, D. (1966): *Pharmacol. Rev.* **18**: 217.
74. STEINBERG, D., P.J. NESTEL, E.R. BUSKIRK, and R.H. THOMPSON (1964): *J. Clin. Invest.* **43**: 167.
75. SVANBORG, A., and L. SVENNERHOLM (1961): *Acta Med. Scand.* **167**: 43.
76. THOMPSON, G.E., and D.M.E. JENKINSON (1969): *Can. J. Physiol. Pharmacol.* **47**: 249.
77. TROUT, D.L., E.H. ESTER, JR., and S.J. FRIEDBERG (1960): *J. Lipid Res.* **1**: 199.
78. VAN HANDEL, E., and D.B. ZILVERSMIT (1957): *J. Lab. Clin. Med.* **50**: 152.
79. VERHEYDEN, J., and J. NYS (1962): *Clin. Chim. Acta* **7**: 262.
80. VINIK, A.I., B.L. PIMSTONE and R. HOFFENBERG (1970): *Metabolism* **19**: 93.
81. WILLIAMSON, J.R., and H.A. KREBS (1961): *Biochem. J.* **80**: 540.
82. YOSHIMURA, H. (1960): Essential Problems in Climatic Physiology. ed. H. YOSHIMURA, K. OGATA, and S. ITOH (eds.), Nankodo, Kyoto, 61.
83. YOSHIMURA, M., K. YUKIYOSHI, T. YOSHIOKA, and H. TAKEDA (1966): *Feder. Proc.* **25**: 1169.

PART IV

SEASONAL AND CIRCADIAN VARIATIONS OF PHYSIOLOGICAL ACTIVITIES

CHAPTER 18

CHRONOBIOLOGY OF THE LIFE SEQUENCE*

MICHAEL SMOLENSKY,[1] FRANZ HALBERG,[2] AND
FREDERICK SARGENT II[3]

[1] School of Public Health, The University of Texas, Houston, Texas
[2] Chronobiology Laboratories, University of Minnesota, Minneapolis, Minnesota
[3] Huxley College for Environmental Sciences, Western Washington State College,
Bellingham, Washington

"The temporal development of happenings is a fundamental characteristic of biological processes." Indeed, "life is finite for the individual, and between birth and death there are circadian and circannual cycles as well as growth, maturation and senility" [206].

For one interested in the ecology of health and disease, population rhythms provide a rich body of data from which to examine interactions between organism and environment. When these rhythms are quantified, a foundation is laid for further work involving phase-shifting and other procedures so that deeper understanding of the time-dimensions of organisms emerges.

One approach to uncovering these interactions is through study of time series summarizing human morbidity and mortality. Statistics on the temporal distribution of death have long been available. More recently, reliable information on the occurrence of cardiovascular and respiratory illness within the span of a day or year has also been published. In addition, data are available on physiologic changes in factors thought to be related to such population rhythms. From statistics reported earlier in tables or graphs summarizing illness and death as well as birth in human populations, bio-periodicities have been documented along two environmental time scales—24 hours and 12 months.

Such information gains in interest from recent findings in keeping with the assumption that certain about-yearly rhythms of man [92] and of an experimental mammal [104] represent at least partly endogenous spectral components with a period near one year. In other words, such rhythms may occur in the absence of those environmental or societal factors acting possibly as forcing functions upon a natural circannual period, i.e., as synchronizers, modulators or influencers [88].

Against the background of renewed interest in circannual rhythms, it seemed desirable to analyze objectively pertinent statistics on certain aspects of human birth and death by least squares spectral and cosinor electronic computer programs [92, 100]. These programs, which already have yielded reliably reproducible endpoints for a number of rhythmic variables of man [171], can reduce raw data from time series to chrono-

*Supported by grants from the CIC Biometeorology Graduate Program (NAPCA Training Grant 5-TI-AP16), the United States Public Health Service (5-K6-GM-13, 981), NASA (NAS 2-2738 and NGR-24-005-006) and the United States Air Force (Contract F29600-69-C-0011).

biologic profiles so that statistically significant [100] rhythms can be detected. Such methods were employed to obtain a complete and objective summary and comparison of several circadian and circannual population rhythms in natality, morbidity and mortality of man using statistics reported in the literature over the last 150 years.

METHODS

1. Data Acquisition

For methods used in collecting the information on population rhythms for this study, the reader must refer to the original articles. Deficiencies in techniques of data collection or medical diagnoses by various authors are real concerns and must not be ignored; but, for our purposes they have been classified as "noise." Noise, in this sense then, represents effects of any and all chance influences—chance being defined as the sum total of sources of variation due to unknown or uncontrolled factors.

One example of the difficulties encountered in interpreting what on the surface appear to be clear-cut diagnoses relates to certain reports dealing with the incidence of acute myocardial infarction confirmed by means of the ECG or, in the event of death, by autopsy. First, not all acute myocardial infarctions are detected by the electrocardiogram. Even the extensive blood enzyme studies now carried out do not detect all infarctions and may fail to reveal one that has been detected by ECG [64, 65, 109, 116, 134, 140, 240, 241, 256]. Second, death certificates are not standardized and vary greatly as a function of locality, century or even decade. Furthermore, the accuracy of such documents vary with the level of competence and motivation of those filling them out and the criteria used for "cause of death."

Further, heterogeneity has been introduced by the circumstance that the original sources of statistics range from government reports to private medical records which include hospital or physicians' files as well as death certificates. The latter documents provide data that are not completely satisfactory for comparative purposes. Statistics on birth or death reported in various publications were collected in geographic areas and over spans of time differing from one study to the next and have been summarized at intervals which range from one to six hours, on the one hand, to one day or longer, on the other. In the case of circannual rhythms, often both time of day and exact calendar date are ignored. With but few exceptions authors report statistics as totals for consecutive individual months over a single year. In a few instances the span of time ranged from 22 to 150 months.

Problems inherent in the utilization of official documents such as birth records have been discussed by Kaiser and Halberg [122]. For instance, bias is introduced into the study of circadian rhythms by the human preference for listing even (rather than odd) hours. Again, births or deaths that occur within a few hours of a new day may not be assigned to the actual clock hour of their occurrence but rather to an hour before or after midnight; thus, secondary crests encountered around midnight in some samples may in part reflect this not uncommon practice.

Statistics from early reports might also be questioned in that reliable timepieces may not have been always readily accessible. Nonetheless, the temporal incidence of birth and death given in reports from the past century agrees surprisingly well, at least in phase, with results of studies carried out as much as 150 years later.

Such agreement is the more noteworthy since clock hours and/or dates on official records serve merely as an approximation of the population system-phase of a circadian or circannual rhythm. Indeed, any change as a function of recorded clock hour or calendar date regarded as statistically significant presupposes that individuals constituting a given sample are more or less synchronized in terms of both the frequency and phase of their rhythms. Unless the given members are so synchronized, differing frequencies and/or phases of the individual rhythms will obliterate the rhythm as a group phenomenon.

This point applies even to events such as birth or death that, for the individual, are unique events revealing rhythmicity solely when approached as group phenomena. This same consideration is equally pertinent for single variables that can be followed on individuals by repeated or even continuous sampling. It can be clearly documented how differences in frequency and/or phase of individual curves representing separate subjects may obscure or at least reduce the extent of any regular change in the average values derived from samples as a whole. Moreover, samples from individuals who are frequency-synchronized can consist of sub-groups with dissimilar phases because of the diversity of social synchronizers. When this is the case, the same time of day may not reflect identical circadian-system-phases in different samples nor a given calendar date signify the same stage of a circannual rhythm. Thus, reliance on external time references—clock hour or calendar day—rather than internal ones, can complicate and confound rhythm detection and quantification.

In addition to the forementioned considerations, differences in antecedents of a given event are equally pertinent. One might indeed presume that among population rhythms those of birth are less "noisy" than rhythms in sickness or death; that is, diagnosis of illness and/or of the cause of death might not always be made without uncertainty. The diagnosis of natural birth obviously is unambiguous; yet, the occurrence of births along the scale of one year may be subject to a bias of a different kind: religious (sexual abstinence during Lent, for example), schedules of taxation and work and other societal factors can drastically influence the times of conception and hence of birth as well.

2. Data Processing

Values found in the literature were first transferred to punched cards. Detection of circadian or circannual rhythms was then explored by fitting cosine curves of appropriate length to individual time series by the method of least squares [92]. If rhythms were demonstrable, an objective quantification and description of their characteristics were attempted by the same curve fitting and, when possible, by added steps.

A rhythm detected by curve fitting can be described by several endpoints. One of these is a rhythm-adjusted level, C_0. For data reported as totals at 30-day intervals, the C_0 is comparable to a monthly average; for data given at hourly intervals, it is comparable to the 60-minute mean.

The amplitude, C, another characteristic of the rhythm, is a measure of the extent of change predictable by the approximation used. Herein, the C obtained by the fit of a 365.25-day or a 24-hour cosine curve approximates the extent of rhythmic within-year or within-day change. The computative acrophase ϕ, in its turn, is an index locating (in time) the peak of the cosine function found to best approximate the rhythm.

Waveform, another aspect of rhythms, was determined in the following manner. Initially amplitude, C, and acrophase, ϕ, values were obtained from separate time series by the method of least squares for each of the first seven harmonics in the case of circadian rhythms and for the first five harmonics in the case of circannual rhythms. Second, amplitude and acrophase pairs [(C, ϕ)'s] from individual time series were tested for statistical significance (P<.05) by cosinor, described below, separately for each harmonic. Third, individual curves, each representing significant harmonics validated by cosinor, were summed over corresponding clock hours or calendar months to give the overall waveform. This methodology differs from the periodic regression technique previously developed by Bliss [19] in which the statistical significance of added harmonics is tested by analyses of variance; each additional harmonic accounting for 90% or more of the remaining variance is included as a component of the waveform. Nonetheless, as it will be seen in later sections, the techniques employed by us adequately represent and reproduce the waveform characteristics of human population rhythms.

Detection and quantification of circannual rhythms were carried out by fitting a set of curves with periods in the region of 365.25 $\pm$ 20 days to time series covering spans of one year or longer by the method of least squares. In these analyses by a Varian 620 electronic computer,* the interval between consecutive trial periods was chosen linear in period and equated to one day. For the case of circadian rhythms, the periods chosen were in the region of 24.0 $\pm$ 4.0 hours, with the interval between consecutive trials chosen linear in period and equated to 0.1 hours. Upon completion of such spectral windows, the parameters C_0, C and ϕ (and their corresponding dispersion indices) were examined at the 365.25-day period for the yearly data and at 24.0 hours for time series covering a single day.

When only a single time series was available, the ratio between the standard error (SE) of the C and the C itself (the SE/C) was used for tentative rhythm detection. Thus, one tested the rhythm by the statistical significance of its amplitude. The SE/C also served to estimate the confidence arc of the acrophase [92].

When three or more comparable time series were available, results of least squares spectral analysis were summarized by cosinor [100]. A cosinor detects a rhythm if, at a given test frequency such as one cycle in 24.0 hours, separate time series constituting a sample exhibit similar acrophases and amplitudes. A rhythm thus substantiated at an acceptable level of statistical significance (P<.05) is described by a sample average level, amplitude and acrophase with 95% confidence limits.

In most cases, the rhythm's amplitude, C, has been expressed as percentage of its rhythm-adjusted level, C_0, in cosinor analyses, as well as in tables and figures in which amplitude is included. Some such transformation became necessary because separate sets of original data were often times given in dissimilar units. For example, some authors listed, as a function of time, the number of cases; while, others presented statistics as a fraction of living persons, deviations from the overall mean or percentages thereof.

Transformation of the C's into relative values further offered statistical advantages such as enabling direct comparison of amplitudes from time series differing in sample

---

*Manufactured by Varian Data Machine, 2722 Michelson, Irvine, California 93664.

size and by making possible a more appropriate weighting, by the relative amplitudes, of acrophases for sets of individual studies summarized by cosinor.

In this paper, the acrophases are expressed as negative values or delays from a chosen phase reference [92]. The period τ of a given single cosine curve, serving to approximate both circadian and circannual rhythms, equals $360°$. Thus when $\tau = 24$ hours $= 360°$, each $15°$ is equivalent to one hour clock time for those phenomena undergoing about one cycle per day. Similarly, when $\tau = 365.25$ days $= 360°$, each $0.986°$ is equivalent to one calendar day for rhythms completing one cycle per year.

In order to compare acrophases for data collected from various geographic sites and on different calendar dates, a suitable phase marker must, at least, compensate for differences in both the geophysical and social schedules of rest and activity in the various populations under study. However, since such information was not included in published reports, of necessity, rather than choice, local midnight (00^{00}) served as reference for circadian acrophases.

The limitations of such a computative acrophase, as compared to values referenced to a more meaningful external phase marker, have been discussed elsewhere [92, 96]. This acrophase, denoted by the symbol ϕ, does not compensate for differences in synchronization patterns. Thus, the use of a clock hour—in this case, local midnight— as a reference for the circadian computative ϕ suffers from the fact that identical values of ϕ may not reflect the same circadian-system-phase in populations adhering to dissimilar rest-activity schedules [96].

The choice of a phase reference for circannual rhythms requires compensation for the inter-hemispheric disparity of calendar date and season. For such compensation, comparable dates on some regular yearly environmental cycles are needed as reference points. Since within-year changes in daily photofraction, hours of daylight to hours of darkness, vary much less from one year to the next than corresponding changes in other environmental factors such as temperature, it seemed reasonable to select for each hemisphere a date approximating, as an average over the years, the day associated with the longest night for the northern hemisphere, i.e., midnight (00^{00}) of December 22, and for the southern hemisphere (00^{00}) of June 22.

Thus referenced, ϕ is denoted as a computative acrophase without implication as to the precise nature of possibly synchronizing external cycles. Whether changes in environmental temperature and/or lighting, among other factors, constitute circannual synchronizers for social man, notably in an urban setting, remains to be investigated. Nonetheless, incorporation of the above calendar dates as references into the computation of the circannual ϕ permits a more direct comparison of acrophases for time series from different hemispheres.

RESULTS

1. Circadian Aspects of Birth

An unequal distribution of spontaneous birth along the 24-hour time scale has been long recognized. Since initial work by Buek [29], Guiette [84], Quetelet [192], Danz with Fuchs [52], and Schneider [213], the circadian periodicity of birth has been rediscovered many times. Indeed, our examination of birth data by the methods of least squares spectral and cosinor analyses represents an extension of earlier investigations, for example, by Kaiser and Halberg [122], in which 600,000 births were evaluated, as well as by Bliss [19], Charles [38], and Malek [146] who approximated their statistics by harmonic functions. In this section, statistics of spontaneous labor [13, 14, 38, 80, 85, 86, 102, 108, 113, 122, 127, 135, 138, 146, 147, 169, 212, 218, 257] and births [13, 14, 19, 29, 34, 36, 38, 40, 51–53, 56, 57, 72, 79, 80, 84–86, 101, 102, 111, 112, 113, 117–119, 122, 126, 129, 131, 136, 138, 145, 149, 160, 161, 179, 181, 190, 192, 201, 202, 213, 219, 225, 230, 244, 252], induced delivery [53, 79, 112, 126, 201] and stillbirths [33, 56, 57, 111, 201] comprise the data analyzed.

The term "induced birth" pertains to those deliveries assisted by chemical, mechanical or operative means. Most time series on this aspect of birth summarize the total number of induced births per interval of time, irrespective of method of induction. Stillbirth refers to those pregnancies terminating in a non-viable neonate

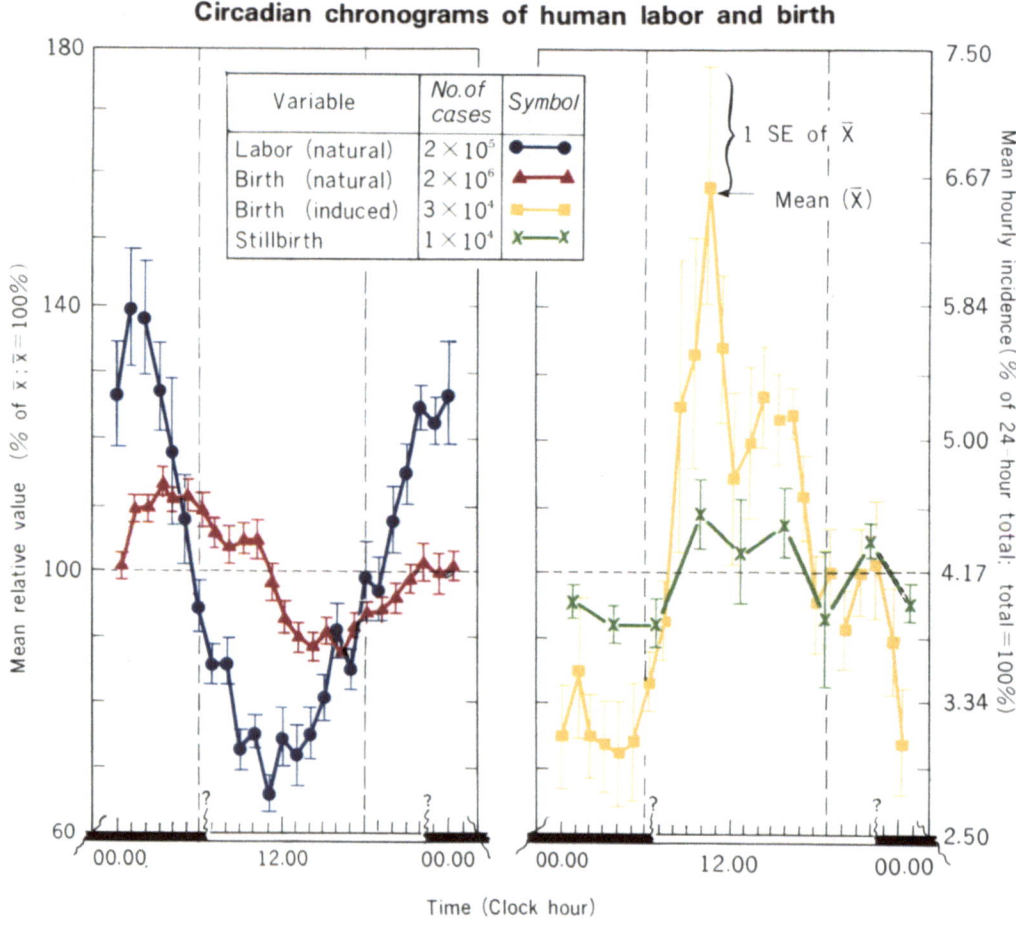

Fig. 134. Circadian Chronograms of Human Labor and Birth. These chronograms reveal circadian population rhythms. Initiation of spontaneous labor and its termination in delivery is greater between 00⁰⁰ and 06⁰⁰; on the other hand, induced birth and stillbirth are more frequent around midday. Note shaded regions at bottom of figure approximate suspected average nocturnal rest span.

following an average gestation. Neonates viable at birth but expiring thereafter usually are excluded from this category.

The hourly incidence of 207,918 spontaneous labors, 2,082,453 natural and 30,493 induced births are shown in Fig. 134. Included in this illustration as well is the average incidence of 12,081 stillbirths summarized for 3-hour spans. For spontaneous labor and natural and induced birth at least 63% of the time series of each category consisted of data given at 60-minute intervals.

Fig. 134 indicates that the commencement of labor—defined as the spontaneous initiation of painful contractions and/or rupture of fetal membranes—as well as natural birth is most frequent between local midnight and 06⁰⁰. Induced delivery and still-births, on the other hand, are more common around midday.

The chronogram (Fig. 134) further demonstrates that only a few hours separate the crest incidence in the initiation of labor from that of birth. Since the mean duration of labor is approximately nine hours [122], a greater difference in timing is expected between the peaks of these rhythms. The disparity between expected and graphed results presumably is due to the variability in the duration of labor among cases and the inclusion, in various time series, of multigravida, who are likely to have labors of shorter duration than those of primigravida. Further, the criteria defining the onset of labor, that is the rupture of fetal membranes or the initiation of contractions, rather than another more pertinent index, may not accurately reflect the exact commence-ment of labor, which physiologically may occur earlier than these indicate.

The curves of human labor and birth reveal that the amplitude of the former is considerably greater than that of the latter. Apparently, this situation reflects dif-ferences in the duration of labor between deliveries. Thus, while the initiation of labor peaks around midnight, its temporal termination in birth is extremely variable. This variability is reflected by a depression of the circadian amplitude for birth. Only if all labors commenced at the same time and were of equal duration would the amplitudes of labor and birth be equal. For this theoretical situation, the rhythms should differ only in phase.

The distribution of the circadian acrophase for each time series is displayed on a polar plot partitioned into units of one hour (Fig. 135). In this figure differently shaded sectors identify the relative amplitudes, acrophases and corresponding confidence intervals of separate periodic aspects of human birth. Blue and red shading identifies labor and natural birth and differently directed single-hatchings colored yellow and green denote induced birth and stillbirth. It may be seen that for labor the acrophases are distributed between $-322°$ (21²⁸) and $-55°$ (03⁴⁰). (It should be realized that an acrophase of $-358°$ differs from one of $-3°$ by 5° rather than 355°.) Those for birth are dispersed within a wider arc; they lie between $-308°$ (20³²) and $-155°$ (10²⁰). Interestingly, 75% of the latter acrophases are found within an arc extending from $-38°$ (02³²) to $-122°$ (08⁰⁸). The acrophase for induced birth and stillbirth differ drastically from the above.

Those for induced birth are found between $-158°$ (10³²) and $-262°$ (17²⁸) and presumably reflect the preferred diurnal working schedules of physicians. The acro-phases of stillbirth lie between $-147°$ (09⁴⁸) and $-289°$ (19¹⁶). All of these differ by nearly 180° from those of natural live birth.

The results of cosinor analyses on acrophases and their amplitudes for each aspect of

Circadian aspects of human birth (360°=24h)

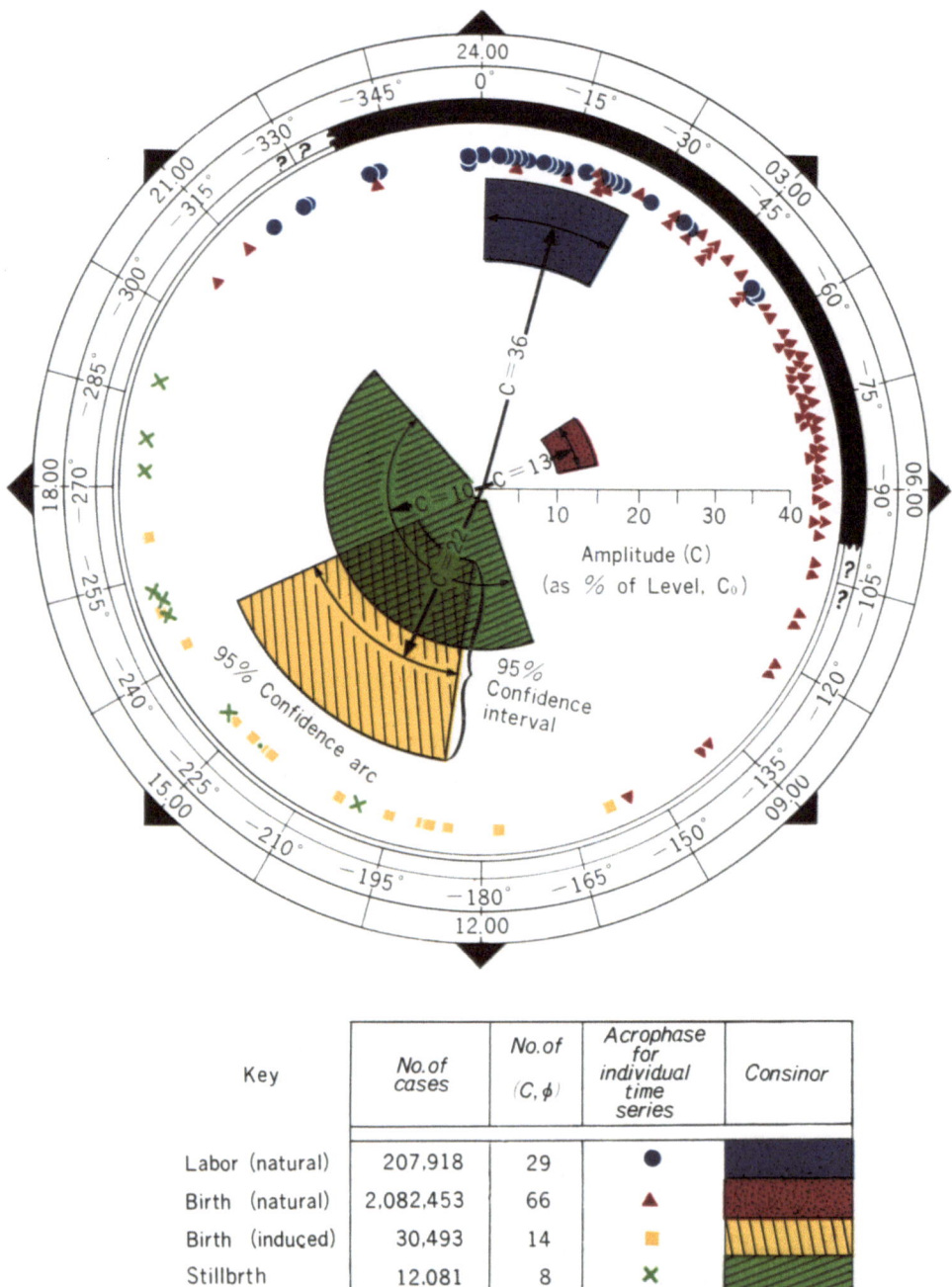

Key	No. of cases	No. of (C, φ)	Acrophase for individual time series	Consinor
Labor (natural)	207,918	29	●	
Birth (natural)	2,082,453	66	▲	
Birth (induced)	30,493	14	■	
Stillbrth	12,081	8	✕	

Fig. 135. Circadian Aspects of Human Birth. Polar plots locate the acrophase of individual time series on natality as well as sample circadian amplitudes and acrophase rhythms in the spontaneous initiation of labor and natural birth crest at −15° and −64° respectively while those for induced birth and stillbirth are differently timed, the acrophases occur at −204° and −257°. Darkened portion of inner border approximates suspected average nocturnal sleep span of pregnant samples.

birth are presented in Table 37. Circadian rhythms were detected for each aspect. The higher incidence of spontaneous labor occurs at $-15°$ (01^{00}), with the 95% confidence arc extending in a clockwise direction from $0°$ to $-27°$. For natural human birth, a circadian acrophase was determined at $-64°$ (04^{16}). Analyses of a small number of time series, separately summarizing the incidence of primigravida and multigravida, indicate an average acrophase for the former at $-41°$, which lags behind the latter at $-27°$ by about one hour ($14°$). Actually, the acrophases of both samples occur earlier than that for the entire sample of time series.

Separate cosinor analysis on the paired C and ϕ values for each of the first seven

TABLE 37 Circadian aspects of human birth

Variable analyzed	No. of cases	No. of samples	Amplitude, C^1	Acrophase, ϕ^2 (.95 confidence limits)
SPONTANEOUS LABOR***	2.1×10^5	29	36(30 to 41)	$-15°(- 0°$ to $-27°)$
NATURAL BIRTH				
Primigravida**	1.4×10^4	12	13(1 to 24)	$-41°(-352°$ to $-139°)$
Multigravida***	2.1×10^4	"	20(11 to 30)	$-27°(-347°$ to $60°)$
All births***	2.1×10^6	66	13(10 to 15)	$-64°(- 51°$ to $-77°)$
Labor***⎫		9	43(22 to 63)	$-6°(-345°$ to $-18°)$
⎬ †	4.5×10^3			
Birth***⎭		"	12(3 to 20)	$-64°(- 51°$ to $-77°)$
INDUCED BIRTH***	3.0×10^3	14	22(9 to 35)	$-204°(-188°$ to $-246°)$
STILLBIRTH				
Incidence of ⎫		8	10(0.5 to 20)	$-257°(-161°$ to $-320°)$
⎬	1.2×10^4			
No./live births⎭		4	15(4 to 27)	$-266°(-185°$ to $-311°)$

1. C expressed relative to C_0 ($C_0 = 100\%$) as a percent value.
2. ϕ reference = local midnight ($15° = 1$ hour).
   † = labor and birth analyses based upon data of the same sample of pregnancies.
   Rhythm detection: ** = $.01 < P < .05$; *** = $.001 < P < .01$.

TABLE 38 Statistically-validated harmonics characterizing waveform of circadian rhythms in onset of natural human labor, birth and death[1]

Variable analyzed /N of single time series/(N of cases)	Period fitted in hours used for cosinor[2]	Amplitude, C^3	Acrophase, ϕ^4 (.95 confidence interval)
LABOR	24***	36.0(30.0 to 41.0)	$-15°(- 0°$ to $-27°)$
/29/	12***	9.4(3.0 to 15.8)	$-89°(- 54°$ to $-113°)$
(2.1×10^5)	8**	4.9(0.1 to 9.7)	$-78°(-352°$ to $-148°)$
	6***	2.9(0.9 to 4.9)	$-206°(-158°$ to $-269°)$
BIRTH	24***	12.5(9.5 to 15.5)	$-64°(- 51°$ to $-77°)$
/66/	8**	1.8(0.1 to 3.5)	$-159°(- 80°$ to $-240°)$
(2.1×10^6)	6***	2.2(0.6 to 3.8)	$-222°(-182°$ to $-293°)$
	4**	2.6(0.2 to 5.0)	$-219°(-164°$ to $-312°)$
DEATH	24***	8.2(2.7 to 13.7)	$-108°(- 72°$ to $-141°)$
/52/	12***	5.7(2.5 to 8.9)	$-131°(- 50°$ to $-164°)$
(4.3×10^5)	4.8**	2.3(0.3 to 4.4)	$-98°(- 50°$ to $-164°)$
	4.0**	2.4(0.1 to 4.7)	$-98°(- 5°$ to $-150°)$
	3.4**	2.0(0.1 to 3.9)	$-127°(- 58°$ to $-212°)$

1. 7 harmonics fitted by least squares to each time series; paired (C, ϕ) for each harmonic summarized by cosinor listed only for rhythm detection at the 5% level or better.
2. Rhythm detection: ** = $.01 < P < .05$; *** = $.001 < P < .01$.
3. Expressed as % of level, C_0.
4. ϕ reference = local midnight ($15° = 1$ hour).

harmonics demonstrates for labor and birth the statistical significance of certain frequencies higher than circadian (Table 38).   Thus, additional periods of six, eight and 12 and four, six and eight hours, respectively, are identified.   These higher-than-circadian frequencies may indicate simply that the waveforms of the population rhythms in labor and birth are somewhat non-sinusoidal.   However, these harmonics may also reflect differences in synchronization schedules of separate occupational or other subgroups in a given sample.   Whatever the origin, these harmonics do reflect the overall waveform of labor and birth as may be seen by comparison of the original data with the synthesized curves (Fig. 136) constructed from the C and ϕ values for each of the statistically significant harmonics shown in Table 37.

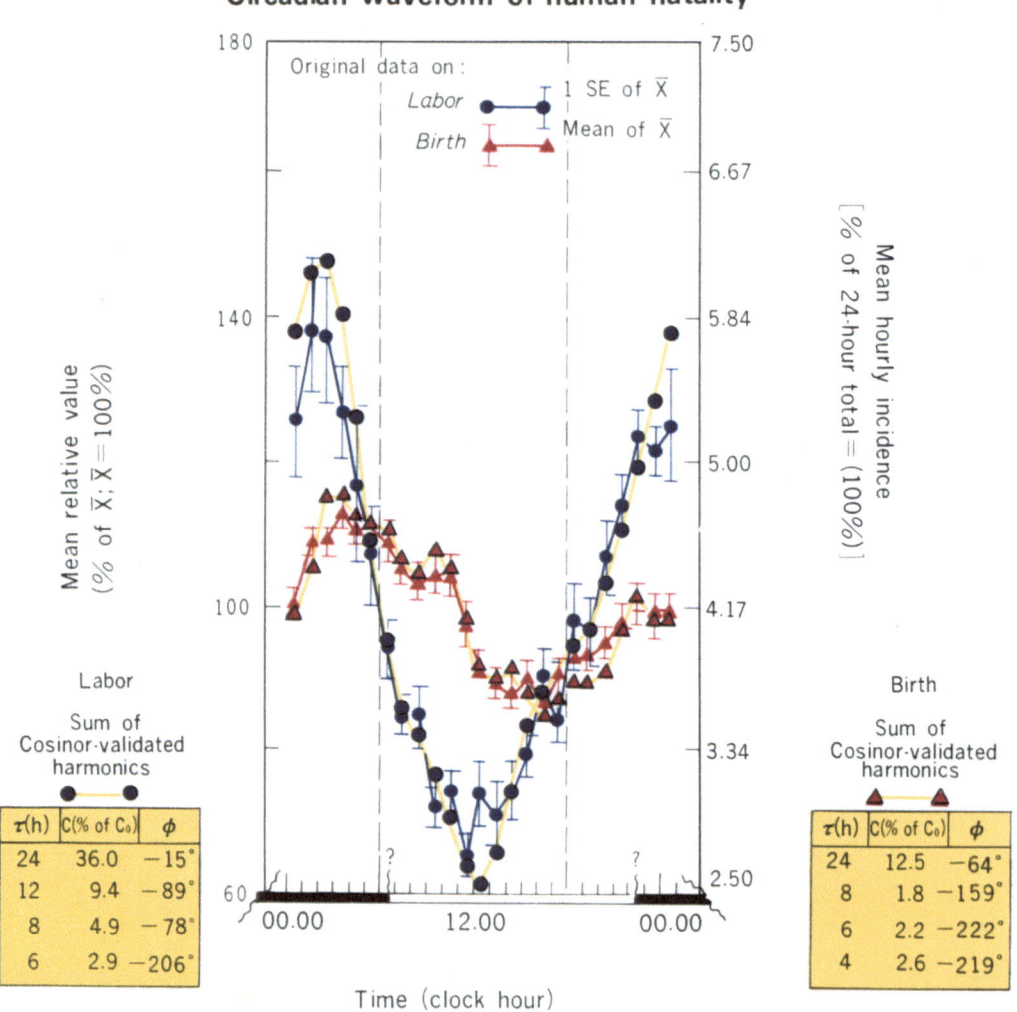

Fig. 136. Circadian Waveform of Human Natality. Chronograms of human natality—spontaneous initiation of labor and natural birth—characterized by high amplitude circadian as well as lower amplitude ultradian frequencies. Comparison of the circadian waveform, constructed from significant periodicities validated by cosinor, with original is good. Note shaded regions at bottom of figure approximate suspected nocturnal rest spans.

The incidence of induced and stillbirth is non-random (Fig. 135, Table 37). Moreover, the phasing of these circadian rhythms differs from that of natural birth. Since only a small number of time series comprise the samples, they were not examined for significant frequencies other than that of 24 hours. Substantiation of a periodicity in induced birth, as well as the timing of its acrophase at $-204°$ (13^{36}), indicates that certain practices associated with the diurnal working schedules of physicians and obstetricians alter the expected biorhythmic patterns.

The detection of a circadian rhythm in stillbirth with an acrophase at $-257°$, differing from that of natural, live birth by almost $180°$, although apparently reflecting those stillbirths following long, difficult labors and others resulting from the side effects of labor inducement, implies an increased neonatal survival for delivery close to the expected acrophase of birth [122]. Evidence for this comes from statistics published by Gulyuk [85] which indicate that deliveries at this time are less often associated with maternal hemorrhaging.

Certain small discrepancies between crest times suggested by chronograms and those detected by least squares spectral and cosinor analyses, especially for induced birth and stillbirth, presumably, are due to the manner in which data were processed. Chronograms shown here are derived by taking simple averages at corresponding clock hours over all time series within each sample category. Thus, the final curve represents a non-weighted, by sample size, expression of temporal events. On the other hand, the cosinor utilizes individual acrophases each weighted by respective time series amplitudes expressed relative to the level, C_0. Therefore, the average sample acrophase and amplitude values determined in this manner reflect such a weighting; thus, differences between crest times suggested by chronograms and those found by cosinor are not unlikely. Moreover, when a sample consists only of a small number of time series, as is the case of stillbirth, the waveform may reflect the influences of certain unknown factors such as errors in reporting. The non-sinusoidal appearance of the average waveform for stillbirth, possibility reflecting a high noise level, does not necessarily imply a random occurrence of the C and ϕ values for time series making up this sample.

2. Circannual Rhythms in Birth

The monthly incidence of birth has long been a topic of interest. Early students reported such numbers to demonstrate seasonal differences in birth or compare the monthly totals of birth and death to population balance. Quetelet [192], who first published in 1825, was one of the earliest investigators. Since then many works have followed [6, 37, 45–49, 59, 183, 185, 186, 204, 231, 243]. The investigations of Cowgill [45–49] are most comprehensive and well documented, containing the monthly incidence of birth summarized for periods ranging from one year to several decades for a number of countries and states. Further, monthly birth totals for each state in America are reported in U. S. Vital Statistics publications [6]. Similar information for certain countries may be located in World Health Organization reports and official governmental tabulations.

Cosinor summary of the paired amplitudes and acrophase values for all time series summarizing human birth reveals a rhythm with an overall sample ϕ at $-50°$ or about 50 days from the chosen phase reference, midnight (00^{00}) of, on the average, the longest nocturnal dark span of the year, June 22 in the northern hemisphere and

TABLE 39 Circannual rhythm in human birth

Sample kind & size	No. of time series	Amplitude, C^1	Acrophase, ϕ^2 (.95 confidence interval)
Using birth control devices** (1.9×10^7)	9	3.9(0.2 to 7.6)	$-120°(- 45$ to $-198)$
Not using birth control devices*** (39×10^6)	20	5.8(1.9 to 9.6)	$- 16°(-320$ to $- 57)$
United States*** (12×10^6)	48	4.8(4.4 to 5.1)	$-218°(-201$ to $-232)$
All† and *** (10.7×10^7)	58	3.2(0.5 to 5.8)	$- 50°(- 4$ to $- 94)$

1. Amplitude expressed relative to C_0 ($C_0 = 100\%$).
2. ϕ reference = 00^{00} of the average longest night of the year, December 22, in the northern hemisphere and June 22 in the southern hemisphere ($1° = 1.01$ days).
   †: 48 time series for U.S. births represented by C & ϕ values from a single cosinor summary.
   Rhythm detection:*** = $.001 < P < .01$; ** = $.01 < P < .05$.

December 22 in the southern hemisphere. Results of least squares spectral analyses on separate time series given in Table 39, however, reveal that the acrophases of birth may differ drastically. For example, in populations unlikely to be using contraceptive devices, mainly consisting of Roman Catholics, the ϕ occurs early in the year; for the United States, on the other hand, its timing is much later. Thus, an average acrophase of $-16°$ is detected for samples not practicing birth control. For countries in which contraceptives are available and their use encouraged ϕ occurs at $-120°$.

A circannual rhythm in birth for regions inhabited mainly by populations relying primarily on natural methods of family planning must not be interpreted as evidence for the timing of an endogenous human fertility rhythm. On the contrary, the timing of a human population periodicity usually reflects the synchronizing, modifying or "influencing" by society, including religious practices. Thus, the not uncommon practices of sexual abstinence and discouragement of marriage during Lent serve to synchronize human circannual birth rhythms. Following Easter the number of marriages increases and sexual abstinence ceases. The calendar date of conception corresponds to April 15th, assuming an average human gestation of 266 days from fertilization and counting backwards from a circannual birth ϕ of $-16°$. On the average, this date varies only slightly from that of Easter, which differs from one year to another between late March and early April.

More concrete evidence that the waveform of birth is at least dependent on societal influences comes from re-examination of statistics presented by Cowgill for York, England from 1538 to 1814 [49] and for Puerto Rico from 1941–1960 [45].

In the case of York, data were originally obtained from baptismal records, and although limited in number and scope, they appear representative, as may be verified by consulting other sources for comparable material [48]. Analyses of these data for separate about 50-year spans from 1538 to 1601 and from 1601 to 1651, reveal a circa-semiannual rhythm in human birth; while the following successive 50-year spans thereafter are characterized solely by circannual rhythms.

In more recent times, the birth curve of Puerto Rico has undergone some rather rapid changes. Analyses of these data indicate that the acrophase has phase-shifted since the end of World War II from $-117°$ (1941–1945) to $-283°$ (1956–1960).

This alteration in phase may be related to certain sociologic and other changes coincident with increased industrialization and urbanization—for example, in seasonal work and vacation schedules and the availability of birth control programs. However, social factors as in the preceding examples may represent only influencers or modifiers of possible as yet non-substantiated intrinsic fertility rhythms.

3. Circadian Mortality Rhythms

Interest in circadian rhythms of human deaths, although not as great as in those of birth, dates back to Virey in 1814 [242]. Since this early study, a large number of

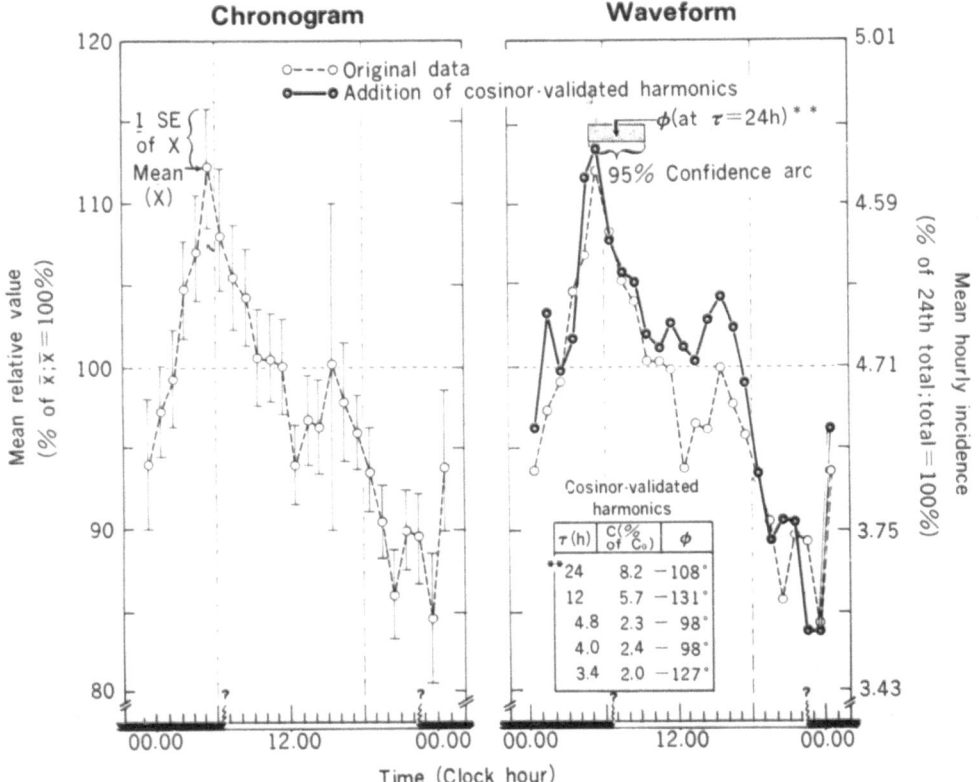

Fig. 137. Circadian Human Mortality Rhythm. The occurrence of human death along the scale of 24 hours suggests circadian rhythmicity with greatest incidence around 06⁰⁰. Irregularities, e.g., secondary crests, may reflect different causes of death, ultradian frequencies and/or synchronization schedules in samples prior to death. Comparison of the circadian waveform (right-hand figure), contructed from significant periodicities validated by cosinor, with original data is good. Note shaded regions at bottom of figures approximate suspected nocturnal rest spans.

follow-up reports have appeared for Europe [17, 24, 25, 28, 29, 31, 35, 36, 39, 50, 73, 76, 77, 81, 87, 107, 114, 1f8, 121, 130, 132, 133, 143, 159, 176, 180, 195, 203, 207, 208, 214, 221, 224, 254], Great Britain [75, 139, 226, 250], United States [17, 20, 21, 32, 43, 44, 151, 154, 155] and other countries [168, 174, 222, 223, 229]. Although in most instances, the temporal incidence of mortality is summarized independently of cause, several time series are available allowing separate evaluation of cardiovascular, pulmonary and pediatric mortalities.

The chronogram in Fig. 137 summarizes the hourly incidence of 432,892 deaths representing statistics collected from 49 separate studies, 26 providing totals for intervals of one hour. Inspection of this figure reveals a major crest in mortality at about 06^{00}; apparent also are several secondary peaks, the most prominent of which occurs at 16^{00}. These latter features may reflect, among other things, 1) synchronization differences among population, 2) frequencies higher than circadian (ultradian), or 3) separate causes of death. The variability introduced by pooling deaths arising from distinctive causes, e.g., general, cardiovascular, pulmonary, pediatric, and post-surgical, is demonstrated in Fig. 138. This figure demonstrates that 78% of the acrophases are distributed between midnight, 00^{00} and midday, 12^{00}. Moreover, 64% lie within a seven-hour span, between $-60°$ (04^{00}) and $-165°$ (11^{00}).

Cosinor analysis of paired acrophases and amplitudes from all time series, reveals a circadian rhythm with sample acrophase at $-108°$ (07^{12}), and 95% confidence limits extending (in a clockwise direction) from $-72°$ to $-141°$ (Fig. 138, Table 40). In addition, rhythms with comparable acrophases are detected separately for male and female deaths, irrespective of age or cause (Table 40).

TABLE 40   Circadian rhythms in human mortality

Group studied	P from cosinor	Amplitude, C^1	Acrophase, ϕ^2 (.95 confidence arc)
Females*	.02	20(4 to 37)	$-118°(- 29$ to $-147)$
Males*	.03	27(3 to 52)	$-112°(-343$ to $-133)$
Adult:			
Lung**	.001	12(6 to 18)	$- 89°(- 15$ to $-131)$
Cardiovascular**	.05	12(.1 to 25)	$-152°(- 75$ to $-234)$
Infants:			
All causes*, **	.04	16(.9 to 32)	$-112°(- 20$ to $-157)$
All groups*, **	.001	9(4 to 13)	$-108°(- 72$ to $-141)$

1.   C expressed relative to C_0 ($C_0 = 100\%$)
2. ϕ reference = local midnight; $15° = 1$ hour.
 *Irrespective of cause.
**Irrespective of sex.

Examination of data for significant periodicities other than 24 hours substantiates additional small amplitude rhythms of 12.0, 4.8, 4.0 and 3.43 hours (Fig. 137). Whether these harmonics reflect differences in synchronization schedules of separate populations or specific causes of death cannot be determined from the information available. Nonetheless, when the waveform of human mortality, constructed from the C and ϕ values of the significant harmonics validated by cosinor, is compared to the original data in Fig. 137, only slight differences are seen. It is readily apparent that the synthesized waveform does account for the overall features of the data, for example, in the characterization of major and minor peaks and troughs.

Circadian rhythm of susceptibility to "death" in human beings

Reveal by 32,892 'natural deaths" over 145 years

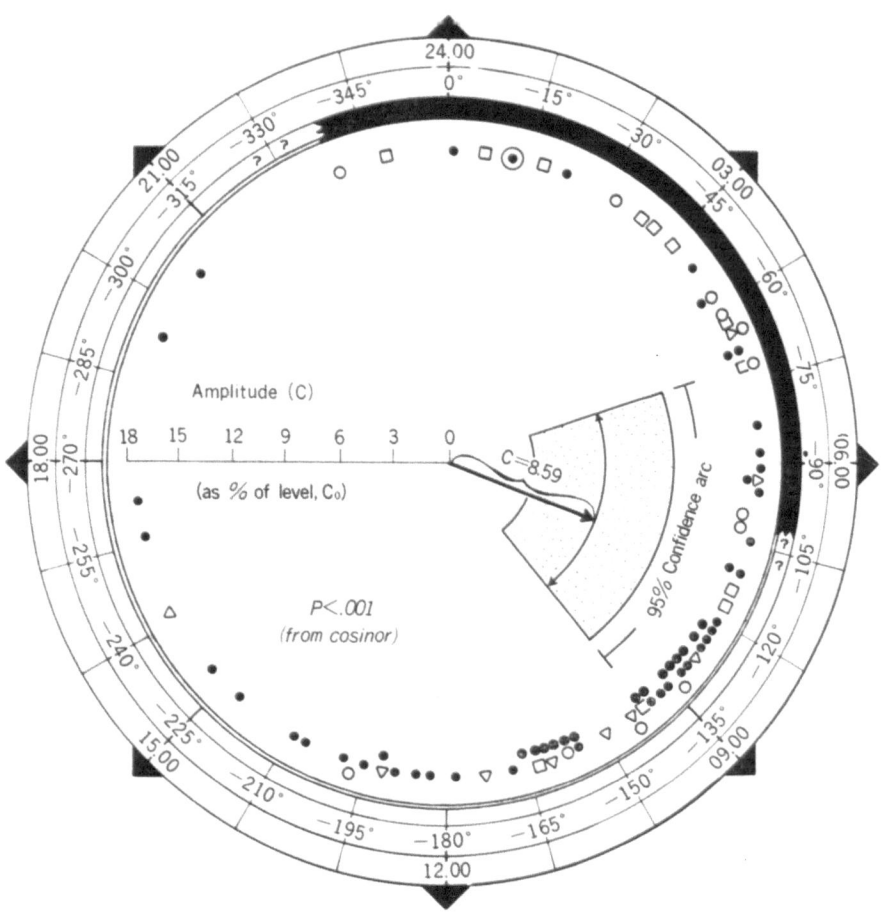

Mortality category	No. of cases	No. of (C, φ)	Symbol for acrophase
Pediatric	21,673	12	○
Postsurgical	500	1	◉
Cardiovascular	7,644	9	△
Pulmonary	9,357	12	□
Cause unspecified	393,718	54	•
Cosinor of above	432,892	88	⊢◁

Fig. 138.   Circadian Rhythm of Susceptibility to "Death" in Human Beings.   Polar plot summarizes the timing of individual acrophases for 88 time series representing nearly 433,000 deaths.   Almost 65% of the φ occurs between 04⁰⁰ and 11⁰⁰.   Greatest overall sample mortality occurs at 07¹². Inner shaded portion indicates suspected nocturnal rest span of sample prior to death.

4. Circannual Mortality and Morbidity Rhythms

Statistics supporting human circannual mortality rhythms have long been available for a number of diseases. Recent analyses by Momiyama *et al.* [163–167] suggest that the amplitude of certain formerly prominent circannual rhythms has gradually decreased. This "deseasonality" [163, 166] of mortality, presumably mirrors social and technological advances such as improved medical care and housing, including the availability of winter heating and summer air-conditioning, which serve to moderate climatic influences upon human mortality patterns. With such a deseasonability in certain causes of human death in mind, cardiovascular and pulmonary mortalities were selected for study: first, they account for a major proportion of deaths in most populations; second, these circannual rhythms are well documented; and third, they continue to persist with only slight modification of amplitude, if any, in most if not all countries.

In many areas of the world, an occurrence of a high incidence of morbidity and mortality from cardiovascular disease has long been noted during the winter months [4, 15, 16, 23, 27, 30, 41, 42, 61, 67, 115, 158, 162–167, 170, 173, 188, 191, 215, 236, 237, 251, 255]. Seasonal differences have been discussed in some studies [15, 16, 27, 30, 41, 153, 236, 237] in relation to the annual cycle of environmental temperature which usually varies inversely with that of heart morbidity and mortality. Seasonal variations in death from acute myocardial infarct, identified as such, or from arteriosclerosis are reported by Momiyama [164, 165, 167] for England, France, Japan, and the United States, by Begg [16], Doring and Loddenkepmer [61], Puffer and Griffith [191], Scheid [207] and Schrire [215] for Wales, Germany, South America, Austria and South Africa, respectively, and by Bundesen and Falk [30], Cohen [42], Petersen [188] and others [27, 55, 110, 115, 162, 170, 220, 251] for the United States. Seasonal differences in occurrence of acute coronary and myocardial infarct are also well documented in the literature [10, 15, 27, 55, 110, 115, 128, 153, 158, 162, 170, 215, 220, 255].

Similar changes in the occurrence of respiratory illness [42, 60, 82, 106, 164, 165, 191, 205, 228] and in the cholesterol concentration in human serum [7, 62, 78, 83, 172, 184, 232, 233, 247] have also been detected and may be related to the temporal incidence of cardiovascular mortality along the time domain of one year.

Cardiovascular Mortality and Morbidity. The highest monthly incidence of cardiovascular disease occurs in January in the northern hemisphere and in June in the southern hemisphere (Fig. 139). The acrophases for individual bodies of data are displayed in Fig. 140. Except for a few time series exhibiting summertime ϕ's, acrophases of cardiovascular morbidity lie between $-308°$ (October 26) and $-69°$ (March 1). Those for mortality are found between $-289°$ and $61°$ (corresponding to October 7 and February 21, respectively, in the northern hemisphere). A circannual rhythm in cardiovascular deaths with the acrophase approximating the average greatest incidence at $-33°$, about 33 days following midnight of the year's longest "average night," also was detected (Fig. 140). When the latter phase reference is used, no differences in the timing for the circannual ϕ are found between regions of the northern and southern hemispheres or between areas with cold winters and warm summers and those with moderate winters and warm or hot summers.

Examination of "heart deaths" for each state in America during 1940, the only monthly tabulation of mortality statistics by state [5], also reveals circannual rhythms with acrophases comparable in timing to those of other time series collected from various

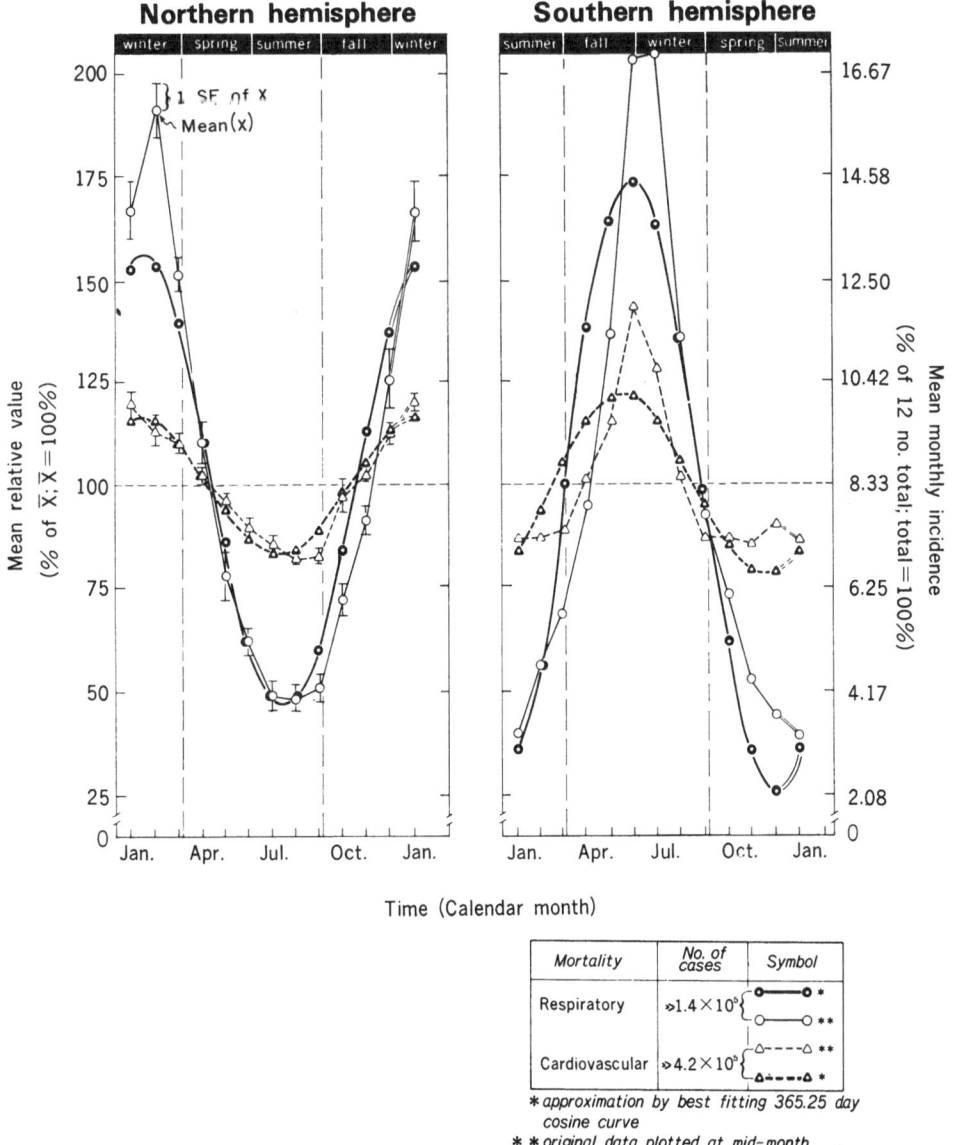

Circannual chronogram of human respiratory and cardiovascular deaths

Mortality	No. of cases	Symbol
Respiratory	≈1.4×10⁹	●——● * / ○——○ **
Cardiovascular	≈4.2×10⁹	△----△ ** / ▲----▲ *

* approximation by best fitting 365.25 day cosine curve

* * original data plotted at mid-month

Fig. 139. Circadian Chronogram of Human Respiratory and Cardiovascular Deaths. Chronograms of human mortality population rhythms reveal highest incidences during winter irrespective of hemisphere. Least squares approximation of the monthly means by a 365.25-day cosine curve accurately reflects waveforms for the northern hemisphere. Slight discrepancies between original data and approximating curve for the southern hemisphere due to small number of samples available.

geographic locations. Results of least squares spectral analysis upon such data originally reported as the number of "heart deaths" per 100,000 inhabitants, are graphically represented in Fig. 141.

Rhythms (P<.05) are found in the data from most states. Failure to detect circannual periodicities for certain ones may reflect inaccuracies in medical diagnosis and statistical reporting. Moreover, the evaluation of time series limited to spans of only

Circannual aspects of human death

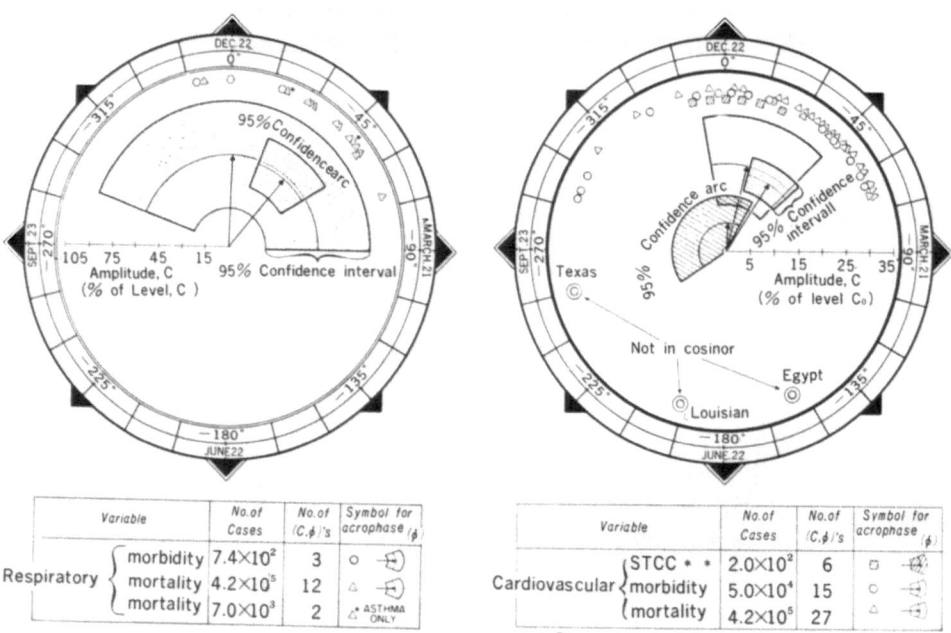

Variable		No. of Cases	No. of (C,φ)'s	Symbol for acrophase (φ)
Respiratory	morbidity	7.4×10²	3	○
	mortality	4.2×10⁵	12	△
	mortality	7.0×10³	2	ASTHMA ONLY

Variable		No. of Cases	No. of (C,φ)'s	Symbol for acrophase (φ)
Cardiovascular	STCC • •	2.0×10²	6	□
	morbidity	5.0×10⁴	15	○
	mortality	4.2×10⁵	27	△

• • Serum total cholesterol concentration

Dec. 22= φ reference for northern hemisphere only ;

Fig. 140. Circannual Aspects of Human Death. Polar plots summarize circannual rhythms in respiratory morbidity and mortality (left) and aspects of cardiovascular mortality (right) revealing a temporal sequences of events. Greatest expected incidence of respiratory morbidity at −2° precedes that for death by −38°. Greatest expected incidence of cardiovascular mortality occurs at −33° which follows highest expected cholesterol concentration at −6° and mortality.

one year restricts rhythm detection and quantification especially in data collected from less populated states or in those with low incidence of heart mortality, in which the influence of "noise" is likely to be considerable. Nonetheless, spot checks of these findings by analysis of more current cardiovascular mortality data, provided through the courtesy of individual state health agencies, confirm findings obtained from analysis of 1941 statistics. In certain cases, analysis of longer time series, for example, for Norte Dakota, substantiates the occurrence of a circannual mortality rhythm with a wintertime acrophase that eluded detection from evaluation of 1940 data only.

Study of Fig. 141 reveals some interesting geographic trends. First, the circannual level, which in this case is comparable to the mean monthly mortality, for states located in the Northern region of the country are of greatest magnitude. Second, states in the North-central and Northeastern areas are characterized by highest amplitudes. Third, the circannual acrophases, although differing but slightly, occur later, 20–40 days, for states in the Midwest and Southeast as compared to those in the Northeast and West, for which the timing is the earliest. Results of t-tests [227] performed on differences between the regional means for the rhythm characteristics C_0 and $φ$ substantiate statistical significance, below the .001% level of probability.

These geographic trends may result from certain local environmental influences

"Month of changing risk" for cardiac death
Summarized by the fit of a 365.25-day cosine curve
to 1940-human mortality from heart disease by state in USA

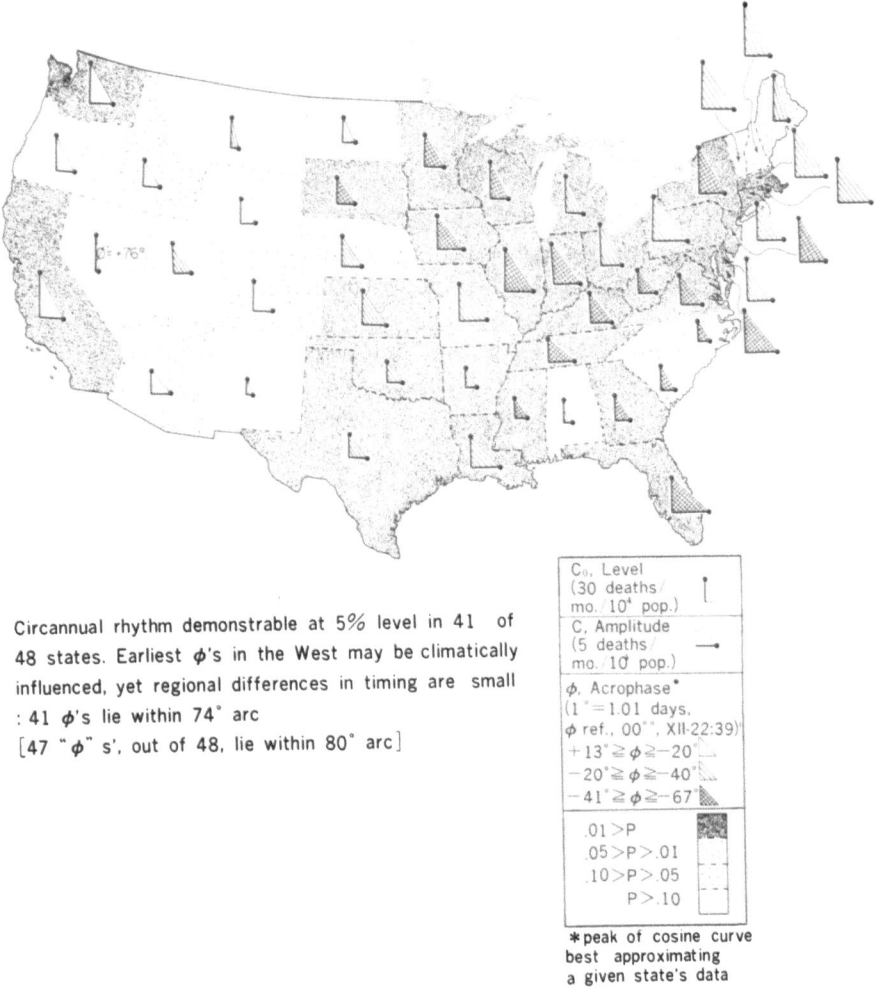

Circannual rhythm demonstrable at 5% level in 41 of
48 states. Earliest ϕ's in the West may be climatically
influenced, yet regional differences in timing are small
: 41 ϕ's lie within 74° arc
[47 "ϕ" s', out of 48, lie within 80° arc]

C_0, Level (30 deaths/ mo./10^4 pop.)	$\uparrow$
C, Amplitude (5 deaths/ mo./10^4 pop.)	$\longrightarrow$
ϕ, Acrophase* (1°=1.01 days, ϕ ref., 00°, XII-22:39)	
+13°≥ϕ≥−20°	
−20°≥ϕ≥−40°	
−41°≥ϕ≥−67°	
.01>P	
.05>P>.01	
.10>P>.05	
P>.10	

*peak of cosine curve
best approximating
a given state's data

Fig. 141. "Month of Changing Risk" for Cardiac Death. Symbols for each state summarize time series on heart deaths. Circannual rhythms demonstrable at 5% level or better in 41 of 48 states. Earliest ϕ's in the west may be climatically influenced, yet regional differences in timing are small: 41 ϕ's lie within 74° arc (47 "ϕ"'s out of 48 lie within 80° arc). Largest C_0's and C's found in northern states possibly reflect climate as well.

such as seasonal patterns in weather. Evidence supporting this hypothesis comes from comparison of C_0's for monthly cardiovascular mortality with those for monthly temperature for each of 48 states. In so doing, a correlation coefficient of −.468 substantiates a statistically significant (P<.01) relationship between states with low mean monthly temperature and high average monthly heart mortality. However, despite such trends, cosinor analysis of (C, ϕ)'s for each state finds a circannual rhythm in "heart deaths" with the acrophase, approximating greatest incidence, at −37° (January

28). This acrophase differs by only four days from that determined for samples collected from all over the world. Such agreement in acrophases for different geographic locations is in itself remarkable considering possible differences in weather from one area to another and from one year to the next.

These statistics indicate circannual rhythms in cardiovascular deaths with greatest incidence during the winter. It has been suggested previously that such deaths might be described by circannual as well as higher frequency components [55, 206]. To study this possibility, monthly mortality data were examined for important harmonics of the one-year period. Separate analyses of data from the northern and southern hemispheres failed to reveal statistical significance (P<.05) for anyone of the first five harmonics of the circannual period, except that of the fundamental.

Circannual rhythms in cardiovascular morbidity and mortality possibly reflect, at least to some degree, rhythms of corresponding period in related or underlying physiologic functions. In this regard, Antonis *et al.* [7], Doyle *et al.* [62], Fyfe *et al.* [78], Green *et al.* [83], Nemeth *et al.* [172], Paloheimo [184], Thomas *et al.* [232], Tochowicz *et al.* [233], and Watanabe and Aoki [247] have studied circannual rhythms in serum total cholesterol concentration (STCC). Since procedures and sampling conditions varied from one study to another, it was decided to examine only those time series consisting of data collected at monthly intervals or less for at least one year upon the same subjects while adhering to a regular routine and diet [62, 184, 232]. Most investigations were made upon prisoners confined to a standardized routine with limited access to the external environment. Although such subjects themselves cannot be described as normal, their setting offers certain advantages—among them an institutional diet which did not vary in fat composition from one season to another. Results of analyses upon these data are shown in Table 41. Rhythms are detected for all samples. Further, the acrophases for STCC differ only slightly between studies and among policemen and prisoners. Despite limited activity (notably during the winter season) and dietary control, prisoners undergo a rhythm in STCC similar to that of policemen with free access to the external environment. The greater circannual amplitude for prisoners possibly reflects their limited activity in confinement, but this point awaits further study.

The distribution of the acrophases of STCC is indicated on the polar plot in Fig. 140; all ϕ lie between $-347°$ and $-22°$. Results of cosinor analysis of the paired C and ϕ values from separate samples substantiates a circannual rhythm for STCC with sample acrophase at $-6°$ (December 28). The ϕ of STCC precedes that of cardiovascular morbidity by $16°$ (16 days) and that cardiovascular death by $27°$ (27 days).

High STCC has previously been associated with increased heart morbidity and mortality [12, 124, 125, 189, 193, 194, 217]. The temporal relationship between peak cardiac morbidity and mortality and high STCC revealed by analyses herein is consistent with this line of thought. The extent, if any, to which this rhythm represents physiologic responses to about yearly changes in its external environment, such as those of temperature, photoperiod, or radiation, remains beyond the scope of this paper. However, since earlier investigations suggest both circadian [22, 26, 150, 187] as well as menstrual rhythms [177, 178] in STCC, an endogenous component for the circannual rhythm in STCC is not inconsistent with prior findings. Moreover,

TABLE 41   Circannual rhythm in serum total cholesterol concentration (STCC) of males

Source of data /location/ (latitude)[2]	Sample size	Level, C_0[6] $C_0 \pm$ S.E.	Amplitude, C[6]	Acrophase, ϕ[1] (.95 confidence interval)
Thomas[3] /Maryland/(39°N)	13***	199 ± 5	12(7 to 17)	− 0°(−340 to − 22)
"	6*	241 ± 6	12(1 to 24)	− 22°(− 34 to −121)
"	4*	296 ± 8	40(.4 to 79)	− 13°(−331 to −117)
Paleheimo[4a] /Finland/(60°N)	45***	225 ± 2	6(2 to 9)	− 4°(−318 to − 43)
" [4b]	35***	212 ± 2	12(8 to 16)	−347°(−326 to − 9)
Doyle[5] /New York/(42°N)	52*	225 ± 2	7(5 to 9)	−354°(−319 to − 29)
Cosinor (STCC)	165**	233 ± 5	14(7 to 25)	− 6°(−240 to − 28)
As relatives	"	100%	6(.3 to 11)	− 6°(−240 to − 28)

1. Acrophase reference = $00°°$ of the average longest day of the year in the northern hemisphere December 22 (1° = 1.01 days).
2. Latitude given constitutes but a rough approximation.
3. Prisoners maintained on institutionalized diet and routine; average age—26 years.
4. (a) Policemen working out-of-doors; average age—33 years; (b) Prisoners same.
5. Group: unspecified composition and occupation; average age—54 years.
   Rhythm detection: ** = $.01 < P < .05$; *** = $.001 < P < .01$.
6. Units in mg/100 ml blood.

although the STCC data here analyzed were collected in geographic regions characterized by moderate to extreme winter conditions, the fact that it persists in prisoners confined mostly to the indoors infers some measure of independence from the external environment, i.e., it suggests a circannual rhythm which is at least independent of seasonal differences in diet or activity [184].

Respiratory Mortality and Morbidity. Since the risk of death by persons susceptible to cardiovascular disease increases with contraction of certain illnesses affecting the cardiopulmonary axis, the temporal relationship between the peak incidence of the cardiovascular and respiratory illness as well as rhythms in the latter are of interest. Information on the monthly incidence of respiratory diseases has been reported by Dingle *et al.* [60], Sargent [205] and Stuart-Harris and Hanley [228]. Statistics summarized by Cohen [42], Gerfeldt [82], Momiyama [164, 165, 167], and Puffer and Griffith [191] as well as others [5, 6] pertain to death from asthma, bronchitis, influenza and/or pneumonia.

Respiratory morbidity, the average monthly incidence of common respiratory infection, for the most part, in the form of "colds" is available from Sargent [205] for a high school population studied for four years. The report by Stuart-Harris and Hanley [228] summarizes the occurrence of respiratory infection—common cold, tonsillitis, influenza, acute bronchitis or pneumonia—in two samples, one composed of 81 presumably healthy persons and the other consisting of 82 individuals with diagnosed organic diseases of the cardiovascular or respiratory system. Monthly incidence of illness is based upon detailed medical records maintained by health inspectors visiting participants at regular intervals. During the three years of study, a total of 273 and 300 cases of respiratory infection was recorded for the samples of healthy and organically diseased subjects, respectively.

The timing of the circannual acrophases of respiratory illness in temperate regions of the northern hemisphere is characterized by a wintertime ϕ. There is close agreement in acrophases for studies conducted in separate countries and during different years. Indeed, when Sargent's data are analyzed as two individual time series, each covering an 18-month span (1935–37 and 1937–39), a difference in ϕ of only four days is detected.

Fig. 142 illustrates the distribution of circannual acrophases for separate time series as well as the relative amplitude, acrophase and 95% confidence interval for the circannual rhythm in respiratory illness as summarized by cosinor. The acrophases lie between $-348°$ (December 10) and $49°$ (January 8); a circannual rhythm is substantiated with sample acrophase at $-2°$ (December 24) or two days following 00^{00} of the longest night of the year.

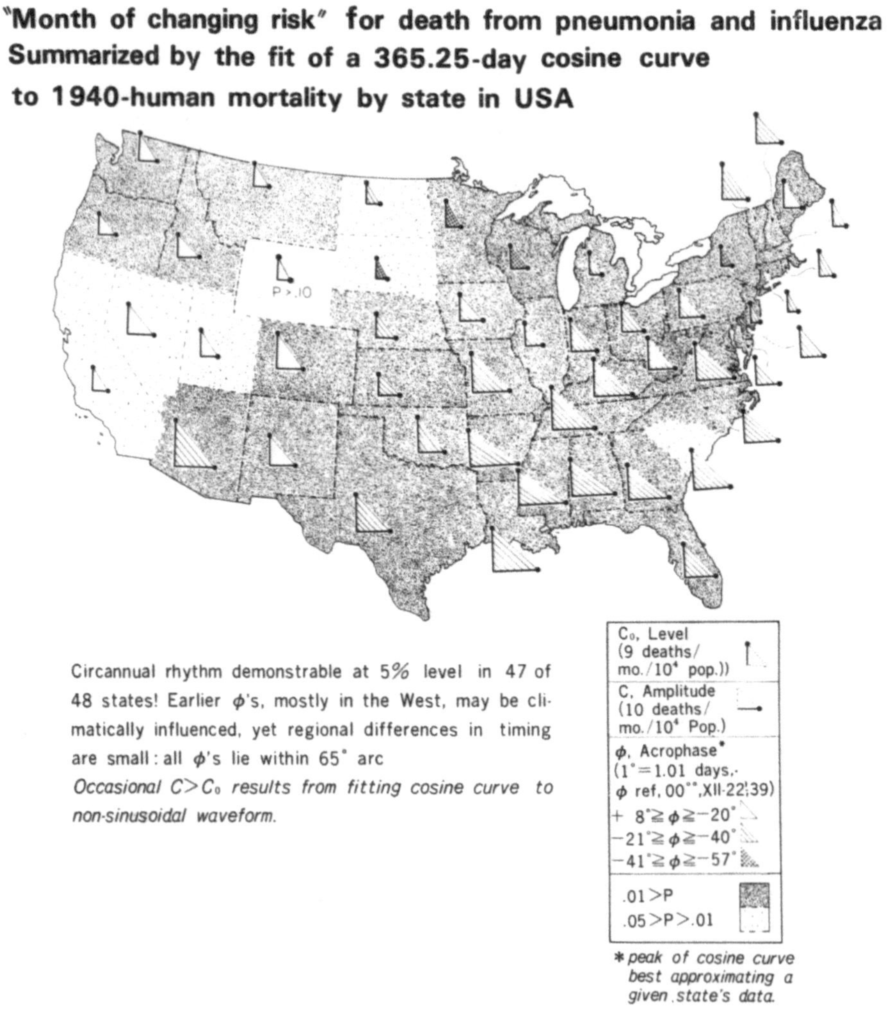

"Month of changing risk" for death from pneumonia and influenza Summarized by the fit of a 365.25-day cosine curve to 1940-human mortality by state in USA

Circannual rhythm demonstrable at 5% level in 47 of 48 states! Earlier ϕ's, mostly in the West, may be climatically influenced, yet regional differences in timing are small: all ϕ's lie within 65° arc
Occasional $C > C_0$ *results from fitting cosine curve to non-sinusoidal waveform.*

C_0, Level (9 deaths/ mo./10^4 pop.))
C, Amplitude (10 deaths/ mo./10^4 Pop.)
ϕ, Acrophase* ($1° = 1.01$ days,· ϕ ref. 00^{00},XII·22|39)
$+ 8° \geq \phi \geq -20°$
$-21° \geq \phi \geq -40°$
$-41° \geq \phi \geq -57°$
$.01 > P$
$.05 > P > .01$
peak of cosine curve best approximating a given state's data.

Fig. 142. "Months of Changing Risk" for Death from Pneumonia and Influenza. Symbols for each state summarize time series on pneumonia and influenza. Circannual rhythms demonstrable at 5% level or better in 47 of 48 states. Earlier ϕ's, mostly in the west, may be climatically influenced; regional differences in ϕ are small: all lie within an arc of 65°. Largest C_0 and C's in the south possibly reflect socio-economic influence. Occasional $C > C_0$ results from fitting cosine curve to slightly non-sinusoidal waveform.

In Fig. 139, the mean monthly incidence of respiratory mortality is separately shown for samples of the northern and southern hemispheres. Most respiratory deaths occur during the winter months; highest mortality takes place during February in the northern hemisphere and during July in the southern hemisphere.

Analysis of time series reporting respiratory mortality for higher frequency rhythms fails to yield statistically significant harmonics (P<.05). Comparison of the mean monthly incidence for the northern hemisphere with its best fitting 365.25-day cosine curve (Fig. 138), shows that the overall trends are closely approximated. Since only two studies of respiratory mortality are known for the southern hemisphere, the best fitting 365.25-day cosine curve was derived by a least squares fit to the mean monthly incidences. Inspection of the graph for the southern hemisphere shows the major features of the curve summarizing the monthly incidence of respiratory mortality are adequately represented.

Examination of 1940 influenza and pneumonia deaths, reported per 100,000 inhabitants, for each state in the U. S. reveals circannual rhythms of similar timing as those found for other samples previously reviewed. As graphically indicated in Fig. 142, geographic trends are reflected by regional differences in level (C_0), amplitude (C) and acrophase (ϕ). The greatest levels and amplitudes are found for states of the extreme Northeast and those of the South. The increased incidence of such mortality in the Northeast is expected and seemingly reflects the temperature and precipitation pattern of the winter season in this region. The high number of cases observed in the mid-Southern states apparently reflects substandard housing as well as inadequate medical and nutritional care for the poor classes, which make up a substantial proportion of the population within this region. Further, it is suggested that in certain regions of the South persons die from respiratory illnesses, possibly at an early age, rather than from other diseases, such as cardiovascular ones, usually contracted later in life.

The acrophases of respiratory mortality for separate states differ only slightly and all lie within an arc of $-65°$. These for states of the Northwest occur somewhat earlier than ones for the Midwest and Southeast, for which they are latest. Results of t-tests [227] performed on differences of regional means for the rhythm characteristics, C_0, C and ϕ, substantiate statistical significance, below the .001% level of probability, for these geographical trends. In spite of these trends a circannual rhythm in respiratory deaths for the United States is detected by cosinor with an average acrophase, approximating highest mortality, at $-30°$ (January 21). This acrophase differs by only $10°$ (10 days) from the average ϕ for other samples collected from various geographic areas as the world.

DISCUSSION

Evidence is presented for rhythms in several aspects of natality and mortality. Least squares spectral and cosinor analyses document circadian and circannual rhythms in birth as well as circadian rhythms in cardiovascular, pediatric and pulmonary deaths. In addition, about-one-year periods in cardiovascular and respiratory morbidity and mortality and in serum cholesterol concentration are demonstrated.

Because few authors have objectively examined human population rhythms, our approach has been to describe rhythmicity in terms of the C_0, C and ϕ using least

squares spectral and cosinor computer programs. Close agreement of waveform parameters between samples is the more noteworthy since in most instances only short,
transverse, time series covering one or slightly more than one period were available
for study and, moreover, the number of different sources of data were gathered from
various geographic areas.

The question of whether the rhythms herein documented represent true biorhythms,
endogenous self-sustaining systems in populations rather than mirror images of geophysical or social cycles of corresponding period, cannot be answered at this time.
Substantiation of these periodicities as true biorhythms requires that three criteria be
met. First, the waveform of the rhythm must be repetitive with the interval of time
between successive tracings being approximately the same. Second, the acrophase
must be phase-shiftable with the change in phase being in the same direction and
ultimately in amount equivalent to that in the synchronizer. (For rodents and
humans, the major synchronizer of circadian rhythms is believed to be the 24-hour
light-dark and rest-activity schedules, respectively. For human circannual rhythms,
several environmental phenomena are suspected [88].) Finally when populations are
completely isolated from environmental and/or societal time cues, a rhythm should
assume its non-entrained, or, so-called, free-running period.

Evidence for biorhythmicity in certain circadian physiologic functions comes from
longitudinal study of separate individuals rather than whole populations. In such
studies, self-measurements on a number of functions are made several times daily
before, during and after phase-shifting (by rapid geographic displacement by airplane)
and/or complete isolation (in underground bunkers or caves).

Similar evidence for biorhythmicity in circadian and circannual human population
rhythms is not easily obtainable. For example, in the case of the circadian ones in
human birth and death, statistics summarizing the hourly incidence of such events
for night versus day workers would be helpful; yet this information is not available.
In the case of circannual rhythms, the ability to substantiate phase-shifting and free-
running characteristics of suspected biorhythms does not appear possible at this time
although such an opportunity may occur when manned orbital space stations become
a reality. Until further information becomes available, results of least squares spectral
and cosinor analyses, providing statistical evidence for at least circadian human
population rhythms in natality and mortality, are presented with the assumption that
such periodicities represent true biorhythms. Additional information is required for
elucidating the relative contributions to human circannual rhythms of similarly periodic
geophysical and social events as well as of rhythms in underlying physiologic
functions.

Circadian and circannual periodicities in natality and mortality may be influenced
by rhythmic processes of corresponding frequency in related or underlying physiologic
mechanisms. For example, reproductive function in the human female, besides revealing an about-30-day period, is organized along the scale of 24 hours as is that of the
male. As shown in Table 42 circadian rhythms have been detected for females in the
excretion of follicle-stimulating hormone, FSH [182], and human chorionic gonadotrophin, HCG [11], and plasma FSH and lutinizing hormone LH [141] and estrogen [216]
concentration as well as the duration of labor according to its time of onset [148] and
the commencement of menstruation [156]. For males circadian rhythms in FSH
[70, 141], LH [141] and testosterone [63, 175, 200] have been reported (Table 43).

TABLE 42   Circadian organization of reproductive function in human females

Variable /subjects/	Level, C_0 $C_0 \pm$ S.E.	Amplitude, C $C \pm$ S.E.	Acrophase, ϕ^7 (.95 confidence arc)
Onset of menstruation[1] (120 NP)***	4.2 ± 0.5	2.7 ± 0.7	$-158°(-131$ to $-186)$
FSH[2] (6 NP)***	15.4 ± 0.9	11.3 ± 1.2	$-111°(-98$ to $-125)$
" (3 BC)**	12.8 ± 2.4	8.1 ± 2.6	$-106°(-88$ to $-113)$
LH[4] (6 NP)***	19.9 ± 2.1	13.2 ± 2.8	$-109°(-81$ to $-136)$
" (3 BC)***	13.4 ± 2.9	14.6 ± 1.1	$-84°(-55$ to $-108)$
Chorionic Gonadotropin[3] (24 P)***	100%	22.2 ± 2.7	$-104°(-91$ to $-117)$
Estrogen[4] (25 P)***	16.7 ± 0.6	3.3 ± 0.6	$-59°(-41$ to $-77)$
Duration of labor from:[5]			
a) Rupture of membranes $(24 \times 10^3 P)$***	9.1 ± 0.3	1.1 ± 0.4	$-111°(-61$ to $-156)$
b) Onset of contractions $(68 \times 10^3 P)$***	10.3 ± 0.4	0.4 ± 0.2	$-121°(-41$ to $-151)$
c) Membranes & contractions $(92 \times 10^3 P)$***	9.7 ± 0.3	0.8 ± 0.3	$-114°(-81$ to $-144)$
Incidence of:			
a) Spontaneous labor[3] $(2.08 \times 10^5 P)$***	100%	36.0 ± 2.6	$-15°(-0$ to $-27)$
b) Spontaneous birth[3] $(2.08 \times 10^6 P)$***	"	13.0 ± 2.6	$-64°(-51$ to $-77)$

Units in: 1. % incidence per hour; 2. FSH (follicle-stimulating hormone) and LH (luteinizing hormone): mIU(2nd IRP-HmG)ml; 3. relatives: %x or C_0; 4. µg/100 ml plasma; 5. hours (ϕ = commencement time for labors of expected longest duration); 6. P = pregnant and NP = non-pregnant females; BC = women taking steroidal-oral contraceptives; 7. ϕ reference = local midnight ($15°$ = 1 hour).
Rhythm detection: ** = $.01 < P < .05$; *** = $.001 < P < .01$.

Interestingly, the acrophases of either the serum concentration or excretion of such reproductive hormones in females and males are comparable in phasing to those of the adrenal cortex [95, 96, 171, 197].   Thus, in diurnally active humans, estrogen and testosterone as well as plasma 17-hydroxycorticosteroids reach greatest concentrations at about the usual time of arousal from nocturnal rest.

The finding of circadian rhythms in several groups of non-pregnant females, including those taking oral contraceptives and in groups of pregnant subjects as well, suggests that circadian organization of endocrine function characterizes not only the non-pregnant state, but pregnancy as well.   The hourly incidence of natural labor and birth along the scale of 24 hours, although dependent on a number of factors, may in part mirror the temporal organization and synchronization patterns of pertinent endocrine secretory functions and/or possible cellular hormone sensitivity rhythms of the same period.

Detection of a 24-hour periodicity in induced birth with a diurnal acrophase reflects recent trends in obstetrical practice.   For example, under the concept of "daylight obstetrics" [3], initiated by Dr. C. I. Csapo, one-half of all deliveries in one St. Louis hospital from 1967 to 1970 were scheduled between 09^{00} and 17^{00}; by 1972, obstetricians at this institution as well as at others expect to induce all births during the day.   The methodology enabling safe daytime delivery, involves continuous

TABLE 43   Circadian organization of human male reproductive function

Hormone (subjects)	Level, C_0 $C_0 \pm$ S.E.	Amplitude, C.	Acrophase, ϕ^3 (.95 Confidence Interval)
FSH[1] (13)**	20.5 ± 4.4	19.7 ± 5.8	$-115°(-78$ to $-152)$
LH[1] (13)**	22.5 ± 3.8	20.3 ± 5.0	$-118°(-86$ to $-149)$
Testosterone[2] (4)***	$.72 \pm .05$	$.11 \pm .04$	$-128°(-61$ to $-210)$
" (9)***	$.62 \pm .05$	$.12 \pm .05$	$-132°(-58$ to $-191)$
" (14)***	$.37 \pm .02$	$.08 \pm .03$	$-112°(-84$ to $-195)$

1. FSH (follicle stimulating hormone) and LH (luteinizing hormone) in units of mIU (2nd IRP-HmG)ml.
2. Units of μg/100 ml plasma.
3. ϕ reference = local midnight ($15° = 1$ hour).
   Rhythm detection: ** $= .01 < P < .05$; *** $= .001 < P < .01$.

regulation of oxytocin infusion in relation to uterine activity, monitored electronically by an extraovular microballon.

The concept of "daylight delivery" is, however, not consistent with the findings on natality: 1) the acrophase of natural birth occurs at $-64°$, 2) a greater incidence of stillbirth is recorded during the daytime, in particular at $-257°$ and 3) deliveries near the antiphase (ϕ $-180°$) of natural birth more often are associated with maternal complications [85]. On the other hand, since serious complications have not been encountered in "scheduled" deliveries, it seems that the increased quality of hospital care provided by carefully trained staff using modern equipment and techniques can override possible risk of danger from delivery during the antiphase of natural birth.

In this regard the finding of a rhythm in stillbirths as well as maternal complications may result in part from inadequate hospital-care systems. Moreover, the temporal incidence of stillbirth may not necessarily represent poorer survival rates for birth during the day; it may reflect circadian fetal or maternal responses to high doses of certain drugs such as anaesthetics sometimes used during delivery. In any event, if one considers the circadian rhythm in natural birth as an expression of underlying or related temporally coordinated reproductive rhythms of the same period, for example, in neural and/or endocrine activity, induction of delivery timed to the expected acrophase of natural birth, when apparently the system is more receptive to birth, may further reduce the duration of labor and, in addition, facilitate more difficult labors. Evidence that the duration of labor, when allowed to proceed without medical intervention, is shorter near the expected acrophase of natural birth is already available [146–148].

Although rhythms in pertinent systems may underlie the incidence of natural birth along the scale of 24 hours, no strong evidence is available suggesting the occurrence of birth along the scale of one year depends upon circannual differences in fertility. A certain number of reports, based mainly on animal experiments, indicate that environment influences, such as high temperatures during the summer, interfere with the viability of sperm. One study [9] finds the monthly incidence of coitus follows a circannual pattern, which suggests the temporal distribution of births is so influenced.

A number of studies [45–49, 231] implicate the importance of various social influences on circannual rhythms in birth. For example, in Roman Catholic samples, religious practices accompanying Lent, such as sexual abstinence, serve to effect the timing of the crest in births during the year. In other populations birth control techniques, schedules of taxation and work as well as important cultural happenings influence the waveform characteristics of this rhythm

Circannual rhythms in birth, found for most samples, are beyond the scope of this review but it should be noted that in animals, fertility rhythms synchronized by photoperiod are known [1, 8, 71, 89, 239]. Possible relationships between latitude and acrophase expressing possible intrinsic fertility rhythms and/or cultural, societal and geophysical factors deserve study.

In addition to rhythms in birth, circadian ones in human mortality were documented for groups of children and adult males and females irrespective of cause of death and for cardiovascular and pulmonary illnesses irrespective of age or sex. Greatest overall mortality, approximated by the acrophase, is expected at $-108°$ (07^{12}). The timing of greatest mortality from specific diseases varied only slightly being $-89°$ and $-152°$ for pulmonary and cardiovascular deaths, respectively.

The phasing of human mortality rhythms, while apparently affected by a number of factors, seemingly depends at least on the nature of the disease and the system(s) attacked. For example, the circadian acrophase of cardiovascular death at $-152°$ coincides in phase with rhythms of reduced heart minute volume [74], expected low systolic and diastolic blood pressure, slow pulse and elevated hematocrit and blood viscosity [100]. The implication of such a physiologic setting in contributing to or precipitating an embolism or thrombosis in persons so disposed has been discussed previously [123, 235]. Whether such phasing of rhythms as these actually underlie the observed periodicity in cardiovascular mortality is not yet certain. While 24-hour rhythms in human mortality may be related to similar frequency rhythms in underlying physiologic functions, the degree to which they indicate the competence and staffing of hospitals from one work shift to another is difficult to assess; although it may be an important contributory aspect.

In addition to circadian rhythms in mortality, circannual ones in cardiovascular, mainly heart, and respiratory (asthma, bronchitis, influenza and pneumonia) illnesses were detected in time series collected from a number of countries located in both the northern and southern hemispheres. Overall, a temporal ordering in the occurrence of peak incidences along the scale of one year became apparent. Thus, for respiratory diseases, highest morbidity occurs at $-2°$ (two days following, on the average, the longest night of the year, irrespective of hemisphere); greatest respiratory mortality is expected at $-40°$, 38 days later. While the acrophase of respiratory mortality might be expected to vary at least slightly from one year to the next, Cohen's [42] data demonstrated that in the monthly incidence of death from influenza and pneumonia in New York City, during a span of 12 successive years, there was a mean difference between the overall acrophase and individual year ϕ's of only 13 days. Furthermore, the occurrence of viral epidemics, for example, such as that of the "Asian" flu of 1969, did not alter the peak incidence of respiratory illness [2]; instead the other rhythmometric parameters, the level and amplitude, reflected it.

For cardiovascular disease, the timing of greatest incidence of morbidity and mortality is displaced slightly later along the scale of one year from that of respiratory disease. Thus, the peak of cardiovascular illness at $-22°$ precedes highest mortality from the same or similar causes by 11 days, at $-33°$. Interestingly, the acrophase of serum total cholesterol concentration, STCC, at $-6°$ precedes the ϕ's of cardiovascular morbidity and mortality by 16 and 27 days, respectively. In human populations, the expected peaking of STCC at $-6°$ along with the greater risk of respiratory infection at $-2°$ may set the stage for the observed increased incidence of cardiovascular morbidity at $-22°$ and/or mortality at $-33°$ or respiratory deaths at $-40°$.

The detection of a wintertime peak in cardiovascular deaths for areas with cold winters agrees for the most part with findings of others. For example, Tromp [206] in summarizing his studies, states "that every year the highest mortality (from arteriosclerotic heart disease) is found in January and February, lowest mortality from heart diseases in summer. The colder January and February are, the greater the mortality. Although July and August have the lowest monthly values, these values are lowest in cool summers, highest in hot summers. The same is found in different biometeorological studies in the northern United States." Continuing, Tromp states that "in Texas it is the reverse, high values in summer, low in the mild winter. Both extreme cold and heat are affecting the cardiovascular function, apparently."

Analyses of mortality statistics for many countries in the temperate zone and each state in America reveal wintertime acrophases. For only one state, Nevada, was such a timing not documented; however, since the fit of the 365.25-day cosine curve was not satisfactory $(SE/C < .33)$ and, in addition, since analyses of data from surrounding states reveal wintertime ϕ's, it seems that the 1940 statistics for this state may have been atypical. Tromp's reference to the occurrence of a summertime crest in cardiovascular deaths for Texas was not substantiated from examination of statistics for 1940, nor for those of 1963 to 1967. In fact, an acrophase, comparable in timing to that for populations residing in regions having cold, harsh winters was found. Further, despite sometimes wide differences in weather, the timing of a higher incidence in cardiovascular deaths is similar from one year to another. Thus, for Texas a total range in ϕ of only 14 days was detected over a five-year span from 1963 to 1967. In connection with this, examination of Cohen's [42] statistics for heart deaths in New York City for a span of 12 successive years reveals a mean difference between the overall acrophase and individual yearly ϕ's of only eight days.

The possibility of semi-circannual rhythms in heart disease has been suggested previously [55, 206] for the Southern United States. In statistics here analyzed, every time series summarizing cardiovascular deaths revealed only a circannual periodicity; tests for significant periodicities other than that of one year did not indicate higher frequency components. However, evidence that heart morbidity may be more prevalent during the hotter months for certain populations living in regions characterized by high summer temperatures comes from studies of small samples by Aviernos [10], DePasquale and Burch [55] and Heyer et al. [110] for Egypt, Louisiana and Texas, respectively.

Although findings on circannual mortality rhythms are based on statistics from populations residing in the temperate regions, climates with large seasonal differences in temperature, circannual rhythms are substantiated for a population of a maritime climate exhibiting only slight seasonal temperature variation. Thus, analysis of current mortality data from Hawaii [234] reveals rhythms in cardiovascular death with an acrophase at $-27°$ ($P<.01$) and respiratory mortality with an acrophase at $-17°$ ($P<.05$). The acrophases of these rhythms agree closely with those found for samples from temperate regions with the former ϕ differing by only $6°$ (six days) from the average sample ϕ of cardiovascular mortality. In a maritime environment with relatively little seasonal changes in temperature as compared to temperate areas, the waveform of circannual mortality rhythms may be expressed with only slight modification; the exact timing of these acrophases possibly reflects the true timing of greatest susceptibility to cardiovascular and respiratory death. In temperate regions, the more extreme seasonal differences in weather possibly influence and modify the waveforms of circannual mortality rhythms.

That circannual rhythms in cardiovascular and respiratory deaths are detected which are comparable in timing for populations situated in different geographic locations and exposed to dissimilar climates suggests that such rhythms are dependent on certain related or underlying similar period rhythms. For example, recent studies by Haus [104] have demonstrated a circannual rhythm in the serum concentration of corticosterone in rodents housed under non-varying 12-hour alternating light (L) and dark (D) spans: L(06^{00} to 18^{00}):D(18^{00} to 06^{00}). For humans, similar period rhythms in endocrine function have been documented on one man studied longitudinally for a number of years [92] and for groups of subjects examined during a single year [246, 249]. Circannual organization for certain constituents of the blood [245, 248] and pulmonary functions [157], among others [59, 237] have been reported as well.

Human mortality patterns possibly dependent on physiologic rhythms of the same period suggest the concept of susceptibility rhythms. A number of studies on rodents [54, 66, 68, 69, 90, 92–94, 97–99, 103, 105, 120, 142, 144, 152, 209–211, 238, 253] document circadian changes in the response to various agents including acetylcholine [120], amphetamines [211], endotoxin [97], ethanol [103, 105], librium [152], noise [90, 91, 94], pentobarbital [54, 66, 209] ouabain [93, 99], and SU-4885 [68, 69].

Greatest susceptibility, approximated by the acrophase, seemingly is independent of states of activity per se and feeding. Such rhythms apparently are a function of the nature of the given agent and the system(s) most effected. Genetically comparable inbred animals subjected to identical conditions at different circadian-system-phases do not respond in the same manner. For example, in groups of mice kept in L(06^{00} to 18^{00}):D(18^{00} to 06^{00}) mortality from an overdose of ouabain [93, 99] was much higher when administered at 08^{00} as compared to administration at 20^{00}. Actually, irrespective of clock hour, one can define the acrophase of mortality from ouabain as occurring about $+60°$ from the middle of the daily light span. On the other hand, death from amphetamines [211] is much greater around 00^{00} than 12^{00}. For this rhythm the acrophase of mortality corresponds to an administration at $-173°$ from the middle of the daily light span (12^{00}).

For humans, Reinberg et al. [196, 198, 199] has documented circadian susceptibilities of a lesser nature in the cutaneous sensitivity of allergic persons to house dust, histamine and penicillin. In addition, DeVries et al. [59] found 24-hour rhythms in the respiratory tract's response to histamine aerosol. The amount of cutaneous erythema or airway resistance following allergen or histamine administration is expected to be greatest about four hours prior to the middle of the subject's nocturnal sleep-span. Not surprising is the fact that the phase of highest sensitivity to allergens correspond in time, and possibly underlies, the observation of a greater incidence of asthma attacks.

That similar circadian and circannual susceptibility rhythms of a more serious nature are related to morbidity and mortality rhythms of the same period certainly deserves further study since the detection of circannual rhythms in cardiovascular and respiratory illness, which are comparable in acrophase for populations differing in geography and climate, is consistent with the concept of endogenous susceptibilities. Further, the observance of but slight geographic trends in other characteristics of mortality rhythms may be considered as evidence that such periodicities may be influenced, modified and perhaps synchronized by certain environmental phenomena rather than directly or indirectly resulting from annual weather cycles.

While it is here suggested that mortality rhythms have endogenous components, environmental phenomena apparently can serve to modify their expression. For example, in graphing the daily mortality for a given area over a span of one or more years, several minor peaks and troughs are present in addition to the major crest of the main frequency. At least some of the minor peaks are believed to result from environmental influences such as the sudden occurrence of extremely hot weather for a prolonged span [137]. In the case of large areas, geographic trends, apparently due to regional weather patterns, are discernable in the waveform characteristics of circannual cardiovascular and respiratory mortality rhythms for individual states of the U. S. The circannual level, C_0, amplitude, C, and acrophase, ϕ, while comparable from one state to the next, vary slightly. In the case of cardiovascular deaths, the monthly incidence approximated by C_0, is much greater in the North than in the South; the amplitude in general varies in a similar manner. The acrophases, all but one lying within an arc of 80°, occur earliest in the West. For respiratory mortality highest values of C_0 and C are found in the South and earliest ϕ's occur in the West.

Since the incidence of heart and respiratory mortality previously has been related to certain meteorologic factors, especially temperature, correlations between the C_0, C and ϕ of time series summarizing the 1940 heart and respiratory death and temperature data of the 48 states have been examined. Table 44 summarizes the relationships between the variables. Most of the findings are consistent with those of earlier reports and the geographic trends previously outlined. For example, a statistically significant negative correlation between mean monthly temperature and mean monthly heart deaths confirms the expectation that a population dwelling in cooler states suffers a higher incidence of heart disease. The significant relationship between the C_0 of heart death and ϕ of temperature apparently results from the situation that higher death rates are found in Northern states in which the onset of winter weather is slightly earlier (a less negative ϕ) than those of the Central or Southern regions of the country.

Many of the correlations between temperature and respiratory mortality while reflecting climate also indirectly suggest societal influences. Thus, the greater C_0 of respiratory death might be expected in the cooler states of the North; yet, the finding of greatest incidence for states with high mean monthly temperature implies that living conditions—apparently poor, crowded housing, inadequate nutrition and poor medical care—in the warmer Southern states contribute to the high risk of such populations. The finding of a significant relationship between the ϕ of temperature and

TABLE 44 Correlations between C_0, C and ϕ of temperature and respiratory and heart mortality for data by states of U.S. for 1940

Environmental temperature			Heart mortality			Respiratory mortality			
C_0	C	ϕ	C_0	C	ϕ	C_0	C	ϕ	
	−.609**	.227	−.468**	−.007	−.153	.646**	.767**	.010	C_0
		−.420**	.125	−.030	−.243	−.379**	−.435**	−.422**	C — Environmental temperature
			−.430**	−.505**	.530**	.216	−.242	.694**	ϕ
				.651**	.090	−.497**	−.601**	−.042	C^0
					−.316*	−.168	−.214	−.328*	C — Heart mortality
						−.072	−.173	−.647**	ϕ
							.023	.879**	C_0
								.027	C — Respiratory mortality
									ϕ

Statistical Significance: *.01 < P < .05; **P < .01

respiratory mortality as well as the former and heart mortality reveals a synchrony in phasing of such circannual rhythms.

Correlations between the C_0, C and ϕ for heart and respiratory death also confirm certain other expectations. For example, a significant negative relationship between the C_0's of these mortality rhythms implies simply death from one disease precludes that from another. The interpretation of the significant relationship between the C_0 of heart mortality and the C of respiratory mortality is less clear; although the high level (C_0) of heart mortality in the states of the North is for the most part associated with low amplitude respiratory mortality rhythms, the reverse situation exists for states making up the South. The positive correlation between the ϕ's for heart and respiratory deaths reflects similarity of phasing in these periodicities.

Although examination of the acrophases for cardiovascular and respiratory mortality for separate states in the U. S. as well as certain countries of the world reveal only small differences, there is some evidence that the acrophase of certain circannual population rhythms may be phase-shifted by extreme environmental conditions. In most regions of the temperate zones, characterized by cold winters and warm summers, greatest cardiovascular morbidity occurs in winter. On the other hand, in some areas having moderate winters and hot summers, for example, Egypt, Louisiana and Texas, highest morbidity is found during the summer. Similarly, the circannual acrophase of human and non-human primate births varies with latitude; the higher the latitude, the later the acrophase. In the latter cases, changes in the ϕ's for birth with latitude may reflect endogenous fertility rhythms, environmental cycles, social influences or interactions among these factors.

SUMMATION

The examples presented herein indicate that in human populations as well as in individuals circadian and circannual rhythms are prominent. These rhythms can be objectively described and quantified by least squares spectral and cosinor analyses. Their genesis is complex and probably the result of interacting internal and external factors.

In the case of circadian and probably circannual rhythms as well, the phasing of such periodicities is apparently synchronized by activity-rest routines along the scale of 24 hours and possibly by a host of other schedules including a relative activity-inactivity sequence along the scale of one year. Since such schedules may vary from one sample to the next and also because statistics are summarized by clock-hour and/or calendar-month rather than by reference to pertinent synchronizer schedules, the same time of day or month does not necessarily indicate similar circadian or circannual phases in populations adhering to different routines. Because of these circumstances the substantiation and quantification of rhythms are often complicated. Yet the ability to document similarly-phased periodicities in separate groups for birth, illness and death is remarkable, reflecting the prominence of human rhythmic phenomena.

The quantification and subsequent interpretation of rhythms is further complicated because a given waveform probably reflects modulation, influence and/or synchronization by environmental and social factors as well as underlying physiologic functions. Moreover, the degree to which a given rhythm is affected by environmental versus social factors is not always apparent and may be dependent on the rhythm itself.

With these difficulties in mind, an attempt has been made to document and quantify human population rhythms in birth, illness and death. In the case of circadian mortality and circannual morbidity and mortality rhythms our approach has been non-classical, as compared to other works in this area, we suggest that such periodicities represent primarily endogenous susceptibility or risk rhythms which are modifiable by environmental phenomena. In the past, circannual morbidity and mortality patterns have been considered as direct or indirect effects of environmental temperature and precipitation cycles of corresponding period. Although it cannot be proven with certainty, the hypothesis that an "internal time structure" is a (not the sole) determinant of human population rhythms is offered for consideration as an alternative to the latter.

Whichever hypothesis one chooses, it is of interest to compare the prominence of the within-day to within-year variation by calculation of circadian/circannual ratios of

TABLE 45   Cosinor summary for circadian and circannual human population rhythms of birth and cardiovascular and respiratory diseases[†]

Period fitted	Endpoint	Variable	Amplitude, C^2	Acrophase, ϕ^3 (.95 confidence interval)
24.0 hours	Natality	Spontaneous***	13(10 to 15)	$-64°(-51$ to $-77)$
		Cardiovascular**	12(.1 to 25)	$-152°(-75$ to $-234)$
	Mortality	Respiratory***	12(6 to 18)	$-89°(-15$ to $-131)$
	Natality	All**	3(.5 to 6)	$-50°(-4$ to $-94)$
		Cardiovascular**	6(.3 to 11)	$-12°(-350$ to $-46)$
365.25 days	Morbidity	Respiratory**	57(23 to 91)	$-2°(-291$ to $-91)$
		Cardiovascular***	17(13 to 20)	$-33°(-15$ to $-48)$
	Mortality	Respiratory***	55(37 to 73)	$-40°(-20$ to $-58)$

1. Rhythm detection: ** $= .01<P<.05$; *** $= .001<P<.01$.
2. Amplitude expressed as % of C_0 ($C_0 = 100\%$).
3. ϕ reference ofr circadian rhythms = local midnight ($15° = 1$ hour); for circannual rhythms $\phi = 00°°$ of the average longest night of the year, December 22 in the northern hemisphere and June 22 in the southern hemisphere ($1° = 1.01$ days).
    † = note circadian/circannual amplitude (within-day to within-year variation) ratio close to unity for cardiovascular mortality (0.923) but not for respiratory deaths (0.207) or birth (4.060).

amplitudes determined by cosinor analyses not only for the rhythms of cardiovascular and respiratory mortality, but birth as well. As shown in Table 45, the circadian/ circannual ratio for respiratory death is much lower than unity (0.207); the extent of rhythmic variation in mortality along the scale of one year greatly exceeds that along the scale of 24.0 hours. On the other hand, a value of more than four for birth indicates that the circadian amplitude is considerably greater than the circannual one. For cardiovascular mortality, a ratio nearly equal to one reflects comparable amplitudes of these circadian and circannual rhythms.

In a similar manner one may compare the amplitudes of cardiovascular and respiratory mortality separately for the periods of 24.0 hours and 365.25 days. In so doing, little difference is found between such circadian amplitudes. On the other hand, examination of the circannual amplitudes of these rhythms reveals that the within-year variation in respiratory mortality is considerably greater than that of cardiovascular mortality.

REFERENCES

1. AMOROSO, E.C., and L.H. MATTHEWS (1955): *Brit. Med. Bull.* **11**: 87.
2. ANONYMOUS (1970): *Metropolitan Life Ins. Stat. Bull.* 9 April.
3. ANONYMOUS (1970): *Med. World News* **11(21)**: 15.
4. Personal comunication, Texas State Health Department, Austin, Texas.
5. ANONYMOUS (1940): Vital Statistics of the United States. U.S. Department Health, Education and Welfare, Table 25, Crude death rates for selected causes by month: United States and each State.
6. ANONYMOUS (1963–6): Vital Statistics of the United States. U.S. Department Health, Education and Welfare. Vol. I. (Tables 1–35 or 36).
7. ANTONIS, A., I. BERSOHN, R. PLOTKIN, D.L. EASTY, and H.E. LEWIS (1965): *Am. J. Clin. Nutr.* **16**: 428.
8. ASCHOFF, J. (1967): *J. Biometeor.* **11**: 225.
9. AUDRY, J.R., and N.M. MORRIS (1967): *Demography* **4(2)**: 673.
10. AVIERNOS, C. (1954): *Congres Mondial de Cardiologie*, Washington, **II**: 876.
11. BAECHLER, C., R. BORTH, and A. MENZI (1966): *Acta Endocr.* **52**: 199.
12. BAJUSZ, E. (1963): Conditioning Factors for Cardiac Necroses. S. Karger, Basel, Switzerland.
13. BARTH, J. (1937): Uber die Ursache für die Jahres- und Tageszeitlichen Schwankungen in der Frequenz des Geburtsbeginns bzw. der Geburtsbeendigung. Würzburg.
14. BASIOR, R. (1934): Die Beziehungen des Geburtsomments zu den Jahres- und Tageszeiten. Basel.
15. BEAN, W.B., and C.A. MILLS (1938): *Am. Heart J.* **16**: 701.
16. BEGG, T.B. (1966): *Brit. Med. J.* **2**: 815.
17. BERENS, J. (1874–5): *Phila, Med. Times* **5**: 420.
18. BERLINSKI, R. (1835): *Froriep Notizen* **45**: 292.
19. BLISS, C.I. (1958): *Conn. Agri. Expt. Stat. Bull.* **615**: pp. 3–53.
20. BOGEN, E. (1930): *Calif. Western Med.* **33**: 473.
21. BOGEN, E. (1941): *Calif. Western Med.* **54**: 260.
22. BOYD, E.M. (1935): *J. Biol. Chem.* **110(1)**: 61.
23. BRADLOW, B.A., and M.M. ZION (1958): *S.A. Med. J.* **32**: 427.
23. BREYER, G. (1932): *Budapesti Or. Ujs.* **30**: 771.
25. BREYER, G. (1937): *Arch. f. Kinderh.* **112**: 34.
26. BRUGER, M., and I. SOMACH (1932): *J. Biol. Chem.* **97**: 23.
27. BROWN, H.R., and R. PEARSON. (1948): *Am. Heart J.* **35**: 763.
28. BRUNING, J. (1935): *Munch. Med. Wschr.* **82(1)**: 510.
29. BUEK, H.W. (1829): Nachrichte von dem Gesundheitszustand der Stadt Hamburg; Gersons und Julius Magazin der Ausländischen Litteratur der Gesammten Heilkunde (Anhang Hamburg), pp. 347–54.
30. BUNDESEN, H.N., and J.S. FALK (1926): *J.A.M.A.* **87**: 1987.
31. BURDACH, C.F. (1830): *L. Voss, Leipzig*, **3**: 498.
32. BURNS, J.F. (1890): *N. Y. Med. J.* **51**: 17.
33. BUTLER, H.R., and D.G. BONHAM (1963): Perinatal Mortality. E. and S. Lingonstone, Ltd., Edingburgh, p. 182.

34. CALHOUN, R., V.K. HARVEY, and J.E. HOLWAGER (1959): *J. Indiana State Med. Assoc.* **52:** 1992.
35. CARAVAGLIOS, F. (1955): *Riv. Ital. d'Ij giene,* **15:** 379.
36. CASPER, J.L. (1846): Der Einfluss der Tageszeit auf Geburt und Tod des Menschen, 1. Kpaitel: Der Einfluss der Tageszeiten auf die Geburt. In: *Denkwurdigkeiten zur Medizinischen Statistik und Staatsarzneikunde.* Buncher und Humblot, Berlin, 740–52.
37. CHANG, K., S. CHAN. W. LOW, and C. NG (1963): *Human Biol.* **35(3):** 366.
38. CHARLES, E. (1953): *Brit. J. Prev. Soc. Med.* **7:** 43.
39. CHIODARELLI, C. (1935): *Giorn. Clin. Med.* **16:** 560.
40. CHRISTENSEN-MOLLER, E. (1937): *Acta Obst. Gynec. Scan.* **17:** 69.
41. COGET, J. WAREMBOURG, J., J. DESRUELLES, and J.F. MERLEN (1962): *La Presse Med.* **70(3):** 119.
42. COHEN, A.E. (1927): *Am. Heart J.:* **2:** 275.
43. COSKERY, O.J. (1877): *N.Y. Med. J.:* **26:** 44.
44. COSKERY, O.J. (1884): *N.Y. Med. J.* **40:** 385.
45. COWGILL, U.M. (1964): *Proc. Nat. Acad. Sci.* **52(5):** 1149.
46. COWGILL, U.M. (1966): *K4oeber Anthr. Soc. Pap.* No. 35, Berkeley, California, Fall.
47. COWGILL, U.M. (1966): *Ecology* **47(4):** 514.
48. COWGILL, U.M. (1966): *Nature* **209(5028):** 1067.
49. Cowgill, U.M. (1970): *Sci. Amer.* **222(1):** 104.
50. CRAMER, M. (1920): *Munch. Med. Wschr.* **47:** 1341.
51. CROWTHER, A.H. (1967): *Times* **63:** 347.
52. DANZ, C.F., and C.F. FUCHS (1848): In: *Schriften der Gesellschaft zur Beforderung der gesammten Naturwissenschaften zu Marburg* **6:** 206.
53. DAVID, J.H.S. (1963): *Gaz. Med. Port.* **16:** 501.
54. DAVIS, W.M. (1962): *Experientia* **18:** 235.
55. DEPASQUALE, N.P., and G.E. BURCH (1961): *Am. J. Med. Sci.* **242:** 468.
56. DEPORT, J.V. (1928): Maternal mortality and stillbirths in New York State, 1915–25, Health Dept. New York State, pp. 38–40.
57. DEPORT, J.V. (1932): *Am. J. Obstet. Gynecol.* **23:** 31.
58. DEVRIES, K., J.T. GOEI, J. BOOY-NOORD, and N.G. ORIE (1962): *Int. Arch. Allergy* **20:** 93.
59. DERUDDER, B. (1952): Grundriss einer Meteorobiologie des Menschen. Springer-Verlag, Berlin, 214 pages.
60. DINGLE, J.H., G.F. BADET, and W.S. JORDAN (1964): Illenss in the Home. Western Reserve University Press, Cleveland, pp. 23–28 and p. 321.
61. DORING, H., and R. LODDENKEPMER (1962): *Zschr. Kriesl. Forsch.* **51:** 401.
62. DOYLE, J.T., S.H. KINCH, and D.F. BROWN (1965): *J. Chron. Dis.* **18:** 657.
63. DRAY, F., A. REINBERG, and J. SEBAOM (1965): *Compte Rec. Acad. Sci.* **261:** 573.
64. DREYFUS, J.C., G. SCHAPIRA, J. RESNAIS, R.V. TAYLOR, and L. SCEBAT (1960): *Rev. Franc. Etud. Clin. Biol.* **5:** 384.
65. DUMA, R.J., and A.L. SILEGEL (1965): *Arch. Int. Med.* **115:** 443.
66. EMLEN, S.T., and W. KEN (1963): *Science* **142:** 1682.
67. ENTERLINE, P.E. (1966): *Arch. Environ. Health* **12:** 467.
68. ERTEL, R.J., F. HALBERG and F. UNGAR (1964): *J. Pharmacol. Exp. Ther.* **146:** 395.
69. ERTEL, R.J., F. UNGAR, and F. HALBERG (1963): *Fed. Proc.*
70. FAIMAN, C., and R.J. RYAN (1967): *Nature* **215:** 857.
71. FARNER, D.A. (1959): In: Photoperiodism and Related Phenomena in Plants and Animals. *Amer. Assn. Adv. Sci.,* Washington, D.C., p. 717.
72. FASLER, S. (1951): *Staatenwissenschaft. Stud.* **10:** 1.
73. FERE, C. (1888): *Compt. Rend. Soc. Biol.* **40:** 742.
74. FINGER, R. (1968): *Deutshe Luft-und Raumfahrt, Rep.* **68:** 31.
75. FINLAYSON, J. (1873–4): *Glasgow Med. J.* **6:** 171.
76. FISCHER, W. (1932): *Munch. Med. Wschr.* **79(2):** 1449.
77. FREY, S. (1929): *D. Zschr. f. Chir.* **218:** 366.
78. FYFE, T., M.G. DUNNIGAN, E. HAMILTON, and R.J. RAE (1968): *J. Atheroscher. Res.* **8:** 591.
79. GAUQUELIN, M.F. (1959): *Population* **14:** 4.
80. GAUQUELIN, M. (1967): *Gyn. Obst.* **66(2):** 229.
81. GEIST, L. (1860): Klinik der Greisenkrankheiten. Erlangen, II Teil, p. 17.
82. GERFELDT, E. (1956): *Archiv. Hyg. Bakt.* **140(7):** 540.
83. GREEN, K.G., W.H.W. INMAN, and J.M. THORP (1963): *J. Atheroscher. Res.* **3:** 593.
84. GUIETTE, M. (1835): *Bull. Soc. Med. Gand.* **1:** 74.
85. GULYUK, N.G. (1961): *Akush. Ginek.* **6:** 45.
86. GUTHMANN, H., and M. BIENHULS. (1936): *Monatsschr. Geburt. Gynakol.* **103:** 337.
87. HAGENTORN, A. (1932): *Munch. Med. Wschr.* **79:** 1181.

88. HALBERG, F. (1969): In: *Ann. Rev. Physiol.* **31:** 675.
89. HALBERG, F.: Body temperature, circadian rhythms and the eye. *Coll. Internat. du C.N.R.S.* Montpellier, 1967. C.N.R.S., 1970. pp. 497–519; Discussion remarks 520–28.
90. HALBERG, F., J.J. BITTNER, and R.J. GULLY (1955): *Fed. Proc.* **14:** 67.
91. HALBERG, F., J.J. BITTNERG, R.J. GULLY, P.G. ALBRECHT, and E.L. BRACKNEY (1955): *Proc. Soc. Exp. Biol. Med.* **88:** 169.
92. HALBERG, ., M. ENGELI, C. HAMBURGER, and D. HILLMAN (1965): *Acta Endocrinol. Suppl.* 103, pp. 54.
93. HALBERG, F., E. HAUS, and A. STEPHENS (1959): *Fed. Proc.* **18:** 63.
94. HALBERG, F., E. JACOBSON, G. WADSWORTH, and J.J. BITTNER (1958): *Science* **128:** 657.
95. HALBERG, F., and A. REINBERG (1967): *J. Physiol* **59(1):** 117.
96. HALBERG, F., and H. SIMPSON (1967): *Human Biol.* **39:** 405.
97. HALBERG, F., W.W. SPINK, P.G. ALBRECHT, and R.J. GULLY (1955): *J. Clin. Endocr. Metabl.* **15:** 887.
98. HALBERG, F., and A.N. STEPHENS (1958): *Fed. Proc.* **17:** 439.
99. HALBERG, F., and A.N. STEPHENS (1959): *Proc. Minn. Acad. Sci.* **27:** 139.
100. HALBERG, F., Y.L. TONG, and E.A. JOHNSON: In : The Cellular Aspects of Biorhythms. H. VON MAYERSBACH, ed. Springer Verlag, Berlin/New York, 1967, pp. 20–48.
101. HAMILTON, A.A. (1890–91): *Indiana Med. J.* **9:** 222.
102. HARST, B. (1935): Besteht ein Einfluss der Gezeiten (Ebbe und Flut) oder des Mondes auf die Geburt? Kiel.
103. HAUS, E., and F. HALBERG (1959): *J. Appl. Physiol.* **14:** 878.
104. HAUS, E., and F. HALBERG (1970): *J. Env. Res.* **3(2):** 81.
105. HAUS, E., E.M. HANTON, and F. HALBERG (1959): *The Physiologist* **2:** 54.
106. HECHTER, H.H., and J.R. GOLDSMITH (1961): *Am. J. Med. Sci.* **241:** 581.
107. HEINEN, G. (1925): *Umschau.* **29:** 848.
108. HENRY, J.R. (1924): *Rev. Franc. Gynec. Obstet.* **19:** 665.
109. HESS, J.W., R.P. MACDONALD, R.J. FREDERICK, R.N. JONES, J. NEELY, and D. GROSS (1964): *Ann. Int. Med.* **61:** 1015.
110. HEYER, H.E., H.C. TENG, and W. BARRIS (1953): *Am. Heart J.* **45:** 741.
111. HILL, A.B. (1937): Principles of Medical Statistics. Lancet, London, p. 90.
112. HOOGENDOORN, D. (1966): *Neder T. Geneesk* **110:** 1039.
113. HORN, J. (1910): *Norsk Mag. Laeg.* **8:** 630.
114. HORN, W. (1843): Zur Charakterisierung der Stadt Erfurt. Erfurt, pp. 363–373.
115. HOXIE, H.J. (1940): *Am. Heart J.* **19:** 475.
116. HVIDT, S., J. ROIN, and K.E. SIMONSEN (1968): *Ugeskr Laeg.* **130:** 42.
117. JENNY, E. (1933): *Mschr. Kinderh.* **56:** 165.
118. JENNY, E. (1933): *Schweiz Med. Wschr.* **63(1):** 15.
119. JENNY, E. (1944): *Schweiz Med. Wschr.* **74(1):** 630.
120. JONES, F., E. HAUS, and F. HALBERG (1963): *Proc. Minn. Acad. Sci.* **31:** 61.
121. JUSATZ, H.J., and E. ECKARDT (1934): *Munch. Med. Wschr.* **81(1):** 709.
122. KAISER, H., and F. HALBERG (1962): *Ann. N.Y. Acad. Sci.* **98:** 1056.
123. KENDELL, R. and E.J. MARSHALL (1963): *Brit. Med. J.* **2:** 344.
124. KEYS, A.B., H.L. TAYLOR, H.W. BLACKBURN, I. BRONZEK, J.T. ANDERSON, and E. SIMONSON (1963): *Circulation* **28:** 381–395.
125. KEYS, A., H. TAYLOR et al.: Coronary heart disease in seven countries. Supplement to *Circulation*, in preparation.
126. KING, P.D. (1956): *Science* **123:** 985.
127. KIRCHHOFF, H. (1935): *Zentr. Gynakol.* **59:** 134.
128. KISHON, Y., and I. KAVIN (1961): *Israel Med. J.* **20:** 259.
129. KLEINWACHTER, L. (1876): *Zeitschr. Geburt Frauen* **1:** 486.
130. KLINKER, L., and W. LEIDREITER (1969): *Zeitschr. Meteor.* **21:** 88.
131. KNAPP, C.B. (1909–10): *Bull. Lying in Hospital* **6:** 69.
132. KREUTZER, J. (1935): Uber die Todesstunden-Verteilung mit Besonderer Berücksichtigung des Kindesalters. Rostock.
133. KNOTH, W. (1952): *Archiv. Phys. Therapie,* **4:** 309.
134. LaDUE, J.S., F. WROBLEWSKI, and A. KARMEN (1954): *Science* **120:** 497.
135. LANKIALA, E. (1935): *Suomalianen Läävaroseura Duodecim Acta* **23:** 1.
136. LANDIS, H.G. (1876–7): *Phila Med. Times* **7:** 559.
137. LANDSBERG, H.E.: Weather and disease. Unpublished rep. U.S. Dept. Commerce, ESSA Tech. Note 33-EdS-1.
138. LAUE, W. (1933): Uber den Tageszeitlichen Beginn und das Ende der Spontangeburt. Leipzig.

139. Lawson, R. (1870): *West Riding Lun. Asyl. Rep.* **4:** 240.
140. Lehmann, V., and S. Raeder (1968): *Nord. Med.* **79:** 50.
141. Leyendecker, G., and B.B. Saxena (1970): *Klin Wschr.* **48:** 236.
142. Lindsay, H.A., and F. Senn (1950): *Acta Pharmacol. Toxicol.* **6:** 181.
143. Linn, T. (1888): De l'habitude et des ses rapports avec l'hygiene et la therapeutique. Paris.
144. Lutsch, E.F., and R.W. Morris (1967): *Science* **156:** 100.
145. Lynch, F.W. (1907): *Surg. Gynecol. Obstet.* **5:** 677.
146. Malek, J. (1948): *Ceskoslov. Gyhaek* **27:** 15.
147. Malek, J. (1962): *Gynaecologia* **133:** 365.
148. Malek, J., J. Gleich, and V. Maly (1962): *Ann. N.Y. Acad. Sci.* **98(4):** 1 ± 42.
149. Magnin, P. (1956): *Lyon Med.* **88(48):** 513.
150. Man, E.B., and E.F. Gildea (1937): *J. Biol. Chem.* **119:** 769.
151. Marsh, H. (1906): *Arch. Phil. Psy., Psy. Sci. Methods* **7:** 9.
152. Marte, E., and F. Halberg (1961): *Feb. Proc.* **20:** 305.
154. Master, A.M., S. Dack, and H.L. Jaffe (1937): *J.A.M.A.* **109(1):** 546.
153. Maschas, H., G. Chilarditis, K. Vasselounis, J. Zahariondakis, and L. Sparros. (1966): *La Presse Med.* **74(40):** 2031.
155. Master, A.M., and H.L. Jaffe (1952): *J.A.M.A.* **148:** 794.
156. McCance, M., C. Luff, and E.E. Widowson (1937): *J. Hyg.* **37:** 571.
157. McKerrow, C.B., and C.E. Rossiter (1968): *Thorax* **23:** 340.
158. McWhinney, I.R. (1968): *Lancet* **2:** 342.
159. Meyer, J.J. (1840): Einfluss der verschiedenen Abschnitte des Tages auf die Sterbefälle. *Meyers Topographia uber Dresden*, Stolberg und Harz, Leipzig, p. 326.
160. Meyer, M. (1935): *Med. Welt* **9(51):** 1856.
161. Meyer, M. (1936): *Med. Welt.* **10(25):** 907.
162. Mintz, S.S., and L.N. Katz (1947): *Arch. Int. Med.* **80:** 205.
163. Momiyama, M. (1969): *Geograph. Rev. Jap.* **42:** 1.
164. Momiyama, M. (1960): *J. Meteor. Soc. Jap.* **38(1):** 46.
165. Momiyama, M. (1961): *J. Meteor. Soc. Jap.* **39(3):** 103.
166. Momiyama, M., and K. Katayama (1969): *J. Meteor. Soc. Jap.* **47(6):** 466.
167. Momiyama, M., and H. Kito (1963): *Pa. Meteor. Geophy.* **14(3-4):** 190.
168. Morgan, R.W. (1968): *Brit. Columbia Med. J.* **16(6):** 163–164.
169. Mulhauser, R. (1935): Uber die Ursachen des Geburtsbeginns. Erlangen.
170. Mullins, W.L. (1936): *Penn. Med. J.* **39:** 322.
171. Nelson, W., and F. Halberg (1966): In: Handbook of Environmental Biology. *Fed. Am. Soc. Exp. Biol.* p. 586.
172. Nemeth, S., R. Stukovsky, and K. Knopp (1965): *Zschr. Inn. Med.* **20:** 500.
173. Nikolaev, I.A., and V.K. Marinov (1959): *Cardiologia* **35:** 179.
174. Niyogi, A.K., and R.G. Dhakappa (1964): *Ind. J. Med. Res.* **52:** 1092.
175. Nieschlag, E., and A.A.A. Ismail (1970): *Klin. Wschr.* **48:** 53.
176. Oesterlen, F. (1865): Handbuch der Medicinischen Statistik. Tübingen, p. 323.
177. Okey, R., and R.E. Boyden (1926): *J. Biol. Chem.* **72:** 261.
178. Okey, R., and D. Stewart (1932–33): *J. Biol. Chem.* **99:** 717.
179. Olivella, J.R. (1940): *Rev. Cubana Obstet. Ginecol.* **2:** 44.
180. Oppenheim, F., and L. Ritter (1920): *Munch. Med. Wschr.* **67:** 1339.
181. Orban, G., and E. Czeizel (1967): *Gynaecologia* **613:** 173.
182. Orlandi, F., G. Abate, B. Ferramosca, P. Bernardi (1966): *Arhciv. Pat. Clin. Med.* **42:** 382.
183. Otto, W. (1960): *Arztl. Forsch.* **14(8):** 404.
184. Paloheimo, J. (1961): *Ann. Med. Exp. Fenn.* **39:** Supl. 8.
185. Pasamanick, B., S. Dinitz, and H. Knoblock (1959): *Pub. Health Rep.* **74(4):** 285.
186. Pasamanick, B., S. Dinitz, and H. Knoblock (1960): *Milbank Mem. Fund. Quart.* **38:** 250.
187. Peterson, J.E., A.A. Wilcox, M.I. Haley, and R.A. Keith (1960): *Circulation* **22:** 247.
188. Peterson, W.F. (1937): The Patient and the Weather. Edwards Brothers, Inc., Ann Arbor, Michigan. Vol. IV, p. 269–302.
189. Pierach, A. (1969): *Herz Kreislauf.* **1:** 179–184.
190. Points, T.C. (1956): *Obstet. Gynecol* **8:** 245.
191. Puffer, R.R., and G.W. Griffith (1967): Patterns of urban mortality. Pan. Amer. Health Organ., Scientific Pub. **151:** 194.
192. Quetelet, M.A. (1842): A treatise on man and the development of his faculties. Translated by R. Knox. In: *Economic and Political Pamphlets* Vol. 99, W. and R. Chambers, Edinburg.
193. Raab, W. (1953): Hormonal and Neurogenic Cardiovascular Disorders. The Williams and Wilkins Co., Baltimore, Md.

194. RAAB, W. (1969): *Ann. N.Y. Acad. Sci.* **147**: 627–686.
195. RASERI, E. (1897): *Riv. d'Ig. San. Publ.* (Torino) **8**: 718.
196. REINBERG, A. (1967): *Per. Biol. Med.* **11(1)**: 111.
197. Reinberg, A., J. GHATA, F. HALBERG, P. GERVAIS, Ch. ABULKER, J. DUPONT, and Cl. GAUDEAU (1970): *Ann. Endocr.* **31(2)**: 277.
198. REINBERG, A., J. GHATA, and E. SIDI (1964): *Ann. Endoc.* **25**: 670.
199. REINBERG, A., E. SIDI, and J. GATA (1965): *J. Allergy* **36**: 273.
200. RESKO, J.A., and K.B. EIK-NES (1966): *J. Clin. Endoc.* **26**: 573.
201. RIPPMANN, E.T. (1964): *Gynaecologia* **158**: 31.
202. ROBLOT, M. (1925): Etude sur l'heure a laquelle accouchent les femmes suivie de commentaires sur l'influence de la lune. Paris.
203. RUMELIS, J. (1936): Uber die Tagesschwankung der Sterblichkeit. Basel.
204. ROSENBERG, H.M. (1966): *Statistrics—Special Reports, Selected Studies* **21(9)**.
205. SARGENT, F. (1940): *Am. J. Pub. Health* **30**: 533.
206. SARGENT, F.S.II (1964): *Proc. Lucknow Sym. Arid Zone* Re:. **24**: 19–32.
207. SCHEID, H. (1959): *Wien. Klin. Wschr.* **71(13)**: 217.
208. SCHNEIDER, E. (1940): *Archiv. Hyg. Bak.* **125**: 65.
209. SCHEVING, L.E. (1968): *Anat. Rec.* **160**: 741.
210. SCHEVING, L.E., and D. VEDRAL (1966): *Anat. Rec.* **154**: 417.
211. SCHEVING, L.E., D.F. VEDRAL, and J.E. PAULY (1968): *Nature* **219**: 621.
212. SCHLEGEL, L.K., STEMBERA, and J. POKORNY (1966): *Gynaecologia.* **162**: 185.
213. SCHNEIDER, C.F. (1859): *Virchow's Arch. Pathol. Anat. Physiol.* **16**: 217.
214. SCHNEIDER, C.F. (1859): *Virchows Arch. Path. Anat. Physiol.* **16**: 95.
215. SCHRIRE, V. (1958): *S. A. Med. J.* **32**: 429.
216. SELINGER, M., and M. LEVITZ (1969): *J. Clin. Endocr.* **29**: 995.
217. SELYE, H. (1958): The Chemical Prevention of Cardiac Necroses. The Ronald Press Co., New York, New York.
218. SHETTLES, L.E. (1960): *Am. J. Obstet. Gynec.* **79**: 177.
219. SIMPSON, A.S. (1952): *Brit. Med. J.* **2**: 831.
220. SMITH, J.F., J.W. KEYES and R.M. DENHAM (1951): *Am. J. Med. Sci.* **221**: 508.
221. SMOLER, M. (1862): *Prag. Vierteljahrsschr. Prak. Heil.* **3**: 134.
222. SOBRINHO, F.R. (1938): *Ann. Paul. Med. Cir.* **35**: 5.
223. SOBRINHO, F.R. (1941): *Arq. Hig. Saude Pub.* **6**: 237.
224. SPANN, W. (1957): *Germ. Med. Monthly* **2**: 116.
225. SPILLER, V. (1940): *Brit. Med. J.* **1**: 435.
226. STEEL, C. (1862): *Med. Times Gaz.* (Jan.) p. 87.
227. STEEL, R.C.D., and J.H. TORRIE (1960): Principles and Procedures of Statistics. McGraw-Hill, New York.
228. STUART-HARRIS, C.M., and T. HANLEY (1957): Chronic Bronchitis, Emphysema and Cor Pulmonale. John Wright, Bristol, pp. 2–9.
229. SUGIHARA, Y. (1954): *Seibutsu-Tokeigaku-Zasshi* **2**: 271.
230. SWAYNE, J.G. (1888): *Bristol M. Chir. J.* **6**: 174.
231. TAKAHASHI, E. (1964): *Tohoku J. Exper. Med.* **84**: 215.
232. THOMAS, C.B., H.W.D. HOLLJES, and F.F. EISENBERG (1961): *Ann. Intern. Med.* **54**: 413.
233. TOCHOWICZ, and L., T. CIBA, J. KOCEMBA, and L. SZOPINSKA (1962): *Polski Tygodnik. Lekarski.* **17**: 587.
234. G.H. TOKUYAMA: State Health Department of Hawaii. Personal communication.
235. TOOLE, J.F.: *Ann. Inter. Med.* **68(5)**: 1032.
236. TROMP, S.W. (1958): *Biometeor. Res. Center, Leiden* **3**: 1.
237. TROMP, W.S., and W.H. WEIHE, eds (1967): Biometeorology. Pergamon Press, Oxford.
238. TSAI, T.H., L.E. SCHEVING, and J.E. PAULY (1970): *Jap. J. Physiol.* **20**: 12.
239. TURNER, D.C. (1964): General Endocrinology. W.B. Saunders Co., Philadelphia, pp. 316–23.
240. VESELL, E.S. (1961): *Ann. N.Y. Acad. Sci.* **94**: 898.
241. VINCENT, W.R., and E. RAPAPORT (1965): *Am. J. Cardiol.* **15**: 17.
242. VIREY, J.J. (1814): Ephemerides de la vie humaine ur recherches sur la revolution journaliere et la periodicite de ses phenomenes dans la sante et les maladies. Paris.
243. WAGGONER, D.E., and J. SCHLACHTER (1947): *U.S. Vital Statistics Special Reports.* **47(4)**: 127.
244. WALKER, M.M. (1882–3): *J. Obstet. Gynecol. Ped.* **4**: 266.
245. WATANABE, G. (1958): *Jap. J. Med. Prog.* **45**: 487.
246. WATANABLE, G. (1964): *Arch. Env. Health* **9**: 192.
247. WATANABLE, G., and S. AOKI (1956): *Jap. J. Med. Prog.* **43**: 301.
248. WATANABE, G., and T. HUYAMA: *Jap. J. Med. Prog.* **43**: 480.

249. WATANABE, G., and S. YOSHIDA (1956): *J. Appl. Physiol.* **9(3):** 456.
250. WATSON, W.W. (1866): Report upon the vital, social and economic statistics of Glasgow for 1865. Glasgow.
251. WEISS, M.M. (1953): *Kentucky State Med. J.* **51:** 14.
252. WEST, R.U. (1853): *Assoc. Med. J.* **1:** 105.
253. WIEPKEMA, P.R. (1966): *Nature* **209:** 937.
254. WIGAND, R. (1934): *D. Med. Wschr.* **60(2):** 1709.
256. WOOD, F.C., and O.F. HEDLEY (1935): *Med. Clin. North Amer.* **19:** 151.
257. WROBLEWSKI, F., and K.F. GREGORY (1961): *Ann. N.Y. Acad. Sci.* **94:** 912.
258. WURSTER, K. (1949): *Zentr. Gynakol.* **71(2):** 159.

CHAPTER 19

CIRCADIAN RHYTHM IN BODY TEMPERATURE

TAKASHI SASAKI

Department of Physiology, Institute of Constitutional Medicine, Kumamoto University
Kumamoto, Japan

It is obvious that the origin of 24-hour rhythm is traced back to the rotation of the earth. Being subject to periodic changes in the environment, organisms will in the long run acquire adaptability to their surroundings. As a natural consequence it follows that they are provided with a sort of biological clock mechanism in the course of phylogeny.

Recent studies of biological rhythms in Japan were presented in the seminar on "Fundamental Problems of the Biological Rhythms of the Human Ecosystem" under the U.S.-Japan Cooperative Science Program in 1967, which was followed by a study group, "Circadian Rhythms in the Human Ecosystem." Rhythms studied by the group covered a wide variety of functions: body temperature regulation, behavior, humoral regulation, metabolic regulation and so forth. In this treatise, however, body temperature was selected as a theme for discussion for the following reasons. 1) Core temperature is an integrative demonstration of temperature regulation and may give more unbiased information about the body as a whole than any single function does. Granting that biological rhythms are not necessarily controlled by the same mechanism that the body temperature is, a better clue to the mechanism of biological rhythm may be obtained. 2) Typical circadian pattern of core temperature can be seen in the patterns of body temperature. It is relatively consistent, although with a few casual fluctuations of short duration. 3) Frequent or continuous observation is possible with ease, which enables us to collect enough data for further mathematical analysis. 4) No elaborate instrumentation is necessary. Observation is easily made in field-work as well.

Continuous recording gives exhaustive detail of the rhythm. In order to fight the flood of information, mathematical analysis of time series should be employed. Serial correlation, harmonic analysis, probability density function, autocorrelation function, power spectra are potential tools to determine the period. In case the period is assumed, calculation of the best fit cosine function to the original observations by the least squares method (the cosinor method by Halberg [6]) is a useful technique to determine the other characteristics of the rhythm—amplitude, phase and wave level. Though circadian pattern of body temperature, which is divided into the four stages of low temperature, morning rise, plateau in the daytime and evening fall, is different from cosine curve, estimation of the parameters proved practically successful.

SITE OF MEASUREMENT

Temperature of the body for the purpose of studying rhythm mechanism should

represent the thermal state of the body.   Since measurement of rectal temperature over
so many days is often restricted by the daily routine of life, the use of xiphoid
temperature and umbilical temperature was proposed.   Ohara [15] compared the
insulated umbilical and xiphoid temperatures with rectal, oral and axillary temperatures.
As long as change in environmental temperature was small, they ran parallel and phase
relationship was maintained.   Coefficients of correlation among a couple of sites were
fairly high (r=0.81—0.85).   But the insulated skin temperature in question was affected
more or less by a sudden change in the environmental temperature and was suggestive
of the original tendency of surface temperature.   Accordingly, if rectal temperature
is not available, oral or axillary temperature with due consideration is recommendable.

NUMBER OF MEASUREMENTS

Since observations in time series form a periodic pattern, it may roughly be approximated by the cosine function

$$y = C_0 + C \cos (\omega t + \phi)$$

where C_0 is wave level; C, amplitude; ω, angular velocity; t, time in hours, and ϕ,
phase.   As the period in this case is assumed to be 24 hours, ω is $2\pi/24$ or 15^0, and
three constants of C_0, C and ϕ are determined by the least squares method.   Fig.
143 shows the daily temperature curves for nine successive days on the same subject.
The range of each constant on successive days was: daily mean of body temperature
36.4—36.7°C, amplitude 0.35—0.63°C, or the difference between the maximal and

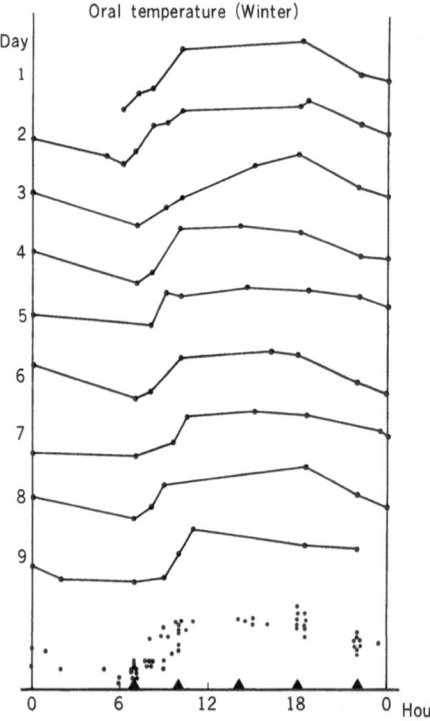

Fig. 143. Day-to-day variation in oral temperature for nine consecutive days. Solid
triangles at the bottom of the page indicate the times recommended for observation.

minimal temperatures ranged from 0.7 to 1.3 °C, and the acrophase −225 — −250°, with the highest temperature occurring at 1500—1630 hours. Therefore the day-to-day variation in the circadian pattern, judged from wave level, amplitude and acrophase, is small and consistent.

In Fig. 144, effect of the number of observations in a day on the constants for

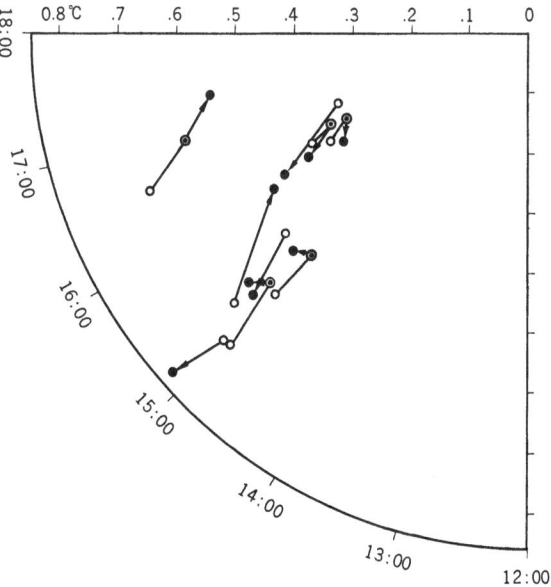

Fig. 144. Effect of number of observations on circadian pattern estimation. Combination of estimated phase and amplitude is plotted.

pattern estimation was shown by plotting the amplitude and phase angle relationship on polar coordinates. A solid circle illustrates the result of ten or more observations, a double circle shows the result calculated from five observations at 700, 1000, 1400, 1800 and 2200 hours taken from the same time series, and an open circle represents the result from four observations excluding the 1400 hours value. In every instance very little difference was shown between solid and double circles, while a considerable difference became manifest between double and open circles. In the case of four observations they all serve to estimate the phase constant, but serve little for amplitude estimation, because 700 and 1000 hours observations are made in the morning rise stage and the 1800 and 2200 hours observations the evening fall stage. By adding the 1400 hours measurement as the fifth observation, which deals with the plateau stage, a better estimation of amplitude is made.

TEMPERATURE RHYTHM IN SHIFT WORKERS

Procedures usually followed to reveal mechanism of biological rhythms are free-running routine in constant environment which is free from every periodic change, inversion of daily routine (12 hour shift), and non-24 hour routine. They all aim at finding a clue through responding changes in biological rhythms which are brought about by disturbing the synchronization of biological rhythm with routine of life and environmental rhythm.

Body temperature of night workers is maintained high at the start of their work, but it gradually falls towards midnight, notwithstanding their physical activities. Thus the morning rise and evening fall in temperature persist irrespective of work schedule, and the temperature level of sleep hours during the day is usually higher than the level of work hours during the night. Accordingly, physical activities and ingestion of food do not result in drastic change in the temperature pattern, but may modify it to some extent.

Watanabe [20] observed temperature patterns of workers in an iron works, which was operating on five-day rotation of three eight-hour shifts. As a shift of eight hours occurred every five days, observation was made for 20 consecutive days to cover four rotation periods. The temperature pattern showed considerable individual variation, but any sign of synchronization of biological rhythm to the routine of living was not observed within a five-day rotation period. Since successive rotation occurred

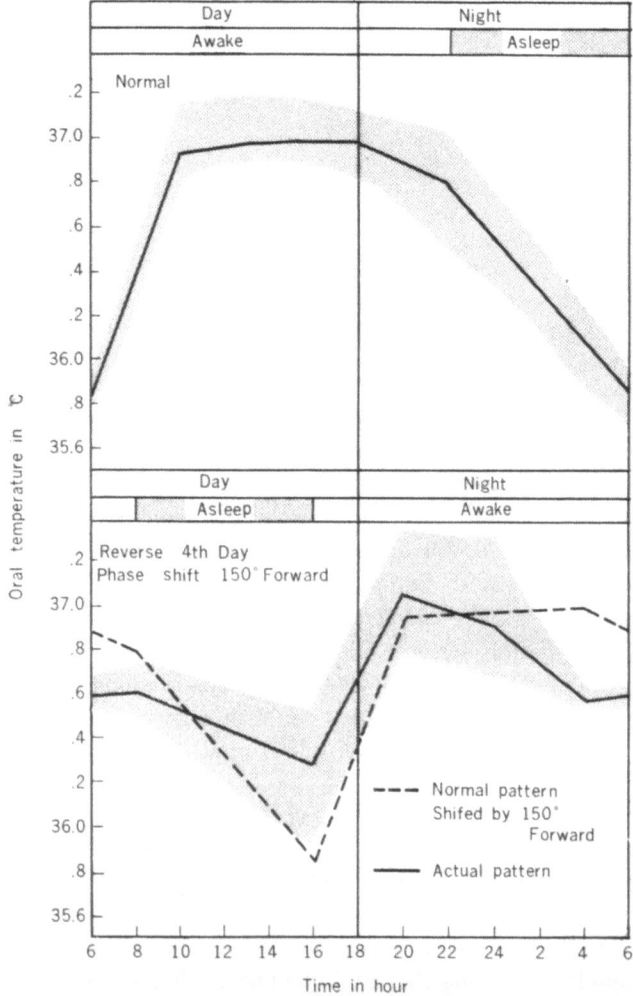

Fig. 145. Circadian pattern of oral temperature on the fourth day after a 10-hour delay in living routine (lower illustration), with the control pattern (upper illustration).

before synchronization developed, the biological rhythm was more and more disturbed, and finally their health was affected. In workers who have engaged in shift work for ten years or more the biological rhythm showed synchronization with their living schedule [19].

In contrast to shift workers, whose circadian temperature pattern resisted various attempts to change its original pattern, intercontinental travelers could adjust their biological clock to a new local time with relative ease in a short period, as will be discussed later. For these conflicting findings, control of experimental conditions—environmental-social as well as meteorological—becomes especially important. Here a missing link between the extreme findings was supplied by Yurugi *et al.* [21], who observed the effect of a 10-hour delay shift in a laboratory (Fig. 145). The experiment corresponded to a laboratory simulation of traveling from New York to Japan. Immediately after the phase shift, the circadian pattern was disturbed, but on the fourth day the temperature pattern showed a tendency to resume the new phase pattern, although the amplitude remained considerably reduced. Synchronization with the new phase, which was found in varying degrees in other functions, too, occurred as early and easily in general as in the case of intercontinental travelers. It is worthy of note that the experiment is in itself analogous to the situation in which night workers or shift workers are placed, but the result is quite different, and this might come from the following difference in control of conditions. The life of workers, except for work and sleep hours, was necessarily exposed directly or indirectly to the non-shift rhythms of home and social life, while in this experiment the laboratory was isolated completely from the outside world and the shift of living routine and environment was designed to be as perfect as possible. To cite an example, at 1700 hours the subject ate a meal which was breakfast in quality as well as in quantity, and which was different from that which his family ate at the same time of the day.

Efforts to establish non-24 hour rhythm in man were made by a number of in-

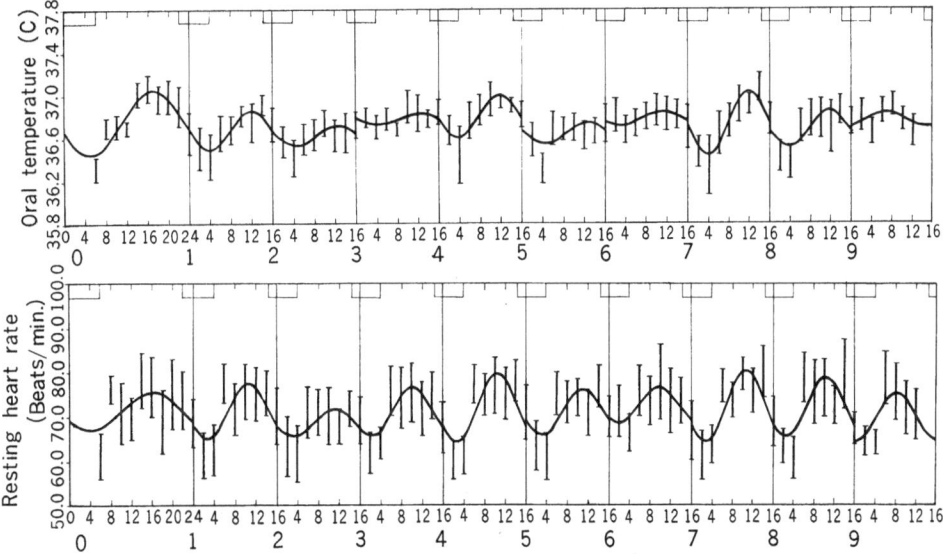

Fig. 146. Effect of 16-hour routine for nine days on oral temperature (top illustration), and heart rate (bottom illustration).

vestigators. Attempts to develop a six-hour, 12-hour, or 48-hour rhythm were not successful and a partial adjustment to the artificial routine was shown only so far as the period was between 18 and 28 hours [9]. Yurugi *et al.* [22] observed the effect of 16-hour routine for nine days and found that the original rhythm of oral temperature was maintained firmly and did not synchronize with the artificial period. The same tendency was shown by other functions too, except for the heart rate, which was coupled more closely with the routine period of meals, activities and sleep (Fig. 146).

From these findings it may be concluded that resynchronization of the biological rhythm following the phase shift of daily routine was achieved more easily than by the non-24 hour routine, and that functions might be classified into three types: those with less adaptability to a new routine, those coupled more closely with routine of living, and intermediate ones.

TEMPERATURE RHYTHM IN TRAVELERS

For a traveler headed eastward or westward, the length of a day becomes shorter or longer than 24 hours. From the age of stage-coach and sail-boat it was recognized that the phase of temperature rhythm varied with local time and did not maintain the time of one's home town. To cross the Pacific took two weeks by boat and 17 hours by airplane at one time, takes nine hours by jet plane now, and will take three hours by S.S.T. Theoretically speaking if a traveler continues to fly westward along the 45th parallel at a speed of 1200 km/hr, which is by no means fantastic now, the sun looks stopped and the length of a day is extended infinitely. A westbound flight along the 70th parallel would result in a day length of 24 hours, with sunrise in the west and sunset in the east.

With such rapid development in the means of transportation, more and more conventions and athletic events are held on a world-wide scale, the biological rhythms of the participants are exposed to quick phase shifts, and the effects on physiological functions and performance are too serious to be overlooked. Under these circumstances observation of the body temperature rhythm during and after the flight is not only of scientific interest in studying the mechanism of phase adjustment, but of practical importance in finding some effective means against "asynchronosis,"—sleeplessness, loss of appetite and feeling of general fatigue.

Fig. 147 is a schematic presentation of adjustment of temperature rhythm to a new local time at different speeds of transposition [17]. Data are taken from reports by previous investigators and average speed of transposition is expressed in terms of deviation of the length of a day from 24 hours. Shift in local time (in other words, position of a traveler) is represented by continuous lines, and phase of temperature pattern by broken lines. So long as the speed of transportation is slow enough and the resulting change in the actual length of a day is less than 30 minutes, as is shown in group A, the circadian pattern follows the local time change without delay. In group B, in which the speed is a little greater, a slight tendency to lag behind the vehicle movement is noticed; and in the case of high speed travel by plane in group C, a considerable amount of phase lag is developed, and it will take several days before complete adjustment is achieved.

Reports of biological clock shift following travel which appeared before 1960 were

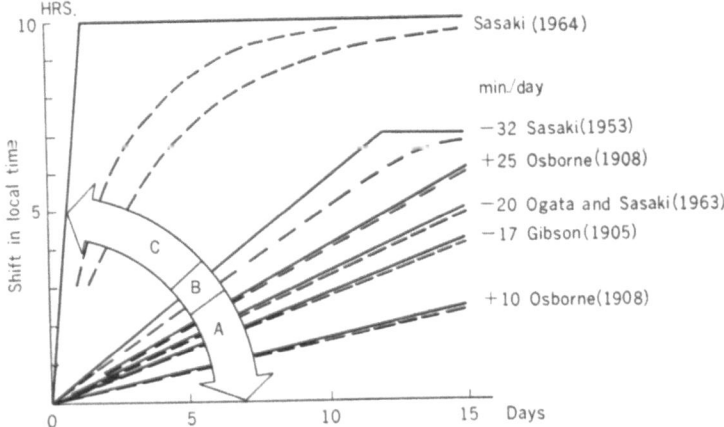

Fig. 147. Schematic presentation of adjustment of circadian temperature rhythm to a new local time at different speeds of transposition.

few in number, and the functions studied were limited to oral temperature, physical performance, and urinary excretion of electrolytes. Considerable numbers of reports were presented in the last ten years [4, 5, 7, 8], and the contributions of groups of Japanese investigators are worth mentioning [11, 13, 14, 17]. As the method of data processing differs with investigators, interpretation of the observations, particularly in ambiguous cases, may be affected by the investigators's subjective point of view. Here the author would like to recommend three different procedures as potential tools for shift evaluation.

The first of these procedures, which lays stress on characteristics of the pattern and subjective judgement, is suitable for drawing an outline of the progress [18]. Fig. 148 illustrates an example of a round trip transpacific flight including a three-week stay in the U.S.A. The progress of resynchronization of biological rhythm to a new local time following intercontinental flight was analyzed on the all-or-none basis; in other words, the phase of temperature pattern on a given day was determined by the alternative to which it had a closer resemblance, the phase of temperature pattern at

Postflight resynchronization

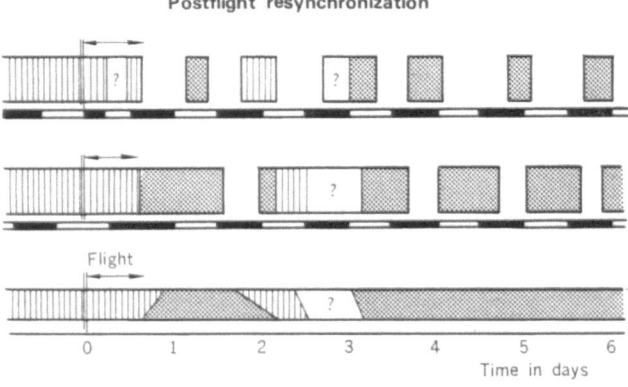

Fig. 148. Qualitative illustration of the progress of phase synchronization.

the start or destination. The hatched area shows dominance of the start phase and the dotted area the destination phase. The day-night cycle is illustrated by a chain of white and black bars. The top row shows the progress of the eastbound flight, and the middle row the westbound one. As there is little difference between them, the common tendency was summarized in the bottom row. For the first 16—20 hours following the take-off, the temperature pattern was maintained at the start phase. Upon awakening from the first sleep, switchover to the destination phase, though ambiguously, was observed. During the period of 40—60 hours after the start, a tendency to transient return to start phase was shown. From the fourth day on, the destination phase became dominant, but a phase lag of some hours still remained and it took several days more before complete synchronization was achieved.

The second of these kinds is in itself a mathematical procedure [6]. By assuming the cyclic pattern to be the cosine function and the period to be 24 hours, wave level, phase and amplitude are estimated by the least squares method (cosinor technique). The procedure was applied to another transpacific case, and progressive changes in the three constants are given in Fig. 149: daily mean of body temperature, time of the highest temperature, and range of temperature in a day.

The third of the procedures, which is performed by comparing the observed pattern with a reference rhythm pattern, is suitable for objective evaluation of the progress [17]. As the reference temperature pattern, the average time course of temperature prior to the trip was taken. The observed pattern was simplified by taking five consecutive readings selected at six-hour intervals (interpolated if necessary). In other words, a simplified circadian curve was formed by connecting five temperature readings, for example at 0000, 0600, 1200, 1800, and 2400 hours local time. Rhythmicity was

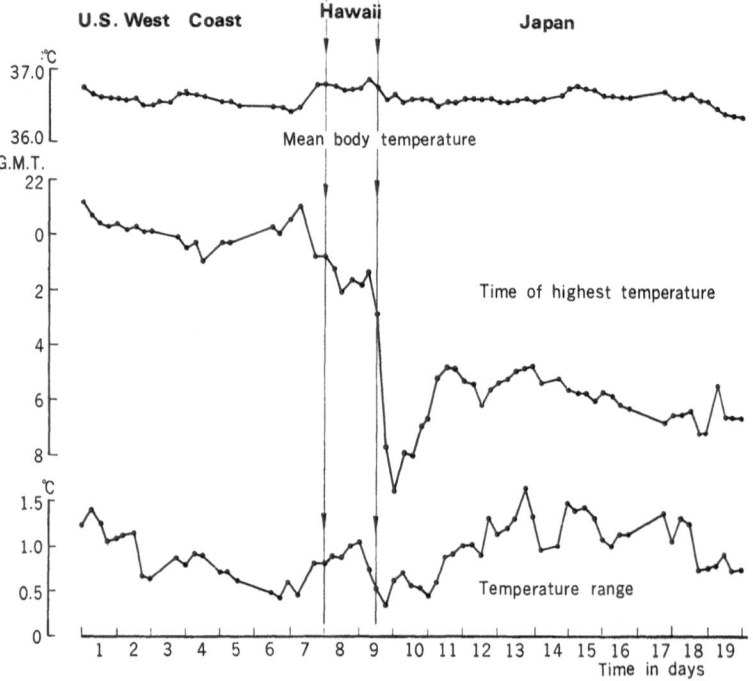

Fig. 149. Quantitative illustration of the progress of phase synchronization.

evaluated on a scale of zero to eight by summing up standardized scores representing four characteristics of the reference pattern: the morning rise, afternoon plateau, evening fall and low night level. By applying the same procedure to the 1-7-13-19-1 hours curve, the 2-8-14-20-2 hours curve, and so on, a series of rhythmicity ratings was obtained. The biological point is represented by the longitude with the highest rating, and the phase lag is defined as the difference in longitudes between the biological point and actual body position. Fig. 150 shows one example of a west-

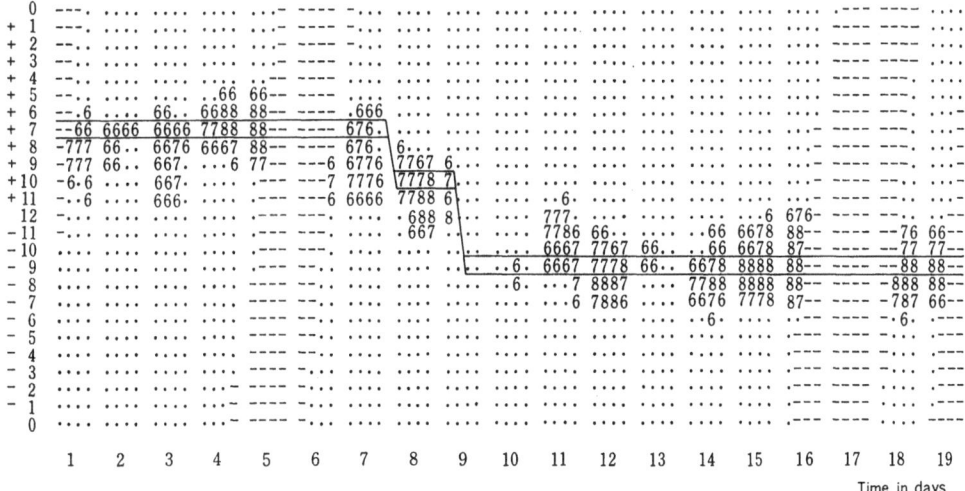

Fig. 150. Combined qualitative and quantitative illustration of the progress of phase synchronization.

bound case. The computer-made map was obtained by repeating the rating procedure at one hour intervals and printing out the rhythmicity rating of zero to eight. Dots represent values less than six and bars missing data. The abscissa represents time and ordinate shows local time zones, or east-west position on the earth. The double line gives the actual body position, and the location of the highest rating on the ordinate represents the position of biological point. Accordingly, the distance between the time course of biological point and the double line is the phase lag, which will be discussed extensively.

As is shown in Figs. 149 and 150, drastic change in daily routine as a result of the flight disturbed the normal pattern of temperature considerably, but the amount of phase lag diminished progressively, though there were occasional fluctuations, and finally the rhythm assumed the new local pattern.

GENERALIZATION [18]

As is obvious from Figs. 149 and 150 the time course appears to approach the zero line asymptotically. The rate of decrease in phase lag to be synchronized becomes smaller with time, instead of being constant as it would be in a linear regression. Therefore the author would like to propose a fundamental assumption that the rate of reduction in phase lag, dy/dt, is proportional to phase lag at time t, and the following equation is derived.

$$\frac{dy}{dt} = \frac{1}{\tau}[f(t) - y]$$

where $f(t)$ is longitude of vehicle position; y is longitude of biological point; $f(t) - y$ is phase lag at time t; t is time in days; and τ is the time constant. By representing an itinerary in the form of $f(t)$, the synchronization process of phase lag resulting from any type of vehicle movement can be calculated. It is easily understood that as a traveler continues to cross the longitudes, local time difference will accumulate, while the effects of this are neutralized in part by shifting the biological clock. The remaining phase lag becomes large as a vehicle gains speed and/or the travel continues longer.

If a traveler starts from a location (λ_0) and moves across the longitudes at a constant speed (v), the vehicle position is expressed by $f(t) = vt + \lambda_0$, and the differential equation for the particular case is

$$\frac{dy}{dt} + \frac{1}{\tau}y = \frac{1}{\tau}(vt + \lambda_0)$$

Solving the equation for y, we find

$$y = (y_0 - \lambda_0 + \tau v) e^{-\frac{t}{\tau}} + (vt + \lambda_0 - \tau v)$$

where y_0 is the initial longitude of biological point; λ_0 is the longitude of the starting point; and v is the angular velocity of a vehicle along latitudes in degrees per day. And it is provided that positive values denote the eastward direction, and vice versa.

If a traveler stays at the same location (λ_0), as is the case in stopovers as well as in arrival at the destination, $f(t) = \lambda_0$ and the solution to the equation would reduce to

$$y = (y_0 - \lambda_0) e^{-\frac{t}{\tau}} + \lambda_0.$$

The empirical values for the time constant, τ, ranged from 2.5 to 4.3 days. Even among travelers in the same party there are some individual differences in the value of the constant. The most distinctive feature is a considerable difference in the constant depending on the direction of the trip. The average eastbound τ was 4.0 days, and the westbound one 2.8 days. The difference was statistically significant at the 0.05 level. This implies that adjustment to a new local time is easier in the case of a westbound flight than an eastbound one. According to Aschoff [2] 22 out of 26

TABLE 46   Estimation of accumulated phase lag of the trips reported by previous investigators

Vehicle speed v deg/day	Trip duration t days	Accumulated phase lag to be synchronized $f(t) - y$		Report of phase lag	Reported by
		degrees	hours		
− 2.47	19	6.9	0.5	No	Osborne
− 4.49	37	12.6	0.8	No	Gibson
− 6.07	14	16.9	1.1	No	Osborne
+ 4.21	24	16.8	1.1	No	Gibson
+ 5.42	24	21.6	1.4	No	Ogata and Sasaki
+ 5.48	21	21.8	1.5	No	Ogata and Sasaki
+ 7.96	12-1/4	30.4	2.0	Yes	Sasaki
+10.54	12	40.1	2.7	Yes	Nohara

subjects had free-running periods longer than 24 hours; this furnishes sufficient evidence for quick and easy adjustment to a longer day as the result of a westbound trip. Observations of a round trip lasting for a few weeks are quite different. As was reported by Hauty and Adams [7, 8] and Ohara [14], adjustment following a home-coming trip was easier than that following an out-going trip. This may be interpreted to mean that the recent phase shift caused by the out-going trip has made the subject sensitive to the shift at the time of the return trip, and that the difference in social and psychological strain between the out-going and home-coming trips strengthened the tendency.

By applying the equation to some reports on east-west trips, the remaining phase lags on arrival at the destination were estimated and are summarized in Table 46. It is to be emphasized that no discrepancies resulting from phase shift are mentioned in their reports so long as the accumulated phase lag is less than 1.5 hours. When the lag exceeds 2.0 hours (30 degrees) an apparent dissociation of circadian rhythm from local time is recognized.

Fig. 151 shows the time course of phase synchronization from different initial phase lags. It is of interest that all curves converge with time around an asymptote. The existence of an asymptote means that the phase lag is always present but the amount neither increases nor decreases so long as the vehicle continues to move at the same speed, and that the amount of asymptotic phase lag is determined by the product of vehicle speed and the time constant of the traveler, as was discussed above.

As an example of application of the equation to a practical problem, the itinerary of the Japanese Team for the Olympic Games in Mexico City in 1968 was analyzed from this point of view. The first party of the team left Japan on September 22 and

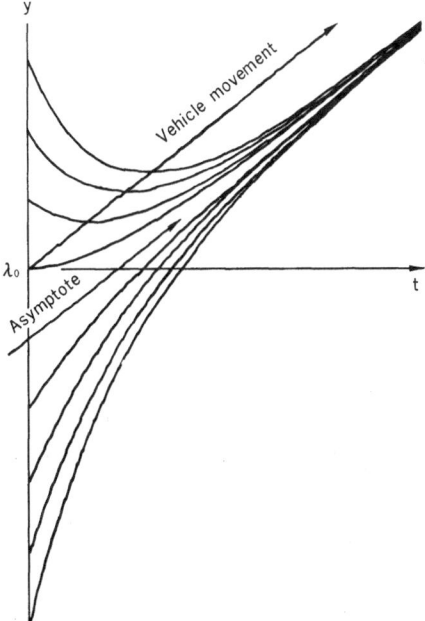

Fig. 151. Theoretical time course of phase synchronization from different initial phase lags. The upper arrow indicates the time course of vehicle movement, and the lower arrow shows the asymptote.

the second party on October 2, 21 and 11 days prior to the Opening Day, respectively. Staying three days at Culver City, Calif., they arrived at Mexico City. The progress of resynchronization is illustrated in Fig. 152 with due allowances for individual differences. As a phase lag of less than one and a half hours is negligible (Table 46), it is considered that synchronization was achieved at that stage. With due consideration for individual differences it was concluded that resynchronization was achieved six to eight days after the flight. In speaking about the performance of athletes exposed to quick phase shift, Rutenfranz and Hettinger [16] advised no hard training for the first three or four days following arrival at the destination,

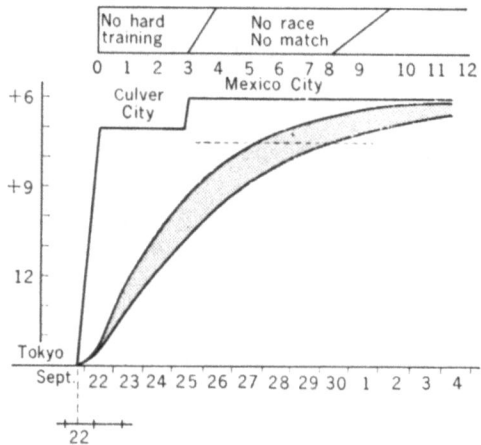

Fig. 152. Estimation of the time course of phase synchronization.

and no participation in races or matches within the first eight to ten days. According to the author's interpretation of phase adjustment process, the third or fourth day corresponds to the stage when a dominant tendency to destination phase was first recognized as is illustrated in Fig. 148, and the eighth to tenth day corresponds to the stage when complete adjustment was achieved and maximum performance of the athletes can be expected. Thus values theoretically estimated are in good agreement with results observed empirically.

CHANGES IN TEMPERATURE PATTERN WITH AGE

No circadian pattern of heart rate was shown by a fetus, while a distinct pattern was presented by its mother. As to temperature the fetus perhaps follows the temperature pattern of the mother. The newborn is monothermic and its temperature is liable to fluctuation. One or two weeks after birth the fluctuation decreases and the temperature level becomes higher than in the preceding week. It is in this stage that perspiration is first observed. These findings are all manifestations of initial development of a regulatory mechanism of temperature. Thus for the first four to nine weeks after birth a baby is primarily monothermic. But Nishimura and Yoshimatsu [12] observed a circadian pattern with the highest temperature at 3 p.m. in six-week-old and 12-week-old babies, when they had a slight fever. Therefore it is

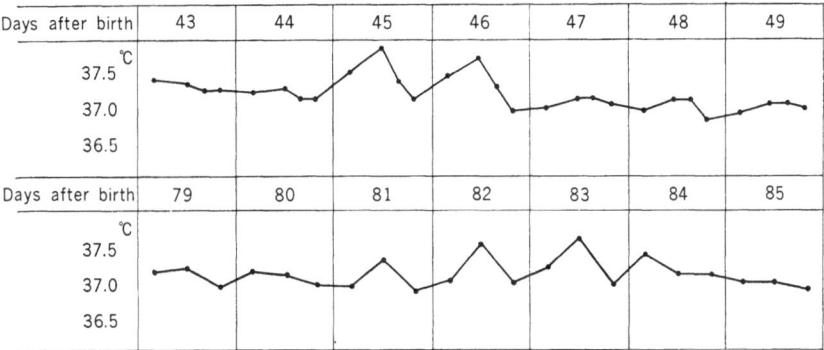

Fig. 153. Manifestation of circadian temperature rhythm in an early stage of childhood.

presumed that the mechanism of circadian rhythm has developed and becomes manifest when the regulatory center is stimulated. According to Benedict circadian rhythm is established in the second year of a child's life, and this is associated with the infant's learning to walk.

Circadian pattern of body temperature in the aged was characterized by an advance of temperature rhythm [10]: the morning rise in temperature occurred earlier and likewise the evening fall. Advance in the time of morning rise developed in every case, while the evening fall shift was not always observed in every case and was subject to variation in the habits and routine of the subject. The level of body temperature in the aged was generally higher in summer and autumn. The seasonal variation as such was to be ascribed to poor stability of the thermostat setting. In regard to the circadian pattern of resting metabolism progressive rise in metabolism in the morning hours was interrupted by a transitory depression in the early afternoon, which was followed by another progressive increase, leading to a maximum in the evening. The biphasic pattern was observed in more than half of the cases. Circadian rhythm of mean skin temperature showed a maximum in the early afternoon, and the pattern had more in common with the body temperature than with the pattern of heat production. In consequence regulatory responses of body temperature in the aged are characterized by an overall lack of stability. Delay, overshoot and roughness of regulatory responses are, therefore, ascribed not only to lowered sensibility to stimuli and reduced function of effector organs, but to poor performance of regulatory network, including feedback pathways.

SUMMARY

As a measure of studying the mechanism of biological rhythms, body temperature was selected for the following reasons: core temperature which is an integrative demonstration of temperature regulation will give more unbiased information than any single function does, and frequent or continuous observation as well as field-work is possible without elaborate instrumentation.

1) As to the site of temperature measurement, the insulated xiphoid and umbilical temperature were studied. They ran parallel with core temperature as long as change in environmental temperature was small, but were affected more or less by a sudden change in the environmental temperature. Accordingly, if rectal temperature

is not available, oral or axillary temperature with due consideration is recommended.

2) In determining the three constants of the circadian rhythm, i.e. mean body temperature, time of the highest temperature, and range of temperature, five observations at 700, 1000, 1400, 1800, and 2200 hours are enough and give as satisfactory results as continuous observations. Since observations at 700 and 1000 hours deal with the morning rise stage, and those at 1800 and 2200 hours with the evening fall stage, they serve to estimate the phase constant, though they serve little for amplitude estimation, which is effectively done by the 1400 hours measurement.

3) Temperature rhythm in shift workers showed considerable individual variation, and quite a few examples showed inadequate adjustment of biological rhythm to the routine of living in a five-day rotation period. But in workers who have engaged in shift work for ten years or more the biological rhythm showed synchronization with their living schedule. The life of workers except during work and sleep hours is necessarily exposed directly or indirectly to the non-shift rhythm of home and social life. If the subject is completely isolated from the outside world and shift of living schedule and environment is designed to be as perfect as possible, synchronization with the new phase occurs within a week.

4) Temperature rhythm in travelers is subject to phase shift resulting from transposition across longitudes. So long as the speed of a vehicle is slow enough and the resulting change of actual length of a day is less than a half hour, the circadian pattern follows the local time without delay. If the speed is a little greater a slight tendency to lag behind the vehicle movement is noticed, and in the case of high speed by plane a considerable amount of phase lag is evidenced. It will take several days before complete adjustment is achieved.

5) Since the rate of decrease in phase lag following a sudden change in local time becomes smaller with time, a fundamental assumption is proposed, that dy/dt, the rate of change in phase lag, be proportional to $f(t)-y$, the phase lag at time t. Accordingly the following equation is derived.

$$\frac{dy}{dt} = \frac{1}{\tau}[f(t) - y]$$

The empirical values for τ, the time constant, ranged from 2.5 to 4.3 days. Application of the equation to observations reported previously revealed that so long as the phase lag was less than 1.5 hours no trouble was noticed and the phase lag was negligible, but when the lag exceeded 2.0 hours an apparent dissociation of circadian rhythm from local time was recognized.

By expressing the itinerary in the form of $f(t)$, the theoretical time course of resynchronization can be illustrated.

6) The newborn is monothermic and its temperature is liable to fluctuation. A regulatory mechanism develops rapidly, and even in a 6-week-old baby a circadian rhythm with a peak at 3 p.m. became manifest when the baby had a slight fever and the regulatory center was therefore stimulated.

Regulatory responses in the aged are characterized by an overall lack of stability. Delay, overshoot and roughness of regulatory responses are ascribed to a lowered sensibility to stimuli and the reduced functioning of effector organs, and also to poor performance of the regulatory network, including feedback pathways.

REFERENCES

1. ASCHOFF, J. (1960): *Cold Harbor Symposia on Quant. Biol.* **25**: 11.
2. ASCHOFF, J. (1965): *Science* **148**: 1427.
3. COLIN, J., J. TIMBAL, C. BOUTELIER, Y. HOUDAS, and M. SIFFRE (1968): *J. Appl. Physiol.* **25**: 170.
4. FLINK, E.B., and R.P. DOE. (1959): *Proc. Soc. Exp. Biol. Med.* **100**: 498.
5. GERRITZEN, F. (1962): *Aerospace Med.* **33**: 097.
6. HALBERG, F., Y.L. TONG, and E.A. JOHNSON (1967): In "Cellular Aspects of Biorhythms." Springer, Berlin, p. 20.
7. HAUTY, G.T., and T. ADAMS (1965): In "Circadian Clocks." Aschoff, J. ed. North-Holland, Amsterdam, p. 413.
8. HAUTY, G.T., and T. ADAMS (1966): *Aerospace Med.* **37**: 668, 1027 and 1257.
9. KLEITMAN, N. (1963): Sleep and Wakefulness. Univ. of Chicago Press, Chicago.
10. MIYAZAKI, M. (1970): *Bull. Inst. Const. Med.* **20**: 271 (in Japanese).
11. NAGASAKA, T., S. ANDO, M. HARA, and K. TAKAGI (1967): *Nagoya J. Med. Sci.* **29**: 369.
12. NISHIMURA, S., and S. YOSHIMATSU. (1951): *Bull. Inst. Const. Med.* **1**: 361 (in Japanese).
13. OGATA, K., and T. SASAKI (1963): *Jap. J. Physiol.* **13**: 84.
14. OHARA, K. (1967): *Nagoya Med. J.* **13**: 143.
15. OHARA, K. (1968): In "Mombusho Kenkyu Hokoku Shuroku." p. 163 (in Japanese).
16. RUTENFRANZ, J., und T. HETTINGER (1957): Sportmedizin **8**: 195.
17. SASAKI, T. (1964): *Proc. Soc. Exp. Biol. Med.* **115**: 1129.
18. SASAKI, T. (1970): *Nihon Rinsho* **28**: 177 (in Japanese).
19. UENO, E. (1962): *Bull. Inst. Const. Med.* **13**: 256 (in Japanese).
20. WATANABE, G. (1968): In "Mombusho Kenkyu Hokoku Shuroku" p. 164 (in Japanese).
21. YURUGI, R., T. TOTSUKA, K. NABA, M. IIZUKA, T. AKIYAMA, and K. KUMURA (1961): *Rept. Aeromed. Lab.* **1(2)**: 1 (in Japanese).
22. YURUGI, R., M. IIZUKA, T. AKIYAMA, C. SAKAKIBARA, N. YUZA, and T. YANAKA (1970): *Rept. Aeromed. Lab.* **11**: 24 (in Japanese).

CHAPTER 20

THERMAL CONDUCTANCE IN MAN: ITS DEPENDENCE ON TIME OF DAY AND ON AMBIENT TEMPERATURE

JÜRGEN ASCHOFF, and AREND HEISE

Max-Planck-Institut für Verhaltensphysiologie, 8131 *Erling-Andechs, Germany*

> Production and loss
> of heat obey the clock's rule —
> creating a rhythm

In 1956, after the International Physiological Congress at Brussels, Rudolf Thauer organized a symposium on problems of thermoregulation. At a happy wine drinking evening, I was lucky to have my place next to Yas Kuno. At this occasion, we founded the 'physiological Haiku-Society.' Unfortunately, no board of editors so far has made up its mind to accept manuscripts written as short as a Haiku. To serve the purpose of our society, of which Yas Kuno is still the president, I have tried to condense the summary of our paper into such a short version.

J.A.

FACTORS CONTRIBUTING TO THE DIURNAL RHYTHM OF CORE TEMPERATURE

In the scientific literature, sporadic references to day-night variations in physiological functions of man first appear at about 1800 (e.g. Autenrieth, 1801). It is, however, not until 40 years later that Gierse (1842) has published quantitative data on measurements of his own oral temperature, covering nearly a full day. In his latin thesis he arrives at the conclusion: "Tempore nocturno igitur calor animalis minor est quam tempore pomeridiano 0.74°R" (= 0.9°C). The temperature curve shown in Fig. 154 is possibly the first ever taken. With regard to causes of this rhythm, later investigators ever and again have stated that 'muscular activity and food appear to be the most important factors' (Pembrey, 1905), or similarily that 'most, if not all, of the diurnal temperature variation is due to ingestion of food and exercise' (Hardy, 1961). This hypothesis has been doubted earlier by Gierse himself, and contradictory experimental results have often been published (c.f. Aschoff, 1947a, 1955). Among the earliest are those of Jürgensen (1867). They demonstrate that the rhythm persists in subjects kept continuously at bedrest, and they also suggest that food intake has little influence on the range (= double 'amplitude') of the rhythm. (c.f. Aschoff 1967a, Fig. 1; see also Figs. 155, 156 and 159 to 162 of the present contribution). Most of the evidence relevant for these two conclusions has

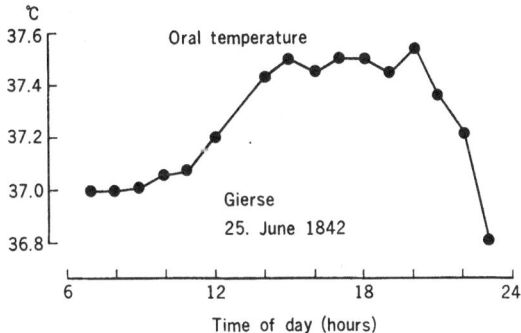

Fig. 154. Diurnal rhythm of oral temperature, according to Gierse (1842), (From Aschoff, 1955).

been discussed extensively in three recent publications (Aschoff 1971; Aschoff and Pohl, 1970a, 1970b).

Deep body temperature is determined by heat production and by heat loss. Rhythmic changes of either or both of these factors, therefore, may be responsible for a rhythm in temperature. So far, the majority of studies on diurnal rhythms in temperature regulation has dealt with measurements of *heat production* only. Despite these efforts, clear demonstrations of a day-night variation in basal metabolism are

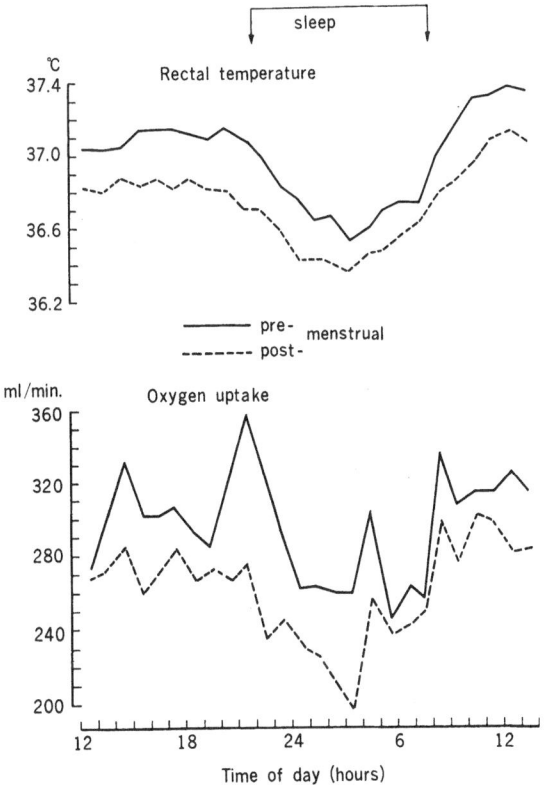

Fig. 155. Rectal temperature and oxygen uptake of a female subject, measured at rest in constant ambient temperature, during premenstrual and postmenstrual periods. According to unpublished data from T. Schmidt. (From Aschoff and Pohl, 1970a).

scarce, and its existence has been denied until recently (Koe *et al.*, 1968). There is, however, ample evidence for such a rhythm in fasting and resting subjects. An example is given in Fig. 155; it demonstrates, in addition, the well known menstrual cycle with higher values for rectal temperature and oxygen uptake after ovulation (Aschoff and Pohl, 1970a). With regard to *heat loss*, only a few attempts have been made to prove a diurnal rhythm (e.g. Benedict and Carpenter, 1918; Metz and Andlauer, 1949/1952; Metz and Sigwalt, 1958), and many investigators have not even discussed its possible contribution to the diurnal rhythm of deep body temperature. This is the more surprising since only two years after Gierse it has been stated by Bergmann (1844) that 'the diurnal rhythm not only depends on the rhythm of CO_2 production ... but that a variation of skin warming is also necessary ... ' (translation from German). In his following important contribution, Bergmann (1845) has developed his model of a homoiothermic 'core' and a surrounding (poikilothermic) 'shell' (although not using these terms). In an educated, impressive discussion he analyzes how blood flow through the shell determines the shell's insulation, and hence determines the amount of heat lost from or stored in the body. In this context, Bergmann mentions the importance of hands and feet which—due to a high surface: volume ratio and also to a high variability in blood flow—are especially suited for the control of heat dissipation. The contribution of heat loss by the hands to the rhythm in deep body temperature, as suggested by Bergmann (1845), is demonstrated in Fig. 156. The data come from two experiments with the first author as the subject, sitting comfortably at a constant room temperature of 24 °C without food intake (Aschoff, 1947a). Heat loss is measured in a calorimeter bath with running water of 32 °C. As can be seen from the diagram, heat loss is small in the forenoon and decreases towards afternoon, such favouring heat conservation. At about 18:00, heat loss suddenly (and without any change in experimental conditions) increases

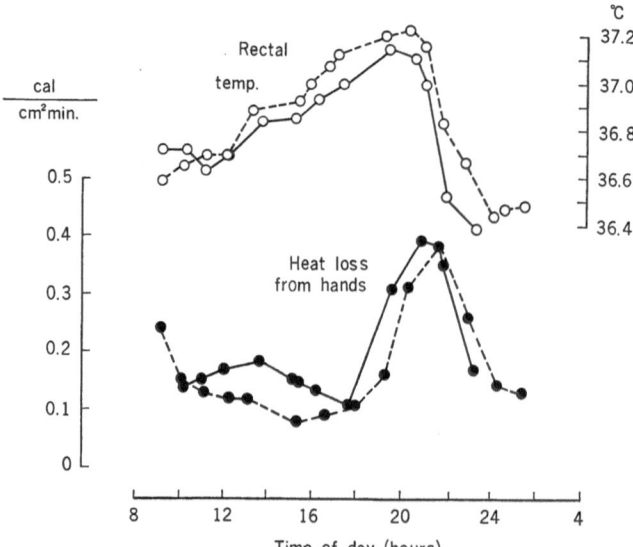

Fig. 156. Rectal temperature and heat loss from hands (in running water of 32 °C) as a function of time of day. Two experiments with the same subject, fasting and seated comfortably at an ambient temperature of 24 °C. (From Aschoff, 1956).

within a few hours to maximal values which surpass the afternoon minimum by 200%. This increase precedes the drop in rectal temperature by about two hours.

Control of heat loss to the environment is mainly based on changes in the shell's insulation. Such changes have profound consequences for the amount of heat drawn out of or stored in the core tissues. (Burton and Bazett, 1936). A decrease in hand blood flow alone, due to cold water immersion, can result in enough heat storage to produce a noticeable increase of rectal temperature (Aschoff, 1944a). It is Bergmann (1945) who again has been the first to discuss the main aspects of an interaction between shell insulation and core temperature and the implications of this interaction for a diurnal rhythm (c.f. Aschoff 1956). He has laid the foundation on which the concept of conductance has been developed (Burton and Bazett, 1936; Winslow *et al.*, 1937a; *Aschoff*, 1943, 1958a). In the following paragraphs, emphasis will be placed on day-night variations of conductance as a main contributing factor to the diurnal rhythm of core temperature.

VARIABILITY OF CONDUCTANCE

Conductance is a coefficient which 'represents the mean heat flux through the skin surface per degree of gradient fall to the skin temperature' (Winslow *et al.*, 1937b). It is obtained by dividing the heat flow per unit surface area by the temperature difference between core and skin. It is possible to compute conductance for parts of the body, e.g. for hand or finger, by measuring the heat lost from that part and dividing it by the difference between core temperature and skin temperature of that part. To get overall conductance, total heat loss from the body's surface is divided by the difference between core temperature and mean skin temperature. (If, in this latter case, heat loss is replaced by heat production in the mathematical equation, several problems arise which have been outlined lastly by Hey and Katz (1970). They are without significance for the present discussion.)

Variability of conductance is the essence of physical temperature regulation. Many investigators have measured the dependence of overall conductance on ambient temperature or on mean skin temperature respectively. The conformity of the published results is surprisingly high. The lower continuous line in Fig. 157, representing conductance for the whole body of resting and starving nude man, is drawn through the data of five groups of workers; they have measured heat loss either in air by partitional calorimetry (open symbols) or in water bath calorimeters (closed symbols). In a warm environment, with mean skin temperature 35 °C or higher, overall conductance may reach values higher than 60 mcal/cm² min °C. With falling temperatures, conductance decreases rapidly and eventually reaches a minimal value of 13 mcal/cm² min °C at a mean skin temperature of about 31° to 30°C. At this point, maximal vasoconstriction of blood vessels (and maximal contercurrent heat exchange in the extremities, c.f. Aschoff and Wever, 1958, 1959) is achieved. The slight increase of conductance at still lower temperatures can probably be explained by an increase in shell blood flow due to shivering. In the range of skin temperature between 36° and 31°, the decrease in overall conductance is adjusted to the increase in temperature gradient between core and skin in such a way that heat loss remains more or less constant (lower dashed line in Fig. 157). If skin temperature falls below this range, heat loss necessarily increases proportional to the further increase of tem-

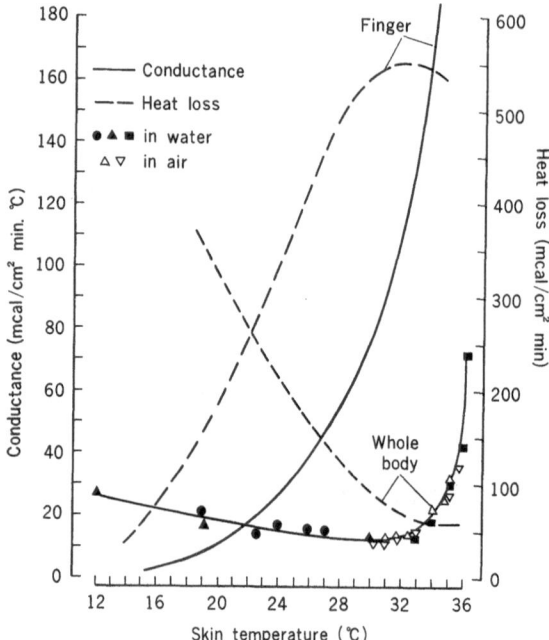

Fig. 157. Conductance and heat loss as a function of skin temperature, for the finger and for the whole body. According to data from: ■ Burton and Bazett (1936); △ ▽ Du Bois *et al.* (1952) ▲ Lefèvre (1898), ● Liebermeister (1869); Finger: Aschoff (1947c). (From Aschoff, 1958a, b).

perature gradient (or more than proportional if conductance is not kept at its minimal value). The point at which heat loss starts to increase is somewhat higher than the critical temperature at which metabolism starts to increase (see below, Fig. 158).

Variability of conductance is based on variability of blood flow. Variability of blood flow (per unit volume of tissue as well as per unit surface area) is especially high in the extremities, increasing from proximal to distal parts (Aschoff, 1947c, 1958b). Therefore, conductance measured for a finger only, reaches higher maximal and lower minimal values than conductance measured at any other part of the body (upper continuous line of Fig. 157). Due to the extremely steep decrease of finger conductance with decreasing skin temperature, heat loss from the finger *decreases* despite the *increasing* temperature gradient (upper dashed line in Fig. 157). The same phenomenon applies to the whole hand (Aschoff, 1947b, 1956; Forster *et al.*, 1946; Bargeton *et al.*, 1959; Clifford, 1965). Since overall conductance of the whole body, on the one hand, is capable only of compensating an increase of temperature gradient over a small range, and since, on the other hand, the extremities (whose conductance is included in the values of overall conductance) can overcompensate, it is clear that other parts of the body, i.e. the trunk and the head, must have a smaller variability of conductance than the body in general. The truth of this conclusion, drawn 20 years ago (Aschoff, 1948), will be demonstrated below.

All data shown in Fig. 157 are based on measurements made in the day-time only. Comparable data from measurements made at night have not been published. There are, however, data from measurements of oxygen uptake, skin and rectal temperature

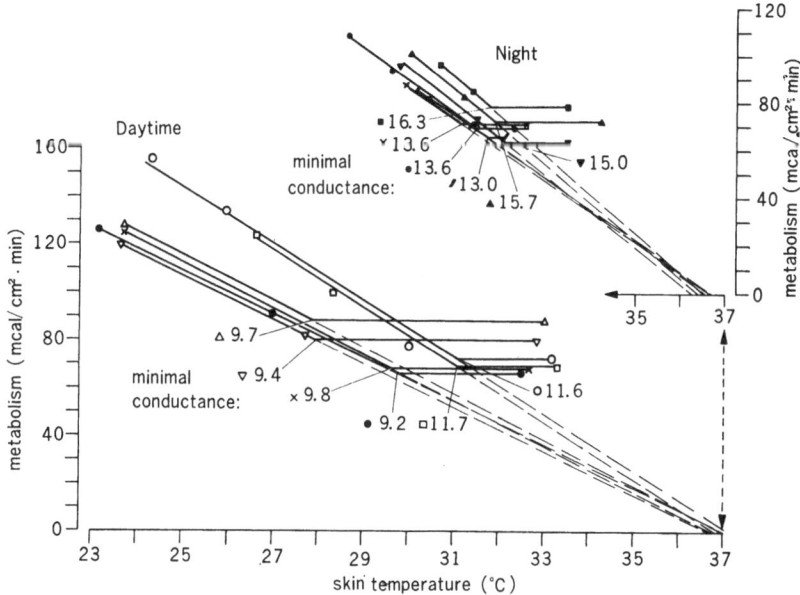

Fig. 158. Metabolism of resting subjects as a function of mean skin temperature. Minimal conductance (core to skin) in mcal/cm² min °C. Experiments in the day-time according to: ● Wezler and Neuroth (1949), □ Iampietro and Burskirk (1960), ▽ Girling (1964); ○ Wyndham et al. (1962), × Budd (1964), △ Hurley *et al.* (1964); Experiments at night according to: ■ Hart *et al.* (1962), × Elsner and Bolstad (1963), ● Andersen *et al.* (1960), ↘ Hammel *et al.* (1959), ▼ Hammel *et al.* (1963), ▲ Irving *et al.* (1960). (From Aschoff, 1967b)

made in the day-time and at night at both, comfortable as well as low environmental temperatures. From these data, the critical temperature can be estimated graphically, if metabolism is drawn as a function of mean skin temperature. This has been done in Fig. 158. The main diagram includes data from six groups of subjects studied in the day-time, the inserted diagram data from six groups of subjects studied at night. The continuous oblique lines, representing the slopes of increasing metabolism on the cold side, extrapolate satisfactory to core temperature on the abscissa (which is drawn at zero metabolism). The critical skin temperatures are given by the points at which the oblique lines cross the horizontal lines representing the basal metabolism. For each group of subjects, minimal conductance can then be computed by dividing basal metabolism by the difference between core temperature and critical skin temperature (c.f. the numbers in Fig. 158). The main results, expressed in mean value and standard deviation, for the experiments made in the daytime (D) and at night (N) are: Metabolism (mcal/cm² min): D 73.8 ± 8.5, N 69.7 ± 5.3; Rectal temperature (°C): D 36.9 ± 0.30, N 36.6 ± 0.15; Critical skin temperature (°C): D 29.60 ± 1.41, N 31.85 ± 0.48; Minimal conductance (mcal/cm² min °C): D 10.20 ± 1.12, N 14.53 ± 1.33. The differences between day and night are statistically significant for critical skin temperature as well as for minimal conductance. (For further details of procedure, and for discussion of approximations and necessary assumptions, see Aschoff, 1967b).

The results summarized in Fig. 158 support the hypothesis of a day-night variation in conductance; however, they are based on measurements made at selected times of day only, and not carried out with the same subjects. Furthermore they are restricted to minimal conductance, leaving open the question of a day-night variation in the whole curve which describes conductance as a function of ambient temperature (c.f. Fig. 157). To demonstrate the temporal course of conductance hour by hour, the second author has recorded heat loss and body temperatures of nude, resting men in a climatic chamber continuously over 27 hours (Heise, 1969). Heat flow has been measured by use of small gradient calorimeters, consisting of round plexi-glass discs with a diameter of 8 mm (Wever and Aschoff, 1957). The discs (below which also skin temperature is taken) have been attached to 11 points on the skin surface. To get mean values for the whole surface of the body, the 11 measurements are weighted according to a system slightly modified from that of Pfleiderer and Büttner (1935). Nine young male subjects have been tested at four ambient temperatures (20°, 24°, 28° and 32°C), with the relative humidity kept between 40% and 50%. Equal amounts of water and of Glucose (Dextroenergen, Deutsche Maizena Werke) have been taken by each subject in hourly intervals. The results, averaged from all measurements made at 20°C chamber temperature, are shown in Fig. 159. As to be expected, there is a decrease in skin temperature and in conductance in the day-time; this decrease turns into a rather steep increase at about 19:00. This in-

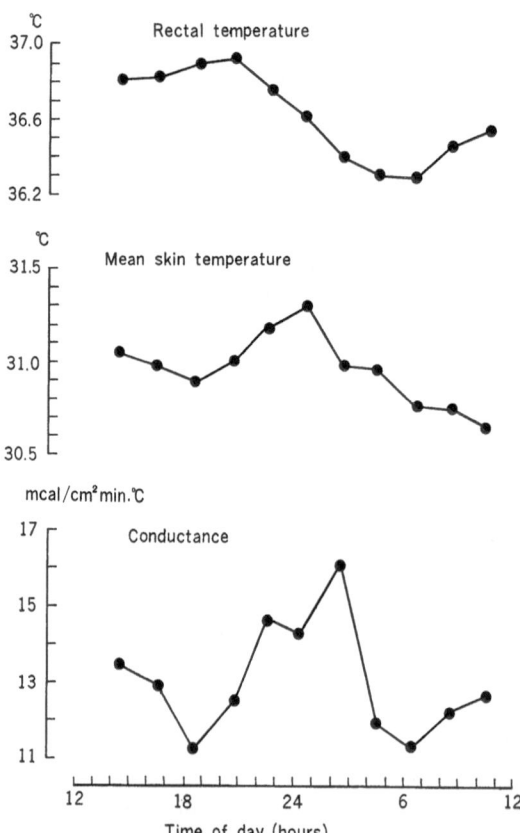

Fig. 159. Rectal temperature, mean skin temperature and internal conductance (core to skin) as a function of time of day. Average data from six subjects, resting in the nude at an ambient temperature of 20°C.

crease precedes the characteristic fall in rectal temperature by two hours. The range of the diurnal oscillation, measured between maximal and minimal values, is 0.64 °C for rectal temperature, 0.60 °C for mean skin temperature, and 5 mcal/cm² min °C for conductance. The mean value of conductance, averaged for 24 hours, is 13.0 mcal/cm² min °C; it agrees with the value for minimal conductance shown in Fig. 154, as expected in a room temperature of 20 °C. When averaged separately for the three measurements made between 18:00 and 24:00 and the three measurements made between 6:00 and 12:00, the values for conductance are 5.8% higher at early night than in the forenoon. This demonstration of an evening increase in conductance is in agreement with observations on differences in the time necessary for skin rewarming after cooling (Hildebrandt, 1957) and on differences in sweat rate (Geschickter et al., 1966; Ogawa *et al.*, 1967) at day and at night.

DEPENDENCE ON AMBIENT TEMPERATURE: TRUNK VERSUS EXTREMITIES

By using heat flow discs at 11 points of the skin surface, we have been able to compute skin temperature and conductance for various parts of the body. In Fig. 160, the one-hour means are shown for one subject, tested at a chamber temperature of 24 °C. The values for skin temperature and conductance at the chest and the upper arm are rather high; they follow more or less closely the curve of rectal temperature. In strong contrast to this, the values for hand and finger decrease to very low values during the first nine to 10 hours of the experiment. From 20.00 on, first finger conductance and, thereafter, conductance measured at the back of the hand, increase sharply; similarly, skin temperature first rises in the finger, thereafter in the back of the hand. This sequence, first observed by Lewis (1929/31), is characteristic of different types of vasodilatation in the extremities (c.f. Aschoff, 1944b). After about 22:00, the high values of skin temperature and of conductance in hand and finger remain constant for six to eight hours. During this time, large variations occur which again are characteristic for the distal parts of the extremities (Honma *et al.*, 1966a). At about 4:00 to 6:00 in the morning, skin temperature and conductance values drop again to the low forenoon level. The pattern of finger temperature shown by this subject, also applies to the majority of the other eight subjects and seems to be similar to that observed by Honma and coworkers (1966b) at room temperatures lower than 20 °C.

From Fig. 160 it is obvious that skin circulation in the distal parts of the extremities behaves quite differently from skin circulation in proximal parts and in the chest. We therefore have computed average values for representative proximal and distal parts of the body. In the following, the term 'Trunk' refers to data averaged from two measurements (chest and abdomen), and the expression 'Hands and feet' refers to data averaged from four measurements (back of one hand, one finger, back of one foot, and one toe). The two-hour means of conductance for these two parts are drawn in Fig. 161 as a function of time of day. The two diagrams include the average values from all nine subjects, tested at 32° and at 20 °C chamber temperature. The main results are: 1) The 24-hour means of rectal temperature and of conductance are lower in 20 °C than in 32 °C; 2) From 32 °C to 20 °C, conductance of the trunk decreases only by about 20%, while conductance of the distal parts of the extremities

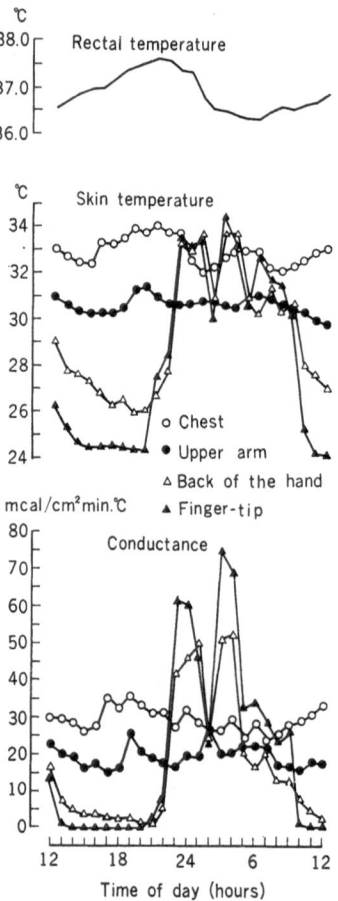

Fig. 160. Rectal temperature, together with skin temperature, and internal conductance at four areas of the body, as a function of time of day. One nude subject measured at 24 °C ambient temperature.

decreases by 90%; 3) The diurnal rhythms of conductance in trunk and in hands and feet are in phase with each other in 20 °C, but are out of phase by 180° in 32 °C.

If varying conductance contributes to the rhythm in deep body temperature, obviously only the rhythm of conductance in hands and feet matches the necessary temporal relationship to the rhythm in rectal temperature in 32 °C as well as in 20 °C chamber temperature. The rhythm of trunk conductance fits to such a functional relationship between core and shell in 20 °C, but works against it in 32 °C. This seemingly inappropriate behaviour of trunk conductance, however, may be over-ridden by the changes of conductance in hands and feet. Lastly, it is not conductance but the heat loss determined by conductance and amount of temperature difference which decides whether rectal temperature falls or rises. In this regard, one has to keep in mind the dependence of the external heat transfer coefficient (determining heat loss from the surface to the environment) on the diameter of the heat dissipating body. Heat loss per degree temperature gradient from skin to the environment is about twice as high from the finger as from the abdomen (Aschoff, 1958a). Due to these special circumstances, and due to other characteristics already mentioned, hands

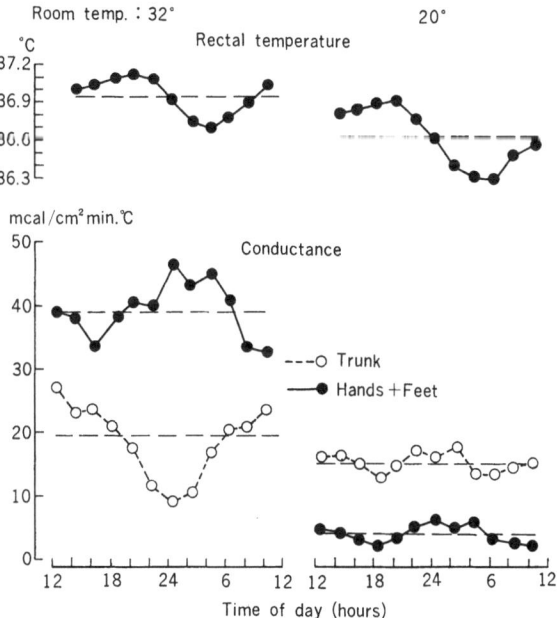

Fig. 161. Rectal temperature and internal conductance at the trunk and at hands and feet as a function of time of day. Average values from nine subjects, resting in the nude at 32 °C and at 20 °C ambient temperature.

and feet are relatively more effective in controlling heat loss, and changes in their conductance contribute relatively more to the diurnal rhythm of overall heat loss than do changes in conductance of the trunk. (Mean values for heat loss at different times of day are given in the last paragraph.)

The striking difference in conductance between the trunk and the distal parts of the extremities relates to the dependence of this difference on ambient temperature: Trunk conductance stays nearly unchanged between 32° and 20 °C chamber temperature, while conductance of hands and feet changes by 90%. These observations support extremely well the conclusion drawn out of a comparison of the two continuous lines in Fig. 157. The 24-hour means for conductance at the four test temperatures (20°, 24°, 28° and 32 °C) are (in mcal/cm² min °C): Trunk 16.0, 14.5, 14.5, 19.5; Hands and feet 4.0, 9.5, 32.0, 39.0. The data demonstrate quantitatively the significance of the extremities for physical temperature regulation, emphasized by Razgha and Szelyonka (1942), Aschoff (1947c), Bazett (1949) and other workers, including most recently Smith (1969). The data also demonstrate that the trunk participates in control of heat loss nearly as little as does the head (c.f. Froese and Burton, 1957). The values for trunk conductance are in agreement with those published by Reader (1952) who has measured heat flow through muscle and skin at the lumber region. From his data it can be computed that trunk conductance decreases from a mean of 26.5 mcal/cm² min °C at local skin temperatures between 30° and 23 °C to a mean of 14.5 mcal/cm² min °C at a skin temperature between 15° and 10 °C (c.f. Aschoff, 1956, Fig. 3).

To draw a general conclusion: For an ambient temperature of 24 °C and above, the statement seems correct that trunk and head more or less belong to the core, while the extremities mainly represent the shell of the body (Aschoff and Wever, 1958a, 1959). However, for lower temperatures (20°C and below), the skin of the frunk seems to belong to the shell.

DEPENDENCE ON AMBIENT TEMPERATURE: RANGE OF DIURNAL OSCILLATION

The range of an oscillation is given by the difference between maximal and minimal value, measured during one period. In studies on diurnal rhythms, often the range has attracted less attention than other parameters of the oscillation, e.g. its phase. It is known that diurnal (or circadian) rhythms have properties of selfsustained oscillations (Aschoff, 1963, 1964), and that range of oscillation can be correlated to other parameters of the oscillation such as level in a characteristic manner (Wever, 1964). It is, therefore, of theoretical interest to know more about the range of temperature oscillation, not to speak of its implications for the mechanisms of thermoregulation at the controlling centers. In the experiments discussed here (Heise, 1969), the range of oscillation in rectal temperature has been proven to depend systematically on ambient temperature. In Fig. 162 are shown the curves of rectal temperature from four subjects, each measured for 24 hours at four different ambient temperatures. With two subjects, the experiment has been started in the morning, with the two other subjects in the evening. In all four subjects, the range of oscillation of rectal temperature is largest at a chamber temperature of 24°C (continuous

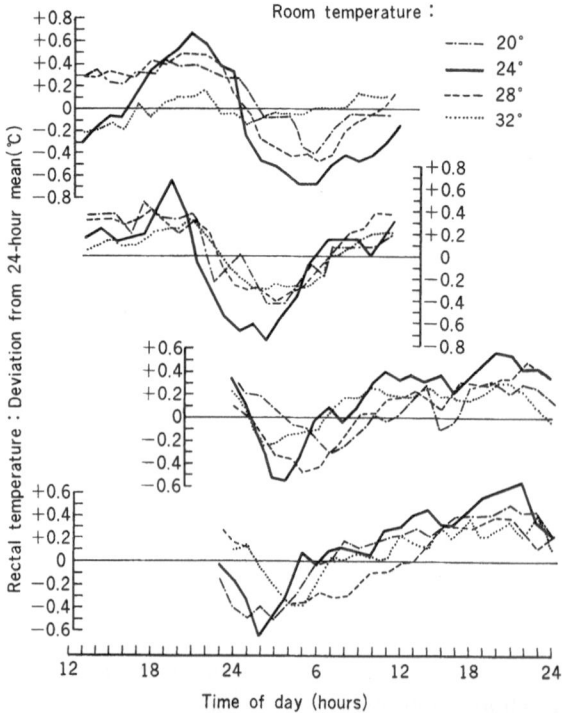

Fig. 162. Curves of rectal temperature of four resting nude subjects, measured at four different ambient temperatures. For two subjects start of the experiments in the forenoon, for the two other subjects in the afternoon.

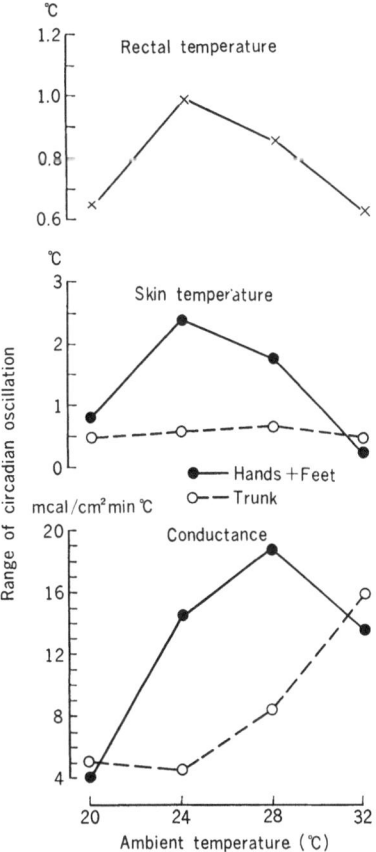

Fig. 163. Range of oscillation of the diurnal (circadian) rhythm in rectal temperature as well as skin temperature and conductance in two parts of the body, as a function of ambient temperature. Average data from nine subjects, computed from the 24-hour means at each ambient temperature.

lines in Fig. 162), and smallest at a chamber temperature of either 32 °C (dotted lines) or 20 °C (dash-dotted lines).

A similar dependence of range of oscillation on ambient temperature, as for rectal temperature, has been observed for skin temperature and for conductance at the distal parts of the extremities. The average results for all nine subjects studied are summarized in Fig. 163. At chamber temperatures of 24 °C and 28 °C, range of oscillation is lower in the trunk than in hands and feet. At 32 °C as well as at 20 °C chamber temperature, the ranges are nearly the same in both parts of the body. Remembering the fact that the distal parts of the extremities are mainly responsible for the control of heat loss, it can be understood that the large ranges of conductance and of skin temperature in hands and feet at 24 °C and 28 °C chamber temperature result in similarly large ranges of rectal temperature. At 20 °C, the need for heat conservation asks for a high vasoconstrictor tone at all times of day, and hence inhibits vasodilatation at night the consequence of which is a decrease in range of oscillation. On the other hand, at 32 °C chamber temperature, the continuous need for heat dissipation does not allow for stronger vasoconstriction in the forenoon, again decreasing the day-night variation of skin temperature and conductance in hands and feet.

Conductance values of the distal parts of the extremities and of the trunk can be combined to compute overall conductance. From the two lines in the lowermost diagram of Fig. 163 it is evident that for this overall conductance the range of oscillation increases from low to high ambient temperatures. Neither the range of oscillation of mean skin temperature (combined from trunk and extremities), nor that of rectal temperature reflects this increase in range of conductance oscillation. The explanation for this behaviour which may appear puzzeling at a first look, is given by the characteristic non-linear function which describes the dependence of skin temperature on blood flow (c.f. Aschoff, 1958a, Figs. 7 and 8; Hertzman, 1953). Due to this function, a large change of blood flow at 32 °C ambient temperature results in the same change of skin temperature (and hence of heat loss) as does a much smaller change of blood flow at 20 °C ambient temperature. In other words: To produce a certain range of oscillation in skin temperature, a larger variation of conductance is necessary at 32 °C than at 20 °C ambient temperature. It is for the same reason that maximal range of oscillation in conductance has not necessarily to occur at the same ambient temperature at which rectal temperature has its maximal range. However, if the hypothesis maintained here is correct, i.e. if variations in heat loss contribute substantially to the diurnal rhythm of core temperature, the temperature dependence of range of oscillation on ambient temperature has to be the same in skin temperature as in rectal temperature; because skin temperature, with the ambient temperature given, determines the external temperature gradient and hence determines the amount of heat loss to the environment. The data for hands and feet shown in Fig. 163 are consistent with this conclusion, emphasizing again their commanding significance for the control of heat loss.

There is no room to discuss in more detail further interesting aspects of the temporal relationship between the rhythm of conductance or of skin temperature on the one hand and the rhythm of rectal temperature on the other hand. The phase-angle difference (for terminology see Aschoff et al., 1965) between the two seems to depend on ambient temperature in a systematic way (Heise, 1969), resulting in changes of time-lag between the variations of heat loss to the environment and the variations of heat storage in the core tissue. According to these observations, the interaction between core and shell is, in its time-course, more complex than assumed so far. To understand these mechanisms fully, the rhythm of heat production and its relationship to the rhythm of heat loss has to be known. It may well be, that the phase-angle difference between the two also varies with ambient temperature, suggesting a multiplicity of circadian oscillators for the whole thermoregulatory system (Aschoff et al., 1967a, 1967b; Aschoff and Pohl, 1970a).

CONCLUSION

There is no doubt about two conclusions which can be drawn out of the data presented here: 1) Internal conductance (core to skin) of man has a profound diurnal rhythm; 2) The distal parts of the extremities, due to large variations in conductance, are especially apt to control heat loss. Most of the observations discussed in the foregoing paragraphs also support the hypothesis that day-night variations in heat loss contribute considerably to the diurnal rhythm of core temperature. To substantiate this conclusion, it is necessary to check the actual difference in heat loss between day and night.

The 24-hour mean of heat loss from the whole body increases from 72 mcal/cm- min at 32 °C chamber temperature to 153 mcal/cm² min at 20 °C. When computed separately for the three measurements made between 6:00 and 12:00 and for the three measurements made between 18:00 and 24:00, the early night values prove to be higher than the forenoon values by an average of 4.5%. Assuming a mean heat loss of 75 mcal/cm² min at comfortable ambient temperature, heat loss before midnight is 1.7 mcal/cm² min higher, and in the morning 1.7 mcal/cm² min lower than the 24-hour mean. Assuming further that the core comprises 50% of the body's volume (Burton, 1935), it can be estimated that, with heat production remaining constant, the core temperature rises or falls respectively by 0.05 °C per hour. (The average size of the nine subjects tested has been 68 kg and 180 cm = 1.85 m² surface area.) If only six out of the 24 hours are used for heating the core, and six hours for cooling, the core changes its temperature from day to night by 0.6 °C. The actual data for the range of oscillation in rectal temperature, averaged from tests with all nine subjects at all four chamber temperatures, is 0.77 °C. Out of this range, 0.6 °C have to be accounted for changes in heat loss.

On the basis of these (conservative) calculations, it seems correct to assume that, in resting man, the diurnal variations of heat loss are responsible for about 75% of the range of oscillation in core temperature, while the variation in heat production contributes 25% only.

REFERENCES

1. ANDERSEN, K.L., Y. LØYNING, J.D. NELMS, O. WILSON, R.H. FOX, and A. BOLSTAD (1960): *J. appl. Physiol.* **15:** 649.
2. ASCHOFF, J. (1943): *Pflügers Arch. ges. Physiol.* **247:** 469.
3. ASCHOFF, J. (1944a): *Pflügers Arch. ges. Physiol.* **248:** 149.
4. ASCHOFF, J. (1944b): *Pflügers Arch. ges. Physiol.* **248:** 183.
5. ASCHOFF, J. (1947a): *Pflügers Arch. ges. Physiol.* **249:** 125.
6. ASCHOFF, J. (1947b): *Pflügers Arch. ges. Physiol.* **249:** 137.
7. ASCHOFF, J. (1947c): *Pflügers Arch. ges. Physiol.* **249:** 148.
8. ASCHOFF, J. (1948): *Naturwissenschaften* **35:** 235.
9. ASCHOFF, J. (1955): *Klin. Wschr.* **33:** 545.
10. ASCHOFF, J. (1956): *Arch. Physik. Ther.* **8:** 113.
11. ASCHOFF, J. (1958a): *Klin. Wschr.* **36:** 193.
12. ASCHOFF, J. (1958b): *Wien. Med. Wschr.* **108:** 404.
13. ASCHOFF, J. (1963): *Ann. Rev. Physiol.* **25:** 581.
14. ASCHOFF, J. (1964): *Arbeitsgemeinschaft Forschg. d. Landes Nordrhein-Westfalen Heft* **138:** 51.
15. ASCHOFF, J. (1967a): In: Life Sciences and Space Research V, A.H. Brown (Ed.), North-Holland Publ., Amsterdam, p. 159.
16. ASCHOFF, J. (1967b): *Pflügers Arch. ges. Physiol.* **295:** 184.
17. ASCHOFF, J. (1971): In: Physiological and Behavioral Temperature Regulation, J.D. Hardy (Ed.) Thomas, Springfield/Ill. (in press).
18. ASCHOFF, J., U. GERECKE, and R. WEVER (1967a): *Jap. J. Physiol.* **17:** 450.
19. ASCHOFF, J., U. GERECKE, und R. WEVER (1967b): *Pflügers Arch. ges. Physiol.* **295:** 173.
20. ASCHOFF, J., K. KLOTTER, and R. WEVER (1965): In: Circadian Clocks, J. Aschoff (Ed.), North-Holland Publ., Amsterdam, p. XI.
21. ASCHOFF, J., and H. POHL (1970a): *Fed. Proc.* **29:** 1541.
22. ASCHOFF, J., and H. POHL (1970b): *J. f. Ornithol.* **111:** 38.
23. ASCHOFF, J., und R. WEVER (1958a): *Naturwissenschaften* **45:** 477.
24. ASCHOFF, J., und R. WEVER (1958b): *Z. ges. exper. Med.* **130:** 385.
25. ASCHOFF, J., und R. WEVER (1959): *Dtsch. Med. Wschr.* **84:** 1509.
26. AUTENRIEHT, J.H.F. (1801): Handbuch der empirischen menschlichen Physiologie, Tübingen, Vol. **1:** p. 209.
27. BARGETON, D., J. DURAND, J. MENSCH-DECHENE, et J. DECAUD (1959): *J. Physiol. (Paris)* **51:** 111.

28. BAZETT, H.C. (1949): In: Physiology of Heat Regulation, L.H. Newburgh (Ed.), W.B. Saunders, Philadelphia, p. 115.
29. BENEDICT, F.G., and Th. M. CARPENTER (1918): Carnegic Inst. Wash-Publ. **261.**
30. BERGMANN, C. (1844): In: Handwörterbuch der Physiologie, R. Wagner (Ed.), Vieweg und Sohn, Braunschweig, p. 273.
31. BERGMANN, C. (1845): Arch. Anat. Physiol. p. 300.
32. BUDD, G.M. (1964): Australian National Antarctic Research Expeditions Reports, Ser. B., Vol. **4:** Physiology, Medicine.
33. BURTON, A.C. (1935): J. Nutrition **9:** 261.
34. BURTON, A.C., and H.C. BAZETT (1936): Am. J. Physiol. **117:** 36.
35. CLIFFORD, J.M. (1965): IAM Report No. 342, RAF Institute of Aviation Medicine, Farnborough, Hants.
36. DU BOIS, E.F., E.G. EBAUGH, and J.D. HARDY (1952): J. Nutrition **48:** 257.
37. ELSNER, R.W., and A. BOLSTAD (1963): Arctic Aeromedical Laboratory Technical Documentary Report 62–64.
38. FORSTER, R.E., B.J. FERRIS, and R. DAY (1946): Am. J. Physiol. **136:** 600.
39. FROESE, G., and A.C. BURTON (1957): J. appl. Physiol. **10:** 235.
40. GESCHICKTER, E.H., P.A. ANDREWS, and R.W. BULLARD (1966): J. appl. Physiol. **21:** 623.
41. GIERSE, A. (1842): Quaeniam sit ratio caloris organici ···, M.D. Thesis, Halle.
42. GIRLING, F. (1964): Canad. J. Physiol. **42:** 319.
43. HAMMEL, H.T., R.W. ELSNER, D.H. LE MESSURIER, H.T. ANDERSEN, and F.A. MILAN (1959): J. appl. Physiol. **14:** 605.
44. HAMMEL, H.T., J.A. HILDES, D.C. JACKSON, and H.T. ANDERSEN (1963): Arctic Aeromedical Laboratory Technical Documentary Report 62–44.
45. HARDY, J.D. (1961): Physiol. Rev. **41:** 54.
46. HART, J.S., H.B. SABENA, J.A. HILDES, F. DECOPES, H.T. HAMMEL, K.L. ANDERSEN, L. IRVING, and G. ROY (1962): J. appl. Physiol. **17:** 953.
47. HEISE, A. (1969): Der Einfluss der Umgebungstemperatur auf verschiedene temperaturregulatorische Grössen beim Menschen mit besonderer Berücksichtigung der Tagesperiodik. M.D. Thesis, München.
48. HERTZMAN, A.B. (1953): Amer. J. physical Med. **32:** 233.
49. HEY, E.N., and G. KATZ (1970): J. Physiol. **207:** 667.
50. HILDEBRANDT, G. (1957): Arch. Physik. Therap. **9:** 292.
51. HONMA, K., K. KIMURA, E. HARADA, and K. SEKINE (1966a): Z. f. Biol. **115:** 287.
52. HONMA, K., K. SEKINE, E. HARADA, and K. KIMURA (1966b): Z. f. Biol. **115:** 209.
53. HURLEY, D.A., E.D. TOPLIFF, and F. GIRLING (1964): Canad. J. Physiol. **42:** 233.
54. IAMPIETRO, P.F., and F.R. BUSKIRK (1960): J. appl. Physiol. **15:** 212.
55. IRVING, L., K.L. ANDERSEN, A. BOLSTAD, R. ELSNER, J.A. HILDES, Y. LøNING, J.D. NøELMS, L.J. PEYTON, and R.D. WHALEY. (1960): J. appl. Physiol. **15:** 635.
56. JÜRGENSEN, T. (1867): Dtsch. Arch. Klin. Med. **3:** 165.
57. KOE, K.F., W. HÖFLER, und K. LÜDERS (1968): Arch. physik. Therap. **20:** 221.
58. LEFÉVRE, J. (1898): Arch. Physiol (Paris), Ser. V. **10:** 1.
59. LEWIS, T. (1929/31): Heart **15:** 177.
60. LIEBERMEISTER, C. (1869): Dtsch. Arch. Klin. Med. **5:** 217.
61. METZ, B., et P. ANDLAUER (1949): C. r. Soc. Biol. (Paris) **143:** 1234.
62. METZ, B., et P. ANDLAUER (1952): J. Physiol. (Paris) **44:** 293.
63. METZ, B., et D. SIGWALT (1958): Arch. Sci. physiol. **12:** 301.
64. OGAWA, T., SATOK, T., and K. TAKAGI (1967): Jap. J. Physiol. **17:** 135.
65. PEMBREY, M.S. (1898): In: Text-book of Physiology, E.A. Schaefer (Ed.), Young J. Pentland, Edinburgh, Vol. **1:** p. 801.
66. PFLEIDERER, H., und K. BÜTTNER (1935): Die physiologischen und physikalischen Grundlagen der Hautthermometrie. Leipzig.
67. RAZGHA, A.V., and L. ZSELYONKA (1942): Z. exp. Med. **110:** 643.
68. READER, S.R. (1952): Clin. Sci. **11:** 1.
69. SMITH, R.E. (1969): J. appl. Physiol. **26:** 554.
70. WEVER, R. (1964): Kybernetik **2:** 127.
71. WEVER, R., und J. ASCHOFF (1957): Pflügers Arch. ges. Physiol. **264:** 272.
72. WEZLER, K., and G. NEUROTH (1949): Z. ges. exp. Med. **115:** 127.
73. WINSLOW, C.-E.A., L.P. HERRINGTON, and A.P. GAGGE (1937a): Amer. J. Physiol. **120:** 1.
74. WINSLOW, C.-E.A., L.P. HERRINGTON, and A.P. GAGGE (1937b): Amer. J. Physiol. **120:** 288.
75. WYNDHAM, C.H., R. PLOTKIN, and A. MUNRO (1962): Proc. 1st Symp. Antarctic Biol. (Paris) p. 535.

CHAPTER 21

INFLUENCE OF LIGHT AND HORMONES UPON CIRCADIAN RHYTHM OF EEG SLOW WAVE AND PARADOXICAL SLEEP

MASAZUMI KAWAKAMI, SADAO YAMAOKA, and TADASHI YAMAGUCHI

2nd Department of Physiology, Yokohama City University School of Medicine, Yokohama, Japan

There is much literature concerned with the many aspects of sleep and its mechanism, but its periodic nature has only recently received attention. A theoretical framework for the sleep mechanism was first constructed by Hess, Magoun and Moruzzi. More recently the late Hernández-Péon (1963, 1964) argued that activity in the "ascending reticular activating system" (Moruzzi and Magoun, 1949) is responsible for arousing the brain, but that the activity itself must be inhibited by a descending inhibitory system, his "vigilance system," in order to prevent a chaotic sensory bombardment of the brain while awake. It is known that the rostral-diencephalic region is essential for wakefulness, since transection of the most rostral pons results in permanent unconsciousness, while a midpontine pretrigeminal transection results in a condition of almost permanent wakefulness, a state capable of perceiving and learning (Moruzzi, 1960). This indicates that a hypnogenic system must exist in the lower bulbopontine structure as well. A contrast to this unitary theory is that proposed by Jouvet (1965), referred to as the "dualistic" theory. According to Jouvet (1967) a possible mechanism might include sleep-inducing structures located in the lower brain stem which act directly on the ascending reticular activating system without generating synchronization. In his system, the orbital cortex is the critical area for regulating the thalamo-cortical synchronizing function. Clemente (1963) also proposed a dual activation of two systems, i.e. the diffuse activating system of the brain stem and the forebrain cortical synchronizing system.

With respect to the mechanism of sleep as a circadian process, however, little has been understood, though there has been speculative discussion as to whether the basis of the mechanism is the intrinsic rhythm of cell activity or rather the rhythmic activation of a hypothetical circuit in the brain. As is well known, the diurnal rhythm is influenced not only by many synchronizing factors such as illumination, temperature, time of feeding and environmental noise and odors, but also by the internal environment of the organism. Sawyer and Kawakami (1959) and Faure and Vincent (1964) have previously reported that there was a close relationship between gonadal hormones and the generation of paradoxical sleep (PS). ACTH suppressed and some adrenocorticoids enhanced the generation of PS (Kawakami, 1960). It was also found that the rhythmicity of PS was profoundly affected by destruction of the hypothalamus and midbrain-pontine reticular formation and by implants of sex hormones into the hypothalamus (Kawakami *et al.*, 1964, 1965, a, b). These results suggest the mediation of endocrine factors as well as neural factors in the generation of sleep.

Thus, our laboratory has studied the effects of pituitary hormones, pineal substances and illumination on the distribution of PS episodes in order to learn about the pacemaker mechanism of sleep rhythm. The following are the results obtained from studies with both animals and men.

SLEEP RHYTHM IN THE RAT AND RABBIT

Continuous EEG recording and behavioral observation was made in 31 female New Zealand white rabbits and 27 female albino rats with the electrodes implanted chronically in the brain. EEG recording was successively classified into three phases of activity, i.e., slow wave sleep (SS) phase, PS phase and awake phase. The duration of each phase in every four hour period was measured and a sliding average was calculated to observe diurnal rhythm of SS and PS as influenced by extirpation of the pineal gland and administration of anterior pituitary hormones. The experiments were performed in a soundproof shielded room maintained at $20 \pm 3°C$ ($26 \pm 1°C$ for hypophysectomized rats) and illuminated from 5:00—19:00 (400 Lux) with complete darkness from 19:00 —5:00 of the next day. In all cases, except for the pinealectomized animals, observation was first made in the control condition for seven to ten days, then in the experimental condition for two to four weeks.

1. SS and PS Rhythm under Light-dark Environment (Control Experiment)

SS and PS patterns were observed in 15 adult female rats (Fig. 164). In a light-dark environment (LD 14–10) the period of maximal SS appearance was 8:00–12:00 or 12:00–16:00 (mean 151.77 mins., max. 173.30 mins. per four hours) and the period of minimal SS appearance was 20:00–0:00 or 0:00–4:00 (mean 49.19 mins., min. 10.65

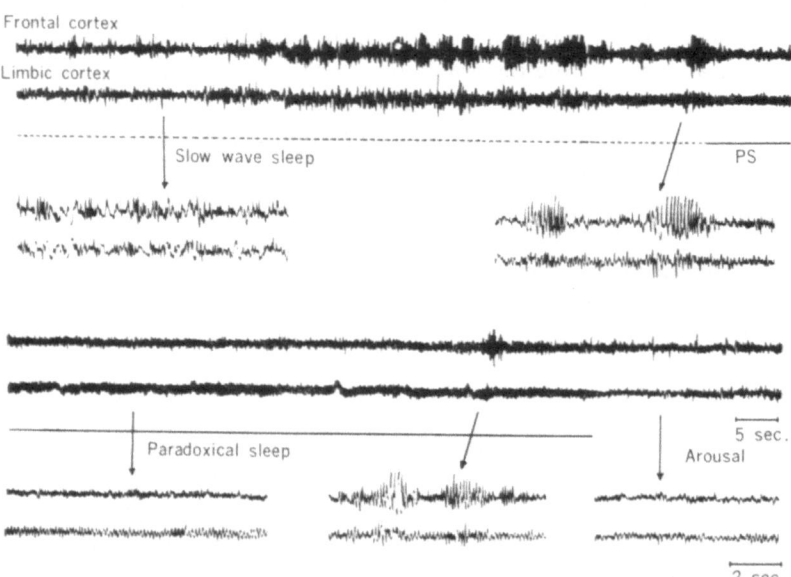

Fig. 164. An example of EEG patterns of frontal cortex and limbic cortex in slow wave sleep (SS), paradoxical sleep (PS) and arousal stages in the rat.
SS stage is indicated by the dotted line and PS stage by a solid line. It is noted that the K-complex wave mingled with the sleep spindle bursts.

mins.). The mean and maximum amount of PS in the PS peak period was 31.97 and 47.40 mins. and the mean and minimum amount of PS in the PS trough was 1.07 and 0 respectively. The total amount of both SS and PS during estrus and diestrus showed no significant difference between the two periods. However, the difference between the peak and trough of the PS and SS rhythm increased during estrus as compared with diestrus (Fig. 165), as Colvin *et al.* (1968) previously reported.

Circadian rhythm of SS and PS was also observed in 10 adult female rabbits. In this experiment it was shown that the periods of maximal and minimal appearance of PS and SS were the same as those in the experiment with rats but that the amount of PS in the rabbit was in general less than that in the rat. Maximal amount of PS appearance was 37.50 mins., while the mean amount was 12.67 mins. .

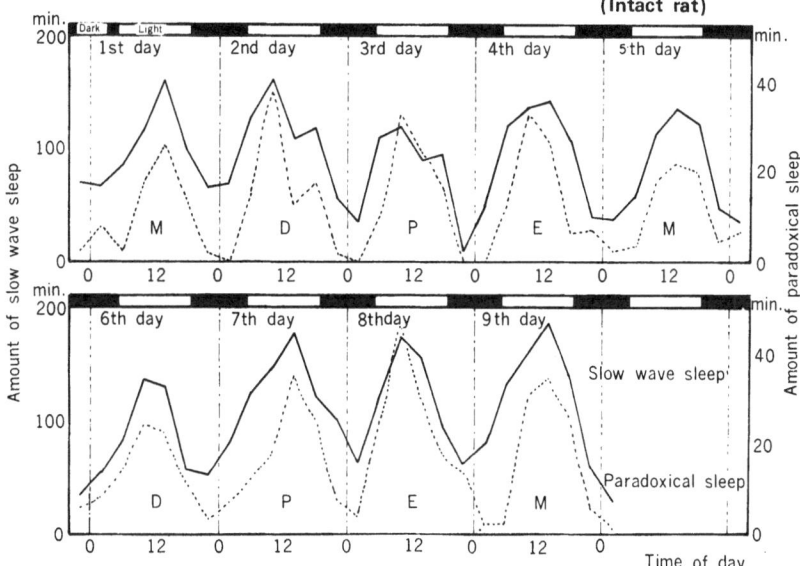

Fig. 165. The graphic representation of sleep rhythm in the intact female rat under light-dark environment.

 The solid line represents changes in the amount of SS and the dotted line that of PS. Changes in vaginal smear were indicated by P (proestrus), E (estrus), M (metestrus), and D (Diestrus).

 SS and PS amounts change synchronously. The peaks of their rhythms was evident in the period from 12:00 to 16:00, the trough in the period from 20:00—24:00 or from 0:00—4:00.

2. SS and PS Rhythm under Constant Dark Environment

The rats which were used in the control experiment were maintained in a completely dark environment for 24 days. It was found that the times of maximal or minimal appearance of PS and SS had the same tendency as was evident in the control experiment; however, the amplitude of the circadian rhythm was slightly decreased. The mean of the SS and PS in the peak period were 131.25 and 28.75 mins., and the mean in the trough period was 45.70 and 6.15 mins., respectively. The pattern of the rhythm showed no significant difference when compared with that of the control light-dark condition. The time of the peak was 8:00–12:00 or 12:00–16:00 and that of trough was 20:00–0:00 or 0:00–4:00 (Fig. 166).

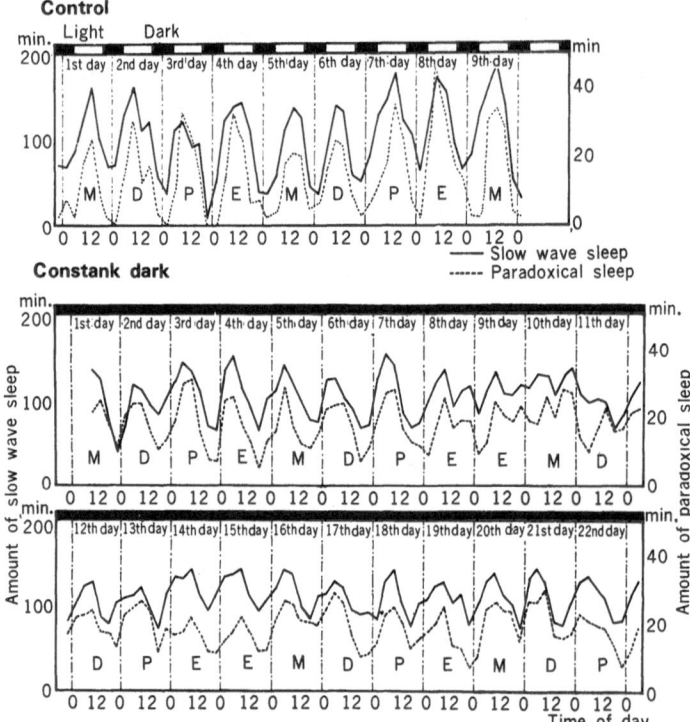

Fig. 166. Sleep rhythm of the rat under constant dark environment. No phase shift occurred after the 15th day after starting continuous dark.

Keeping mature rabbits in complete darkness revealed somewhat different results. While the total amount of PS and SS showed no significant change, the rhythm first appeared to lose periodicity, with deviations from the normal 24 hour period ranging from 20 to 28 hours, and gradually the period of a cycleshortened. The phase advanced about half a day between the 15th and 18th day of experiment; however, the amplitude of the rhythm did not change.

3. SS and PS Rhythm under Constant Illumination

Continuous illumination (400 Lux) failed to induce any change in the SS and PS rhythm until the fourth day of the experiment. The peak of SS and PS was 12:00–16:00, the trough 20:00–24:00 or 0:00–4:00. Then the periodicity began to be affected. Disorders such as two-peak rhythm or a decrease in amplitude was observed. By the eighth or nineth day the rhythm with one peak and trough reappeared. However, the peak and trough tended to show delay and the period was extended on the 15th day; at that time the peak was 0:00–4:00, and the trough was 12:00–16:00, which was a complete phase reversal of the control (Fig. 167).

Reviewing all of the above experiments, the results seem to show a synchronizing action of external light-dark changes, influencing the organism in the establishment of a periodicity of around 24 hours. Thus, it was found that PS as well as SS has a free-running rhythm, and that this rhythm, though regulated by illumination, tends to maintain its former pattern in spite of environmental changes for a considerable number of days. It is a well-known fact that constant illumination causes persistent estrus in

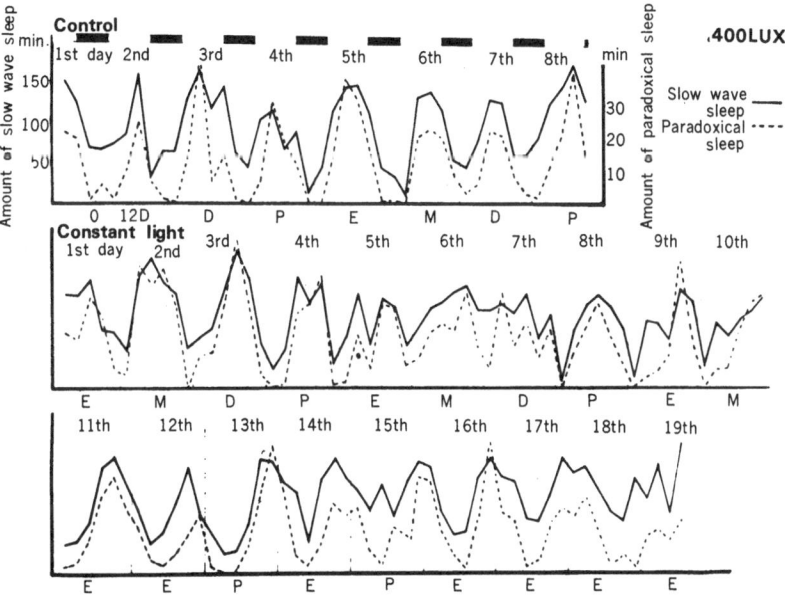

Fig. 167. Sleep rhythm of the rat under constant light environment.
It is noted that 180° phase shift occurred on the 15th day after the onset of continuous illumination. The tendency began to show on the eighth day after starting continuous illumination, and vaginal smear test showed persistent estrus on the 11th day and thereafter.

the female rat (Hemmingsen and Krarup, 1937; Everett, 1940). In the present experiment the estrous cycle began to be disturbed from the eighth or nineth day of constant illumination. The vaginal smear revealed a gradual shifting to prolonged estrus. 10–14 days of continuous light were necessary for the achievement of persistent estrus in female rats and to induce prolonged estrous behavior in female rabbits. Exposing rabbits to repeated immobilization stress could also induce changes in the circadian rhythmicity of adrenocorticoid biosynthesis in the adrenal cortex and in that of the corticosterone level in the plasma on the first day of the stress. These rhythms recovered gradually (Kawakami *et al.*, in press); according to Orth *et al.* (1967) it took six to 12 days to form a new pattern of sleep rhythm in man. After a trip by airplane from Minneapolis to South Korea it took nine days for urinary hormones to synchronize to the new local time (Flink and Doe, 1959). It is interesting that the diurnal animal, and the nocturnal animal, man as well as rat and rabbit, need approximately the same amount of time to change from one rhythm to a new one.

4. SS and PS Rhythm of Adrenalectomized Female Rats under Light-dark Environment

Kawakami *et al.* (1965) have pointed out the close relationship between stress and PS. To be specific, during immobilization stress for a period of four hours after release from this stress, PS did not appear in the adult animal. Yet, in the immature animal (25 to 27 days old), the PS appeared as usual after release from immobilization stress. This fact may be attributed to the immaturity of the hypothalamus and some other brain regions.

Among hormones, ACTH had the effect of blocking PS. As for the adrenocortical hormones, desoxycorticosterone facilitated PS, while corticosterone proved ineffective in doing this. Insulin decreased the appearance of PS.

These results suggested that the neuro-humoral factor in stress had an important role in PS appearance as well.   This agreed with the recent results of Okuma *et al.* (1968), that is that after 24 hours of sleep deprivation the plasma corticosterone level was significantly low prior to the initiation of sleep, and rose significantly soon after the onset of sleep.

The activity of corticotrophin releasing factor (CRF) in the hypothalamus rose slightly from early morning until afternoon in parallel with the change of the serum corticosterone level, but when serum corticosterone level reached its maximum in the evening, the activity of CRF fell rapidly to return to its control level within three hours (David-Nelson and Brodish, 1969, Seiden and Brodish, 1970).   On the other hand, Itoh *et al.* (1969) reporting about the diurnal rhythm in rats stated that the high level of CRF activity in the hypothalamus led by four hours that of serum corticosterone level, and that the diurnal rhythm of CRF-ACTH system was not apparent until three weeks of age. It might, therefore, be worthwhile to examine the diurnal rhythm of CRF further.

The diurnal rise of plasma corticosterone disappeared after electrolytic lesion of the anterior hypothalamus or median eminence, while lesioning the posterior tuber cinereum had no such effect (Ganong *et al.*, 1961; Slucher, 1964).   The diurnal pattern of plasma corticosterone disappeared after the implantation of cortisol into the arcuate nucleus, median eminence, ventral hippocampus or midbrain reticular formation (Slusher, 1966).   The diurnal rhythm in plasma corticosterone level was quite different in the rat with a frontally isolated hypophysiotrophic area from that of the normal rat (Halász *et al.*, 1967).   From those results, it would seem that the anterior hypothalamus and some extra-hypothalamic areas participate in the generation of diurnal rhythm in plasma corticosterone through regulation of ACTH release.

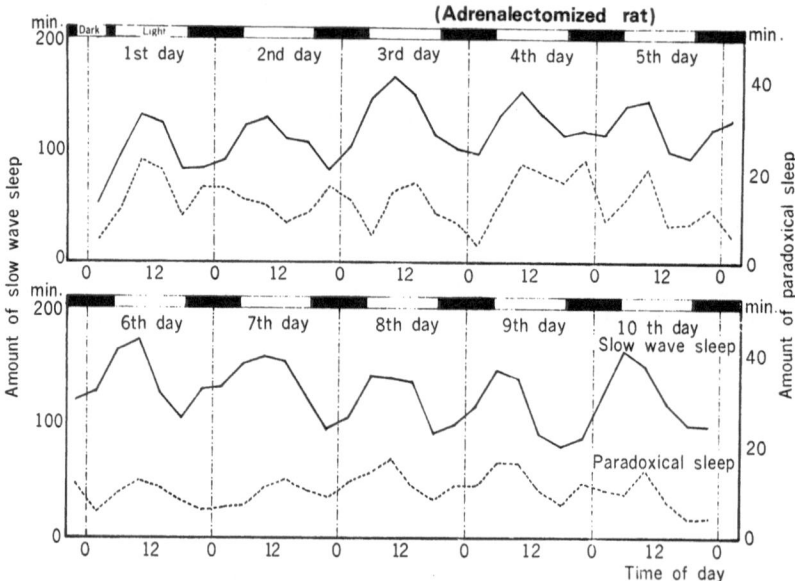

Fig. 168.   The graphic representation of sleep rhythm in the adrenalectomized rat under light-dark environment.
No difference between the period in which the peak and trough appear was observed between sleep rhythm in intact and adrenalectomized rats.   It is noted that total amount of SS increased but that of PS decreased, and that the amplitudes of both sleep rhythms were reduced.

Therefore, the effect of adrenalectomy was observed under a light-dark environment, seven days after recovery from the postoperative shock. The periodicity of SS and PS rhythm was maintained but the amplitude of these rhythms was suppressed. To be specific, the time zone of maximum and minimum appearance of SS or PS was the same as in the experimental control. The mean amount of SS and PS in the peak period was 163.56 mins. and 17.31 mins., and the mean SS and PS in the trough period was 113.29 and 4.13 mins., respectively. As compared with the intact animal, the total amount of SS increased but that of PS decreased and the diurnal fluctuation of both the SS and PS episode was reduced (Fig. 168). Generally speaking, the total amount of PS increased or decreased in parallel to that of SS in intact rats, whereas the dissociation between the changes in total amounts of each sleep was characteristic of the adrenalectomized rats.

5. SS and PS Rhythm of Hypophysectomized Rats under Light-dark Environment

The close relationship between pituitary hormones and PS appearance was presumed because of the alteration of spontaneous PS in the estrous cycle, the change in the induced-threshold of PS by electrical stimulation, and from the induction of PS by the administration of gonadotrophin, ACTH or growth hormone.

Thus sleep rhythm in hypophysectomized rats was observed under light-dark condition. The experiments were started seven days after hypophysectomy. The rhythm of both SS and PS showed an unsettled period of maximal or minimal appearance of SS and PS. This result was the same as reported in the rabbit by Spies and Sawyer (1970). Pituitary hormones, therefore, seem to be related to the pacemaker mechanism of sleep rhythm.

The mean duration of SS in the peak period was 122.30 mins. and in the trough period 47.55 mins., while the mean of PS in the peak was 24.77 and 7.07 mins. in the trough.

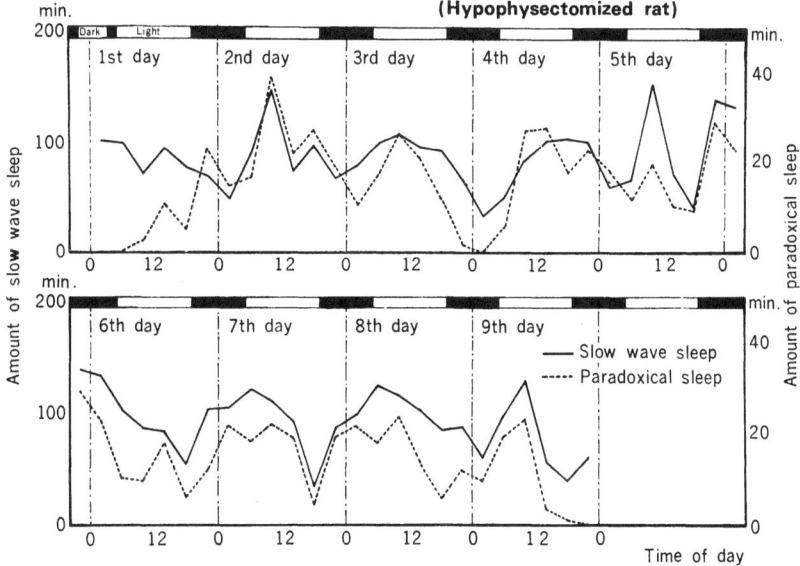

Fig 169. The graphic representation of sleep rhythm in the hypophysectomized rat under light-dark environment.

SS and PS are indicated as in Fig. 164. The disturbed rhythmicity and reduced amplitude was noted.

In the hypophysectomized rat the total amount of SS was reduced, as was the amplitude of the SS and PS rhythm (Fig. 169).

6. PS and SS Rhythm in Pinealectomized Rats under a Controlled Lighting Schedule

The pineal gland is known to be related to melatonin synthesis and sexual motivation, its influence correlated with level of illumination (Fraschini *et al.*, 1968). Pinealectomized rats were observed with respect to sleep rhythm patterns, under light-dark environment, from 10 to 20 days after the operation. The period of maximal SS was between 8:00–12:00 or 12:00–16:00, and that of minimal SS was between 16:00–20:00 or 0:00–4:00. In addition, a small peak of SS was observed between 20:00–24:00. The rhythm of PS showed bimodal circadian rhythm, one between the 8:00–12:00 period and another between 20:00–24:00. The pineal gland seems to exert an important influence on PS rhythm as regulated by the changes in light and darkness. Furthermore, the two peaks might be understood in terms of another neural or humoral factor. The amplitude of the SS or PS rhythm in the pinealectomized rats decreased in comparison with that of the intact rats. The mean duration of SS in the peak period was 152.65 mins. and that of the trough period was 90.30 mins. .

Regarding the rhythm of pinealectomized rats in continuous darkness: the two PS peaks reduced to one during the first two to three days of darkness, then returned to

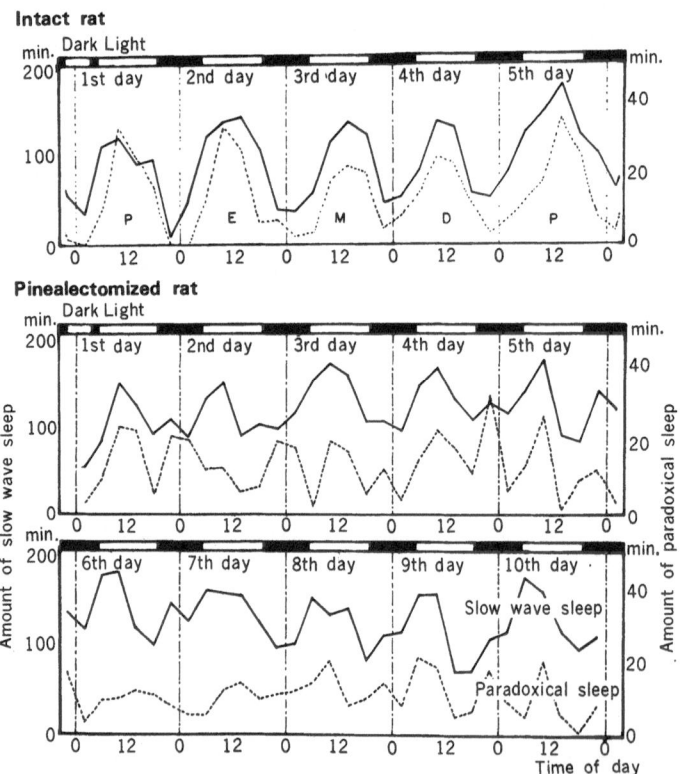

Fig. 170. The graphic representation of sleep rhythm under light-dark environment in the pinealectomized rats. SS and PS are indicated as in Fig. 164.

Biphasic diurnal rhythmicity was observed in both SS and PS. The peaks were in the periods from 8:00—12:00 and from 20:00—24:00. It is noted that the diurnal distribution of PS episode is dissociated from that of SS.

two peaks, and persisted thereafter. The amplitude of the rhythm was remarkably reduced. Observation of the SS rhythm revealed entirely different changes: a complete loss of regularity and a great reduction of the amplitude of the rhythm (Fig. 170).

7. The influence of Melatonin on the PS Rhythm of Pinealectomized Rats

In order to understand the origin of the two peaks in PS rhythm, the influence of melatonin on PS appearance was examined in pinealectomized rats. Melatonin was administered intraperitonealy in the amount of 1 mg per kg. The times of administration were 10:00 and 22:00, when PS appearance was at its maximum, and 2:00 and 16:00, i.e., three hours before the change in illumination. The second PS peak disappeared upon injection at 22:00; the suppression was observed for about two hours. However, little change was observed in SS appearance. After melatonin administration at 10:00 or 16:00, both SS and PS appearances markedly increased; however, the second peak of PS disappeared with the increase in the amplitude of the first peak. Melatonin administration at 2:00 did not affect either PS or SS appearance. Sham-operated rats, with venous plexus cut by ligation above the pineal gland, showed a decrease in PS appearance upon melatonin injection at 10:00, but no change following injection at other times. From this experiment it may be concluded that the pineal body is related to the formation of PS rhythm correlated with illumination. Quay (1963) reported that studies of serotonin level in the pineal gland revealed diurnal fluctuation and that the highest level was shown at 13:00 and the lowest at 23:00. It is well known that melatonin is formed within the pineal gland by N-acetylation of serotonin and O-methylation of this product. According to the report by Axelrod et al. (1965) melatonin level in the pineal gland showed a diurnal variation, lower level in the day time and a higher level at night. These facts do not explain the present experimental results, but it is interesting to note that the pinealectomized rats reestablished a normal PS rhythm upon administration of melatonin.

Serotonin, a precursor of melatonin, has been considered to have some significant role in sleep mechanism. Jouvet (1965) reported that in cats given reserpin to suppress SS and PS, a 5-hydroxytryptamine (5-HTP) injection immediately initiated SS but not PS. Also, DOPA administration facilitated the restoration of PS. On the basis of these results, Jouvet concluded that serotonin induced SS, but needed the participation of catecholamine for PS induction.

Quay (1968) reported the regional differences in diurnal rhythm of serotonin content in the brain. Scheving et al. (1968) reported on the diurnal change of serotonin concentration in the brain, finding maximum between 11:30 and 17:30 and minimum between 20:30 and 21:30. A figure in this paper shows a small peak between 23:00 and 2:30, showing, on the whole, a two peak rhythm. Our results coincide with the two-peak rhythm observed in this figure. Krieger and Rizzo (1969) showed that a change in brain serotonin affected other aspects of biological rhythm. For instance, they observed the extinction of the elevating phase of plasma 17-OHCS at night by injection of four agents which affected the serotonin level in the central nervous system.

8. Sleep and Wakefulness Rhythm and Brain Lesion

Massive destruction of the hypothalamus or midbrain reticular formation induces coma (Ranson, 1930; Bremmer, 1936; Morruzi and Magoun, 1949; French and Magoun, 1952). Batini et al. (1959) reported that midpontine pretrigeminal transection in cats resulted in arousal, as observed both behaviorally and electroencephalographically, and he suspected the existence of a sleep inducing center in the region extending from the middle of the pons to the medulla. The lesion of either retropontine or medial pontine tegmentum abolished the occurence of PS (Jouvet, 1961). Therefore, it is suggested that pontine tegmentum plays an important role in the control of PS. On the other hand, Hess (1944) and Akimoto (1956) observed the induction of sleep by low frequency stimulation of the hypothalamus or non-specific nuclei of the thalamus. Favale *et al.* (1961) reported that low frequency stimulation of the midbrain reticular formation resulted in EEG slow waves with behavioral sleep.

The genesis of sleep seems to be regulated by neural factors. However, the neural mechanism related to the diurnal variation of SS and PS is not yet known.

Kawakami *et al.* (1964) reported on the influence of brain destruction on SS and PS rhythm in cases treated with sex hormones. Ovariectomized rabbits did not show the diurnal variation of SS and PS under constant illumination and showed an increase in PS appearance following the administration of sex hormones. Bilateral massive lesions in the medial basal hypothalamus, including the posterior tuberal region, the ventromedial hypothalamus, or the premammillary region, were found to block PS appearance which was facilitated by administration of sex hormones. Giannazo *et al.* (1969) reported that fastigial lesions affected sleep-wakefulness rhythm. Such a lesion induced an increased wakefulness and decreased SS in the early stage (first to third day after operation) and an increased SS and decreased wakefulness in the later stage (from the fourth day after operation). However, PS did not show such changes.

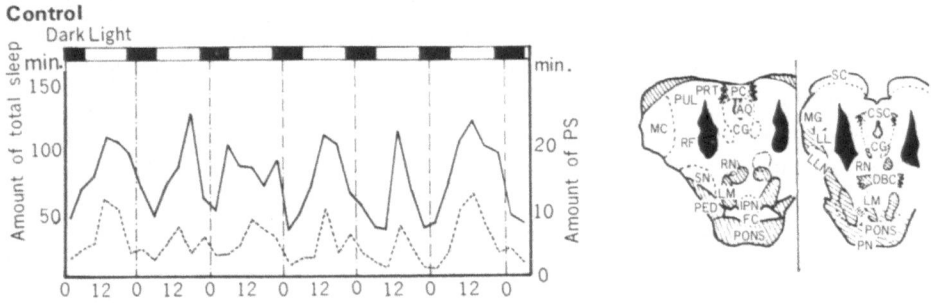

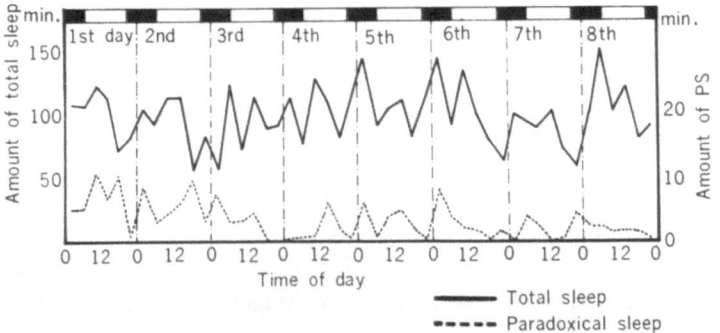

Fig. 171. (continues on next page.)

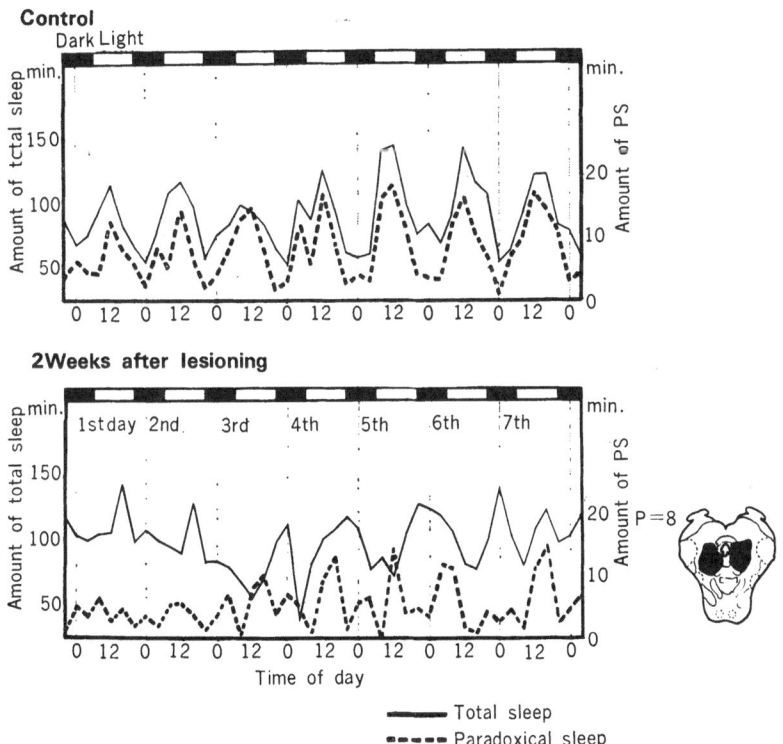

Fig. 171. Two examples of changes in sleep rhythm in rats with bilateral distruction of the midbrain reticular formation.

The sites and size of the brain lesions are represented schematically in the frontal section. Irregular rhythms of SS and PS are observed with an increase in SS amplitude and a decrease in
PS amplitude.

In our experiment, bilateral lesions were made in a part of the midbrain reticular
formation and the posterior hypothalamus and the influence on the distribution of the
PS episode was examined. EEG recording was started under a light-dark environment
two weeks after lesioning either one of these two regions. The results showed irregularity
of SS rhythm, though the total amount per day was unchanged. PS also showed this
irregularity as well as marked decrease in the total amount per day. SS and PS rhythms
ceased to be parallel with each other (Fig. 171, A, B).

From these facts, it was supposed that brain lesions, particularly in the midbrain
reticular formation and posterior hypothalamus, were concerned in the formation of
PS and SS circadian rhythm.

PS RHYTHM IN IMMATURE ANIMALS AND MEN

In the newborn infant the sleep-wakefulness episodes are polyphasically distributed
within a day. However, this polyphasic rhythm changes into a monophasic circadian
rhythm as he grows. This phenomenon is a spontaneous rhythm which will later be
synchronized by the light and dark stimuli with a 24 hour rhythm. Sleep at night
is reduced from 15 hours to seven to eight hours per 24 hours (Kleitman, 1963). The
aquisition of 24 hours' cycle is a gradual process. On the other hand, PS, in human

beings, can be observed at an early stage of sleep in the infant and patients of narcolepsia in daytime sleep, but not in the normal adult.

In general the rate of thermogenic sweating is closely associated with deep sleep in daytime sleep, but the association of phenomena is not so close in night sleep, especially in later sleep cycles (Takagi, 1970).

The duration of PS is generally 20–30 minutes except for the first PS in the sleep period. The average PS duration does not change from early childhood to adulthood. In the newborn infant, the total amount of sleep is longer than child and adult, and subsequently the frequency of PS is also increased. The ratio of PS to total sleep is 70% at birth, then gradually decreases to 50% at 50 days of age.

The ratio of PS to SS differs according to species; the tortoise completely lacks PS and in birds very little PS is observed. In mammals the ratio is about 30%. Klein reported the ratio to be 30% in the adult cat, 80% in kittens. In young animals PS occurs more frequently than in the adult.

PS is currently assumed to be regulated by some biochemical mechanisms which synthesize and metabolize particular substances at an appropriate rate. Consequently, activation of the mechanisms (to synthesize and discharge the active substances) is surmised to occur in a more sporadic and random way in infant animals than in the adult.

In our experiment with the immature New Zealand white rabbit, EEG recording and EMG recording of M. Scapuloauricularis superior commenced 10 days after birth. Rhythmicity was not observed in EEG at 10 days of age and the amount of PS was the same during the day and night. At 30 days of age a peak of PS appeared at a fixed hour of the day and rhythmicity was relevant. The rhythm was irregular, though a peak could be seen between 15 to 25 days of age. The adult rhythmicity was attained at 40 days of age. On the other hand, SS rhythm showed a different course of development. At 10 days of age a characteristic bimodal rhythm appeared. As the animal grew, the interval between the two peaks decreased and finally the one-peak rhythm of the adult was attained between 35 to 40 days of age. These results may suggest that the SS and PS rhythms were controlled by different regulatory mechanisms of the nervous system or humoral system.

SLEEP RHYTHM OF MAN

EEG recordings were made during sleep in 12 women during the menstrual cycle and four men on five occasions at intervals of one week. The environmental conditions of daily life in the subjects were held constant as much as possible. Basal body temperature of the female subjects was measured every day. EEG was recorded in a sound-proof room at the normal sleep time of the subjects. Nystagmus, EMG, ECG, GSR and respiratory movement were recorded polygraphically to judge the depth of sleep.

The period of circadian rhythm of sleep and wakefulness in the human being was reported to be between 24.52 and 25.9 hours by Aschoff, Mills, Siffre, Kleitman, Okuma and Koga. Our results coincided with those already reported.

The course of sleep depth throughout the night was represented graphically as shown in Fig. 172. The male and female showed essentially similar courses of sleep depth. Sleep gradually deepened for one hour after falling asleep, then showed SS which shifted to PS continuing 10–30 mins. (20–30 mins. by Dement, Kleitman, Okuma and Koga). Directly before PS a short period of SS appeared. This sequence was repeated four to

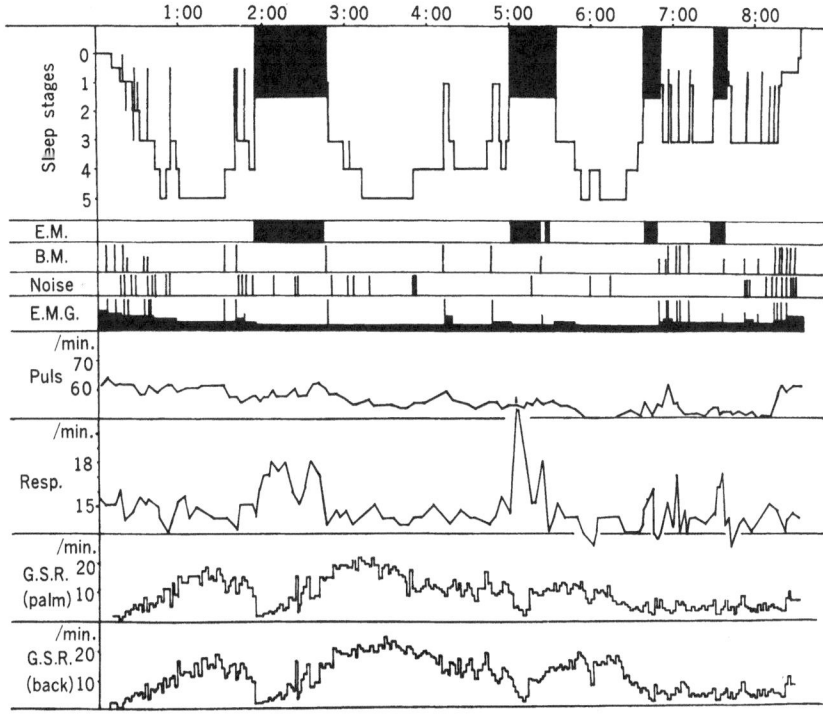

Fig. 172. An example of sleep diagram in a 34 year old woman.

The abscissa indicates the time of day. Sleep depth is indicated by number (0—arousal stage; 1—drowsiness; 2—very light sleep; 3—light sleep; 4—moderately deep sleep; 5—deep sleep). PS is represented by a black bar. The period in which eye movement (EM), body movement (BM) and noise occurred is indicated by a black bar in each column. Activity of surface EMG was recorded from the neck. Pulse rate, respiratory rate and GSR was represented in numbers per minute.

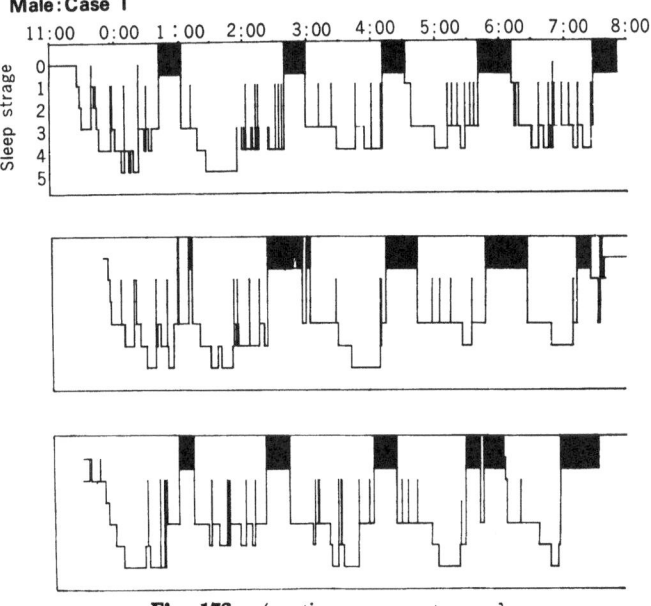

Fig. 173. (continues on next page.)

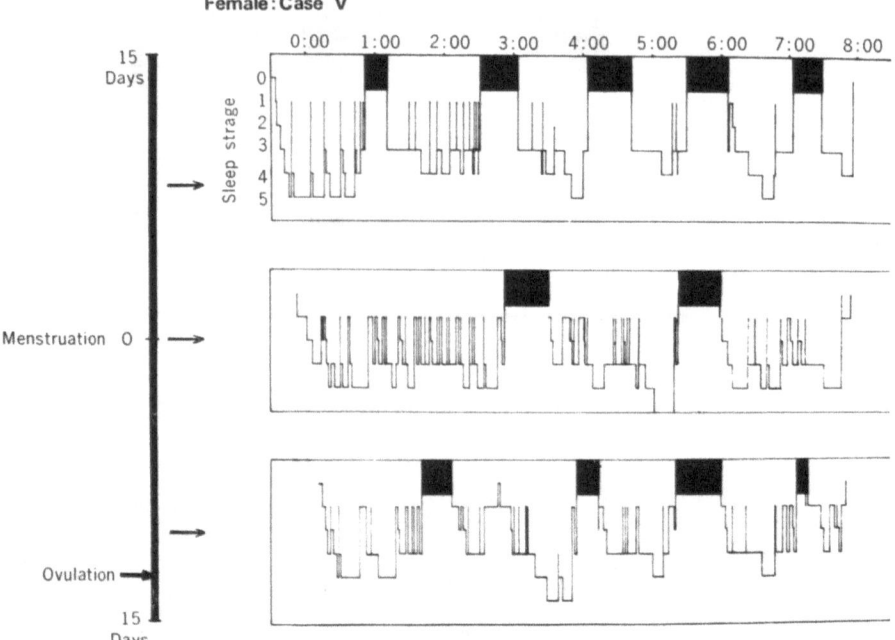

Fig. 173. The pattern of night sleep in a man (26 years old) and a woman (27 years old).
The abscissa shows time of night and the ordinate shows the depth of SS. The black bar indicates PS.
Recordings were made once every week, and also before, during, and after menstruation in the
case of the woman. The regularity of distribution of PS episode in the man is noted.

five times during one night's sleep. Arousal was sometimes preceded by PS, but sometimes by SS. Time of the first appearance of PS did not seem to be related to time
passage after falling asleep but it did tend to appear at a relatively definite time of night
(1:00–3:00) and to show ultradian rhythm (Fig. 173). Even in the four male cases
where a relatively irregular course of SS depth was observed, the first appearance of
PS occurred at 1:00–3:00, showing thereafter a similar ultradian rhythm of SS and PS
was seen. The alternative appearance of SS and PS was also observed in these cases.

EEG recording was performed during menstruation in 12 female subjects whose menstrual cycles were generally regular. The change in basal body temperature showed
that nine of the 12 menstrual cases were ovulatory, while the rest were non-ovulatory.
In the nine ovulatory cases, sleep depth increased after falling asleep until a moderately
deep SS appeared; a very deep SS was not achieved. A short course of drowsy to moderately deep SS preceded PS. The interval between the 2 PS episodes in the menstrual
phase is 1.5 to 1.8 times as long as those in the other phases (Fig. 173). However, the
length of PS phase itself did not change, thus, the total amount of PS decreased. On
the other hand, in the three non-ovulatory menstruation cases, alteration in rhythm
as such was not observed.

COMMENT

Aschoff (1960), Pittendrigh (1960) and other researchers have reported in detail about
the circadian rhythm under continuous illumination or constant darkness. Aschoff

reported that the period of activity in diurnal animals was shortened under continuous illumination and was extended under continuous dark. This is "Aschoff's Rule." However, if other factors besides light and dark are taken into account, Aschoff's Rule is shown to be not comprehensive enough itself to explain the genesis of the circadian rhythm (Pittendrigh, 1960).

Kawakami and Yoshida (1965), based upon the idea that an PS genesis is closely related to humoral factors, hypothesized that PS is regulated by the oxidizing and reductive system and energic metabolism of the brain, and supposed that activation of the TCA cycle and ATP storage might be the main humoral factors involved.

We observed the circadian rhythm of SS and PS under artificial light-dark condition and under continuous light and continuous dark conditions. As was already observed by Sawyer *et al.* (1959), SS and PS alternated parallel to each other under light-dark conditions. In the rat, a periodically ovulating animal, the amplitude of the rhythm was large at proestrus and estrus while small at metestrus and diestrus. This fact shows that differences in the balance of sex hormones at different stages of the estrus cycle affects the alternation of sleep rhythm.

Kawakami *et al.* (1964) reported on the influence of localized destruction of the brain and of sex hormones on PS genesis in ovariectomized rabbits under continuous illumination. Rhythmicity was rarely observed before or after brain destruction.

Progesterone administration in the ovariectomized estrogen primed rabbit caused a biphasic alternation of the SS/PS ratio. Destruction of the medial basal hypothalamus blocked this biphasic alternation. Thus, it was concluded that PS genesis is influenced by both sex hormones and by the basal hypothalamus.

Rats in these experiments showed little alteration from normal conditions in the form, phase, and amplitude of rhythm under constant darkness. The inconsistency with "Aschoff's Rule" might be related to an insufficient period of continuous recording. On the other hand, the period of SS and PS was reduced in the mature rabbit. The rabbit, as a nocturnal animal, demonstrates "Aschoff's Rule."

SS and PS rhythm in the rat gradually extended under continuous light conditions, and on the 15th day of recording a phase reversal of $180°$ was observed. This tendency coincides with "Aschoff's Rule." It was reported by Hemmingsen and Krarup (1937) and Browman (1937) that the estrous cycle under continuous light condition became persistent. Everett (1942) demonstrated that mature rats showing normal 20 to 40 day cycles showed a tendency toward persistent estrus within 10 days of the onset of constant illumination. The present experiment was performed at a temperature of $20 \pm 3°C$. After the ninth day of constant illumination the vaginal smear preparations began to show cornified cells persistently. Persistent estrus induced by constant illumination may be explained in terms of over-secretion of gonadal estrogen and other hormones due to the changes in the Hypothalamus-Hypophysis-Gonadal axis regulatory mechanism caused by the constant illumination. The rhythm of SS and PS also reacted sensitively to the change, first showing a transient irregularity of rhythm, accompanied by restoration of balance and regularity of rhythm.

In rabbits, continuous light induced irregularity in the total rhythm of SS and PS. This indicates a destruction of the balance between humoral and neural factors. The sleep rhythm of rabbits under continuous light condition did not coincide with "Aschoff's Rule." The species difference appeared to be important in explaining this.

The secretion of CRF, ACTH and ACH is known to show diurnal rhythm. In man, the maximum secretion of ACTH and ACH was observed shortly before wakefulness in the morning, and is therefore supposed to be an important factor in sleep-wakefulness rhythm. Cortisone has been found to promote PS genesis (Kawakami *et al.*, 1965), however, in the present experiment bilateral adrenalectomy caused only alternation in amplitude and not in phase and periodicity of SS and PS. The rabbit shows a nocturnal rhythm of SS and PS. However, it is important that blood corticosterone is minimum at 0:00 and maximum at 6:00, which is typical in man, a diurnal animal. Thus, it is suspected that only the amplitudes of SS and PS rhythms are influenced by the adrenal gland. The rhythm of corticosterone sectetion and the SS and PS rhythms do not necessarily run parallel; they seem to be influenced independently by external and internal environment.

After hypophysectomy, both SS and PS showed an irregularity in rhythm, although the diurnal rhythm survived. Thus, pituitary hormones promoting or suppressing SS and PS are apparently only indirect regulators of the periodicity and amplitude of the rhythm, acting through the cooperative functioning of the pituitary and target organs.

The pacemaker of sleep rhythm could be anything other than hormones of the pituitary gland and its target organs. These hormones are only one of many factors influencing the pacemaker of sleep rhythm, including light, temperature, sound, odor, feeding time, etc.

The pineal gland, through which light impulses activate 5-hydroxytryptophan decarboxylase (5-HTPD) to facilitate serotonin synthesis and inhibit 5-hydroxyindole-0-methyltransferase (5-HIOMT) activation to block melatonin production from serotonin, seemed to be related to the genesis of diurnal rhythm. Thus, the pineal gland is suspected to influence sleep genesis through diurnal changes in serotonin and melatonin levels.

In pinealectomized rats, PS showed a two-peak rhythm under light-dark and continuous dark conditions. However SS rhythm was irregular in the continuous dark condition. The observation two peaks in PS rhythm coincides with the results reported by Scheving *et al.* (1968) concerning the diurnal change of serotonin concentration in the brain. Therefore, the two-peak rhythm of PS in pinealectomized rats may be related to serotonin genesis in the brain. In other words, the pineal gland may be involved in making the two-peak rhythm into one-peak rhythm by the cooperative functioning of melatonin and light stimulus. This hypothesis is supported by the experiment in which melatonin was administered to the pinealectomized rat. Elevation of the melatonin level during darkness resulted in disappearance of a PS peak in darkness. Melatonin administered during light increased the PS duration in light. Furthermore, the fact that the serotonin storage level is raised during light conditions or that melatonin increases and is activated in darkness, suggests the involvement of certain enzymes in serotonin genesis or the cooperative functioning of catecholamine and light stimulus.

Thus, it may be concluded that sleep rhythm is regulated by various humoral and neural factors; the details of such mechanism should be studied in the future.

ACKNOWLEDGEMENTS

The authors would like to thank Mrs. Hagino for her kind help with English Dr. Ishida, and Dr. Yoshida, Dr. Fujii and Dr. Konda for their kind assistance in this work.

A part of this article was presented at the US-Japan Seminar on Fundamental Problems of Biological Rhythms and the Human Ecosystem (1967) and of Sleep (1968).

The investigations herewith reported were supported by grants from the Japan Ministry of Education, and the U.S. National Institutes of Health, U.S. Public Health Service (NB-03860-5).

REFERENCES

1. AKIMOTO, H., N. YAMAGUCHI, K. OKABE, T. NAKAGAWA, I. NAKAMURA, K. ABE, H. TORII, and K. MASAHASHI (1956): *Folia Psychiat. Neurol. Jap.* **10**: 117.
2. ASCHOFF, J. (1960): *Cold Spring Harbor Symp. Quant. Biol.* **25**: 11.
3. ASCHOFF, J. (1967): *Ann. Rev. Physiol.* **25**: 581.
4. BATINI, C., G. MORUZZI, M. PALESTRINI, G.F. ROSSI, and A. ZANCHETTI (1959): *Arch. Ital. Biol.* **97**: 1.
5. BATINI, C., F. MAGUT, M. PALESTRINI, G.F. ROSSI, and A. ZANCHETTI (1959): *Arch. Ital. Biol.* **97**: 13
6. BROWMAN, L.G. (1937): *J. Exp. Zool.* **75**: 375.
7. CLEMENT, C.D., and M.B. STERMAN (1963): *Electroenceph. Clin. Neurophysiol. Suppl.* **24**: 172.
8. COLVIN, G.B., R.D. WHITMOYER, R.D. LISK, D.O. WALTER, and C.H. SAWYER (1968): *Brain Res.* **7**: 173.
9. DAVID-NELSON, M.A., and A. BRODISH (1969): *Endocrinology* **85**: 861.
10. DEMENT, W., and N. KLEITMAN (1957): *Electroenceph. Clin. Neurophysiol.* **9**: 673.
11. DEMENT, W. (1965): *Amer. J. Psychiat.* **122**: 404.
12. EVERETT, J.W. (1940): *Anat. Rec.* **76**: Suppl. 21.
13. FAURE, J., and D. VINCENT (1964): *C. R. Soc. Biol.* **158**: 515.
14. FAVALE, E., C. LOEB, G.F. ROSSI, and G. SACCO (1961): *Arch. Ital. Biol.* **99**: 1.
15. FLINK, E.B., and R.P. DOE (1959): *Proc. Soc. Exp. Med.* **100**: 498.
16. FRASCHINI, F., B. MESS, and L. MATINI (1968): *Endocrinol.* **82**: 919.
17. GANONG, W.F., A.M. NOLAN, A. DOWDY, and J.A. LUETSCHER (1961): *Endocrinol.* **68**: 169.
18. GIANNAZO, E., T. MANZONI, R. RAFFAELE, S. SAPIENZ, and A. URBANO (1969): *Arch. Ital. Biol.* **107**: 1.
19. HALÁSZ, B., M.A. SLUSHER, and R.A. GORSKI (1967): *Neuroendocrinol.* **2**: 43.
20. HEMMINGSEN, A.M., and N.B. KRARUP (1937): *Kgl. Danske. Vidensk. Selsk. Biol. Med.* **13**: 1.
21. HERNÁNDEZ-PEÓN, R. (1963): *Electroenceph. Clin. Neurophysiol. Suppl.* **24**: 188.
22. HERNÁNDEZ-PEÓN, R. (1964): *Acta Neurol. Lat. Amer.* **10**: 18.
23. HESS, W.R. (1944): *Helo. Physiol. Acta* **2**: 305.
24. HIROSHIGE, T., M. SAKAKURA, and S. ITOH (1969): *Endocrinol. Japon.* **16**: 465.
25. HIROSHIGE, T., and T. SATO (1970): *Endocrinol. Japon.* **17**: 1.
26. JOUVET, M. (1961): In "The Nature of Sleep" p. 188 G.E.W. WOLSTENHOLME, and M. O'CONNOR, eds. Churchill, London.
27. JOUVET, M. (1965): In "Progress in Brain Research" 20 K. Akert, C. Bally and J.P. Shade, eds. American Elsevier, New York.
28. JOUVET, M. (1967): *Physiol. Rev.* **47**: 117.
29. KAWAKAMI, M., and C.H. SAWYER (1959): *Endocrinol.* **65**: 631.
30. KAWAKAMI, M., and C.H. SAWYER (1959): *Endocrinol.* **65**: 652.
31. KAWAKAMI, M. (1960): Sex Hormones and Brain. Kyodo-isho, Tokyo (in Japanese).
32. KAWAKAMI, M., S. ISHIDA, K. YOSHIDA, K. IBUKA, E. TERASAWA, and H. NEGORO (1964): *Gunma Symposia on Endocrinol.* **1**: 221.
33. KAWAKAMI, M., and C.H. SAWYER (1964): *Exp. Neurol.* **9**: 470.
34. KAWAKAMI, M., H. NEGORO, and E. TERASAWA (1965): *Jap. J. Physiol.* **15**: 1.
35. KAWAKAMI, M., and K. YOSHIDA (1965): *Jap. J. Physiol.* **15**: 140.
36. KAWAKAMI, M., and S. ISHIDA: *Jap. J. Physiol.* in press.
37. KLEITMAN, N. (1963): Sleep and Wakefulness. Revised and England Edition, The Univ. of Chicago Press.
38. KRIEGER, D.T., and F. RIZZO (1969): *Amer. J. Physiol.* **217**: 1703.
39. MILLS, J.N. (1964): *J. Physiol.* **174**: 217.
40. MILLS, J.N. (1966): *Physiol. Rev.* **46**: 128.
41. MORUZZI, G., and H.W. MAGOUN (1949): *Electroenceph. Clin. Neurophysiol.* **1**: 455.
42. MORUZZI, G. (1960): Electroenceph. Clin. Neurophysiol. Suppl. 13.
43. ORTH, D.N., D.P. ISLAND, and G.W. LIDDLE (1967): *J. Clin. Endocrinol.* **27**: 549.
44. PITTENDRIGH, C.S. (1960): *Cold Spring Harbor Symp. Quant. Biol.* **25**: 159.
45. QUAY, W.B. (1968): *Amer. J. Physiol.* **215**: 1448.
46. SAWYER, C.H., and M. KAWAKAMI (1959): *Endocrinol.* **65**: 622.
47. SCHEVING, L.E., W.H. HARRISON, P. GORDON, and J.E. PAULLY (1968): *Amer. J. Physiol.* **214**: 166.

48. SEIDEN, G., and A. BRODISH (1970): *Proc. 52nd Meeting of Endocrinol. Soc., U.S.A.*
49. SIFFRE, M., A. REINBERG, F. HALBERG, J. GHATES, G. PERDRIEL, and R. SLIND (1966): *La Presse Medicale* **74**: 915.
50. SLUSHER, M.A. (1964): *Amer. J. Physiol.* **206**: 1161.
51. SLUSHER, M.A. (1966): *Exp. Brain Res.* **1**: 184.
52. SPIES, H.G., D.I. WHITMOYER, and C.H. SAWYER (1970): *Brain Res.* **18**: 155.
53. TAKAGI, K. (1970): Physiological and behavioral temperature-regulation. p. 669. J.B. HARDY, A.P. GAGGE, and J.A.J. STOLWIJK (eds.), Thomas, Springfield, Illinois.
54. TAKAHASHI, S., Y. HONDA, K. TAKAHASHI, and T. OKUMA (1968): *Folia Psychiat. et Neurol. Jap.* **22**: 347.

CHAPTER 22

CIRCADIAN RHYTHM IN PITUITARY-ADRENO-CORTICAL FUNCTION

KAZUO TAKEBE, and MUNEKI SAKAKURA

Second Department of Medicine, Hokkaido University School of Medicine, Sapporo, Japan

Since the original observation of the diurnal rhythm in the activity of the adrenal cortex was first presented by Pincus in 1943 on the basis of estimation of urinary 17-ketosteroids, this phenomenon has been well demonstrated by many investigators. The diurnal rhythm in the adrenocortical activity is reflected in the plasma cortisol levels and in the urinary excretion of 17-hydroxycorticosteroids (17-OHCS) and this rhythm is regarded as the results of diurnal variation in ACTH secretion of the pituitary. Recently, the role of the central nervous system in the regulation of ACTH secretion via corticotropin-releasing factor (CRF) has been coming to light and circadian rhythm in CRF activity was shown to exist [14, 37]. This review deals with the circadian rhythm in the pituitary-adrenal axis from physiological as well as clinical view-points.

CIRCADIAN RHYTHM IN PITUITARY-ADRENAL FUNCTION IN BASAL STATE

Most workers agree that plasma cortisol levels in man follow a definite pattern throughout the day and night. The cortisol levels increase before the time of awakening, being highest from 6 a.m. to 10 a.m., and then fall gradually from morning to evening, being lowest from midnight to 4 a.m. The rate of urinary excretion of corticosteroids lags behind the plasma concentration by about two or three hours. The pattern of the circadian rhythm in adrenocortical activity is different with each species of animal. Monkeys and dogs show similar patterns to that of man, while mice, rats and hamsters show a rhythm almost exactly opposite in phase, as they are active at night.

However, it has recently become evident in man that the circadian cycle of the plasma cortisol level is not a smooth curve when analyzed at short time intervals [3, 11, 28, 33]. This would suggest that cortisol is secreted intermittently rather than continuously. Hellman *et al.* [11] reported that cortisol was secreted episodically throughout the sleeping and waking day in eight periods of activity which were separated by quiescent periods. Approximately half the day's cortisol production was achieved in the early morning hours during sleep and the secretory episodes were temporally related to rapid eye movement sleep.

The presence of a rhythmic variation in ACTH concentration in the plasma was first shown by Liddle *et al.* [19]. Further confirmation of this was made by Demura *et al.* [7] and Berson *et al.* [3] by using a sensitive radioimmunoassay technique. These variations in ACTH level were accompanied by parallel changes in plasma 17-

OHCS [3, 24]. Therefore, the circadian rhythm of corticosteroid secretion appears to be under the influence of rhythmic changes in ACTH concentration. Furthermore, the release of ACTH is considered to be controlled by peptide, CRF. Up to this date, very few reports have been made on the question of whether a circadian rhythm in CRF in the median eminence exists or not. Ungar [37] reported a daily variation of CRF activity in the mouse hypothalamus. On the other hand, Retiene et al. [30] failed to demonstrate circadian rhythm in the CRF activity of the rat hypothalamus. Recently Hiroshige et al. [13] reported that there was a circadian rhythm of CRF activity in extracts of the rat median eminence and that this rhythm was in parallel with certain phase shifts of the diurnal rhythm in peripheral plasma corticosterone. We also found the same phenomenon. In our study, male rats of Wistar strain were housed at a constant ambient temperature of $22 \pm 2\,^\circ$C under artificial light, light on from 8 a.m. to 7 p.m. Extracts of the median eminence were sampled at 8 a.m., 1 p.m., 3 p.m., 5 p.m., 6.30 p.m. and 9 p.m. CRF activity in crude extracts of the median eminence was estimated by the method of intrapituitary microinjection in rats [12] (Table 47). The results

TABLE 47   Assay procedures for CRF activity by direct intrapituitary microinjection. Change in plasma corticosterone level was taken as a measure for endogenous ACTH release and given as $\triangle 20$ in the following figures

Assay Procedures for CRF Activity by Direct Microinjection
Female rats, Wistar strain 160∼190 g.

6:00 pm	Dexamethasone 50 µg/100 g.B.W. i.p.
10:00 am	Dexamethasone 100 µg/100 g.B.W. i.p.
11:00 am	Chlorpromazine 1 mg/100 g.B.W. i.p.
1:30 pm	Nembutal 5 mg/100 g.B.W. i.p.
1:50 pm	Exposure of the pituitary gland
4:00 pm	Femoral cannulation
4:30 pm	1st blood sampling I
4:35 pm	Microinjection of test material 0.4 µl
4:55 pm	2nd blood sampling II

Plasma corticosterone
response = II − I = $\triangle 20$ (µg/100 ml)
Autopsy

obtained are shown in Fig. 174. There were observed definite diurnal variations. The peak value observed at 6.30 p.m. was approximately three and a half times higher than the minimal value at 8 a.m. It is well known that hypothalamic tissue contains considerable amounts of posterior pituitary hormones and several biogenic amines such as catecholamines, histamine and serotonin, and these substances induce the secretion of ACTH upon systemic administration. However, Hiroshige et al. [13] suggested that it was most unlikely that the daily rhythm in the hypothalamic CRF activity was due to amines and posterior pituitary hormones present in the hypothalamic tissue.

Few reports have appeared in the past about the postnatal development of circadian rhythm in the hypothalamo-pituitary-adrenocortical axis. Allen and Kendall [2], who systematically examined this problem, reported that the adrenocortical circadian rhythm in rats became evident at 30 to 32 days of age. However, Ader [1] showed that the circadian variation in rats began to appear between 21 and 25 days old. More recently, Hiroshige et al. [14] demonstrated that the circadian rhythm of plasma cor-

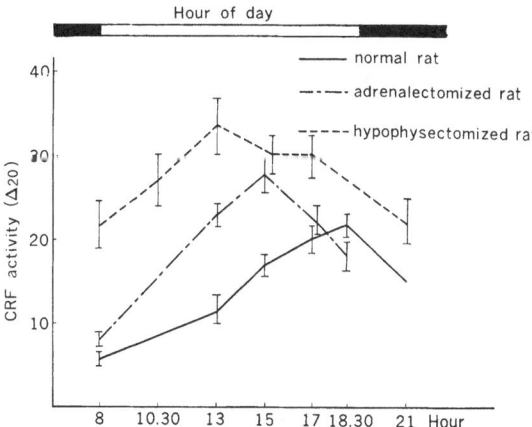

Fig. 174. Circadian rhythms of CRF activity in the hypothalamus in normal rats, adrenalectomized rats and hypophysectomized rats. Each CRF activity is the mean of six to nine determinations, accompanied by its standard error.

ticosterone level became evident during the third week of life. The hypothalamic content of CRF activity was not detectable till the end of the second week after birth. A significant increase of CRF activity in the evening became manifest during the third week of postnatal life, whereas the CRF activity in the morning remained undetectable. They showed that the rhythmical postnatal appearance time of CRF rhythmicity coincided with that of plasma corticosterone level. In human infants an abnormal rhythm was reported; the plasma corticosteroids rose gradually from 4 a.m. until 8 p.m. and then rapidly declined in 12 infants aged five to 12 months [26].

Endogenous rhythms are not necessarily related to day-night variations in illumination, temperature, atmospheric pressure, etc., but are synchronized or regulated by such exogenous or external rhythms as light and dark, or habits. It is said that if the timing of an external signal is altered but remains within the range of about 20 to 28 hours, a circadian bio-rhythm often becomes synchronized with the new signal. Light acts as a synchronizer of circadian rhythms and appears to be of primary importance in synchronizing circadian rhythm. Orth *et al.* [27] examined the influence of dark-light cycles on the plasma cortisol rhythm in man by dissociating insofar as possible the timing of dark-light cycle from the timing of sleep-wake cycle. They concluded that the dark-light may be an important synchronizer of the pituitary-adrenal cycle in man. Meanwhile, constant light was associated with a diminution of ACTH in the plasma [4]. As to habits, Perkoff *et al.* [29] found that an eight-hour shift in the timing of the sleep-wake schedule of normal subjects resulted in a corresponding eight hour shift in the timing of the 17-OHCS cycle. It appeared that the circadian rhythm of cortisol level was controlled by the sleep-wake activity. In an attempt to ascertain whether the pituitary-adrenal cycle of normal man necessarily has a 24-hour period or whether it has such a period merely because it is linked to a habitual sleep-wake cycle of 24 hour duration, Orth *et al.* [28] tried to alter sleep-wake schedule. They found that the period of the pituitary-adrenal cycle was not necessarily 24 hours in length, but was rather a function of the duration of habitual sleep-wake cycle of the subjects. If subjects abruptly reversed their habits in an Arctic summer, i.e. sleeping in darkened tents [31], it was eight days before corticoid excretion showed a near normal morning peak, and even then the peak was later than on a normal routine before reversal. When the subjects again reversed their habits and returned to a normal routine, adrenal excretion restored itself to normal only after another eight day delay. The other common form of phase shift occurs on flight into a different time-zone. A complete phase shift of nine hours in all external periodicities was achieved in a subject flying from Mineapolis to Korea [8]. His corticoid excretion took about a week to acquire the new phase. It is said that contact with other people living a normal diurnal-nocturnal existence is much more important as a "Zeit-geber" than are the habits of the subjects themselves. It was reported that the rhythm in plasma corticosteroids completely disappeared in a man who spent three months alone under ground, even though he followed a regular circadian cycle of activity, meals and sleep [22].

It is considered that adrenocortical hormones and ACTH may have some influence on the circadian rhythm of the pituitary-adrenal axis. We tried to demonstrate circadian variations of CRF activity in bilaterally adrenalectomized rats and hypophysectomized rats (Fig. 174). Adrenalectomized male rats were killed two weeks following the surgery. There were observed definite diurnal rhythms. The daily variation of CRF activity in the median eminence displayed maximum concentration at 3 p.m. with mean value of 26.7 $\pm$ 1.8 (S.E.) and minimum at 8 a.m. with 8.6 $\pm$ 0.6. There was a phase shift; the peak in intact rats which occurred around 6.30 p.m., was shifted to 3 p.m. in the adrenalectomized rats. The peak value was approximately three and a half times that seen at 8 a.m. The levels of maximal and minimal concentrations of CRF activity were slightly higher ($p < 0.05$) than those in the intact group. Next, male rats were hypophysectomized by the transauricular method and killed two weeks after the operation. In these animals CRF activity level in the median eminence was considerably elevated. The peak value was observed at 1 p.m. with mean value of 34.2 $\pm$ 2.9 (S.E.) and the minimal value was seen at 8 a.m. with mean value of 21.7 $\pm$ 2.5. The peak value was approximately one and a half times that seen at 8 a.m. The maximal and minimal values in these rats were significantly greater ($p < 0.01$) than those in intact rats. The circadian rhythm and phase shift in CRF activity were distinctly demonstrated in these animals. However, the amplitude in the circadian rhythm of CRF activity was less than that in intact rats. It is well known that CRF activity in the median eminence is suppressed by ACTH via a short feedback mechanism. We confirmed this phenomenon by using our assay method of CRF activity; the level of CRF activity in rats two weeks following hypophysectomy and adrenalectomy was suppressed by four day administrations of ACTH-zinc. It is considered that the production of CRF may be regulated by higher centers in the brain. The presence of a circadian rhythm of CRF activity in the absence of the adrenal gland or the pituitary gland suggests that the circadian variation of ACTH is controlled by higher centers. Support for this view comes from observations of subjects with brain damage. In patients with suprasellar tumours in which there was displacement of the hypothalamus, or in patients with central nervous system diseases affecting the pretectum and the temporal lobe, the circadian rhythm in plasma 17-OHCS was lost [17, 18]. Furthermore, Mason [21] suggested, on the basis of studies involving stimulation and artificial lesions of limbic structures in the monkey, that the hippocampus-fornix system appears to be involved in the maintenance of normal diurnal rhythm in ACTH secretion. Slusher [32] reported that bilateral anterior hypothalamic lesions which bilaterally destroyed the periventricular zone and arcuate nuclei were associated with inhibition of the normal 5 p.m. rise in plasma corticosterone in male rats and she suggested that the integrity of anterior hypothalamic areas appeared essential for normal diurnal rise in plasma corticoid levels. Nauta [23] demonstrated in rodents that a massive projection from the fornix bundle was distributed to the medial and periventricular regions of the anterior and infundibular levels of anterior hypothalamus. Therefore, it is possible that the anterior hypothalamus may be related to factors modulating the diurnal variation in corticoid level. In mice a circadian rhythm of corticosterone persisted after suprathalamic brain ablations, but more extensive brain ablations, including the removal of the thalamus and the hypothalamus interfered with the demonstration of a circadian rhythm in pituitary ACTH content [9]. These observations suggested that the important site of circadian rhythm in ACTH secretion existed between the suprathalamic and the suprapontine regions.

CIRCADIAN RHYTHM IN THE PITUITARY-ADRENAL
RESPONSE FOLLOWING VARIOUS STIMULI

It is well known that there is circadian rhythm in the pituitary-adrenal response to various

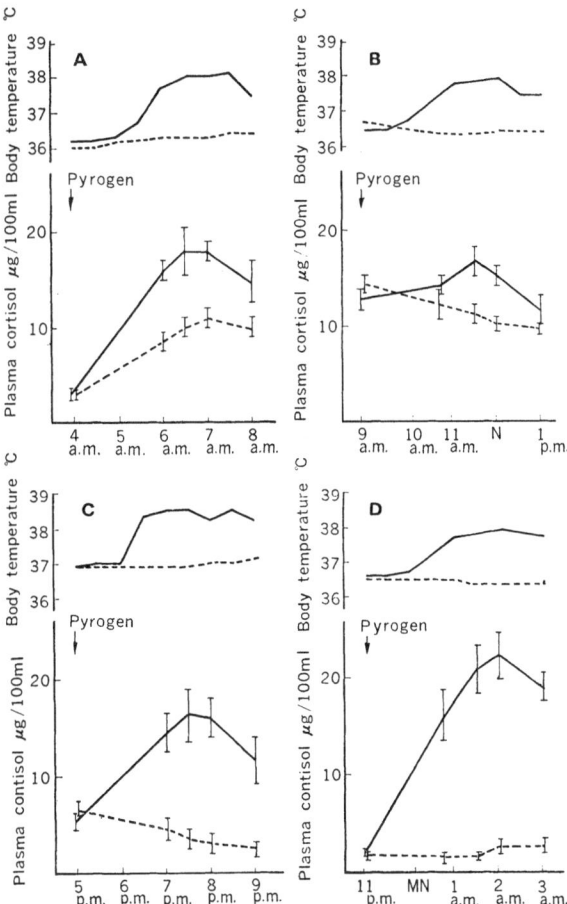

Fig. 175. Effect of pyrogen on plasma cortisol level and body temperature in the subjects who were injected at 4 a.m. (A), 9 a.m. (B), 5 p.m. (C), and 11 p.m. (D). Solid line indicates plasma cortisol and body temperature on the pyrogen injected day. Dotted line indicates plasma cortisol and boxy temperature on the saline injected day. Horizontal bar indicates standard error.

stimuli.   Clayton *et al.* [5] indirectly showed a circadian rhythm of ACTH secretion in man by the determination of plasma 17-OHCS, using a synthetic analog of vasopressin.

1.   Circadian Rhythm in the Pituitary-adrenal Response to Pyrogen

We found a circadian rhythm in the pituitary-adrenal response to pyrogen [35, 36]. Bacterial pyrogen (Organon Laboratories) was given intravenously to normal subjects after diluting it in 5 ml of normal saline.   An equivalent volume of saline was intravenously administered as a control in the same subjects on another day.   Fig. 175 shows the effect of pyrogen on plasma cortisol level and body temperature in the subjects who received the drug at 4 a.m., 9 a.m., 5 p.m. and 11 p.m.   All mean peak values of plasma cortisol in response to pyrogen showed approximately the same levels.   The maximal increase of plasma cortisol from the value before pyrogen was 15.7 $\pm$ 1.3 μg/100 ml at 4 a.m., 4.5 $\pm$ 1.4 at 9 a.m., 12.4 $\pm$ 1.7 at 5 p.m. and 21.8 $\pm$ 2.8 at 11 p.m.   Thus, pyrogen administered at 11 p.m. provoked the greatest response of plasma cortisol and the injection at 9 a.m. the least.   Fig. 176 shows the relationship between the plasma cortisol level before pyrogen and the maximal increase of plasma cortisol after pyrogen. There was a highly significant negative correlation (r = -0.81.   p<0.01) between these values.   Plasma ACTH response following the administration of pyrogen at 11 p.m. was greater than that at 9 a.m.   Meanwhile, there was no significant correlation between the maximal increase of plasma cortisol and body temperature from the value before pyrogen (Fig. 177).   The febrile response to pyrogen at night was similar to that in the morning, but the plasma cortisol response to pyrogen at night was greater than in the morning.

2.   Circadian Rhythm in the Pituitary-adrenal Response to Insulin

We also reported a diurnal variation in the piuitary-adrenal response to insulin [34]. It has been established that insulin provokes the release of cortisol, probably by way of hypoglycemia.   It is said that the adrenocortical response to insulin is related to both

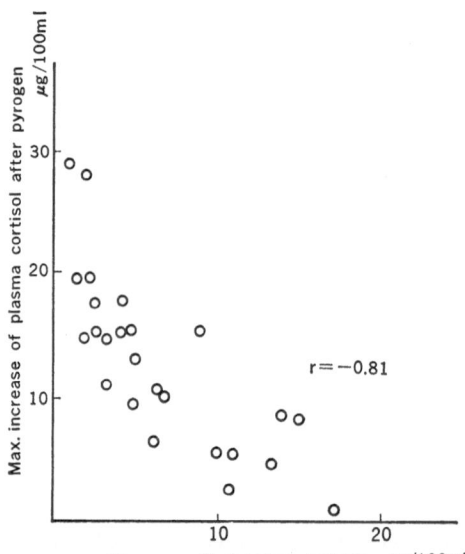

Fig. 176.   Relationship between the plasma cortisol level before pyrogen and the maximal increase of plasma cortisol after pyrogen.

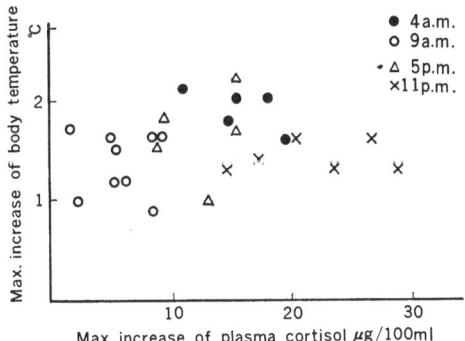

Fig. 177. Relationship between the maximal increase of plasma cortisol and body temperature after pyrogen from the value observed before pyrogen in subjects who received it at 4 a.m., 9 a.m., 5 p.m., and 11 p.m.

the duration and the degree of the induced hypoglycemia, and is usually absent if the blood sugar fails to fall below about 40 mg/100 ml. Six healthy male college students served as test subjects in this study. All were hospitalized in our clinic. They received a single intravenous injection of insulin 0.1 U/kg body weight at 10 a.m. and midnight after a 12 hour-fast. An equivalent volume of saline was administered intravenously as a control on another day. The mean resting levels of blood sugar at 10 a.m. and at midnight were 77.0 ± 1.1 and 75.0 ± 1.9 mg/100 ml, respectively. Blood sugar levels fell maximally 30 minutes after insulin in both cases. The mean minimal value of blood sugar induced by insulin was slightly lower (p<0.05) in the morning than at midnight (18.0 ± 1.3 (S.E.) vs. 22.0 ± 0.8 mg/100 ml) (Fig. 178). When insulin was given at 10 a.m., plasma free fatty acids (FFA) decreased from a mean fasting level of 447.3 ± 32.8 μEq/l to a mean minimal value of 321.3 ± 21.7 μEq/l 30 minutes after the injection. When injected at midnight, plasma FFA fell from 432.5 ± 39.5 to 292.1 ± 41.9 μEq/l 30 minutes after the administration. The mean maximal decrement after the injection at midnight was somewhat greater than that at 10 a.m., though the differ-

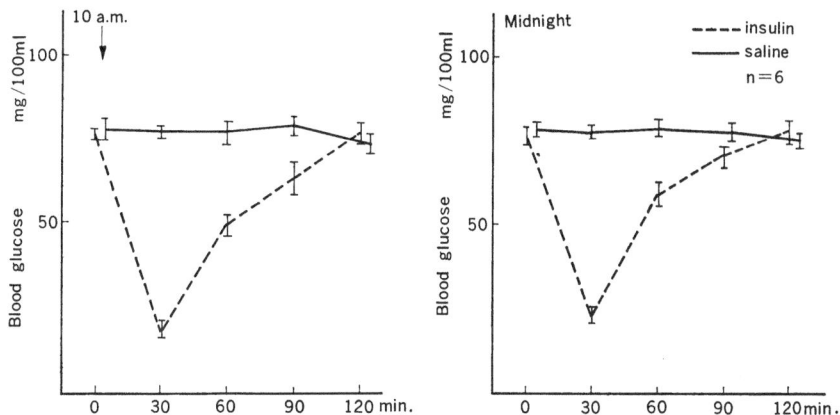

Fig. 178. Effect of insulin on blood glucose following the drug administrations at 10 a.m. and midnight. Dushed line indicates blood glucose on the insulin injected day. Solid line indicates blood glucose on the saline injected day. Horizontal bar indicates standard error.

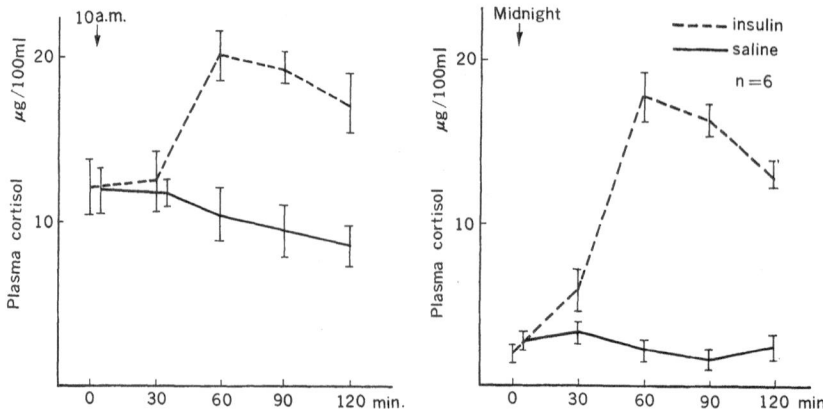

Fig. 179. Effect of insulin on plasma cortisol following the drug administrations at 10 a.m. and midnight. Dashed line indicates plasma cortisol on the insulin injected day. Solid line indicates plasma cortisol on the saline injected day. Horizontal bar indicates standard error.

ence was not significant. Meanwhile, insulin provoked a definite increase in plasma cortisol (Fig. 179). Following the injection of insulin at 10 a.m. or midnight, the plasma cortisol level rose from mean basal values of 11.9 ± 1.8 or 2.0 ± 0.5 µg/100 ml to mean maximal values of 20.1 ± 1.4 or 17.5 ± 1.7 µg/100 ml 60 minutes after the administration. The maximal response of plasma cortisol to insulin from the value before the injection was significantly greater ($p < 0.01$) at midnight than at 10 a.m. (15.9 ± 0.6 vs. 8.4 ± 0.8 µg/100 ml). The pattern of circadian rhythm in response to insulin was in keeping with those patterns of vasopressin and pyrogen. It is established that there is a circadian rhythm in the increment of plasma cortisol in response to various stimuli. This is probably dependent upon the variation in ACTH secretion by the pituitary. This is because the rate of removal of cortisol from plasma was shown to be the same at various times of the day and plasma cortisol binding capacity did not show any diurnal variation. This conclusion is also supported by the fact that the adrenal response to ACTH at night was less than in the morning. The latter finding suggests that in the present experiments a greater amount of ACTH must have been released from the pituitary at night than in the morning in order to achieve this plasma cortisol response at night. This assumption is supported by estimating plasma ACTH levels after pyrogen injection. In the interpretation of the difference in ACTH responses to various stimuli at least two possible explanations should be considered; first, the sensitivity of CRF or ACTH release to stimuli vary at different times, and second, significantly high levels of cortisol in the plasma may have an inhibitory effect on the ACTH releasing effect of the administered stimuli. In this regard, Critchlow *et al.* [6] have demonstrated that the pituitary ACTH content in male rats was highest when plasma corticosterone levels were lowest.

3. Circadian Rhythm in the Response of CRF Activity to Stress

Recently, Hiroshige *et al.* [15] reported that the response of CRF activity in the median eminence to a stressful stimulus, i.e., laparotomy under ether anesthesia, was significantly greater in the morning when the plasma corticosterone level was lowest, than in the evening when the level was highest. We also found the same phenomenon (Fig. 180).

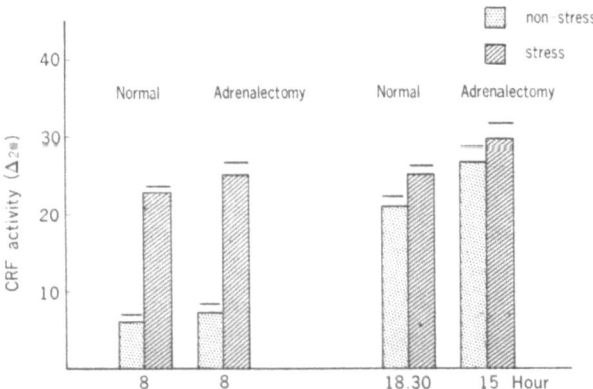

Fig. 180. Response of CRF activity in the hypothalamus in normal rats and adrenalectomized rats to stress. Each time shows the peak and the lowest in the circadian rhythm of CRF activity. Stippled columns represent CRF activity in basal stage. Hatched columns represent the response of CRF activity to stress. Each CRF activity is the mean of six to nine determinations, accompanied by its standard error.

These findings may suggest that the significantly higher level of plasma corticoids before stimulus have an inhibitory effect on the ACTH release following stimulus. Thus we examined how much the response of CRF activity in the median eminence to stimulus was influenced by the corticoids from the adrenal gland. We used laparotomy under ether anesthesia as stimulus. We found that there was a circadian rhythm in the response of CRF activity of male adrenalectomized rats to the stimulus; the response to the stress at 8 a.m., when the level of CRF activity was lowest, was significantly greater (p<0.01) than that at 3 p.m. when the level was highest. This phenomenon was similar to that in intact rats. The pre-existing plasma corticoids before stress were not related to the magnitude of the response of CRF activity to stress. It is likely that the circadian rhythm in the response of ACTH release to stress was only barely influenced by the circadian variation of plasma corticoids from the adrenal gland. This finding is supported by the following reports; Hodges *et al.* [16] demonstrated that the secretion of ACTH induced by stress was independent of changes in blood corticoids level within the physiological range. Furthermore, Slusher [32] reported that anterior hypothalamic lesions bilaterally destroying the periventricular zone and arcuate nuclei were associated with inhibition of the normal 5 p.m. rise in plasma corticoid levels and were also associated with normal rise in response to sound or to a one-minute electrical stimulation of the posterior diencephalon. On the other hand, in rats with posterior tuber cinereum lesions the normal 5 p.m. rise in plasma corticosterone was observed, but the response of plasma corticoid to sound was not observed. The integrity of anterior hypothalamic areas appears essential for normal diurnal rise in plasma corticosteroid levels, while more posterior areas are involved in mediation of the pituitary-adrenal response to acute sound stress. Thus, it is likely that the circadian rhythm in the response of ACTH release to stimulus is not related to the diurnal rhythm of plasma corticosteroid, but is related to other factors such as sensitivity in the brain to stress.

CIRCADIAN RHYTHM IN THE PITUITARY-ADRENAL RESPONSE
TO NEGATIVE FEEDBACK MECHANISM

Investigations of the hypothalamo-pituitary system have been greatly extended by the discovery of several different tests. Metyrapone (Su-4885) is used as an assessment of the integrity of the negative feedback control of ACTH secretion. Gold *et al.* [10] and Martin *et al.* [20] observed the adrenocortical response to ACTH and metyrapone given intravenously at different times in 24 hours. The rise in 17-OHCS excretion induced by metyrapone was greatest at the time of day when adrenocortical activity was maximal and least when adrenal secretory activity was minimal. We also studied the response to metyrapone given at different times in normal subjects and patients with Cushing's syndrome due to bilateral adrenal hyperplasia. Metyrapone in a dose of 2 g was given orally at 10 a.m. and 10 p.m. in six normal subjects. Urine samples for the estimation of 17-OHCS were collected in serial six-hour periods for two days before and after administration of the drug. The 9 a.m. plasma cortisol level of 11.7 $\pm$ 1.2 (S.E.) μg/100 ml before the 10 a.m. administration decreased to 1.1 $\pm$ 0.3 at 1 p.m. (in the control period plasma cortisol was 8.6 $\pm$ 0.2) and then gradually increased to 4.6 $\pm$ 1.0 at 9 p.m. (2.8 $\pm$ 0.6). On the other hand, the 9 p.m. plasma cortisol level of 2.8 $\pm$ 0.6 before the 10 p.m. administration decreased to 0.2 $\pm$ 0.1 at 1 a.m. (in the control period plasma cortisol was 2.2 $\pm$ 0.2) and then gradually increased to 10.6 $\pm$ 1.7 at 1 p.m. (8.6 $\pm$ 0.2). The pattern of difference between the plasma cortisol levels in the control period and after the drug administration at 10 a.m. was similar to that after the administration at 10 p.m. Fig. 181 shows excretions of urinary 17-OHCS before and after metyrapone at 10 a.m. and 10 p.m. The administrations at 10 a.m. and 10 p.m. were followed by a rise in 17-OHCS excretion from the first six-hour period which lasted for about 42 hours. The maximal rise in response to the 10 a.m. administration of the drug was observed early on the next morning (4 a.m.–10 a.m.), while that of the 10 p.m. administration occurred in the period 10 a.m.–4 p.m. in the next day. The

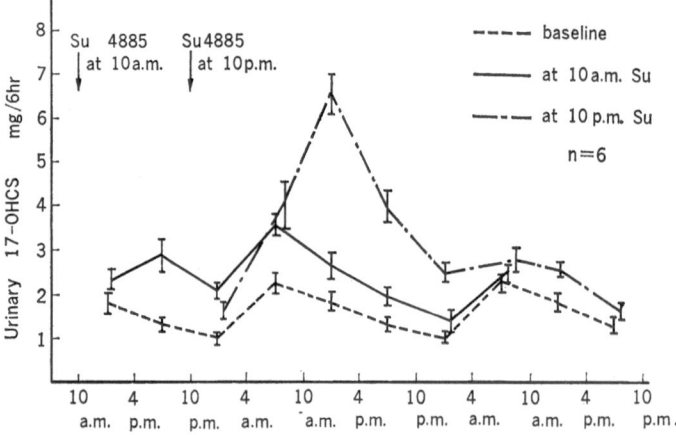

Fig. 181. Effect of methyrapone on urinary 17-OHCS following the drug administrations at 10 a.m. and 10 p.m. in normal subjects. Dash line indicates urinary 17-OHCS in basal stage. Solid line indicates urinary 17-OHCS after the administration of methrapone at 10 a.m. Chain line indicates urinary 17-OHCS after the administration of metyrapone at 10 p.m. Horizontal bar indicates standard error.

maximal increment and peak value of urinary 17-OHCS after the 10 p.m. administration was significantly greater (p<0.01) than after the 10 a.m. administration. The response to metyrapone showed a circadian variation. The rise in urinary 17-OHCS excretion induced by the drug was greater during the period before adrenocortical activity was maximal than during the period before adrenocortical activity was minimal. This finding suggests that the response to metyrapone may be related to the magnitude of adrenocortical activity during the effective concentration of the drug in the plasma. Thus, it is interesting to examine whether or not the response to metyrapone shows a circadian rhythm in patients with Cushing's syndrome due to bilateral adrenal hyperplasia who do not show a circadian rhythm in plasma cortisol or urinary 17-OHCS. Fig. 182 shows changes of plasma cortisol levels before and after the administrations at 10 a.m. and 10 p.m. in these patients. The administration at 10 a.m. and 10 p.m. provoked an immediate fall in plasma cortisol concentration at 1 p.m. and 1 a.m., respectively, followed by a gradual increase. The minimal level or the pattern of difference between the plasma cortisol in the control period and after the administration at 10 a.m. was similar to those at 10 p.m. On the other hand, the rise in urinary 17-OHCS

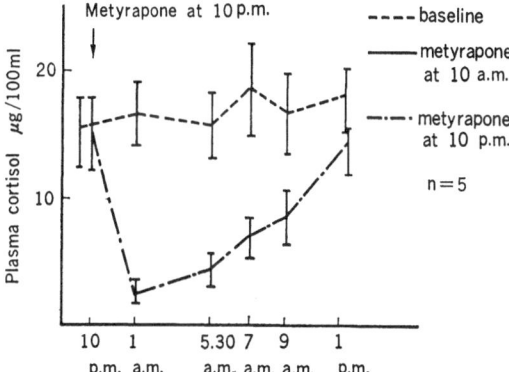

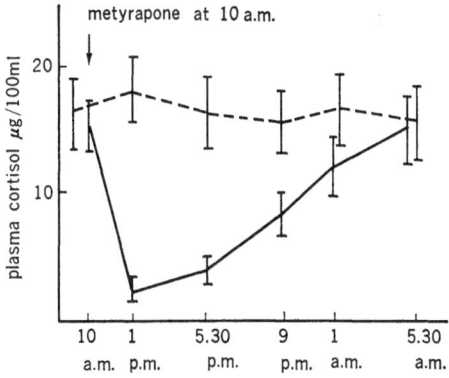

Fig. 182. Effect of metyrapone on plasma cortisol following the drug administrations at 10 a.m. and 10 p.m. in patients with Cushing's syndrome due to hyperplasia. Dash line indicates urinary 17-OHCS in basal stage. Solid line indicates urinary 17-OHCS after the administration of metyrapone at 10 a.m. Chain line indicates urinary 17-OHCS after the administration of metyrapone at 10 p.m. Horizontal bar indicates standard error.

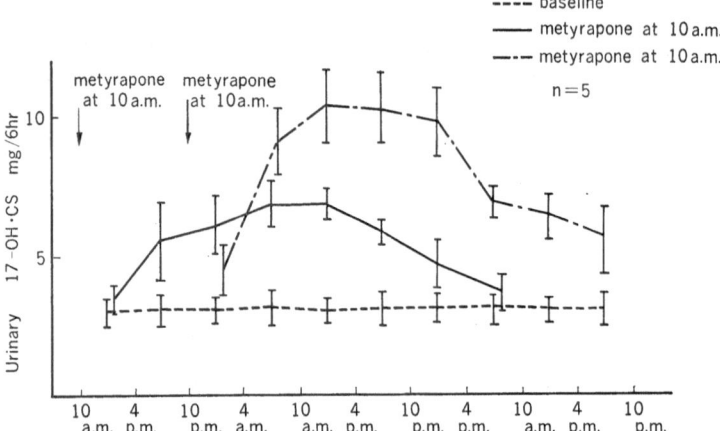

Fig. 183. Effect of metyrapone on urinary 17-OHCS following the drug administrations at 10 a.m. and 10 p.m. in patients with Cushing's syndrome due to hyperplasia. Dash line indicates urinary 17-OHCS in basal stage. Solid line indicates urinary 17-OHCS after the administration of metyrapone at 10 a.m. Chain line indicates urinary 17-OHCS after the administration of metyrapone at 10 p.m. Horizontal bar indicates standard error.

excretion after metyrapone at 10 p.m. was greater than that at 10 a.m. (Fig. 183). The circadian rhythm in response to the drug was also demonstrable in these patients. In the interpretation of the circadian rhythm in the pituitary-adrenal response to the administration of metyrapone, at least the following three possibilities should be considered; first, circadian rhythm in absorption from the intestines or disappearance from the plasma of metyrapone, second, circadian rhythm in the effect of it on selectively inhibiting 11-β-hydroxylation of the steroid nucleus, and third, difference in sensitivity of the negative feedback center to the fall of plasma cortisol level at different times of a day. The first and second possibilities could be eliminated, because the maximal decrease of plasma cortisol level and the pattern of difference between the plasma cortisol in the control period and after the drug administration were the same at different times when the drug was administered. As for the third possibility, the fall of plasma cortisol after the administration at the time of the circadian rise of cortisol in normal subjects provoked larger increments in ACTH release as compared with that at the time of circadian decrease of cortisol. On the other hand, ACTH secretion induced by the drug occurred independent of the plasma cortisol concentration in patients with Cushing's syndrome. Therefore, the circadian rhythm in response to metyrapone was not related to the circadian rhythm of plasma cortisol in the control period, but might be related to the different sensitivity of the negative feedback center. This interpretation is also supported by a report establishing the temporal variation in suppression of pituitary-adrenal function by glucocorticoids [25]. 0.5 mg of dexamethasone given at midnight was found to halt almost completely corticoids production for 24 hours but the same dose at 8 a.m. or 4 p.m. merely suppressed corticoids production temporarily.

CONCLUSION

We found a definite circadian rhythm in the CRF activity in rat hypothalamus; the peak was seen at 6.30 p.m. and the minimum at 8 a.m. The peaks of CRF activity in adrenalectomized and hypophysectomized rats were shifted to 3 p.m. and 1 p.m., respectively, and CRF activity in hypophysectomized rats was significantly greater than that in the intact rats. However, the circadian rhythms in these operated animals still existed. This finding suggests that the daily variation of ACTH release is controlled by higher centers, perhaps on or above the hypothalamus.

Furthermore, circadian rhythms were observed in the pituitary-adrenal response to pyrogen, insulin and metyrapone in man; the response was significantly greater at night when the plasma cortisol level was lowest than in the daytime when the level was higher. The same phenomenon was also observed in intact rats. These findings may suggest that the significantly higher level of plasma corticoids before stimulus has an inhibitory effect on the ACTH release following stimulus. However, there was still observed a circadian rhythm in the response of CRF activity to stimulus in male rats two weeks following adrenalectomy. Furthermore, a circadian rhythm in the response of ACTH release to metyrapone was also demonstrable in patients with Cushing's syndrome who did not show a circadian rhythm in plasma cortisol and urinary 17-OHCS. These findings suggest that the circadian rhythm in the response of ACTH release to these substances will be only barely influenced by the circadian variation of plasma corticoids.

REFERENCES

1. ADER, R. (1969): *Science* **163**: 1225.
2. ALLEN, C., and J.W. KENDALL (1967): *Endocrinology* **80**: 926.
3. BERSON, S.A., and R.S. YALOW (1968): *J. Clin. Invest.* **47**: 2725.
4. CHEIFETZ, P., N. GAFFUD, and J.F. DINGMAN (1968): *Endocrinology* **82**: 1117.
5. CLAYTON, G.W., L. LIBRIK, R.L. GARDNER, and R. GUILLEMIN (1963): *J. Clin. Endocr.* **23**: 975.
6. CRITCHLOW, V., R.A. LIEBELT, M. BAR-SELA, W. MOUNTCASTLE, and H.S. LIPSCOMB (1963): *Amer. J. Physiol.* **205**: 807.
7. DEMURA, H., C.D. WEST, C.A. NUGENT, K. NAKAGAWA, and F.H. TYLER (1966): *J. Clin. Endocr.* **26**: 1297.
8. FLINK, E.B., and R.P. DOE (1959): *Proc. Soc. Exp. Biol. & Med.* **100**: 498.
9. GALICICH, J.H., F. HALBERG, L.A. FRENCH, and F. UNGAR (1965): *Endocrinology* **76**: 895.
10. GOLD, E.M., V.C. DiRAIMONDO, and P.H. FORSHAM (1960): *Metabolism* **9**: 3.
11. HELLMAN, L., F. NAKADA, J. CURTI, E.D. WEITZMAN, J. KREAM, H. ROFFWARG, S. ELLMAN, D.K. FUKUSHIMA, and T.F. GALLAGHER (1970): *J. Clin. Endocr.* **30**: 411.
12. HIROSHIGE, T., H. KUNITA, K. YOSHIMURA, and S. ITOH (1968): *Jap. J. Physiol.* **18**: 179.
13. HIROSHIGE, T., M. SAKAKURA, and S. ITOH (1969): *Endocrinol. Japon.* **16**: 465.
14. HIROSHIGE, T., and T. SATO (1970): *Endocrinol. Japon.* **17**: 1.
15. HIROSHIGE, T., T. SATO, R. OHTA, and S. ITOH (1969): *Jap. J. Physiol.* **19**: 866.
16. HODGES, J.R., and M.T. JONES (1963): *J. Physiol.* **167**: 30.
17. HOKFELT, B., and R. LUFT (1959): *Acta endocr. (Kbh)* **32**: 177.
18. KRIEGER, D.T., and H.P. KRIEGER (1966): *J. Clin. Endocr.* **26**: 929.
19. LIDDLE, G.W., D. ISLAND, and C.K. MEADOR (1962): *Recent. Progr. Hormone Res.* **18**: 125.
20. MARTIN, M.M., and D.E. HELLMAN (1964): *J. Clin. Endocr.* **24**: 253.
21. MASON, J.W. (1958): In "Reticular Formation of the Brain" p. 645 H.H. JASPERS, ed. Little Brown Co., Boston/Toronto.
22. MILLS, J.N. (1964): *J. Physiol.* **174**: 217.
23. NAUTA, W.J.H. (1958): In "Reticular Formation of the Brain" p. 3 H.H. JASPERS, ed. Little Brown Co., Boston/Toronto.
24. NEY, R.L., N. SCHIMIZU, W.E. NICHOLSON, D.P. ISLAND, and G.W. LIDDLE (1963): *J. Clin. Invest.* **42**: 1669.
25. NICHOLS, T., C.A. NUGENT, and F.H. TYLER (1965): *J. Clin. Endocr.* **25**: 343.
26. OLIVI, O., and R. GENOVA (1962): *Folia Endocrinol. (Pisa)* **15**: 421.
27. ORTH, D.N., and D.P. ISLAND (1969): *J. Clin. Endocr.* **29**: 479.
28. ORTH, D.N., D.P. ISLAND, and G.W. LIDDLE (1967): *J. Clin. Endocr.* **27**: 549.
29. PERKOFF, G.I., K. EIK-NES, C.A. NUGENT, H.L. FRED, R.A. NIMER, L. RUSH, L.T. SAMUEL, and F.H. TYLER (1959): *J. Clin. Endocr.* **19**: 432.

30. Retiene, K., E. Zimmerman, W.J. Schindler, J. Neuenschwander, and H.S. Lipscomb (1968): *Acta endocr. (Kbh)* **57**: 615.
31. Sharp, G.W.G., S.A. Slorach, and H.J. Vipond (1961): *J. Endocrinol.* **22**: 377.
32. Slusher, M.A. (1964): *Am. J. Physiol.* **206**: 1161.
33. Takahashi, Y., D.M. Kipnis, and W.H. Daughaday (1968): *J. Clin. Invest.* **47**: 2079.
34. Takebe, K., H. Kunita, S. Sawano, Y. Horiuchi, and K. Mashimo (1969): *J. Clin. Endocr.* **29**: 1930.
35. Takebe, K., C. Setaishi, M. Hirama, M. Yamamoto, and Y. Horiuchi (1966): *J. Clin. Endocr.* **26**: 437.
36. Takebe, K., C. Setaishi, M. Yamamoto, and Y. Horiuchi (1968): *J. Clin. Endocr.* **28**: 924.
37. Ungar, F. (1964): *Ann. N. Y. Acad. Sci.* **117**: 374.

Chapter 23

SEASONAL AND CIRCADIAN VARIATIONS IN BODY FLUID

Hisato YOSHIMURA, and Taketoshi MORIMOTO

Department of Physiology, Kyoto Prefectural University of Medicine, Kyoto, Japan

In our previous monograph (1960), seasonal variations of water and electrolytes in body fluid were described and important possible physiological meanings were pointed out. The mechanism of these seasonal variations was also discussed and it was demonstrated that metabolism of water and electrolytes in body fluid is affected by changes in climate through stimulation of neuro-humoral context, e.g. thirst sensation, sweating, ADH secretion etc. Water and electrolyte content under hormonal control undergo some adaptation to changes in metabolism caused by climate.

There remain, however, some unsolved problem with respect to seasonal variations in body fluid. It is well known that the water and electrolyte contents of body fluid are maintained constant in accordance with the principle of homeostasis. Sargent and Weinman (1966) pointed out that there is a ranking or hierarchy of the precision of physiological regulation of physico-chemical properties of the internal environment, i.e. extracellular fluid. Among these, the osmolality and electrolyte concentrations in serum are included in the top ranks, because they are essential for the proper functioning of the organism presenting little intra- and inter-individual variation. On the other hand, these properties of blood are known to present seasonal variations. How are these changes due to climate to be explained in view of the principle of homeostasis? This is the first problem to be dealt with in this chapter.

Among types of biological variation, two kinds of rhythm, are classified, i.e., long-term and short-term. The long-term variation is apt to be influenced by environmental factors, and in some case can be explained in view of the ecosystem. The short-term variation is more physiological in origin. The seasonal variation in body fluid belongs to the former category, and the circadian variation may belong to the latter under standardized conditions. In an attempt to better understand the biological variation in body fluid, the circadian variations and seasonal variations in body fluid are both dealt with in this chapter, and environmental factors or living habits and habitats possibly influencing the biological variation will be discussed.

SEASONAL VARIATION OF WATER AND ELECTROLYTE IN SERUM WITH RESPECT TO HOMEOSTASIS

In an attempt to clarify the meaning of seasonal shift of electrolyte content in body fluid in view of homeostasis, Morimoto *et al.* (1969) performed a series of experiments using 10 college student volunteers. Blood samples were collected from the subjects who stayed in the laboratory on the night preceding the experiment. Two out of the ten subjects stayed in the laboratory for about one month, eating a standardized diet of 2400–2600 Cal (protein content 75 g) daily. Blood sampling and measurement was repeated in all 10 subjects at three day intervals. The control values of blood thus measured were not significantly different from the values of these subjects on a free diet. The ten subjects underwent a three day test, three days and nights in the laboratory. The control test was performed on the first day, water loading test on the second day and sweating test on the third day. On each day, blood sample were collected five times from 8:00 a.m. until 12:30 at interval of 60–90 minutes. The subject did not eat or drink until the last sampling was over. On the day of the water loading test, the subjects drank water (20 ml per Kg of body weight) just after the first blood sampling, and hemodilution was initiated. On the third day, sweating was induced by having the subject stay for exactly one hour in a climatic chamber 30 °C DBT and 20 °C of WBT, where his feet were dipped in 45 °C hot water. The water lost through sweating was about 10–20 ml/Kg·hr. The sweating test was performed between the first and the second blood samplings, and hemoconcentration was then initiated. On three out of ten subjects, the ADH level of plasma was determined by the bioassay method of Share and Yoshida (1963). All the experiments were repeated in winter (February and March) and in summer (August and September). In winter, however, an additional experiment was performed with two of the aforementioned subjects, who stayed for three weeks in the 30 °C climatic chamber after the three days' test was over.

The principal results obtained with the serum collected under basal conditions are summarized in Table 48. The results in the table almost exactly coincide with previous

TABLE 48   Comparison of results between summer and winter

	Winter	Summer	P**
Osmolality (mOsm/Kg H_2O)	287.2 ± 3.6*	282.9 ± 4.5	<0.001
Sodium (mEq/l)	139.6 ± 4.5	129.8 ± 3.1	<0.001
Chloride (mEq/l)	104.7 ± 3.5	103.6 ± 2.3	n.s.
Potassium (mEq/l)	4.0 ± 0.1	3.9 ± 0.2	<0.05
Hematocrit (%)	44.2 ± 2.4	43.7 ± 3.3	n.s.
A D H (μU/ml)	5.8 ± 0.8	12.6 ± 1.6	<0.001
Blood volume (ml/Kg)	85.5 ± 7.4	86.2 ± 9.1	n.s.
Na/K ratio	34.8 ± 2.9	33.8 ± 2.1	n.s.

*Means and standard deviations of 30 measurements except for ADH which are calculated on nine measurements.
**Percent level of statistical significance of the differences between winter and summer. Blood volume means the circulating blood volume which was measured by RISA method (Shiraki et al., 1968).

results (Yoshimura, 1958) and confirm that osmolality, sodium, potassium and ADH concentrations show highly significant seasonal changes, while plasma chloride concentration and the Na/K ratio do not change significantly. Previous reports concerning climatic effect on serum potassium level show conflicting results. Our previous report (1958) and Harashima (1953) demonstrated a depression in plasma potassium caused by hot climate. On the other hand, Henrotte (1967) reported that the plasma potassium level of Indian and European students in a tropical climate is higher than that found in cold climates in Europe. The reason for this discrepancy is unknown. Probably the plasma potassium level is influenced by many factors other than climate. In our previous paper (1958), seasonal variation of the Na/K ratio in plasma was explained by seasonal variation of aldosterone excretion. As the present data of Na/K ratio does not coincide with the previous results, it follows that this ratio may be a function of many factors, not simply an indication of aldosterone as was thought previously.

Though the tendency of the present data is definitely indicative of hemodilution in summer, i.e. a decreased hematocrit and increased circulating blood volume, the seasonal change is not statistically significant. Even those characteristics of the serum that did not show statistically significant differences, however, showed seasonal change when the data was examined for each individual. Nevertheless, the degree of seasonal change is less in this experiment than was previously reported by one of the present authors about 10 years ago (Yoshimura, 1958). Among the factors contributing to this decrease in seasonal variations, improved and more widespread air conditioning and heating in Japanese houses and an overall improvement in nutritional standards may be mentioned. It follows that seasonal changes in blood properties will be affected by changes in habitat.

A part of the results of the three days' test is presented in Fig. 184 where the time courses of osmolality are summarized in group means and standard deviations (vertical lines).

The upper curves represent the control test in winter and summer. The middle curves are those of the water loading test. The arrow indicates the time of water intake. The lowest curves show the results of the sweating test. Horizontal shaded band represent the time of sweating. Winter and summer are characterized by the fixed levels of

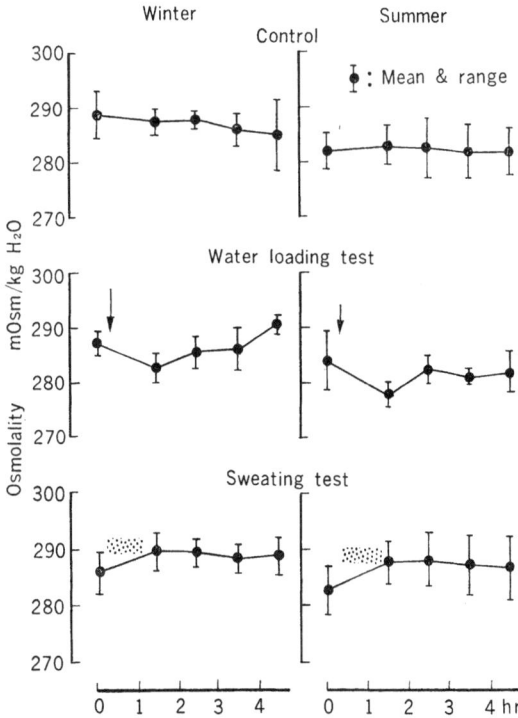

Fig. 184. Time course of osmolality change after water loading test and sweating test together with control test. Each circle and bar represents a mean of ten subjects and the standard deviation.

osmolality in which the regulatory processes are directed. The hemoconcentration resulting from sweating and the hemodilution resulting from water loading occur relative to the fixed level, and the changes in osmolality tend to recover gradually. Although the recovery from the hemoconcentration after sweating took longer in summer than in winter, the magnitude of the responses is otherwise not significantly different. Thus, it is clearly demonstrated that the set point of homeostasis of osmolality shifts to a lower level in summer than in winter. The most remarkable seasonal changes and responses to stress were observed in the plasma ADH level. In Fig. 185, means and ranges of plasma ADH level from three subjects are presented. The ADH level decreased after the water loading test and increased after the sweating test, but the initial levels were regained within four hours. Furthermore, plasma ADH level was significantly higher in summer than in winter and changes induced by water loading and by sweating were observed in both summer and winter levels, respectively.

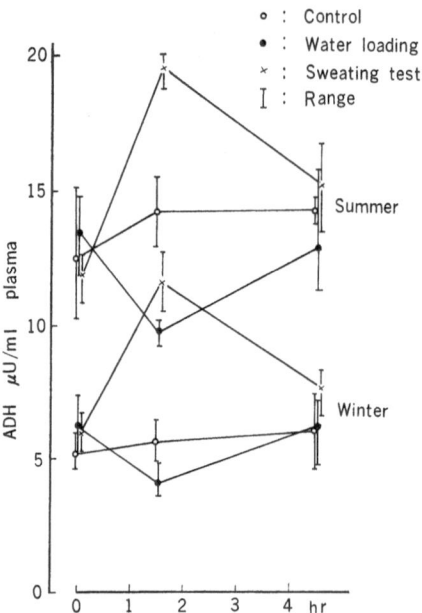

Fig. 185. ADH level of plasma in summer and winter and its responses to water loading or sweating. Each point and bar represents mean of three subjects and variation range.

In Fig. 186, the ADH level in plasma is plotted against serum sodium concentration determined from the same blood sample. Open circles represent control data obtained under basal conditions and closed circles that obtained after the sweating test or water loading test. Both the serum sodium concentration and plasma ADH level show remarkable seasonal variation, so two distinct clusters of points may be seen here. The three closed circles at the top of each group are results obtained after sweating tests, while the three closed circles at the bottom of each group are the results after water loading tests. From the point of mean value for the control data under basal conditions, two vectors can be drawn: one to the mean of the upper three points in each respective clusters of plots, and the other to the mean of the lower three points. With these two

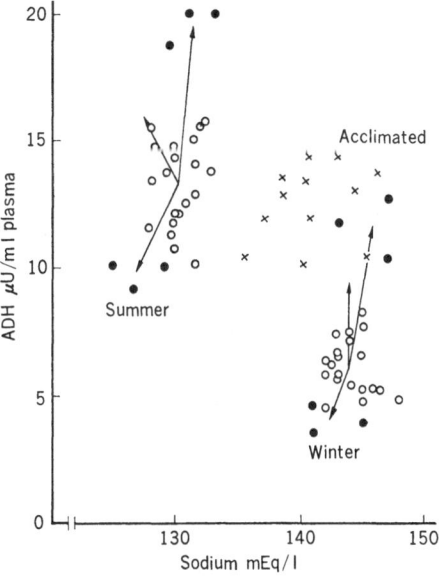

Fig. 186. Shift of internal environment with respect to ADH and sodium. Open circles are results obtained under basal conditions and closed circles are those obtained after sweating test (three closed circles at the top of each group) and after water loading test (three closed circles at the bottom of each group).

vectors as components, a resultant vector can be drawn. This was done with the data clusters for both seasons. The cross points in the central part of the figure represent the results obtained from the two subjects undergoing acclimation to heat in the winter experiment. Six measurements were made in both the second and the third weeks of acclimation on respective subjects. The ADH levels in this acclimated state are the same as the summer levels, while the sodium levels lie between those of summer and winter. Interestingly, it is noted that the third vector drawn for the winter data points in the direction of acclimation. It is suggested that the set point of homeostasis may be moved along this vector.

From the above results, it is presumed that the seasonal changes in serum electrolytes are caused by repeated heat exposure, leading to sweating and thirst, and therefore to repeated drinking of water. The change of water and salt metabolism induced by these repeated heat exposures may initiate the shift in the set point of water and salt balance.

Koshitani (1957) performed a similar acclimation on four subjects in winter. The subjects stayed in the laboratory for three to five weeks. In the first week, the control measurements of water metabolism and water and electrolytes in body fluid were made, and then the subjects entered a climatic chamber of DBT 30 °C and WBT 26 °C. Two of the subjects stayed there for two weeks, the remaining two subjects for four weeks. Sweating test were made by the aforementioned method after the second and the third week. The results obtained are summarized in Table 49. The total perspiration indicated in the table means the sum of insensible water loss and sweat water loss. Water intake and water loss were calculated from daily measurements of food and water intake, weight of feces and body weight. Total body fluid was measured by the antipyrine method, and the extracellular fluid by measuring thiocyanate space. The blood volume was measured by the congored method in this experiment. The data from control and

TABLE 49   Changes in water metabolism and body fluid during heat acclimation

	Control	Acclimation in hot chamber. (D.T. 30°C ± 2.0, W.T. 26°C ± 4.0)			
	Period (one week)	1st week	2nd week	3rd week	4th week
Total water intake (g/day)	2680	3046* (+13.5%)	3251* (+21.1%)	3557 (+28.3%)	3755 (+35.4%)
Total perspiration (g/day)	1179	1975** (+68.0%)	2074* (+76.2%)	2631 (+115.7%)	2539 (+111.9%)
Total water loss in urine and feces (g/day)	1752	1166** (−31.0%)	1257* (28.4%)	1059 (39.1%)	1281 (−26.3%)
Total circulating serum volume (ml/kg)	44.0	48.5* (+11.3%)	46.9* (+8.2%)	49.8 (+8.3%)	49.9 (+8.2%)
Extra cellular fluid volume (ml/kg)	217.8	229.2 (+5.2%)	228.8* (+5.1%)	245.3 (+6.3%)	247.6 (+7.3%)
Total body water content (ml/kg)	582.1	526.9 (−3.4%)	579.2 (−0.6%)	639.9 (+3.5%)	643.1 (+4.0%)
Serum Na concentration (mM/l)	143.1	138.7 (−3.0%)	140.3* (−1.9%)	137.6 (−3.8%)	137.5 (−3.9%)
Serum Cl concentration	107.6	106.1 (−1.4%)	106.0* (−1.5%)	106.9 (−1.9%)	105.8 (−2.9%)
Serum K concentration (mM/l)	4.69	4.38 (−6.7%)	4.22** (−10.3%)	4.05 (−13.6%)	4.19 (−10.6%)

*Change is statistically significant at 5% level as compared with the control.
**Significant at 1% level.
The values in the 3rd and 4th weeks are not subjected to the statistical examination (see the text). % value in the parentheses indicates percentage change from the control value (+increase, −decrease).

from first and second week of acclimation in the table are the mean values of four subjects. The difference between the values obtained after acclimation and the control values were statistically examined. The results in the third and fourth week of acclimation, however, were not statistically examined because the subjects numbered only two. The percentage change of data in each week of acclimation was calculated with each respective subject by taking the value obtained in the control period as the standard. The percentage change thus calculated was averaged and the mean value is presented in parentheses. It is demonstrated in the table that the water intake increased gradually in a hot room, rising to +35% in the fourth week. The water loss through perspiration increased while the urinary water loss decreased. As these measurements of water intake and water loss are not very exact due to a technical error, the water balance was not calculated, though relative tendency of water metabolism in acclimation to heat may be seen in the table. The extracellular fluid volume increased in the first week of acclimation, while the total body water content decreased. This fact indicates that the extracellular fluid increased at the expense of the intracellular fluid level. In the advanced stage of acclimation to heat, i.e. in the third and fourth week, however, both the extracellular fluid and the total body fluid increased. This increase in body water is believed to be caused by a positive water balance. Koshitani (1957) verified that the ADS level of plasma determined by Birnie's method showed an increase in heat acclimation, and he explained the retention of water in the body by the increase of plasma ADH level.

Decrease of serum electrolyte concentrations in acclimation which is shown in the table can also be explained by this increased water retention in body fluid. Thus, the above presumption as to the mechanism of seasonal changes in serum electrolytes was experimentally verified. As was pointed out in the previous monograph (1960), seasonal change in water and electrolytes in body fluid in summer is a feature of the attempt by an organism to prepare for possible dehydration and salt loss in the heat. Thus seasonal changes in serum electrolytes and water are an outcome of the adaptation to change in climate. In other words, the seasonal change of set point for homeostasis is a result of repeated changes in internal environment induced by change of climate, i.e. external environment. It follows that the homeostasis does not fix the internal environment at a constant set point but maintains it at the condition most effective against external stress.

CIRCADIAN VARIATION OF BODY FLUID

Although circadian variations have been studied in various fields, studies concerning the circadian variations in body fluid are few (Mills, 1966). Tamura (1957) studied the circadian variation of blood water content, which shows low value in the morning and keeps almost a constant value in the daytime, while it increases in the evening, especially during sleep at night. The increase in blood water content during sleep was analyzed and it was found that it was due to the increased water content of the plasma and the decrease of hematocrit, but the mechanisms which cause the increase in the water content in blood and the diurnal change of the blood volume or the plasma volume have not been dealt with. Cranston and Brown (1963) measured circulating blood volume at 09:00 and 16:00 and found an insignificant increase of 2.5% from 09:00 to 16:00 in normal subjects while hypertensive patients showed a significant increase of 8.5% from morning to eveing. Parry and Dollery (1968) also found 8.4% increase of plasma volume from 09:00 to 16:00 in hypertensive patients. A similar study on healthy young adults was reported by Finlayson et al. (1964). They measured blood volume and hematocrit three times i.e. in the morning just after arising, at midday approximately 20 minutes after lunch, and at bedtime at least three hours after supper. According to our calculations of their results, the blood volumes and hematocrits of the 12 subjects expressed as the percentages of the daily means are $97.6 \pm 4.6\%$ and $101.6 \pm 2.4\%$ in the morning, $99.2 \pm 2.4\%$ and $99.9 \pm 1.9\%$ at noon and $103.2 \pm 3.9\%$ and $98.4 \pm 2.2\%$ at bedtime. Their results indicate that blood volume is significantly ($P<0.01$) higher at bedtime than in the morning or at midday, while hematocrit decreases progressively from morning to bedtime.

Because none of these three reports deals with midnight levels, one of the authors and his colleague (Morimoto and Shiraki, 1970) measured the blood volume and the hematocrit of 8 healthy male subjects at 12:00 and 24:00. Diet and fluid intake were unrestricted and daily activities were as usual for this group except for a 30 minute bed rest period before measurement. As a result, the circulating blood volume was almost identical between 12:00 and 24:00, the difference being 0.5% and not significant. The hematocrit decreased by 3.6% ($P<0.001$) and the body weight increased by 0.9% ($P<0.005$) from 12:00 to 24:00. The circulating erythrocyte volume and circulating plasma volume were calculated from the circulating blood volume and hematocrit.

The circulating erythrocyte volume decreased 3.2% (P<0.05) and the circulating plasma volume increased 1.6% (not significant) from 12:00 to 24:00.

From these reports, it may be concluded that the circulating blood volume is lowest in the morning and increases gradually up to a peak value in late evening and again diminishes to the low morning value. The circadian variation of hematocrit shows a somewhat different pattern: the hematocrit shows high value on waking and the level stays rather constant during the daytime. The value starts to decrease in the evening to a minimum value at midnight, and gradually increases to the high value in the morning. Together with this rhythm of hematocrit, water content in blood or serum shows highest value in midnight.

The mechanism underlying the circadian variation of body fluid is very complex because the homeostasis of body fluid is controlled by a number of interlinked systems. To study circadian variation in body fluid, the inflow and outflow of water, electrolytes and plasma protein together with changes in circulation should be taken into consideration.

From this point of view, Morimoto and Shiraki (1970) studied circadian variation of body fluid under strictly controlled conditions.

Ten healthy male subjects were confined to bed for a 24-hour period. Water and food intake was evenly distributed throughout the 24 hours by giving 200 ml of milk every three hours, freshly prepared from 18 gm of skimmed milk, 6 gm of sugar, 1.3 gm of NaCl and adding water to 200 ml. The room temperature was maintained at 22 ± 1 °C, with constant artificial illumination throughout the experiment. Under these experimental conditions, the circulating blood volume was measured at 12:00, 18:00, 24:00 and 06:00 with the RISA-^{131}I method. The hematocrit and concentrations of plasma protein and serum sodium and potassium were determined with one and the same sample. The body weight, urinary volume and sodium and potassium concentrations were measured every three hours for 24 hours.

In Fig. 187, the circadian pattern of the circulating blood volume is shown together with that of the hematocrit and circulating erythrocyte volume and circulating plasma volume calculated from the circulating blood volume and the hematocrit. To analyze the circadian pattern excluding individual variation as much as possible, the percentage changes derived from the mean of the four measurements in the 24-hour period were calculated for each subject. The means and standard deviations for the 10 subjects are shown in the figure. The circulating blood volume is rather steady during the day (12:00 and 18:00) but shows a significant decrease at night (P<0.001) of 6.1% (12:00 vs. 24:00) or of 5.8% (18:00 vs. 24:00), and increase in the morning (06:00).

The hematocrit showed no significant change throughout the 24-hour period. The circulating erythrocyte volume and circulating plasma volume both showed a circadian pattern similar to that of the circulating blood volume which decreases towards midnight, but the differences between values in the day and those at midnight were bigger for the erythrocyte volume and smaller for the plasma volume: the difference between the circulating erythrocyte volume at 12:00 and 24:00 was 6.0% (P<0.005) and between that at 18:00 and 24:00 was 6.8% (P<0.001), while the circulating plasma volume decreased by 5.9% (P<0.001) from 12:00 to 24:00 and by 5.0% (P<0.005) from 18:00 to 24:00.

Under these experimental conditions, the circadian variation of circulating blood was somewhat different from the variation seen during the normal activity of every day

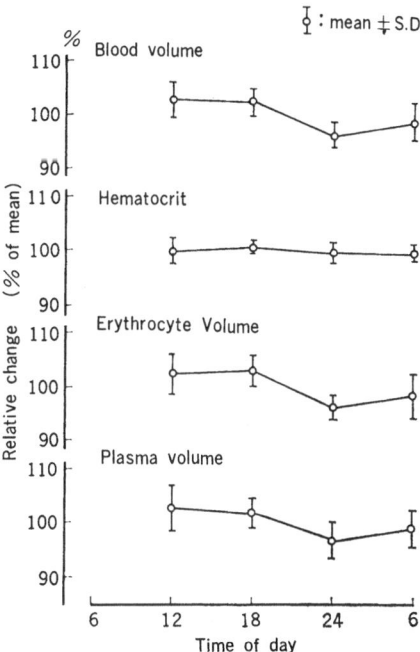

Fig. 187. Changes in blood volume, hematocrit, erythrocyte volume, and plasma volume of 8 subjects during 24 hours. Values are means ($\pm$S.D., n = 10) as percentages of the mean for the whole period.

life. The maximum circulating blood volume observed in the evening with normal activity is absent in these experimental conditions, and the blood volume is rather stable during the daytime with a trough at 24:00. Hematocrit, which shows a remarkable decrease at midnight under normal conditions showed a constant value throughout the day in this experiment. Because circulating blood volume decreases at 24:00 without any change in hematocrit, circulating erythrocyte volume and circulating plasma volume decrease at 24:00, though less in degree in the latter. These results may indicate the presence of two factors underlying the circadian variation in the circulating blood volume. One is the circadian variation of circulating erythrocyte volume, which is high during the day and minimal at night. The other is the circadian change in the water content of the blood with a higher value at night.

To investigate the circadian variation in erythrocyte volume in more detail, and to determine the amount of erythrocytes stored in the blood reservoir, the total blood volume and circulating blood volume were determined simultaneously using ^{51}Cr, and RISA ^{125}I on two subjects, under similar experimental conditions.

In Table 50, the total blood volume determined with ^{51}Cr, the circulating plasma volume determined with RISA ^{125}I, together with the circulating erythrocyte volume, total erythrocyte volume and erythrocytes in depots obtained from calculations are shown.

For these calculations, two assumptions were made: first that the blood volume determined with ^{51}Cr labelled erythrocytes injected 16 hours before the first measurement is the total blood volume including that in the blood reservoir, and second, that the plasma volume determined with RISA ^{125}I injected 10 minutes before blood sampling is the total

TABLE 50   Circadian variations in erythrocytes in depots

Time of day (hr.)	12	18	24	6
Circulating blood volume (ml/Kg)	77.0	75.2	70.5	73.8
Circulating plasma volume (ml/Kg)	47.6	45.6	42.2	44.0
Circulating erythrocyte volume (ml/Kg)	29.4	29.6	28.3	29.8
Total erythrocyte volume (ml/Kg)		36.3		
Erythrocytes in depots (ml/Kg)	6.9	6.7	8.0	6.5

Note: The results are means of two subjects.

circulating plasma volume.   The first assumption may be justified by the facts that the total blood volume measured with ^{51}Cr labelled erythrocyte remains constant for at least five days (Gray and Sterling, 1950) and that ^{51}Cr labelled erythrocyte can be mixed with more than 95% of the blood in the spleen within 30 minutes (Kraintz et al., 1958). On these assumptions, the circulating blood volume (CBV) was calculated from the circulating plasma volume (CPV) and hematocrit (Ht) as follows: CBV = CPV/ (1 — Ht).   The circulating erythrocyte volume (CEV) was calculated from the circulating blood volume and the circulating plasma volume (CEV = CBV — CPV). The total erythrocyte volume (TEV) was calculated by subtracting the circulating plasma volume from the total blood volume (TBV) (TEV = TBV — CPV), and the volume of erythrocytes in depots (EID) was obtained as the difference between the total erythrocyte volume and the circulating erythrocyte volume (EID = TEV — CEV).   The mean of four measurements within a day of the total erythrocyte volume was used for the calculation because the total erythrocyte volume did not show any consistent circadian variation and also because theoretically it should be constant throughout a day.   These calculations show that the volume of erythrocytes in depots is largest at 24:00.

This finding explains a decrease in the hematocrit during the night observed during normal everyday life.   However, under the strictly controlled conditions of this experiment, the hematocrit remained constant throughout the 24 hours, and as shown in Table 50, erythrocytes retained in the erythrocyte depots were highest at 24:00.   Accordingly, the constancy of the hematocrit may be explained by presuming that erythrocytes and water are excluded from the circulation at the same rate as the hematocrit.   On the other hand, during the routine of everyday life, the circulating plasma volume remained constant or increased slightly at night, causing a significant decrease of the hematocrit at night.

Fig. 188 shows the circadian patterns of change in serum sodium and serum potassium concentrations, plasma protein, and water content in plasma.   The difference between the sodium concentrations at 12:00 and 24:00 was not significant, while the decrease from 18:00 to 24:00 of 1.1% was barely significant (P<0.02).   Potassium decreased by 5.72% (P<0.01) from 12:00 to 24:00 and by 3.58% (P<0.02) from 18:00 to 24:00.   Plasma protein measured in six of the 10 subjects decreased by 4.7% and water content in plasma increased by 0.45% from 18:00 to 24:00 (P<0.025, respectively).   These results indicate that the circulating plasma volume decreases at 24:00, and that it is also diluted around midnight.

Under these controlled experimental conditions, water and salt intake was evenly distributed throughout the 24 hours.   Accordingly, water and salt balance can be analyzed from urinary output.   In Fig. 189, the circadian variation of urine volume, sodium output and GFR are shown.   The results are mean values taken from 4 subjects on whom

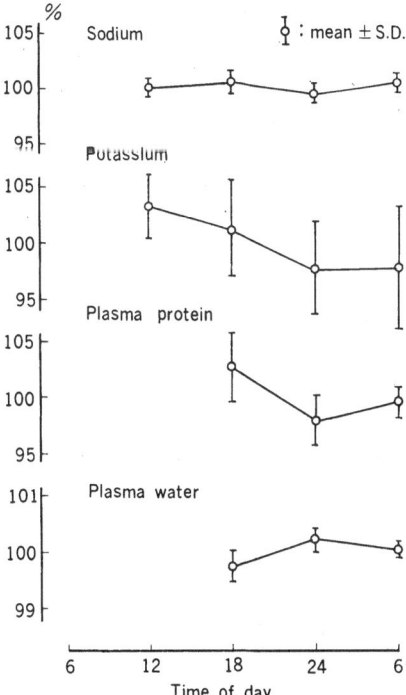

Fig. 188. Changes in serum sodium and potassium, plasma protein and plasma water of six subjects, during a 24-hour period. Values are means ($\pm$S.D., n = 6) as percentages of the mean for the whole period.

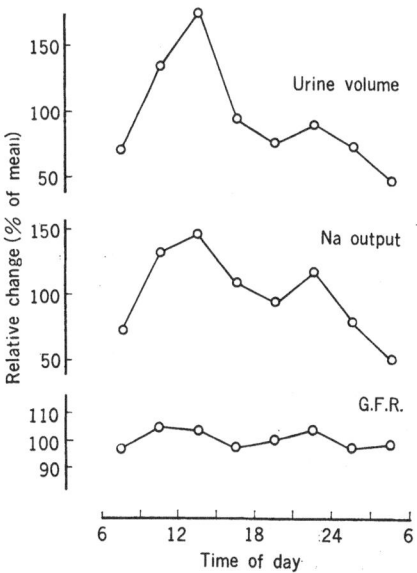

Fig. 189. Changes in mean values of urine volume, urinary sodium output and GFR of four subjects during a 24-hour period. The results are expressed as percentages of the mean value for the whole period.

GFR's were determined as endogenous creatinine clearance. As shown in the figure, urine volume shows about 100% difference in day and night, while GFR varies only about 10%. But the contour of the circadian variations are similar to each other, except in that higher variations of urine volume and sodium output are seen during the daytime. This fact might suggest that the circadian variation of urine is partly under the influence of the cirdadian variation of GFR. Furthermore, the circadian variation of urine is influenced by the known circadian variation of ADH (Zsótér and Sebök, 1955), because the increase in urinary output is much higher during the day as compared with the increase in GFR. The circadian variation of ADH can be attributed at least in this experiment, to the circadian variation of blood volume, as the urine volume is high during the day when the blood volume is high, and is low during the night when the blood volume is low. Sodium output also differs by about 100% between day and night like the urine volume. The output is high during the day and low during the night when hemodilution is observed. Circadian variation in aldosterone is known to be regulated mainly by posture (Balikian et al., 1968, Wolfe et al., 1966). During this experiment, the subjects remained in bed, so the circadian variation of aldosterone may have been diminished or abolished by this constancy of posture, and the variation in urinary output of sodium may be attributed to the variation of urine volume.

As is obvious from these results, kidney functions and their controlling factors are working to maintain homeostasis and not to cause variations, even circadian variation. Hemodilution, which was observed at midnight, can not be explained by the water and salt balance results and may possibly be explained by hemodynamic factors.

Finnerty et al. (1958) reported that adrenergic drug induced hypertension caused a decrease in plasma volume and an increase in hematocrit and plasma protein, and they attributed this cause to increased hydrostatic capillary pressure. Weil and Chidsey (1968) observed plasma volume expansion together with decrease in hematocrit and plasma protein during the reduction of adrenergic function by the administration of guanethidine. As reported by Richardson et al. (1964), arterial blood pressure shows circadian variation with a high value during the day and a low value during the night. These findings explain well the increased plasma volume and the decreased plasma protein during the night.

Summarizing these results, it may be concluded that the factors which cause the circadian variation of circulating blood volume under conditions involving controlled food intake and posture are the circadian variation of erythrocyte deposition in blood depots and the changes of capillary permeability caused by the circadian variation of blood pressure or catecholamine. With regards to the circadian variation of circulating blood volume during normal living conditions, the process may be essentially the same as that of the circadian variation observed under the controlled experiment, but with modification due to variations in water intake. The different conditions controlled in these experiments were posture, water and food intake. Finlayson et al. (1964) attributed the progressive hemodilution during daytime to orthostatic decrease of intrathoracic blood volume accompanying the erect position, but this explanation is contradicted by the high urine volume observed during the day and also by the reported circadian variation of ADH. If that were the case, the erect position, acting through left atrial stretch receptors, should increase ADH secretion and diminish urine volume.

The amount of water intake may well be assumed to be highest around evening, and this assumption explains the peak plasma volume around bed time and continued high plasma volume at midnight together with the remarkable decrease of hematocrit observed during everyday life.

For more detailed explanations of the circadian variation of body fluid, simultaneous measurements of interstitial fluid and intracellular fluid are needed. More complete information on the circadian variation of body fluid will facilitate investigations in various fields including body temperature regulation and body water regulation.

SUMMARY

1) Seasonal variation of water and electrolyte in serum was discussed with respect to homeostasis. It was confirmed that the seasonal changes in serum electrolytes and water are the outcome of the adaptation to the changes in seasonal climate. Thus the set point of homeostasis is shifted by the adaptation to climate. This change of set point of homeostasis was verified to be a result of repeated changes in internal environment induced by the climate change.

2) The magnitude of the seasonal variation has become less recently compared to about ten years ago. The reason for this decrease in seasonal variation was discussed in relation with changes in living conditions of Japanese.

3) The principle of homeostasis is not to fix the internal environment to a constant set point to maintain it at the constant state but to maintain it in the condition which is most effective for tolerating external stress.

4) Among biological variations, two kinds of rhythms are classified, i.e. long-term and short-term. The seasonal variation in body fluid belongs to the former, while the circadian rhythm belongs to the latter.

5) Seasonal changes in blood properties are apt to be affected by changes in living habit and habitat. The circadian variation in the volume of circulating blood, i.e. low in the morning and high in the evening was investigated under the well-controlled and standardized living conditions as well as under the conditions of normal everyday life. The two were essentially the same. In the former experiment, the circadian variation in the circulating blood was initiated by circadian changes in physiological functions proper to the organism, i.e. retention of red cells in blood depot, and change in capillary permeability caused by blood pressure or catecholamine secretion. In daily life, the circadian variation is modified by circadian variation in water intake and other living conditions. But these influences are far less than those found in the seasonal variation of blood properties.

REFERENCES

1. BALIKIAN, H.M., A.H. BRODIE, S.L. DALE, J.C. MELBY, and J.F. TAIT (1968): *J. Clin. Endocr.* **28:** 1630.
2. CRANSTON, W.I., and W. BROWN (1963): *Clin. Sci.* **25:** 107.
3. GRAY, S.J., and K. STERLING (1950): *J. Clin. Invest.* **29:** 1604.
4. FINLAYSON, D.C., F.J. DAGHER, and L.D. VANDAM (1964): *J. Surg. Res.* **4:** 286.
5. FINNERTY, R.A., JR., J.H. BUCHHOLZ, and R.L. GUILLAUDEU (1958): *J. Clin. Invest.* **37:** 425.
6. HARASHIMA, S. (1953): *Jap. J. Med. Progr.* **40:** 574 (in Japanese).
7. HENROTTE, J.G. (1967): *Biometeorology* **2:** 115, S.W. TROMP and W.H. WEIHE eds., Pergamon Press, Oxford.
8. KOSHITANI, J. (1957): *J. Physiol. Soc. Jap.* **19:** 1148 (in Japanese).
9. KRAINTZ, L., J. DEBOER, E.L. SMITH, and R.A. HUGGINS (1958): *Am. J. Physiol.* **195:** 628.

10. Mills, J.N. (1966): *Physiol. Rev.* **46**: 128.
11. Morimoto, T., K. Shiraki, T. Inoue, and H. Yoshimura (1969): *Jap. J. Physiol.* **19**: 801.
12. Morimoto, T., and K. Shiraki (1970): *Jap. J. Physiol.* **20**: 550.
13. Parry, E.H.O., and C.T. Dollery (1968): *Clin. Sci.* **35**: 373.
14. Richardson, D.M., A.J. Honour, G.W. Fenton, F.H. Stott, and G.W. Pichering (1964): *Clin. Sci.* **26**: 445.
15. Sargent, F., II, and K.P. Weinman (1966): *Ann, N.Y. Acad. Sci.* **134**: 696.
16. Shiraki, K., T. Inoue, T. Morimoto, M. Sweki, and T. Okamoto (1968): Proc. 8th Con. Redio-isotopes, Japan Atomic Industrial Forum, Inc., Tokyo, p. 371, (in Japanese).
17. Tamura, M. (1957): *Shikoku Acta Med.* **10**: 423 (in Japanese).
18. Weil, J.V., and C.A. Chidsey (1968): *Circulation* **37**: 54.
19. Wolfe, L.K., R.D. Gordon, D.P. Island, and G.L. Liddle (1966): *J. Clin. Endocr.* **26**: 1261.
20. Yoshida, S., K. Motohashi, H. Ibayashi, and S. Okinaka (1963): *J. Lab. and Clin. Med.* **62**: 279.
21. Yoshimura, H. (1958): *Jap. J. Physiol.* **8**: 165.
22. Yoshimura, H. (1960): In Essential Problems in Climatic Physiology, p. 61, H. Yoshimura, K. Ogata, and S. Itoh, eds, Nankodo, Kyoto.
23. Zsótér, T., and S. Sebök (1955): *Acta med. scand.* **152**: 47.

CHAPTER 24

SEASONAL VARIATION OF BASAL METABOLISM IN JAPANESE

RYOHEI YURUGI,[1] TAKASHI SASAKI,[2] and MANABU YOSHIMURA[3]

[1] *Airomedical Laboratory, JASDF., Tachikawa, Japan*
[2] *Department of Physiology, Institute of Constitutional Medicine, Kumamoto University
Kumamoto, Japan*
[3] *Department of Physiology, Kyoto Prefectural University of Medicine, Kyoto, Japan*

There have been many conflicting reports on the seasonal variation of basal metabolism (BM) in man since around 1920. Some authors [12, 13] have failed to find such seasonal changes, while other investigation have obtained results showing some definite seasonal patterns. Most Japanese investigators [17, 18, 22, 29] have supported the view that the BM is higher in the winter and lower in the summer. However, most American authors support the view that the BM is almost constant throughout the year. The inconsistencies in these reports may derive from the wide variety of factors affecting the results. The fact that almost all experiments performed on Japanese subjects have consistently shown a winter-high-and-summer-low pattern suggests that BM is apparently affected not only by season but also by indirect factors as diet, habit, and activity, which change seasonally in a relatively homogenous population.

The purpose of this paper is to discuss how and why Japanese people show seasonal variation in their BM, what is its role in thermal adaptability and how their habitual diet may relate to it and to their thermal tolerance and thyroid activity. The discussions are shared by all authors, the analysis and follow-ups of annual periodicity are by Sasaki, the role of dietary composition is discussed by all the authors, the section on the relation to thermal tolerance is by Yurugi, and that on dietary effect on thyroid activity and thermal adaptability is by Yoshimura.

ANNUAL PERIODICITY OF BASAL METABOLISM IN JAPANESE

A great deal of research [5, 9, 15, 16, 17, 18, 21, 22, 26, 34] has been done on the seasonal variation of BM over the last twenty-five years in Japan. It seems well established that Japanese subjects show a winter-high-and-summer-low pattern. Among these results, a typical pattern and the results of its detailed pattern analysis will be introduced first. Monthly observation of BM was performed on nine males and six females in Kumamoto, located in the southwest part of Japan, during the period 1949–52 by Sasaki [22]. The metabolism presented a typical seasonal periodicity with a maximum of 8% in January and a minimum of −9% in the July–September period for males and −11 to −13% for females. The annual range, 17% for males and 21% for females, is extremely wide when compared with the 10% range which is generally considered normal in Japan. The pattern is characterized by two distinctive features: a wide annual range and a marked drop in summer. In order to follow the annual course of metabolism in relation to temperature, a total of 766 determinants were analyzed. The BM was expressed in the following equation:

y (%) = 8.83 sin (t + 64°16′) + 2.21 sin (2t + 187°52′) + 0.22 sin (3t + 257°28′)...

where y is the percentage of deviation of metabolism from the annual mean and t is the number of days (or more exactly 360/365 times the number of days) after January 1. Harmonic analysis was applied to the daily mean of outdoor temperature as well.

x (°C) = 15.47 + 11.06 sin (t + 244°16′) + 0.87 sin (2t + 314°25′) + 0.51 sin (3t + 146°19′) + ... where x stands for temperature in centigrade. Fig. 190 illustrates

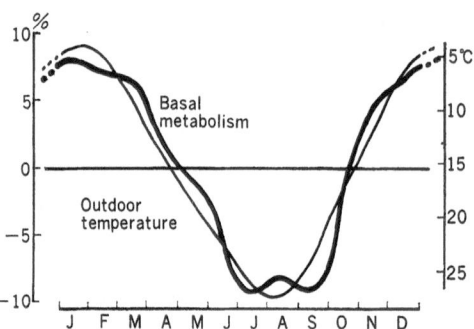

Fig. 190. Annual periodicity of BM in relation to mean outdoor temperature. The observations, performed on adult males in Kumamoto, Japan, were characterized by a wide annual range and marked drop in summer.

seasonal changes in BM along with mean outdoor temperature. For a direct comparison between them, the curves are drawn in such a way that amplitudes for one cycle per year in each function are equal. The temperature scale is reversed for ease of follow-up. In the spring BM, when compared with the rising tendency of temperature, stayed relatively high, and followed the change in environmental temperature after three weeks. Likewise in late September, the change in BM followed that of temperature after a week or two. But in October the phase lag recovered and in November a rise in BM preceded a fall in temperature by about two weeks. Accordingly when the functions, temperature (x) and BM (y), operating at a particular time of year (t) are plotted on an x-y plane, the relation between them forms a hysteresis. This shows that the BM is dependent not only on the current environmental temperature condition but also on the past condition, and depends very little on the temperature of the room in which the subject actually lives. From the stand point of heat production it may be concluded that man's body readies itself to meet the cold season, while it is slow to adjust to the hot season.

Statistical analysis of the relation of BM to room temperature or to a daily mean of outdoor temperature revealed that day-to-day variation in BM was dependent neither on the mean outdoor temperature (r = 0.41) nor room temperature (r = −0.24). Analysis of the relationship between the monthly mean of BM (M) in terms of percentage deviation from the annual mean and monthly mean of outdoor temperature (T) gave a significant correlation of −0.877 and a regression equation:

M = 0.86T − 11.7

Namely, BM is inversely proportional to outdoor temperature; a rise in temperature by 10°C corresponds to a fall of 8.6% in BM in both sexes. It is note worth that the BM is related more closely to the monthly mean of outdoor temperature than to room temperature and thus may serve as a good indication of season.

Suzuki [21] also reported that the BM of Japanese changes inversely to monthly atmospheric temperature in the living place at a rate of 3–4% per 10°C change. Similar results were reported by Oshiba [18]. The BM of four male adults was measured monthly in Kyoto under a standard condition of 25°C throughout a year. After completing the one year experiment, the BM of the same subject was again measured monthly during the next year in a natural environment, i.e. at basal conditions in bed in the subjects usual place of residence. The results were actually the same, and the BM showed remarkable seasonal variation in both first and second years. The mean extent of variation from maximum to minimum was about 18% of the annual mean. The monthly mean atmospheric temperature showed a variation of 22.3°C in a year. During the same experiment, Oshiba also found that the level of PBI in the serum presented a seasonal variation parallel with that of the BM. He presumed that this seasonal variation results from adaptation of the BM to seasonal variations in climate, probably due to changes in thyroid activity.

Sasaki [22] investigated the relationship between the BM of groups of young adult males (18–25 years of age) living in different parts of Japan and the monthly mean temperature. Within the temperature range of 10–25°C a rise of 10°C was accompanied by a fall of 2.5–3.0 kcal/m²·hr in metabolism. The temperature coefficient was almost identical to the one given above. Below 10°C the metabolic increase was slight and negligible. As to the temperature range above 25°C, very little data was available in Japan. It may, however, be presumed that over the higher temperature range no further drop in BM will occur and that the metabolism will maintain the same level as is seen at 25°C. If the seasonal variation of BM depended exclusively on monthly mean outdoor temperature, the annual range of metabolism would be small in the polar zones and the tropics and considerably wider in the temperate zones. To cite an example, observations at Little America V in the Antarctic by Milan *et al.* [13] showed no change in the BM. But the wide range between the upper and lower limits of BM at any temperature level in Japan suggests the participation of some other factors. The factors affecting the seasonal variation in BM are many and complex. Wilson [27, 28] observed the BM of subjects in the Antarctic, and found a significant seasonal trend with peaks in the autumn and in the spring and a drop during the polar night. He says that this periodicity is attributable to the fact that outdoor activity, cold exposure and other factors affecting BM change seasonally with the Antarctic climate.

FOLLOW-UPS ON THE ANNUAL PERIODICITY OF BM AND THE INFLUENCE OF DIETARY COMPOSITION

Annual periodicity in BM has been observed over the last 20 years. These observations are summarized in Table 51, showing changes in the annual range of BM and in dietary composition. A winter-high-and-summer-low pattern was common to all of these observations. The annual range showed a tendency towards gradual reduction during succeeding years. Since a drastic change in climate over such a short period of time is unlikely, this reduction may be ascribed to factors other than climate; such as habit, activity, diet and the like.

The subjects used in these experiments were students, laboratory workers, and soldiers,

TABLE 51   Progressive change in annual range of BM and dietary composition in the Japanese

		Basal Metabolism			Dietary Composition					
Series	Year	No. of Subject	Sex	Annual Range	Total Caloric Intake	Protein	Fat	Carbo-hydrate	F/C Ratio	Author
				%	kcal	%	%	%		
A	1949–	9	M	17.3	2204	13.4	8.7	77.9	0.112	Sasaki (22)
	1950	6	F	21.2	2425	12.5	10.6	76.9	0.138	
B	1950	8	M	19.8						Sasaki (22)
C	1951	4	F	15.2						Sakamoto (20)
D	1952–	9	M	12.2						Fukuda (6)
	1953	3	F	12.4						Masuko (11)
E	1953–	9	M	17.6						Oshiba (18)
	1955									
F	1956–	29	M	16.1						Koga (8)
	1957									
G	1957–	4	M	9.9						Tashiro (25)
	1958									
H	1958	total	M	15.9	2858	15.0	12.4	72.7	0.171	Miyazaki (15)
	1959	201			2860	14.0	12.4	73.6	0.168	
I	1961	5	M	11.3	2743	14.9	14.8	70.2	0.211	Masuda (9)
	1962				2735	16.5	16.2	67.3	0.241	
J	1966–	5	M	9.6						Sasaki et al. (24)
	1967									
K	1967	7	M	7.7	3255	14.6	18.3	67.1	0.277	Yurugi et al. (34)

and their daily activities varied.   As Fujimoto and Watanabe [5] reported that the intensity of work did not cause any substantial difference in the annual range.   Race factors are usually closely associated with dietary habits.   Of the 11 groups, personnel of the Self Defense Force were used in the series F, H, I and K.   Higher energy intake was due to their high level of activity.   It was clearly demonstrated that as the percentage of carbohydrate decreased or that of fat increased in relation to total food intake, seasonal range of metabolism decreased.   The relationship was accentuated more in the last series by a sharp drop in the carbohydrate rate to 67%, by a sharp increase in fat rate from 8.7% to 18.3% and by the reduction of the annual range from 17.3 to 7.7%. The gradual change in the fat/carbohydrate ratio (F/C) is not restricted to the subjects studied in these series but represents a general trend among the Japanese.   Based on the nationwide survey on nutrition conducted quarterly by means of random sampling

TABLE 52   Annual survey of nutrition in Japan (male adults)

Year	Total Caloric Intake	Protein	Fat	Carbo-hydrate	Protein	Fat	Carbo-hydrate	F/C Ratio
	kcal	g	g	g	%	%	%	
1946	1963	59	14	400	12.0	6.4	81.6	0.078
1948	2047	63	13	419	12.3	5.7	81.9	0.070
1952	2109	69.9	20.1	412	13.3	8.6	78.1	0.110
1956	2092	69.1	21.8	405	13.2	9.4	77.4	0.121
1960	2096	69.7	24.7	398.8	13.3	10.6	76.1	0.139
1964	2223	74.4	34.3	398	13.5	14.0	72.5	0.194
(1970)	2300	75.0	38.0	(414.5)	13.0	14.9	72.1	0.207
(1975)	2500	75.0	56.0	(407.7)	12.3	20.8	66.9	0.311

Note: Figures for 1970 and 1975 are target figure for a dietary improvement program now under way.

at a rate of 1:1000 by the Ministry of Health and Welfare of Japan since 1946, percentages of energy sources and F/C ratio were calculated and are given in Table 52. Except for the first few years no change in the total energy intake was seen, while substantial changes were found in the composition of foodstuffs; total protein intake was maintained almost unchanged, while the proportion of calories derived from carbohydrate showed a steady decrease from 81.6 to 72.5% with a compensatory rise in fat from 6.4 to 14.6% for the last 20 years. The change looks small and slow, but consumption of fat was doubled.

Table 53 shows the monthly mean BM in seven Japanese Self Defense Force members and their average daily dietary intake in each month during 1967. The annual range of BM of that year was represented in series K in Table 51. As was described above, the annual range of BM was 7.7%, which had lowered progressively since inception of the study. In Table 53, it is also demonstrated that the composition of the diet was maintained almost unchanged throughout the year. Fat intake was slightly higher in the summer season. Japanese people have a distaste for fatty foods in the hot and humid summer months, but this habit was ameliorated in this series of experiments. In summary, it is suggested that continuous high rate of fat intake may inhibit the seasonal variation in BM in Japanese people.

TABLE 53   Monthly mean BM in 7 Self Defense Force personnel and their daily dietary intake averaged in each month of 1967

Month	BM ± SD kcal/m²·hr	Total Intake kcal/day	Protein g/day	Animal Protein Ratio %	Fat g/day
JAN	36.7 ± 2.8	3173	109	45	56
FEB	38.1 ± 2.9	3253	113	36	62
MAR	35.9 ± 3.0	3232	130	46	61
APR	36.1 ± 2.8	3304	112	38	65
MAY	35.9 ± 2.8	3224	110	40	67
JUN	36.1 ± 3.2	3411	112	41	67
JUL	34.1 ± 2.7	3142	111	44	61
AUG	35.7 ± 3.1	3148	114	45	62
SEP	36.4 ± 3.0	3179	114	47	67
OCT	36.4 ± 2.7	3333	123	42	66
NOV	38.0 ± 1.9	3205	116	41	63
DEC	38.3 ± 2.7	3358	124	40	67
Average	36.5	3255	116	42	64

The Japanese, and many other people in the Far East and in Southeast Asia, are generally heavy carbohydrate eaters. Americans consume an enormous amount of fat. Peculiar dietary habits are observed in Eskimos [2]. In this case observers admit to considerable differences between groups as well as between individuals, and furthermore, to variation in day-to-day intake in the same individual, however it is obvious that carbohydrate intake is extremely small and that the majority of energy comes from fat and protein. Rodahl [19] demonstrated that the basal metabolism of the Eskimo was higher in the winter, when the protein intake increased. The tendency agrees with the observations by Brown et al. [2] who reported a high protein intake in their subjects but who are reluctant to simply ascribe the high metabolic rate to protein. It should be commented, in fairness to the former, that Rodahl's subjects consumed a tremendous amount of protein (over 300 g a day). Adolph [1] found that the Chinese in southern China, subsisting mainly on rice usually had a lowered BM, and pointed to the composition of their food and the climatic conditions as potential causes.

The race factor in BM is related so closely to dietary habits that an attempt to isolate and there upon generalize and interpret this factor correctly has met with great difficulty. Furthermore dietary habits also depend on the way of living and the social and economic status of a family, a community, or a nation. Ultimately, with progress in the control of environmental conditions and food resources, man will be able to eat a more balanced diet and differences due to dietary habits will be reduced a great deal.

As was described above, the annual range of BM has lessened progressively; there have also been changes in composition of the diet characterized by a steady increase in the rate of fat intake with a compensatory decrease in carbohydrate consumption. In order to study whether or not there exists a definite cause and effect relationship between these facts, the effect of food composition on BM was observed by Sasaki *et al.* [23] in each season of the year on three adult subjects (two males and one female) by giving a test diet composed of different foodstuffs. The standard diet consisted of 15% protein, 10% fat and 75% carbohydrate—a typical Japanese diet composition. A high carbohydrate diet which drived 85% of its calories from carbohydrates 10% from protein and 5% from fat corresponds to the diet of Koreans. For a high fat diet, two different levels of fat content were given, 20% and 40%, respectively, the former corresponding to the fat content of Italian or French food and the latter roughly to that of American food. The high protein diet contained 25% protein. The total calories of each experimental diet were kept equal and daily intake on protein was never below 1.25 g/kg body weight. Table 54 shows the result. Changes in BM following the test diet were ex-

TABLE 54   Effect of diet composition on basal metabolism

Season	Subject	High protein	High fat	High carbohydrate	Control
		%	%		%
Spring	A	−0.7	−1.8	−1.2°	.0
	B	—	—	—	—
	C	—	—	—	—
Summer	A	0.0	−0.1	−6.2	.0
	B	−2.6	+1.4	−5.5	.0
	C	−5.9	+3.2	+4.9	.0
Autumn	A	−1.0	+3.0	+3.2	.0
	B	+1.1	+1.9	+2.4	.0
	C	+0.9	+4.5	−4.7	.0
Winter	A	+6.0	+6.1	+0.7	.0
	B	+7.2	+9.0	−0.1	.0
	C	+7.8	+7.0	−3.9	.0

pressed as a percentage of control level (standard diet). The high protein diet showed no effect except during the winter experiment. The amount of protein intake was not enough to expect any substantial influence on the BM. The noticeable rise in metabolism in winter was ascribed to an enhanced fat intake which was incidental to high protein food in this season. The protein content of the other test diets being almost equal, the high fat diet, high carbohydrate diet, and standard diet with an intermediate F/C ratio come into the same category and will be discussed from a standpoint of F/C ratio. In the spring experiment the change in the ratio exerted no effect in either direction, although the number of subjects was not sufficient to draw a definite conclusion.

In summer when the F/C ratio was high the BM was maintained above the control level, in other words, the drop in metabolism during the summer months was suppressed; when the F/C ratio was low a sharp drop in BM was observed in all of the subjects. Among them Subject C, a female subject, was found susceptable to changes in diet composition in either direction. This finding coincides with the fact that the summer fall in the BM is greater in females. In autumn the F/C ratio did not cause any change in the BM level of the male subjects, as was the case in the spring experiment. But in the female subject the summer pattern was maintained, though to a smaller degree. These results suggest that in women responses of some metabolic functions to change of season lag behind those of men. In winter, a high fat diet resulted in a rise in metabolism but a high carbohydrate diet did not affect the metabolic level. To summarize, the effect of change in diet composition on basal metabolic level is evident in summer and winter, and small in spring and autumn. This series of experiment proves the participation of diet composition in reducing the annual range of seasonal periodicity in BM, observed in Japan over the last 20 years.

THE ROLE OF SEASONAL VARIATION OF BM IN HUMAN THERMAL ADAPTABILITY

In an attempt to differentiate between climatic, racial and dietary factors in the seasonal variation of BM and thermal adaptability, another series of observations were made. Yoshimura, M. [33], one of the present authors, went to Santa Barbara, USA, and measured his own BM. He found that his BM increased somewhat in the USA as compared with that observed in Kyoto, Japan, and that the seasonal variation of the BM which appeared in Japan was abolished in the USA. The thyroid activity was estimated with ^{131}I, and it was found that ^{131}I uptake and ^{131}I conversion ratio increased considerably as compared with the values determined in Japan. These results are given in Fig. 191. Among the living conditions which differed from those of Japan, the climate and habitual diet were most striking. As the climate in Santa Barbara did not show remarkable seasonal variation, the disappearance of seasonal variation in his BM may be related to this change of climate, however an elevation of BM accompanied by an increase in thyroid activity cannot be explained by difference of climate. Analysis of his diet revealed that the western diet he consumed daily contained abundant fats as compared with his habitual diet in Japan.

A similar experience was reported by Sasaki [17]. He measured his BM himself during a stay in Lexington, Ky., USA in 1962–1964, and compared the results with those obtained in Kumamoto, Japan during the period 1949–1950. The results are given in Fig. 192. In Lexington the annual mean outdoor temperature was 13.1 °C. The temperature extremes experienced during the two years were 36.7 °C and −29.4 °C, respectively. It should be mentioned here that in the the United States the subject stayed during the daytime in a room controlled at 22 °C throughout the year, and that the night temperature during October–April period was maintained higher than usual, i.e. 27 °C, for research purposes. In Japan the subject evidenced the annual pattern of BM with a winter rise of 10.4% and a summer fall of −11.8%, extending the range to 22.3%. In the United States the pattern of a winter high and a summer low was maintained, and was characterized not only by a higher level of BM, in spite of the subject being more than ten years older, but also by a reduced annual range of 7.7%,

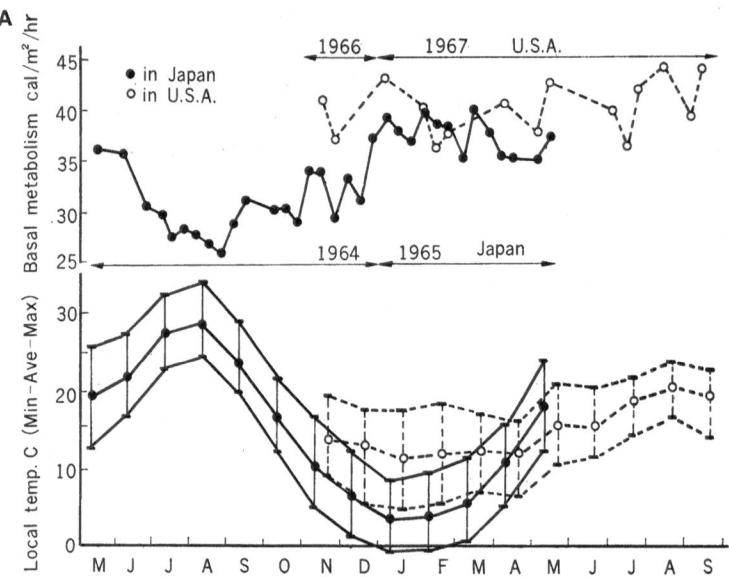

Fig. 191 A. Seasonal variation of BM at Santa Barbara, U.S.A., compared with that in Kyoto, Japan.

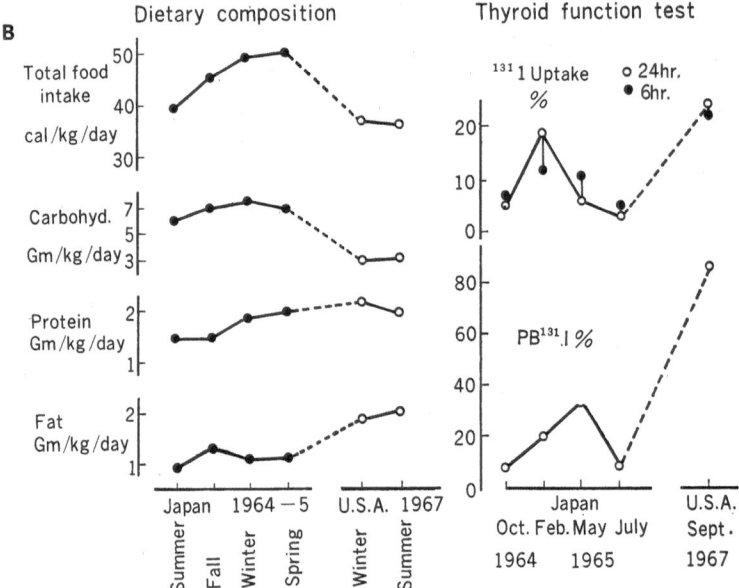

Fig. 191 B. Dietary composition during four seasons in Kyoto compared with that in U.S.A.

which was ascribed not to the winter high but mainly to the moderate summer depression. With regard to temperature coefficient, a rise in temperature by 10°C in Japan resulted in a decrease in metabolism by 3.5 kcal/m²·hr or 9.5%, while in the United States the coefficient, though reduced only to 1.0 kcal/m²·hr or 2.6%, was still highly significant. Since in the United States the subject lived in an environment which was

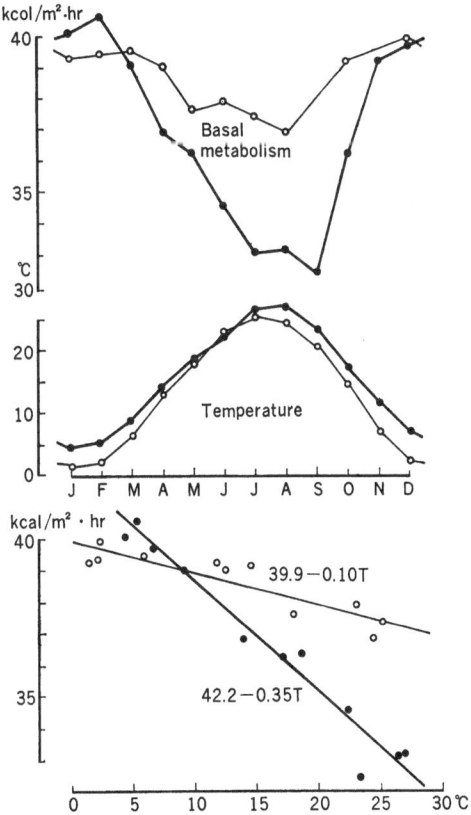

Fig. 192. Annual periodicity of BM in the same subject at different locations; Kumamoto, Japan (solid circle) and Lexington, Ky., U.S.A. (open circle).

largely independent of outdoor temperature, the very small but significant temperature coefficient suggests participation of innate periodicity of body function synchronized with season rather than temperature dependence. The fact that the seasonal variation of his BM was very much reduced may also due to the increased fat intake in his diet in the United States.

From the experience of Yoshimura and Sasaki, it was suggested that thyroid activity was closely related to the composition of habitual diet, especially its fat content, and that the annual mean BM of people who are eating rice without enough fatty foods is a little lower than that of peaple eating a high fat diet.

According to the Oshiba's [18] climate chamber experiment in the winter season, BM decreased gradually a few days after entering the hot chamber (29.5 °C), and attained the minimum level (about 10% lower than the control) after seven to 10 days with no further decrease. The PBI level was also lower than that of the control. Oshiba concluded from these facts that some adaptive mechanism is provoked by exposing the subject to heat in summer and cold in winter, and that the seasonal variation of BM is thus initiated. Thyroid activity, which may be related to dietary fat intake, seems to be involved in this adaptive mechanism.

In an attempt to verify this supposition, Yoshimura et al. [30, 31] measured the monthly variation in BM of five Canadian missionaries living in Kyoto in a Japanese style house

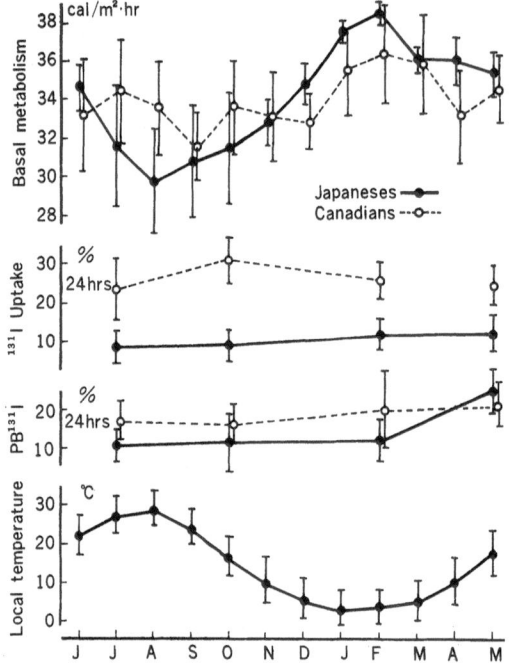

Fig. 193. Seasonal variation of BM and thyroid activity of Japanese and Canadian living in Kyoto, Japan.

which was not equipped for temperature control and compared the results with those of Japanese controls living in similar house. Results are summarized in Fig. 193. The BM of Japanese control presented a clear sesonal variation, rising in winter, falling in summer. On the other hand, the BM of the Caucasian did not show any such consistent variation. A slight tendency towards a lowering of the BM is seen in summer, but it is not statistically significant as compared with the values in winter. Thyroid activity measured with ^{131}I was higher in the Caucasian than in the Japanese. A dietary survey was made and it was demonstrated that the Canadians consumed considerably more fat than the Japanese through the year, while Japanese intake of carbohydrate was somewhat higher than that of the Caucasians. From these measurements, it is suggested that the seasonal variation in the BM of the Canadian may be inhibited by their high fat intake. This suggestion is also supported by Table 51 in which it is seen that the seasonal variation in BM of the Japanese decreased year by year as their fat intake increased.

Yurugi et al. [35] performed another series of experiments on the relationship between seasonal variation of the BM and adaptive mechanism to cold in Japanese Air Self Defense Force personnel. Subjects were exposed to cold of $5\,^\circ C$, with clothes of about 1.7 clo of insulation, for 60 minutes; decrease in mean skin temperature (ΔTs) and increase in metabolism (ΔM) during exposure were measured and compared with those of a warm comfortable resting control. The value of $\Delta M/\Delta Ts$ was in harmony with the cold tolerance estimated by their experiences. Prior to this experiment, their monthly BM had been measured for one year and annual range (ΔBM) was calculated. It was found that a positive relation between $\Delta M/\Delta Ts$ and ΔBM may exist in this series of experiments. However, additional experiments performed later showed a decreased tendency in this relation, probably due to the decrease in the ΔBM and increase in fat intake.

These findings support the supposition that metabolic adaptation to cold exposure may decrease parallel with decreasing annual range of BM, probably due to increased fat intake, in consequence of which cold tolerance may elevate.

ANIMAL EXPERIMENTS REGARDING THE EFFECT OF DIET ON THERMAL ACCLIMATIZATION

In an attempt to analyze the effect of fat intake in suppressing the seasonal variation in the BM, effect of dietary composition on thyroid activity and climatic acclimation was investigated in the rat by Yoshimura et al. [31, 32].

Animal experiments were made in four series, I, II, III, and IV. In series I, 120 rats initially weighing about 150 g were divided into two groups of 60 rats each. One group was placed in a cold chamber at 5 °C, the other group in a heated chamber at 30–34 °C. The temperature of the chambers were regulated automatically. Each group was subdivided into three subgroups and the subgroup were fed high fat, high carbohydrate and high protein diets, respectively. Table 55 shows the composition of these three diets.

TABLE 55   Composition of purified diets

Type of diet	Experiment I			Experiment II & III	
	High-fat (A)	High-CHO (A)	High-protein	High-fat (B)	High-CHO (B)
	gm%	gm%	gm%	gm%	gm%
Casein	18	18	42	25	25
Flour	—	—	51	—	—
Starch	28	78	—	6	66
Lard	50	—	—	60	—
Cottonseed oil	—	—	—	2	2
Whole liver oil	—	—	3	1	1
Salt	4	4	4	4	4
Multi-vitamin*	0.4	0.4	0.4	2	2

*Multi-vitamin powder; Panvitan powder from Takeda Chemical Industries, Ltd.

Fat content of high fat food (A) was too high to maintain the normal growth of rat. Thus the fat content was reduced reasonably in high fat food (B) in the experiment II and III.

After Six weeks, the resting oxygen consumption was measured. Then 1 μc of ^{131}I was injected intraperitoneally, and the rat was not fed for 15 hours. Blood was collected from the femornal vein and the thyroid gland was excised. PB[131]I conversion ratio was measured with the blood sample, and ^{131}I uptake was measured from the thyroid gland. Fig. 194 illustrates the results of the experiment. In this figure, data obtained from two other subgroups of 10 rats each which were fed high fat and high carbohydrate food, respectively, in a chamber of 25 °C for about 5 weeks are included as the control temperature group. The most striking results shown in the figure are that all of the heat acclimated rats had lower mean resting oxygen consumption and lower FFA concentration in the plasma than any of the control or cold acclimated rats, regardless of food

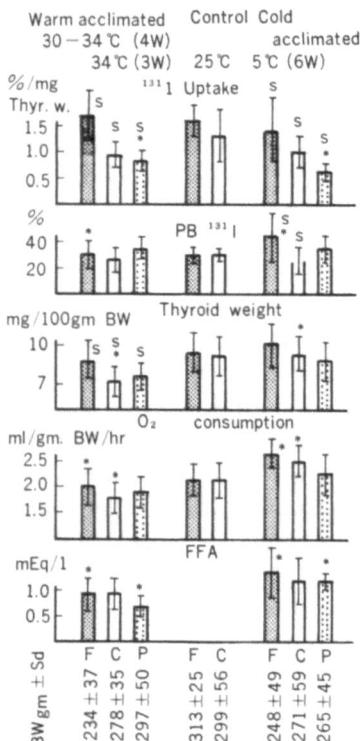

Fig. 194. Thyroid activity, O_2 consumption and FFA in three environmental temperature condition. F: high fat, C: high carbohydrate, and P: high protein subgroup.

composition, and further that high fat subgroups showed, in general, higher thyroid activity, O_2 consumption and plasma FFA than those of other food subgroups, regardless of their acclimated temperature. The asterisk in the figure indicates the presence of a statistically significant difference between different temperature groups fed one and the same food. S means significant difference between different food subgroups. Thus it was verified that heat acclimation results in lowering of thyroid activity and resting metabolism both in O_2 consumption and FFA level, while reverse changes are brought about by cold acclimation. A high fat diet increases the thyroid activity and resting metabolism. In these experiments it was verified that high fat food affects the resting metabolism inversely to the effect of heat acclimation. Thus it is suggested that the effect of heat acclimation on the resting metabolism may be abolished by high fat foods.

In an attempt to verify this suggestion, another series of experiments II were designed. Two groups of rats were kept in a room with a constant temperature of 20°C as a control, and in a heat chamber at 30°C for 5 weeks, respectively. Each group was divided into two subgroups and was fed a high fat and high carbohydrate food, respectively. The diet composition is shown by B on the right hand side of Table 55. The number of heat acclimated rats was 30, and those of the control temperature group 20. Results are shown in Fig. 195. The resting oxygen consumption was measured for both groups in chambers of 30°C and 20°C. The resting O_2 consumption at the experimental temperature of 30°C was much lower than that at 20°C. Under both these experimental conditions, a higher rate of O_2 consumption was noticed in the high fat subgroup as

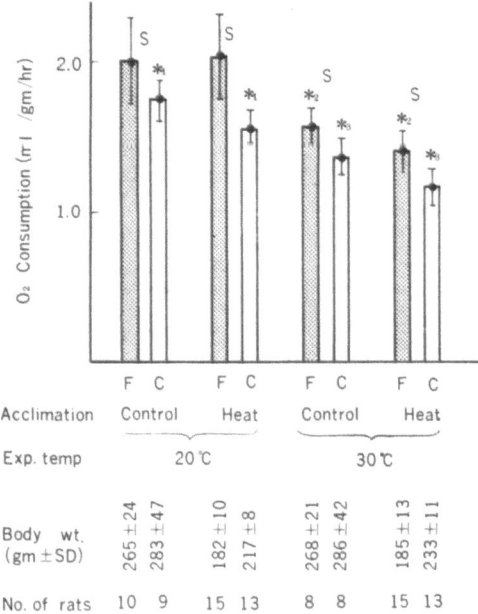

Fig. 195. Effect of diet on thermal acclimation of O_2 consumption
in high fat (F) and high carbohydrate (C) diet.

compared with the high carbohydrate subgroup.

In comparison with the control, heat acclimated rats presented a lower rate of O_2 consumption in both carbohydrate and fat subgroups. However, the reduction rate of O_2 consumption in the heat acclimated group is striking in the carbohydrate subgroup and less so in the heat acclimated high fat subgroup. In the measurement taken at 20 °C, the difference in O_2 consumption between the high fat subgroup at the control temperature and the heat acclimated high fat subgroup is not clear and is insignificant, while the difference between the two high carbohydrate subgroups at the two temperatures is statistically significant.

In the measurements taken at 30 °C, the difference between the two high fat subgroups at control and with heat acclimation is statistically significant, but it is far less than the difference between two high carbohydrate subgroups. Thus it may be verified that the reduction of resting metabolism by heat acclimation is inhibited by taking high fat food. It is inferred that this inhibition is due to an enhanced thyroid activity caused by high fat feeding.

The above experimental results suggest that seasonal variation of BM may appear among Japanese and other people in East Asia who eat rice as their main food and consume insufficient fat, and that this seasonal variation is due to acclimatization to changes in climate with the seasons. On the other hand, this variation of the BM does not appear among Caucasian who eat a high fat diet, because the reduction in the BM due to heat is inhibited by increased thyroid activity caused by the high fat intake.

The third series of experiments was designed to clarify the effect of high fat intake on thyroid activity. About 100 rats were divided into four groups. The first three groups were placed in a 20 °C chamber, and each group was divided into two subgroups fed high fat and high carbohydrate foods for five weeks, respectively. One group was

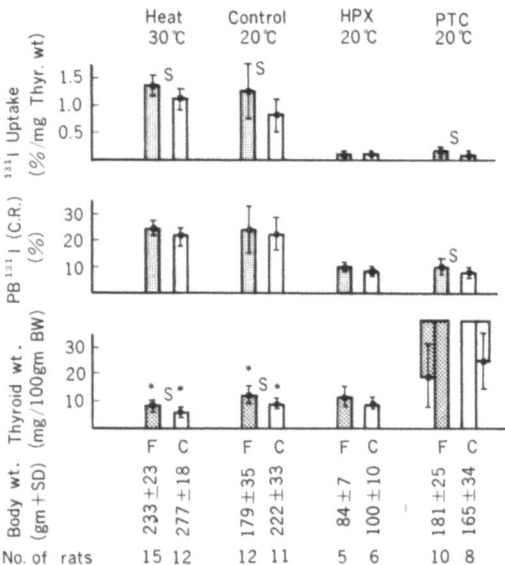

Fig. 196. Thyroid function in heat acclimated, control, hypophysectomized and prophyl-thiouracil feeding rats. F: high fat and C: high carbohydrate subgroup. Difference between F and C was statistically examined.

the control group of 30 rats, the second group was the hypophysectomized 20 rats and the third the propyl-thiouracil 20 rats whose food contained 0.1% of propyl-thiouracil. The fourth group were 30 normal rats acclimated to heat in a 30°C cage and fed on high fat or high carbohydrate food (B). After five weeks, the thyroid activity was examined as in the previous experiments. The results are illustrated in Fig. 196. It is demonstrated in this figure that the propyl-thiouracil rats (PTC) showed goiter, while the difference in thyroid gland weight between the high fat group and the high carbohydrate group was not significant. On the other hand, the difference is significant in the ^{131}I uptake and the PB^{131}I conversion ratio with PTC. As seen in Fig. 196, the difference is significant in the ^{131}I uptake and thyroid weight with the control group as well as with the heat acclimated normal rats. No significant difference between high fat and high carbohydrate group was found, however, with hypophysectomized rats. Thus it is suggested that TSH may be involved in the influence of dietary composition on thyroid activity. According to Hegsted's group, high cholesterol intake may accelerate the excretion of thyroxin in the bile and may initiate a reduction of thyroxin in plasma, which may stimulate TSH secretion by a feedback mechanism. Overshooting of this feedback mechanism may result in increased thyroid activity. This is the author (Yoshimura)'s working hypothesis and should be a subject for future study.

To test the physiological role of dietary effect on metabolism, another animal experiment (IV) was designed. Three groups of rats were fed high fat, high carbohydrate and high protein foods, respectively, for five weeks and were then placed in a very cold −10°C room for five hours. The body weight of all the rats was about 300 g. Rectal temperature was measured and it was found that the rate of decrease in rectal temperature in a −10°C chamber was highest in the high carbohydrate group, smallest in the high fat group. Adaptation and strong resistance to cold in the fat feeding animal were already noticed by Mitchell *et al.* [14], Dugal *et al.* [4] and others. Masoro [11] supported the view that some other factor than a higher insulation of subcutaneous fat is responsible for the superiority of high fat group in preventing a drop in deep body temperature. An increased thyroid activity upon acute cold exposure was demonstrated by Yamada. Since the utilization of body fat during cold exposure may differ from the case of shivering and non-shivering thermogenesis, whether this adaptation results from changes in metabolism induced by a high fat diet or from an alteration in insulation or from a combination of these factors remains to be established.

Turning to the problems of the role of thyroid activity in heat adaptation, the results of animal experiments and observations in man reported above suggest that metabolic adaptation to heat may be increased by high carbohydrate intake or low fat intake, probably due to inhibited thyroid activity. Collins and Weiner [3] also support the view that lowered thyroid activity reduces the BM and increases heat tolerance. Thus the heavy carbohydrate eater may possess an inhibited thyroid activity and a superior heat adaptability by reducing BM in hot environments.

In conclusion, metabolic adaptation to heat may be accelerated with a high carbohydrate diet through an acclimatization of thyroid activity to heat, while a high fat diet may contribute to increased cold tolerance. It may be an evidence that the Japanese, a heavy carbohydrate eater, possesses a considerable range of seasonal variation in the BM, high in winter and low in summer, and that the Caucasian, a high fat eater, shows a constant BM throughout the year.

REFERENCES

1. ADOLPH, W.H. (1925): *Acta Med. Scand.* **81:** 249.
2. BROWN, G.M., G.S. BIRD, L.M. BOAG, D.J. DELAHAYE, J.E. GREEN, J.D. HATCHER, and J. PAGE (1954): *Metabolism* **3:** 247.
3. COLLINS, K.J., and J.S. WEINER (1968): *Physiol. Rev.* **48:** 785.
4. DUGAL, L.P., C.P. LEBLOND, and M. THERIEN (1945): *Can. J. Res. Sect. E.* **23:** 244.
5. FUJIMOTO, S., and T. WATANABE (1965): *Acta Med. Nagasaki* **10:** 1.
6. FUKUDA, M. (1953): *J. Physiol. Soc. Jap.* **15:** 68 (in Japanese).
7. INOUE, G. (1954): *J. Physiol. Soc. Jap.* **16:** 326 (in Japanese).
8. KOGA, Y. (1959): *Bull. Res. Inst. Diath. Med.* **10:** 180 (in Japanese).
9. MASUDA, G. (1967): *Bull. Inst. Constit. Med.* **17:** 68 (in Japanese).
10. MASORO, E.J. (1966): *Physiol. Rev.* **46:** 67.
11. MASUKO, K. (1958): *J. Physiol. Soc. Jap.* **20:** 204 (in Japanese).
12. MCCLENDON, J.F., and P. OLSEN (1940): *Endocrinol.* **27:** 160.
13. MILAN, F.A., R.W. ELSNER, and K. RODAHL (1961): *Arctic Aeromed. Lab. Tech. Rep.* **60-9.**
14. MITCHELL, H.H., N. GLICKMAN, E.H. LAMBERT, R.W. KEETON, and M.K. FAHNESTOCK (1946): *Am. J. Physiol.* **146:** 84.
15. MIYAZAKI, M. (1970): *Bull. Inst. Constit. Med.* **20:** 292 (in Japanese).
16. NAKAMURA, M., S. USUTANI, R. ISHIDA, and Y. OGINO (1964): *Hirosaki Med. J.* **16:** 137 (in Japanese).
17. OGATA, K., T. SASAKI, and N. MURAKAMI (1966): *Bull. Inst. Constit. Med.* **16** (Supplement): 36.
18. OSHIBA, S. (1957): *Jap. J. Physiol.* **7:** 355.
19. RODAHL, K. (1952): *J. Nutr.* **48:** 359.
20. SAKAMOTO, A. (1953): *Bull. Res. Inst. Diath. Med.* **4:** 452 (in Japanese).
21. SUZUKI, S. (1959): World Review of Nutrition and Dietetics, Vol. 1. BOURNE, G.H.; Hafner; New York; 103.
22. SASAKI, T. (1954): *Bull. Res. Inst. Diath. Med.* **4:** 439 (in Japanese).
23. SASAKI, T., M. TANIGUCHI, and I. YASUMOTO (1966): *J. Physiol. Soc. Jap.* **28:** 76 (in Japanese).
24. SASAKI, T., I. YASUMOTO, M. MINAKAMI, T. INOUE, A. ISHIHARA, and M. TANIGUCHI (1969): *Bull. Inst. Constit. Med.* **20:** 72 (in Japanese).
25. TASHIRO, Y. (1961): *Bull. Res. Inst. Diath. Med.* **12:** 589 (in Japanese).
26. UETA, T., Y. DAIKOKU, K. SENNO, and K. ETO (1954): *Med. and Biol.* **32:** 282 (in Japanese).
27. WILSON, O. (1956): *Metabolism* **5:** 531.
28. WILSON, O. (1956): *Metabolism* **5:** 543.

29. YOSHIMURA, H. (1960): Essential Problems in Climatic Physiology. H. YOSHIMURA, K. OGATA, and S. ITO; Nankodo, Kyoto; 61.
30. YOSHIMURA, M., K. YUKIYOSHI, T. YOSHIOKA, and H. TAKEDA (1966): *Fed. Proc.* **25:** 1169.
31. YOSHIMURA, M. (1969): *J. Jap. Soc. Food Nutr.* **23:** 394 (in Japanese).
32. YOSHIMURA, M., H. TAKEDA, and H. YOSHIMURA. (1969): *J. Physiol. Soc. Jap.* **31:** 178.
33. YOSHIMURA, M., and H. YOSHIMURA. (1970): *Nippon-Rinsho* **28:** 1988 (in Japanese).
34. YURUGI, R., M. IIZUKA, T. AKIYAMA, H. IKEGAMI, and C. SAKAKIBARA (1968): *Rep. Aeromed. Lab. JASDF.* **8:** 142 (in Japanese).
35. YURUGI, R., M. IIZUKA, T. AKIYAMA, F. KAWASHIMA, and C. SAKAKIBARA (1968): *Rep. Aeromed. Lab. JASDF.* **8:** 150 (in Japanese).

INDEX